MELANOMA - FROM EARLY DETECTION TO TREATMENT

Edited by **Guy Huynh Thien Duc**

Melanoma - From Early Detection to Treatment
http://dx.doi.org/10.5772/50853
Edited by Guy Huynh Thien Duc

Contributors

Lee Cranmer, Sherif Morgan, Joanne Jeter, Evan Hersh, Sun Yi, Paul Mosca, Paul Speicher, Douglas Tyler, Hinrich Abken, Jennifer Makalowski, Laura Hutchins, Konstantinos Arnaoutakis, Dorothy Graves, Jianli Dong, Lester Davids, Kazuya Murata, Hideaki Matsuda, Megumi Masuda, Yumi Abe, Akemi Uwaya, Palmieri, Maria Colombino, Paolo Antonio Ascierto, Amelia Lissia, Corrado Rubino, Antonio Cossu, Jose Neptuno Rodriguez-Lopez, Luis Sanchez-del-Campo, Magali Saez-Ayala, Maria F. Montenegro, Maria Piedad Fernandez-Perez, Juan Cabezas-Herrera, Gloria Ribas, Maider Ibarrola-Villava, Maria Peña-Chilet, Lara P. Fernandez, Conrado Martinez-Cadenas, Andrea Zangari, Elisabetta Cerigioni, Annachiara Contini, Mercedes Romano, Federico Zangari, Maria Giovanna Grella, Ascanio Martino, David Weber, Kira Hartman, Ruth Prichard, Denis Evoy, Zahraa Al-Hilli, Enda McDermott, James Geraghty, Yasuhiro Nakamura, Rizos, Roger Chammas, Guilherme Francisco, Priscila Cirilo, Fernanda Gonçalves, Tharcisio Tortelli Jr, John Ogden Mason, Emine Kilic, Mario Santinami, Roberto Patuzzo, Roberta Ruggeri, Carlotta Tinti, Giulia Baffa, Gianpiero Castelli, Andrea Maurichi, Alexeev, Miriam Jasiulionis, Jonathan Castillo Arias, Duane Miller, Victoria De Los Ángeles Bustuoabad, Lucia Speroni, Arturo Irarrázabal, Storkus, Sakuhei Fujiwara, Yoshitaka Kai

Published by InTech

Janeza Trdine 9, 51000 Rijeka, Croatia

Notice

Publishing Process Manager Ana Pantar
Technical Editor InTech DTP team
Cover InTech Design team

Additional hard copies can be obtained from orders@intechopen.com

Melanoma - From Early Detection to Treatment, Edited by Guy Huynh Thien Duc
p. cm.
ISBN 978-953-51-0961-7

For EU product safety concerns:
IN TECH d.o.o., Prolaz Marije Krucifikse Kozulić 3, 51000 Rijeka, Croatia,
info@intechopen.com or visit our website at intechopen.com.

Meet the editor

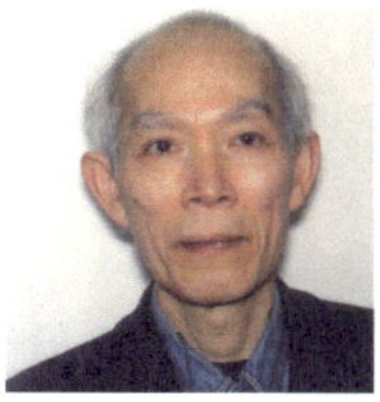

Guy Huynh Thien Duc is Research Director emeritus from the CNRS (Centre National de la Recherche Scientifique). He started his career in the Pasteur Institute where he prepared his Ph.D in the field of Immunopathology. Thereafter, as researcher in the CNRS, he has been mainly involved in fundamental aspects of Immunology, focusing on Transplantation Immunity and Immunomodulation. In the last two decades, his work at the University Paris XI in the southern of Paris, presently inside the structure of INSERM U-1014 Groupe Hospitalier Paul Brousse – Villejuif, is essentially devoted to Cancer Immunotherapy.

Contents

Preface

The link of melanoma risk to ultraviolet (UV) radiation exposure is widely recognized, but UV radiation independent events account also for a significant number of cases which highlights the need for analysing further the mechanism(s) underlying melanomagenesis. Therefore, the essential aspects to be considered would be related to the balance between Mc1R (melanocortin 1 receptor)-inherited background and the mutated BRAF (BRAF V600E) conveying stresses caused either by UV radiation or oxydative damage in the context of defined pheomelanin/eumelanin ratio.

Concerning the treatment of metastatic melanoma, overall results so far obtained still remained poor, although significant response rate has been observed with vemurafenib (PLX4032). However resistance to this remarkable small molecule is beginning to emerge and it is known that only patients with relevant mutation respond to this agent.

In this context, it is worth noting the development of new technologies, following the advent of human genome sequencing allowing to identify important somatic driver mutations that harness most aggressive cancer types. Progress gained in sequencing thousands of individual cancer genomes has already provided an invaluable insight into activating mutations and surrogate signalling pathways sustaining deregulated proliferation, invasiveness and resistance to apoptosis as well as to inhibitors. On the other hand, the throughout deep sequencing will also help development of other active inhibitors like PLX4032 specifically adapted for targeting defined activating mutations. Needless to say that personalized medicine based on patient's genetic background represents also important aspect for taking in consideration. Overall, the huge effort provided by scientists in many areas along with that of physicians recently will open, beyond doubt, the ways to development of appropriate and efficient strategies in the treatment of metastatic melanoma in particular and other cancer types in general.

As such, the book "Melanoma - From Early Detection to Treatment" assembles data and knowledge from most experienced experts in the field. It covers sections from fundamental aspects of the melanoma biology to various treatment approaches including melanoma related features.

Acknowledgements: We thank Chaobin Zhu for his helpful assistance.

Guy Huynh Thien Duc
Research Director emeritus from the CNRS (Centre National de la Recherche Scientifique),
INSERM, U-1014, Université Paris XI – Groupe hospitalier Paul-Brousse,
Villejuif, France

Section 1

Fundamental Aspects of the Melanoma Biology

Chapter 1

Overcoming Resistance to BRAF and MEK Inhibitors by Simultaneous Suppression of CDK4

Jianli Dong

Additional information is available at the end of the chapter

http://dx.doi.org/10.5772/53620

1. Introduction

Melanoma is one of the most prevalent malignancies and has a very poor prognosis. Mutations in v-raf murine sarcoma viral oncogene homolog B1 (*BRAF*) occur in approximately 50% of melanomas [4]. While the response to selective BRAF inhibitors (BRAFi) in *BRAF*-mutant melanoma is encouraging, virtually all patients rapidly develop secondary resistance [6, 7]. Based on the finding that the mitogen activated protein kinase/ERK kinase (MEK)-extracellular signal regulated kinase (ERK) pathway is frequently reactivated by various BRAFi resistance mechanisms, a combination trial of a selective mutant BRAF inhibitor (dabrafenib, GSK2118436) with a MEK inhibitor (trametinib, GSK1120212) is underway and has achieved clinical responses in 17% and disease control in 67% in patients who failed prior single-agent treatment with a BRAF inhibitor [9]. While these results are promising, there is a critical need to overcome resistance to BRAF and MEK inhibitors. The clinical efficacy of BRAFi and MEKi therapy is believed to rely on a functional retinoblastoma (RB) axis to inhibit cell proliferation. The inhibitor of cyclin-dependent kinase 4A (*INK4A*) gene encode the p16 protein, a critical cell cycle regulator that interacts with cyclin dependent kinase (CDK) 4, inhibiting its ability to phosphorylate and inactivate RB [12, 13]. Genetic disruption of *INK4A* occurs in approximately 50% of melanomas irrespective of *BRAF* mutation and has been detected in melanoma cells that developed resistance to BRAFi. Of note, cyclin D is still expressed even in the setting of maximum tolerance dosing of BRAF inhibitor [7]. We have reported that combination of BRAFi or MEKi with the expression of wild-type *INK4A* or a CDK4 inhibitor (CDK4i) significantly suppresses growth and enhances apoptosis in melanoma cells [1-3]. Currently, CDK4 inhibitors are in active clinical development (http://clinicaltrials.gov/). Based on our previous work and recent insights into molecular mechanisms of resistance to BRAF and MEK inhibitors, we hypothesize that simultaneous suppression of

CDK4 is an effective strategy to overcome resistance to BRAF and MEK inhibitors. BRAF mutation assays have been used to guide treatment with BRAF and MEK inhibitors, development of sensitive and specific INK4A/p16 assays may serve as predictive biomarkers for treatment with CDK4 inhibitors.

2. Body

Constitutive activation of RAS-RAF-MEK-ERK signaling pathway in melanomas.*NRAS* and *BRAF* mutations were found respectively in 10-20% and 60-80% melanomas [4]. NRAS and BRAF are components of the RAS-RAF-mitogen activated protein kinase/ERK kinase (MEK)-extracellular signal regulated kinase (ERK) signaling pathway (Fig. 1) [5]. This signaling pathway plays an essential role in cell proliferation, differentiation and survival [5, 14, 15]. Constitutive activation of the ERK pathway has been shown to mediate the transforming activity of mutant BRAF in melanoma cells [16-18]. Suppression of mutant *BRAF* expression has been shown to inhibit ERK pathway activation and subsequent suppression of melanoma cell proliferation and survival *in vitro* and *in vivo* [19-21]. Our previous data revealed that the inhibition of mutant BRAF decreased levels of phospho-ERK (p-ERK), a marker of ERK pathway activation in melanoma cells [5, 14, 15].

The high frequency of *BRAF* mutation in melanomas makes it an ideal target for therapy. Because normal cells require wild-type *BRAF* for survival [22], specifically inhibiting mutant, but not wild-type *BRAF* in tumor cells could avoid toxic side effects generated by targeting normal cells. The finding that mutations in v-raf murine sarcoma viral oncogene homolog B1 (*BRAF*) occur in approximately 50% of melanomas led to extensive investigation of targeting BRAF for melanoma treatment, resulting in the first approved mutant specific BRAF inhibitor for treatment of advanced melanoma.

Combine BRAF and MEK inhibitors with chemotherapeutic agents. Intrinsic therapy resistance is a major limitation in the treatment of malignant melanomas. The mechanisms involved in the resistance of melanomas are largely unknown [23, 24]. It is believed that apoptosis and cytostasis (growth arrest/differentiation) are two of the main cellular responses to anticancer agents and loss of either process promotes treatment failure [25-27]. Activating *BRAF* mutations could drive cell proliferation and increase the cell death threshold through ERK pathway or alternative mechanisms [28-30], resulting in the blockage of both cytotoxic and cytostatic effects of therapeutic drugs [14, 31, 32]. It has been shown that inhibition of ERK pathway sensitizes melanoma cells to apoptosis induced by DNA damaging agents including cisplatin and ultra-violate (UV) irradiation [32, 33]. Rational combination of BRAF and MEK inhibitors with selective chemotherapeutic agents, for example, dacarbazine (DTIC), may generate additive/synergistic therapeutic effects.

ERK pathway activation and p16 in melanocytic lesions. Melanocytic lesions can be grouped into two main categories: nevi and melanomas. Nevi are divided into several different types based on histology. These include acquired melanocytic nevi, congenital melanocytic nevi, blue nevi, Spitz nevi, and dysplastic nevi. Melanoma can be further divided based on clinical and traditional histological methods as superficial spreading melanoma, lentigo maligna melanoma, acral lentiginous melanoma, and nodular melanoma. In early stages of melanomas, neoplastic cells are confined to the epidermis or with microinvasion into the dermis. In advanced melanomas, cancer cells expand in the dermis and generate tumor nodules and have a high potential for metastatic spread. In the metastatic phase, cancer cells disseminate to lymph nodes or distant organs [34, 35]. For the early diagnosed and localized melanomas, surgery is the choice of treatment. But there is currently no effective treatment for invasive and metastatic melanomas. Patients with late stage melanomas have a high mortality rate and life expectancy averages approximately 6-8 months after diagnosis.

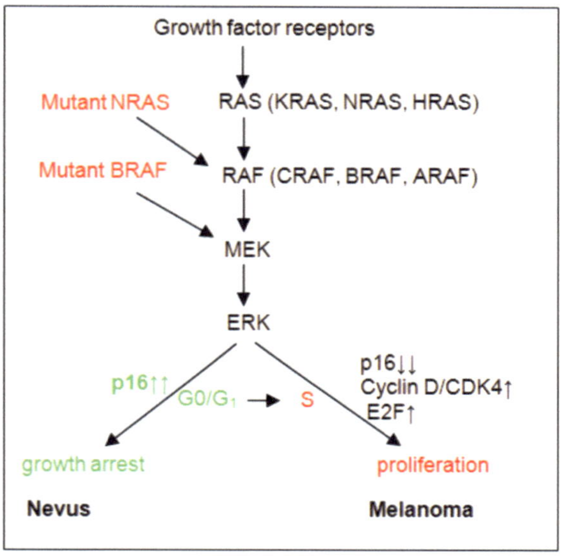

Figure 1. p16-cyclin D/CDK4 modifies the outcome of RAS/RAF/MEK/ERK signaling activation. RAF relays RAS signals through MEK to ERK. The activation of this pathway has multiple effects on cell proliferation, differentiation, and survival depending on the cellular contexts [5]. Constitutive activation of growth factor signaling pathways or NRAS and BRAF activating mutations can trigger over-expression of p16 leading to proliferative senescence, which manifest as benign nevus [10, 11]. Loss of p16 by genetic and epigenetic changes allows activation of cyclin D/CDK4 and inactivation of RB, leading to E2F activation, cell cycle progression from G1 to S phase, cell proliferation and tumor formation [12, 13]. Further genetic changes cause tumor progression to malignant melanoma. Of the three *RAS* and three *RAF* genes, *NRAS* and *BRAF* are mutated in melanoma [4].

Of note, in addition to melanomas, *BRAF* mutations are found at high frequencies (70-80%) in benign melanocytic nevi [36, 37]. There are a large numbers of melanocytic nevi in the general population compared to the relatively low incidence of melanomas [34, 35]. Clinically, it is known that nevi often regress over time. This suggests that BRAF mutations alone are insufficient to induce malignant transformation in nevus cells. The growth arrest of nevi is believed to result from oncogene-induced senescence, which is known as a protective mechanism against unlimited proliferation that could result from *BRAF* mutations and activation of the ERK signaling pathway (nevus in Fig. 1) [10, 11]. Tumor suppressor genes have been found to be involved in senescence process. For example, p16 is one tumor suppressor found to be induced by ERK activation and telomere attrition involving cell senescence [8, 10, 11, 38]. The tumor suppressor p16 is encoded by *INK4A* (Fig. 2) and is often inactivated in a variety of human cancers, including 30-70% in melanomas [39, 40]. Most melanomas, but not nevi, have lost the expression of wild-type *INK4A*, either through DNA deletion/mutation or promoter hypermethylation [41-45]. It is possible that the loss-of-function of p16 in melanomas may make it possible to bypass the cellular senescence mechanism and function as an anti-tumor mechanism against ERK signal activation triggered by *NRAS* and *BRAF* oncogenic mutation (Fig. 1) [11, 46, 47].

Indirect evidence from cultured cells and animal models reveal that there may be a cooperative role between the constitutive activation of ERK pathway and the loss of p16 in tumor progression. Daniotti et al. [48] reported the co-existence of *BRAF* mutations and *INK4A* mutations/deletions/loss-of-expression in 26 of 41 (63%) short-term cell lines obtained from melanoma biopsies. Recent evidence suggests that growth arrest in benign nevi is due to cell senescence and that p16 at least partially contributes to the process of senescence in nevi [11, 46, 47].

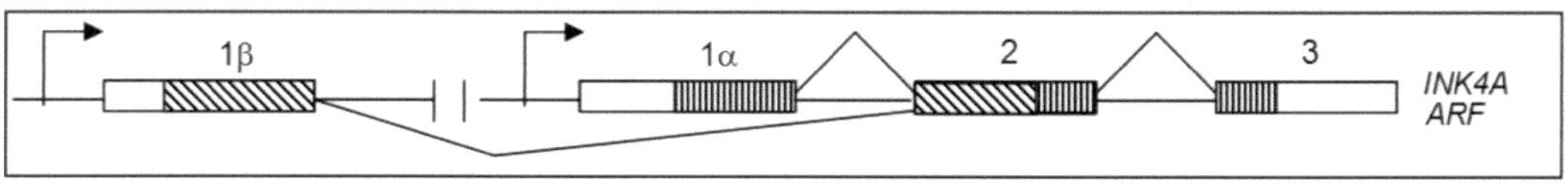

Figure 2. *INK4A* and *ARF* share sequences in the *CDKN2A* locus. Exons are shown as rectangles. Alternative first exons (1α and 1β) are transcribed from different promoters (arrows). Exons 1α and 1β are spliced to the same splicing acceptor site in exon 2 but are translated in alternative reading frames. *INK4A* coding sequences in exons 1α, 2, and 3 and *ARF* coding sequences in exons 1β and 2 are indicated by different shading patterns. Adopted from Sherr [8]. *INK4A* lesions detected by FISH and Sanger sequencing may also affect *ARF*.

Resistance of melanoma to BRAF and MEK inhibitors. The finding that mutations in *BRAF* occur in melanomas led to extensive investigation of targeting BRAF for melanoma treatment. While the response to selective mutant BRAF inhibitors (BRAFi) in *BRAF*-mutant melanoma is encouraging, virtually all patients rapidly develop secondary resistance. Based on the finding that the mitogen activated protein kinase/ERK kinase (MEK)-extracellular signal regulated kinase (ERK) pathway is frequently reactivated by various BRAFi resistance mechanisms, the first combination trial of a selective BRAF inhibitor (dabrafenib, GSK2118436) with a MEK inhibitor (trametinib, GSK1120212) is underway and has achieved clinical responses in 17% and disease control in 67% in patients who failed prior single-agent treatment with a BRAF inhibitor [9]. While these results are promising, again, the treatment response is short-lived; there is a critical need for additional strategies to overcome this deadly disease [49, 50].

There is evidence that treatment response to BRAFi and MEKi relies on a functional p16-cyclin D-CDK4-retinoblastoma (RB) axis. *INK4A* mutations/deletions occur in most of the melanoma cells that demonstrated resistance to BRAFi (e.g.; 451Lu, Mel1617, WM983, WM902, A375, M238, SKMEL28, and A2058) [51-57]. Over-expression of cyclin D and deletion of *RB* confer treatment resistance to BRAFi [56, 58]. Unlike other components of the p16-cyclin D-CDK4-RB axis that harbor genetic changes at low frequency in melanomas (e.g., *CDK4* and *RB* each approximately 3%) [59], and may not overlap with *BRAF* mutation (e.g., amplification of cyclin D1 gene *CCND1* and *CDK4*) [60], *INK4A* lesions are frequently detected in melanomas (~50%) irrespective of *BRAF* mutation [59-61]; therefore, abnormal p16 is a major mechanism of RB-axis attenuation in *BRAF*-mutant melanoma cells. p16 binds to and inhibits the catalytic activity of CDK4, representing a crucial gatekeeper at the G1>S checkpoint [62, 63]. The relative abundance of CDK4-cyclin D and p16 can determine the activity of the CDK4 kinase, thus regulate RB and cell-cycle progression [62, 63]. BRAF-MEK-ERK signaling pathway upregulates/activates the cyclin D-CDK4 enzyme, which phosphorylates and inactivates RB leading to cell cycle progression in melanoma cells; such an effect can be blocked by tumor suppressor p16 [2, 3, 61]. Several pathways that confer BRAFi resistance, including COT, RAF splicing variants, RAF dimerization, NRAS, IGF-1R, and RTK can reactivate cyclin D-CDK4 through signaling pathways including MEK-ERK as well as PI3K-AKT [51-53, 55, 56, 64]. Although the addition of MEKi to BRAFi may suppress reactivation of MEK-ERK-cyclin D-CDK4, alternative resistance mechanisms, including growth factor receptors and PI3K-AKT pathway can activate cyclin D-CDK4 [52, 55, 64-66] *in the absence of a functional p16*, adding CDK4 inhibitor may help overcoming resistance to BRAFi and MEKi (Fig. 3). *BRAF* mutation assays have been used to direct BRAFi treatment. There is significant genotypic heterogeneity of *INK4A* including bi- and mono-allelic deletions, nonsense and missense mutations, and also different levels of epigenetic modification by promoter hyper-methylation. Characterization of whether these *INK4A* changes correlate with different treatment resistance to BRAFi/MEKi/CDK4i may lead to companion molecular tests to better manage melanoma patients under BRAFi, MEKi, and CDK4i therapy.

As shown in Fig. 4, in addition to BRAF and MEK inhibitors, several drugs designed to inhibit the activity of CDK4 are in active clinical trials for melanoma and other cancers including LEE011 (Novartis Pharmaceuticals), LY2835219 (Eli Lilly and Company), PD-0332991 (Pfizer) (http://clinicaltrials.gov/).

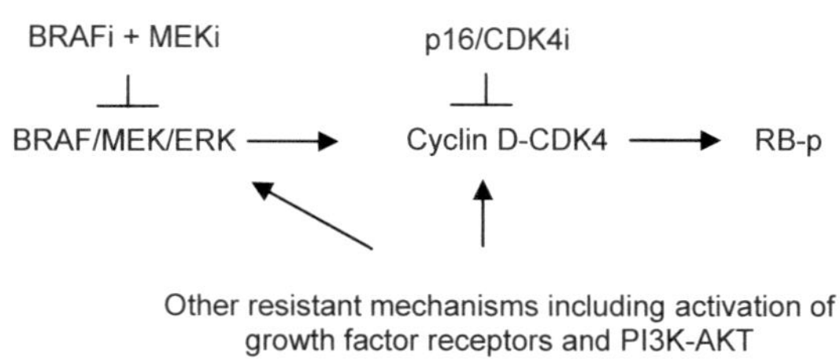

Figure 3. The presence of functional p16 may offset resistance mechanisms that lead to activation of cyclin D-CDK4 in melanomas that progressed under BRAFi/MEKi treatment, whereas abnormal p16 may predict treatment failure in melanomas that develop resistance mechanisms un-opposed by BRAFi + MEKi treatment.

Combined inhibition of CDK4 potentiate the effect of MEKi. In order to design better strategies for the treatment of this devastating disease a better understanding of melanoma biology is necessary. Multiple genetic and environmental factors have been linked to the development and aggressive behavior of melanomas [49, 50]. *BRAF* mutations have been identified in approximately 60–80% of human melanomas, while *NRAS* mutations occur in about 10% of melanomas [4, 67]. Both NRAS and BRAF are components of the RAS-RAF-mitogen activated protein kinase/ERK kinase (MEK)-extracellular signal regulated kinase (ERK) signaling pathway. Apart from *NRAS* and *BRAF* mutation, other factors have been identified leading to constitutive activation of the ERK signaling, for example, amplification and somatic mutations of KIT and constitutive expression of hepatocyte growth factor (HGF) and fibroblast growth factor (FGF) [49, 50]. ERK signaling pathway controls cell proliferation, differentiation, and survival, and has been shown to be a targetable pathway in melanoma treatment [5, 14, 15, 68].

Deregulation of the p16-cyclin D:cyclin-dependent kinases (CDK) 4/6-retinoblastoma (RB) pathway is a common paradigm in malignancy including melanoma [12, 13, 39] and represents another attractive target in melanoma treatment. The great majority of melanoma cells have lost or reduced expression of wild-type *INK4A* caused by genetic and epigenetic changes including mutation, deletion, and promoter hypermethylation [69, 70]. Loss of p16 leaves cyclin D:CDK4 unoppressed to phosphorylate and inactivate RB and cell cycle progression [8, 13, 49, 50, 69, 70]. Amplification of cyclin D1 and CDK4 genes have also been identified, mostly in melanomas that harbor wild-type *NRAS* and *BRAF* [58]. A germ-line Arg24Cys (R24C) mutation in CDK4 was identified in familial melanoma patients [40, 58]. This mutation abolishes CDK4 inhibition by p16 and thus is believed to be a functional equivalent to p16 loss. Both ERK signaling and CDK4 kinase have been shown to regulate RB protein and cell cycle progression [58, 61]. Activation of BRAF-MEK-ERK signaling pathway can cause upregulation of cyclin D resulting in the activation of CDK4 [61]. Activated CDK4 phosphorylates and inactivated RB proteins result in the liberation of E2F transcription factors and cell cycle progression. It has been shown that in advanced melanoma cells, RB is highly phosphorylated and inactive, and E2F transcriptional activity is constitutively high ([5, 12].

Various resistance mechanisms have been identified that contribute to treatment failure of melanoma patients to BRAFi and MEKi therapy. Loss of p16 may represent a common gateway permitting the phenotypic expression of several resistance mechanisms to BRAFi and MEKi (Figs. 1 and 3), a hypothesis that has not been and is waiting to be tested in clinical trials. We reported that simultaneous expression of *BRAF* siRNA and *INK4A* cDNA in melanoma cells leads to dramatically increased apoptosis (17), suggesting that correcting the two most common genetic lesions could be effective in melanoma treatment. It is unclear whether the effect is specific to *BRAF* and *INK4A* or can be generalized to other components of the ERK and RB pathways. It has been shown that *BRAF* and *INK4A* may have activities independent of the corresponding canonical ERK and RB pathways, and the two pathways also mediate cellular signals independent of aberrant *BRAF* and *INK4A*. For example, RAF can act through apoptosis signal-regulating kinase-1 (ASK1)/c-Jun-NH2-kinase or mammalian sterile 20- like-kinase 2 (MST2) pathways ([71]; cyclin D:CDK4 can be activated by enhanced phosphatidylinositol 3-kinase (PI3K) and wingless (WNT) signaling pathways in melanomas [27, 72]. Therefore, we tested PD98059 and 219476, commercially available inhibitors of MEK and CDK4, respectively, in human melanoma cells.

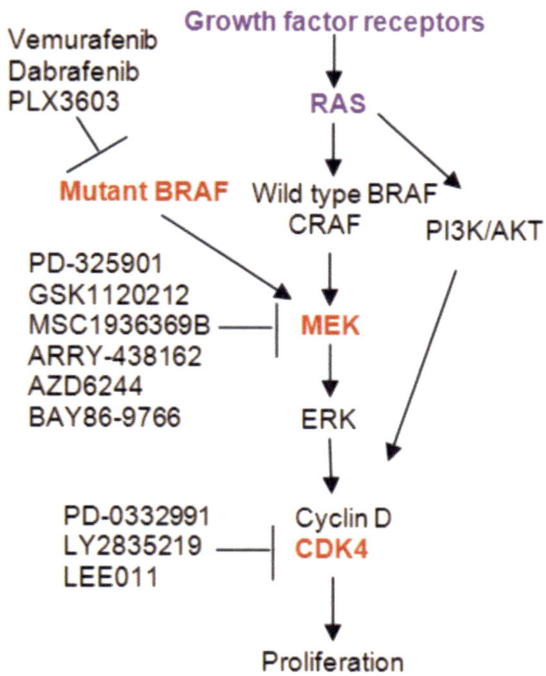

Figure 4. BRAF, MEK and CDK4 inhibitors are in active clinical development and may be used in combination to increase treatment efficacy. Melanoma cells acquire resistance to BRAF and MEK inhibitors by mechanisms including activation of growth factor receptors and RAS signaling pathways. Activation of growth factor receptors and RAS pathways can cause overexpression of cyclin D and activation CDK4 kinase, leading to cell cycle proliferation, which is believed to play major roles in the emergence of treatment resistance. Adding CDK4 inhibitors may overcome resistance to treatment targeting BRAF and MEK. Apart from Vemurafenib (PLX4032, RO5185426) (Hoffmann-La Roche) that has been U.S. Food and Drug Administration (FDA) approved for treatment of melanoma, other mutant BRAF inhibitors including PLX3603 (RO5212054) (Hoffmann-La Roche) and GSK2118436 (dabrafenib) (GlaxoSmithKline) are in active clinical trials. There are clinical trials of MEK inhibitors PD-325901 (Pfizer), GSK1120212 (GlaxoSmithKline), MSC1936369B (EMD Serono), ARRY-438162 (MEK162) (Array BioPharma), AZD6244 (AstraZeneca), and BAY86-9766 (Bayer). Several drugs designed to inhibit the activity of CDK4 are also in active clinical trials for melanoma and other cancers including PD-0332991 (Pfizer), LY2835219 (Eli Lilly and Company), LEE011 (Novartis Pharmaceuticals) (http://clinicaltrials.gov/).

MEK inhibitor PD98059 (Calbiochem, San Diego, CA) was dissolved in dimethyl sulfoxide (DMSO) as a 50 mM stock solution, aliquoted and stored at -20C. CDK4 inhibitor 219476 (Cat. # 219476, Calbiochem, San Diego, CA) was dissolved in DMSO as a 2 mM stock solution and stored at 4C. Human melanoma cell lines 624Mel, A101D, and OM431 were kindly provided by Dr. Stuart Aaronson (Mount Sinai School of Medicine, New York, NY). Cells were maintained in Dulbecco's modified Eagle medium (DMEM) (Mediatech, Herndon, VA) supplemented with 10% fetal bovine serum (FBS; Sigma, St. Louis, MO) and 50 units/mL penicillin–streptomycin (Invitrogen, Carlsbad, CA) in a humidified incubator at 37C with 5% CO2. CellTiter 96® R AQueous One Solution Cell Proliferation Assay (MTS) kit (Promega Corporation, Madison, WI) was used to measure dehydrogenase enzyme activity found in metabolically active cells. Melanoma cells were seeded in a 96 well plate at a density of 2 $\times 10^4$ cells/well in DMEM with 5% FBS. On the second day, the culture medium in each well was changed to 150 μL DMEM without phenol red and supplemented with 0.5% FBS. Cells were treated in triplicate for 24 and 48 hr with either vehicle solvent (control), 25 μM PD98059, 1 μM 219476, or their combination for 624Mel; control solvent, 50 μM PD98059, 1 μM 219476, or their combination for A101D; and control solvent, 50 μM PD98059, 2 μM 219476, or their combination for OM431 cells. CellTiter 96® AQueous One Solution Reagent (30 μL) was then added per well and cell cultures were returned to the incubator for another 4 hr. Subsequently, the absorbance of each well was measured at 450 nm with a Vmax Kinetic Microplate Reader (Molecular Devices, Sunnyvale, CA). The absorbance of the well with only medium and CellTiter 96® AQueous One Solution Regent was background and subtracted from each sample well. The average and standard deviation of three wells with the same treatment were calculated.

Apoptosis was assessed by terminal deoxynucleotidyl transferase-mediated dUTP-biotin nick end labeling of DNA fragments (TUNEL) method using *in situ* Cell Death Detection Kit, Fluorescein (Roche Applied Science, Indianapolis, IN). Melanoma cells were seeded in triplicate in a 6 well plate at a density of 2 × 10^5 cells/well in DMEM with 5% FBS and antibiotics. On the second day, cells were treated with PD98059 and 219476 under the same conditions as the MTS assay. After treatment with the respective chemicals for 48 hr, cells were harvested to detect apoptotic cells using the TUNEL assay according to the manufacturer's instructions (Roche Applied Science, Indianapolis, IN). Using a cytospin, cells were placed onto Polysine glass slides (Fisher Scientific, Fair lawn, NJ), fixed in 4% paraformaldehyde (Fisher Scientific, Fair lawn, NJ) at room temperature for 1 hr, then permeabilized with a fresh prepared mixture of 0.1% Triton X-100 (MP Biomedicals, Inc. Solon, OH) and 0.1% sodium citrate (Fisher Scientific, Fair lawn, NJ) for 5 min at room temperature. Slides were rinsed with phosphate buffered saline (PBS), air dried, and incubated with 50 μL of TUNEL reaction mixture, containing terminal deoxynucleotidyl transferase (TdT)- and fluorescein isothiocyanate (FITC)-labeled dUTP, in a dark humidified atmosphere at 37C for 2 hr. For nuclei counterstaining, slides were cover-slipped with Vectashield mounting medium containing DAPI (Vector Laboratories, Burlingame, CA). Fluoresce positive cells were viewed with a Nikon Eclipse TE 2000-U inverted microscope (Nikon Corp., Tokyo, Japan) equipped with a FITC filter and a DAPI filter. The percentage of apoptotic cells was determined for each sample in a blind fashion by counting the number of green fluorescent nuclei (TUNEL positive) among a total of 300 or more 4'-6-diamidino-2-phenylindole (DAPI)-stained blue nuclei in three random fields at magnification of 20/0.5 (objective) as described previously [1-3].

For Western blotting, 1 × 10^6 melanoma cells were seeded in a cell culture dish (10 cm) in DMEM containing 5% FBS and antibiotics. On the second day, cells were treated with PD98059 and 219476 at the same concentration as described in the MTS assay. For cell cycle regulators cyclin-dependent kinase inhibitor p27 kinase interacting protein 1 (KIP1) and RB, cells were treated with the chemicals in medium with 5% FBS for 24 hr and then harvested. For apoptosis-related protein B-cell chronic lymphocytic leukemia (CLL)/lymphoma 2 (BCL2), BCL2-like 1 (BCL2L1 or bcl-xL), inhibitor of apoptosis family (IAP) protein baculoviral IAP repeat-containing 5 (BIRC5 or survivin), apoptosis facilitator BCL2 interacting mediator (BIM), cysteine-aspartic acid protease (caspase) 3, and poly (ADP-ribose) polymerase (PARP), cells were treated with the various chemicals in DMEM with 5% FBS for 48 hr and then harvested. For phospho- and total-ERK, cells were treated with the chemicals in medium with 0.5% FBS for 18 hr and then harvested. Western blots were performed as described [1-3]. Briefly, harvested cells were lysed in Lysis Solution (Cell Signaling, Danvers, MA) supplemented with Complete Mini Protease Inhibitor Cocktail Tablets (Roche Diagnostics Corporation, Indianapolis, IN). Protein concentration of lysates was determined using the Quick Start Bradford 1 × Dye Reagent (Bio-Rad, Hercules, CA). Lysates were separated in either 12 or 15% SDS-polyacrylamide gel, electrophoretically transferred to Immobilon-P membrane (Millipore Corp, Billerica, MA), and probed with primary antibodies followed by incubation with horseradish peroxidase-conjugated secondary antibodies. The following antibodies were used: BCL2 and tubulin, beta (Sigma-Aldrich, St. Louis, MO); BCL2L1 and BIRC5 (Santa Cruz Biotechnology, Santa Cruz, CA); phosphor-ERK, total ERK, Caspase 3, PARP, and PhosphoPlus(R) RB (Ser780, Ser795, Ser807/811) Antibody Kit (Cell Signaling, Boston, MA); p27KIP1 (BD Biosciences, San Jose, CA); and peroxidase-conjugated antimouse and antirabbit secondary antibodies (Calbiochem, San Diego, CA). Immunoreactive bands were visualized with SuperSignal chemiluminescence substrate (Pierce, Rockford, IL). The blots were exposed to blue sensitive blue X-ray film (Phenix Research, Candler, NC) [1-3].

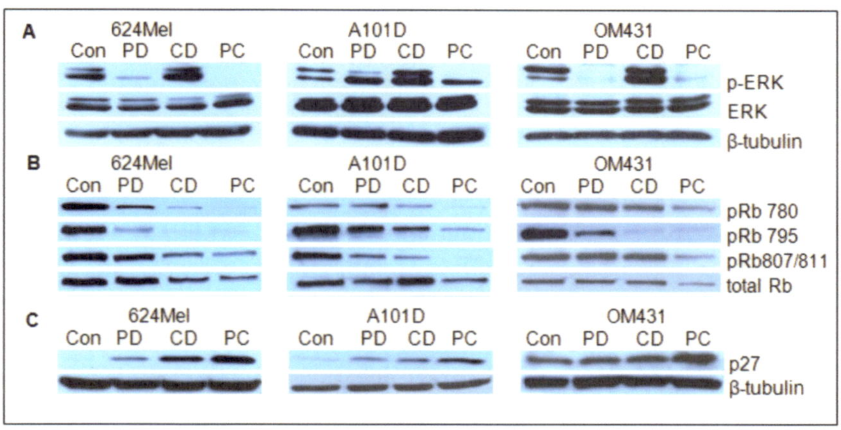

Figure 5. Regulation of ERK phosphorylation, RB phosphorylation, and p27KIP1 expression by PD98059 and 219476, alone and in combination. Human melanoma cell lines 624Mel, A101D, and OM431 were treated with either vehicle solvent (Con), PD98059 (PD), 219476 (CD), or PD98059 plus 219476 (PC) as described in Materials and methods. Western blot was performed using 20 μg total cell lysates, tubulin was used as loading control, as described previously [1-3].

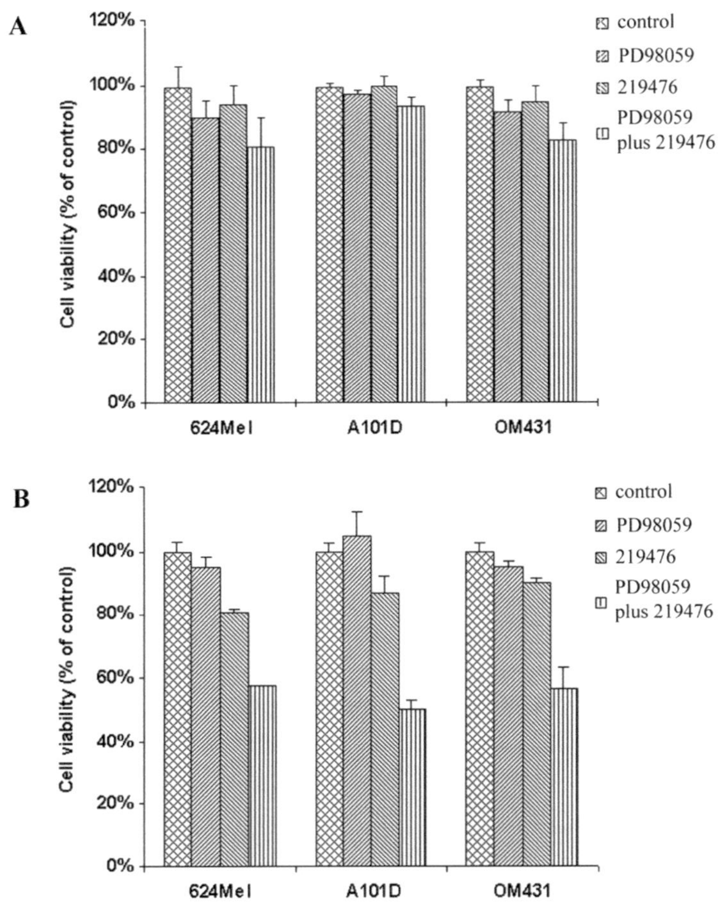

Figure 6. Cytotoxicity by PD98059, 219476, and combinatorial treatment. MTS cytotoxicity assay was performed in 624Mel, A101D, and OM431 cells after (A) 24-hr and (B) 48-hr treatment in medium supplemented with 0.5% FBS. The results are given as means ± SD from three independent tests, as described previously [1-3].

We have shown previously that human melanoma cell lines 624Mel, A101D, and OM431 cell lines harbor heterozygous *BRAF* T1799A mutation and loss of wild-type *INK4A* [1, 61]. Cells were treated, alone or in combination, with MEK inhibitor PD98059 (22) and CDK4 inhibitor 219476 (23). As anticipated, ERK phosphorylation was reduced in cells treated with PD98059, and PD98059 plus 219476 (Fig. 4A). Phosphorylation of S780, S795, and S807/811 of RB, known cyclin D:CDK4 and cyclin E:cyclin dependent kinase 2 (CDK2) targets (7),was decreased in cells treated with either PD98059 or 219476 (except S780 and S807/811 in OM431 cells), and further reduced in cells with combinatorial treatment (Fig. 4B). Of note, total RB was decreased under combinatorial treatment with PD98059 and 219476 in all three melanoma cells (Fig. 4B). Levels of p27KIP1, a negative regulator of cyclin E:CDK2, were increased in cells treated with either PD98059 or 219476, and further increased in cells with combinatorial treatment (Fig. 4C).

PD98059 and 219476 inhibit tumor cell growth in a dose dependent manner [1, 2]. In order to make it possible to monitor the additional therapeutic effects of the combinatorial treatment, both chemicals were used at dosages lower than that which would lead to maximal effect by either agent. The cytotoxicity of PD98059 and 219476 was examined 24 and 48 hr after treatment using the MTS assay that measures the dehydrogenase enzyme activity found in metabolically active cells. After 24-hr treatment, there was no significant difference in cell viability between control, single, and combined treatment groups of 624Mel cells (p = .05, R-square 0.57320, ANOVA). Small but significant differences were observed in A101D and OM431 cells (p = .05, R-square 0.7136 and 0.8091 in A101D and OM431 cells, respectively, ANOVA); the differences were between the combined treatment vs. control and PD98059 in A101D cells, and between the combined treatment vs. control and single treatment of either PD98059 or 219476 in OM431 cells (Figure 2(a), HSD Test at 0.05 significance level). After 48-hr treatment, a significant difference in MTS counts existed for the control, PD98059, 219476, and PD98059 plus 219476 groups in all the three cell lines (p <.0001, R-square 0.981444, 0.956956, and 0.991102 in 624Mel, A101D, and OM431, respectively, ANOVA). Further analysis showed that simultaneous treatment with PD98059 and 219476 after 48-hr treatment resulted in significantly reduced numbers of cell survival than control-treatment or monotreatment as measured by MTS in all the three cell lines (Fig. 6B, HSD Test at 0.05 significance level).

Next, we performed the TUNEL DNA fragmentation assay to identify loss of viability due to programmed cell death after 48-hr treatment. As shown in Figure 3, at the drug concentrations used, significantly different levels of apoptosis exist among control for PD98059, 219476, and combinatorial treatment groups (p < .0001, R-square 0.973862, 0.990697, and 0.987900 in 624Mel, A101D, and OM431, respectively, ANOVA). Treatment with PD98059 alone resulted in no difference in apoptosis over controls in all three cell lines; 219476 enhanced apoptosis in OM431 but not in the other two cell lines; However, combined treatment dramatically increased apoptosis over that seen for the control-treatment and monotreatment (Fig. 7. HSD Test at 0.05 significance level).

As apoptosis was the major effect observed when melanoma cells were exposed simultaneously to MEK and CDK4 inhibitors, we examined the expression of several pro-apoptotic and anti-apoptotic proteins. Mono-treatment with PD98059 or 219476 caused a decreased or no change in the expression of anti-apoptotic proteins BCL2, BCL2L1, and BIRC5. While there were variations in the patterns of expression of BCL2, BCL2L1, and BIRC5 among the different cell lines (Fig. 8), combinatorial treatment caused a comprehensive down-regulation of the proteins in all three cell lines (Fig. 8). In addition, apoptosis facilitator BIM-EL was increased following treatment with PD98059 and PD98059 plus 219476 in all three cell lines. It was also increased in OM431 cells following treatment with 219476. Consistent with increased apoptosis, caspase 3 was activated by simultaneous treatment with PD98059 plus 219476 in all three cell lines, as shown by decreased procaspase 3, increased levels of the active form of caspase 3 (cleaved caspase 3), and degradation of PARP, a direct substrate of active caspase 3 (Fig. 8).

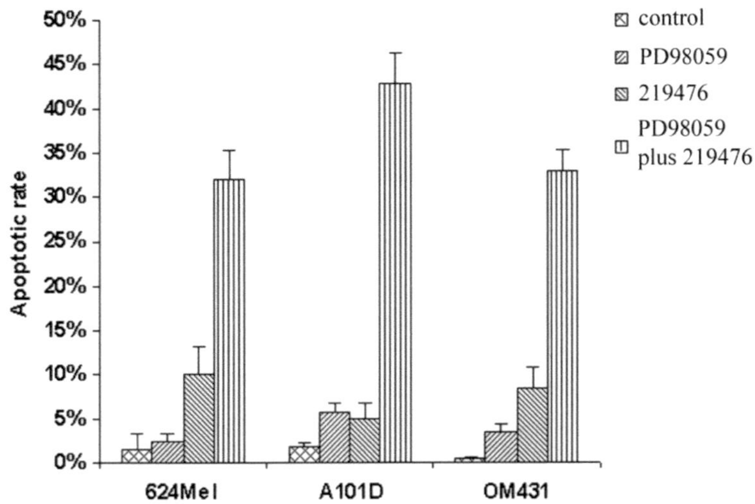

Figure 7. MEK and CDK4 inhibitors induce apoptosis of melanoma cells. TUNEL Assay was performed in 624Mel, A101D and OM431 cells after 48h treatment with vehicle solvent, PD98059, 219476, or PD98059 plus 219476 in medium with 0.5% FBS. The results were given as means ± SD from three independent assays, as described previously [1, 2].

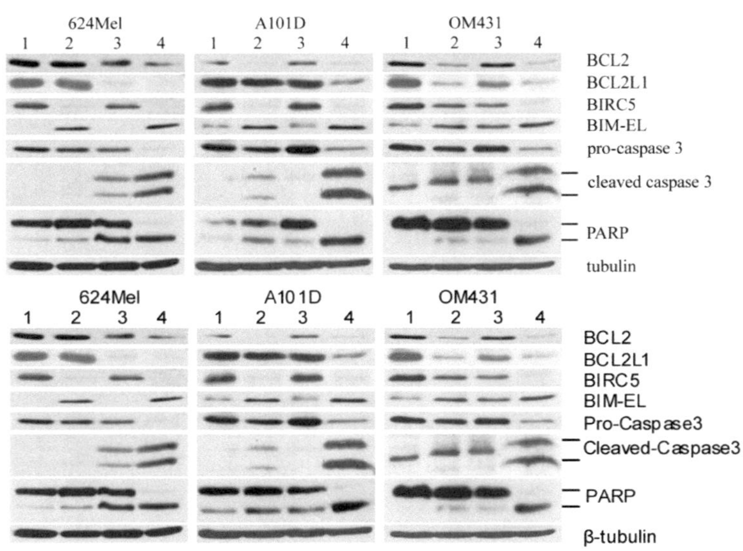

Figure 8. Changes in the expression of pro-survival and pro-apoptotic proteins. Cells were treated with solvent vehicle control (1), PD98059 (2), 219476 (3), and PD98059 plus 219476 (4) for 48 h in medium containing 5% FBS. Western blotting of 20 μg total cell extracts from 624Mel, A101D and OM431 cells using BCL2, BCL2L1, BIRC5, BIM, caspase-3, and PARP antibodies; tubulin was used as loading control, as described previously [1, 2].

In this study, we simultaneously inhibited MEK and CDK4 kinases using pharmacological inhibitors PD98059 and 219476 and observed significantly increased apoptosis compared to control and single agent treatment. This is consistent with our previous report that simultaneous knockdown of BRAF using small interfering RNA (siRNA) and expression of *INK4A* cDNA in melanoma cells leads to a significant increase in apoptosis [1, 3]. These results demonstrate that an increase in apoptosis can be achieved through combinatorial targeting of ERK and RB pathways. It has been well established that constitutive activation of the ERK signaling induces the expression of cyclin D [1, 2, 61], which binds to and activates CDK4 leading to the phosphorylation of RB protein facilitating cell cycle entry [1, 2, 61]. Consistent with an epistatic regulation between ERK pathway and cyclin D:CDK4, amplification of cyclin D1, and CDK4 genes have been identified mainly in melanomas that harbor wild-type *NRAS* and *BRAF* [58, 60]. Additionally, cyclin D:CDK4 mediates resistance to inhibitors of the ERK signaling pathway [58]. Therefore, the enhanced apoptosis and decreased proliferation by simultaneously inhibiting ERK and RB pathways could result from the double hitting of ERK-cyclin D:CDK4-RB that regulate cell cycle progression and cell survival. Alternatively, in support of our previous results that *BRAF* and *INK4A* have a nonlinear functional interaction [1, 61], additional cellular processes could be affected when cells are exposed to both PD98059 and 219476. ERK pathway has pleiopotent activities that regulate cell proliferation, survival, and differentiation through both cyclin D:CDK4 dependent and independent routes [5, 61]. Likewise, cyclin D:CDK4 can be regulated and converges multiple cellular signals. For example, while PI3K signaling can activate CDK4 through downregulation of *INK4A* and upregulation of cyclin D [73], WNT signaling can turn on CDK4 through suppression of *INK4A* transcription [72], It is conceivable that inhibition of MEK and CDK4 not only affects ERK and RB pathways, but also PI3K, WNT, and other ERK signaling activities not mediated through the RB pathway. Therefore, simultaneous targeting of both ERK and RB pathways can generate enhanced effects by targeting both linear and non-overlapping activities.

Apoptosis resistance is a critical factor for therapy failure in melanoma patients. Encouragingly, combined treatment with PD98059 and 219476 leads to significant apoptosis in all the three melanoma cell lines studied (Fig. 7). The apoptotic rate caused by the combined treatment is higher than the combined apoptosis by monotreatment, suggesting that MEK and CDK4 kinases mediate each other's pro-survival effect. The apoptotic effect is associated with changes of apoptosis-related proteins (Fig. 8). PD98059 and 219476 combined treatment leads to significant down-regulation of the pro-survival proteins BCL2, BCL2L1, and BIRC5, and up-regulation of the pro-apoptotic protein BIM. We showed previously that BCL2 and BIM were regulated by *BRAF* and *INK4A* [1, 61]. BCL2L1 and BIRC5 are highly expressed in melanoma cells, and increased expression correlates with tumor progression [74, 75]. A straightforward explanation for the observed apoptosis is that the changes in the pro-apoptotic and anti-apoptotic factors offset the balance and lead to apoptosis [1]. Sequencing analysis of TP53 cDNA [1, 3] showed that 624Mel and OM431cells respectively harbor a T1076G (Cys275Trp) and a G1048A (Gly266Glu) mutations in the DNA binding domain that is likely to compromise the transcription and apoptosis function of p53 [76]. No TP53 mutation has been detected in A101D cells. Although apoptosis is enhanced in all the three cell lines, it is more pronounced in A101D than 624Mel and OM431 cells (Fig. 7), suggesting that TP53 status may influence the magnitude of apoptosis. Combinatorial-treated cells have further inhibited phosphorylation of ERK and RB, reduced total RB, and increased expression of p27KIP1 (Fig. 5). We observed similar effects on ERK and p27KIP1 in a previous report of simultaneous expression of *BRAF* siRNA, and *INK4A* cDNA in melanoma cells [1, 3]. Yu et al. demonstrated that loss of Rb causes apoptosis without effect on cell proliferation [77], and Wang et al. found that overexpression of p27KIP1 leads to apoptosis in melanoma cells [78]. The mechanisms of these changes in relationship to each other and to the observed cooperative effects need to be further investigated. To our knowledge, this study is the first to demonstrate that combined inhibition of MEK and CDK4 using pharmacological inhibitors can cooperate to trigger significant apoptosis in melanoma cells. Deregulation of the RAS-RAF-MEK-ERK and p16-cycylin D:CDK4-RB pathways are common in human malignancies and appears to be important for melanoma development. There has been significant effort to target components of these pathways in cancer treatment. Pharmacologic agents targeting components of the ERK and RB pathways have been developed. However, clinical studies as monotherapy showed that the clinical responses have failed expectations and maximum tolerated doses are often reached before reaching clinical efficacy. Our current study further reinforces the notion that combination targeting of ERK and RB pathways is a promising strategy for melanoma treatment and should encourage further in-depth investigations.

Development of biomarkers to predict treatment response to BRAF, MEK, and CDK4 inhibitors. Apart from *BRAF* mutation, there is no other validated molecular assay to direct BRAFi and MEKi treatment. Comprehensive and standardized *INK4A* molecular assays have not been established in the context of BRAFi and MEKi treatment. Technical and clinical validation of *INK4A* molecular assays may lead to the clinical use of new molecular companion biomarkers to accurately predict clinical response to BRAF and MEK inhibitors, and may also direct future combination treatment that includes CDK4 inhibitors for metastatic melanoma. Because CDK4 is important in both normal and cancerous cells, CDK4 inhibitors are expected to decrease the ability of the bone marrow to make white blood cells, platelets, and red blood cells. Although these effects are expected to be reversible, they can increase the risk of infection, bleeding and fatigue. Like BRAF inhibitors, these drugs are also expected to be expensive. Therefore, development of predictive molecular markers, as in the case of *BRAF* mutation assay for BRAFi, should help selecting patients that are likely to response to the treatment, therefore to maximize efficacy and avoid unnecessary side-effect and treatment cost [79, 80].

Genetic and epigenetic changes of *INK4A* have been identified in 30-70% of melanomas irrespective of *BRAF* mutation [59, 70, 81]. Bi-allelic deletion of *INK4A* (p16 null) occurs in 10-27% of melanomas [60, 82]. Other changes include mono-allelic deletion, point mutation, or promoter hypermethylation, resulting in various levels of p16 expression/activity (Table 1) [57, 60, 81-83]. It is believed that the acquisition of p16 lesions allows melanoma cells to bypass senescence/growth arrest during melanoma development [84]. Although preliminary results with combination therapy of BRAFi and MEKi are encouraging with better clinical response over single agent BRAFi treatment [9], levels of treatment responses vary under the combination treatment [9]. We hypothesize that clinical response to combination therapy of BRAFi and MEKi correlates with status of *INK4A*/p16 (Table 2). The development of clinically useful *INK4A* assays requires an understanding of the underlying biology and access to technology that allows high quality assay performance. Recent advances in molecular technology enable accurate, rapid, and cost-effective *INK4A* molecular testing that can be performed routinely on tumor specimens. However, validation of the technical performance characteristics of *INK4A* assays and understanding of assay limitations are necessary for the accurate interpretation of test results.

***INK4A* status**	**p16 protein sequence and expression**
Wild-type	Normal sequence
Various mutations	Heterogeneous sequence changes
Bi-allelic deletion	Protein null
Promoter hypermethylation	Lower levels of p16

Table 1. Heterogeneity of *INK4A* and p16 in melanoma specimens

As examples, Table 2 is a list of molecular assays to comprehensively examine *INK4A*/p16 lesions in melanoma specimens. Technical and clinical validation studies are necessary before the routine use of these assays in the clinic.

Test	Method	Reference
INK4A deletion	fluorescent *in situ* hybridization (FISH) (p16 SpectrumOrange/ chromosome 9 centromeric probe (CEP9) SpectrumGreen Probe, Abbott Molecular, Des Plaines, IL)	[85, 86]
INK4A mutation	Sanger sequencing	[86, 87]
INK4A promoter methylation	Pyrosequencing (PyroMark Q24 CpG p16 Kit, Qiagen, Valencia, CA)	[82, 88, 89]
p16 expression	Immunohistochemical staining (IHC)	[90, 91]

Table 2. Summary of molecular assays

These assays need to be validated both technically and clinically with defined cut-off values. There should be correlation of results among assay methods; for example, cells with bi-allelic *INK4A* deletion show negative p16 IHC staining and cells with mono-allelic *INK4A* deletion show mutations with loss of heterozygosity (LOH), and p16 expression inversely correlates with levels of *INK4A* promoter methylation. The major obstacles in testing tumor specimens are the presence of non-tumor cells in the samples, the cellular heterogeneity within tumor specimens, and degradation/damage of nucleic acid and protein during sample processing. To ensure accurate testing results, SOPs need to be established with clearly defined instructions on the selection and handling of tumor specimens. For example, FISH assay requires fixation time between 6-48 hrs [92]. Alterations in *INK4A* may also affect the overlapping *ARF* gene (Fig. 2). Although the proposed study focuses on *INK4A*, changes in *INK4A* may also affect *ARF*, which may also be analyzed. Assay clinical sensitivity, clinical specificity, positive predictive value, and negative predictive value of *INK4A* biomarkers for a given treatment response can be calculated as described in Table 4.

INK4A result	**Treatment resistant case**	**Treatment sensitive case**	
Lesion +ve	A	B	Positive predictive value = A / (A + B)
Lesion -ve	C	D	Negative predictive value = D / (C + D)
	Sensitivity = A / (A + C)	Specificity = D / (B + D)	

Table 3. Calculation of clinical sensitivity, clinical specificity and predictive values

3. Conclusion

Patients with metastatic melanoma have a median survival of 6-8 months [93]. Recently, ipilimumab (Yervoy, Bristol-Myers Squibb), an inhibitor of cytotoxic T-lymphocyte antigen 4 (CTLA-4) and vemurafenib (PLX4032, Zelboraf, Plexxikon/Roche), an inhibitor of mutant BRAF, gained FDA approval to treat patients with metastatic melanoma. Although both drugs offer new approaches to the treatment of advanced melanoma, their therapeutic efficacy is limited. Both drugs typically lengthen life by only several months in patients that initially responded to the treatment [94, 95]. There is mounting evidence that acquired resistance to BRAFi frequently correlates with reactivation of the RAS-RAF-MEK-ERK signaling pathway [52, 53, 64]. This finding led to clinical trials combining BRAFi and MEKi in patients with *BRAF*-mutant metastatic melanoma who progressed on a prior BRAFi treatment regimen [94]. Dabrafenib (GSK2118436, GlaxoSmithKline) is a potent and selective inhibitor of mutant BRAF and is comparable in safety and efficacy to vemurafenib. In phase I testing, it achieved a 67% response rate in metastatic melanoma patients with BRAF V600 mutations [96]. Trametinib (GSK1120212, GlaxoSmithKline) is a potent and selective inhibitor of MEK1/2, achieved a clinical response of 40% in patients with an activating *BRAF* mutation in phase I study [97]. A multicenter phase I/II trial of combined treatment with dabrafenib and trametinib demonstrated a disease control rate of 67% (12/18) in patients who failed prior single-agent treatment with a BRAFi [9]. We hypothesize that although reactivation of MEK-ERK-cyclin D-CDK4 in tumors previously treatment with BRAFi may be suppressed by the combination of dabrafenib and trametinib, cyclin D-CDK4 can also be reactivated by alternative resistance mechanisms that cannot be suppressed by the addition of MEKi (e.g.; activation of growth factor receptor and PI3K-AKT pathway) [51-53, 55, 56, 65, 66], if unopposed by p16, can lead to resistance to the BRAFi and MEKi combination therapy (Fig. 1). It has been shown that melanoma cells that harbor abnormal *INK4A* are more sensitive than *INK4A* wild-type cells to the growth inhibitory effect of a p16-mimicking pep-

http://dx.doi.org/10.5772/53620

tide [98] or of flavopiridol, a pan-CDK inhibitor [99], and combination of BRAFi or MEKi with the expression of wild-type *INK4A* or a CDK4 inhibitor significantly suppresses growth and enhances apoptosis in melanoma cells [2, 3]. Therefore, melanoma combination treatments that include CDK4 inhibitors may overcome treatment resistance and enhance efficacy. There is a critical need to identify predictive markers for therapies not only to improve treatment outcomes, but to help avoid ineffective toxic therapies, also because of the likely high cost of combination regimens. Like *BRAF* mutation assay, testing of *INK4A*-p16 may predict which patients will response to BRAF, MEK, and CDK4 inhibitors. Therefore, *INK4A* biomarkers may also have great potential to guide future melanoma combination treatments that include CDK4 inhibitors.

Nomenclature

ASK1: apoptosis signal-regulating kinase-1

ARF: alternative open reading frame

BCL2: B-cell chronic lymphocytic leukemia/lymphoma 2

BCL2L1: BCL2-like 1

BIM: BCL2 interacting mediator

BIRC5: baculoviral IAP repeat-containing 5, also known as survivin

BRAF: v-raf murine sarcoma viral oncogene homolog B1

BRAFi: BRAF inhibitor

Caspase: cysteine-aspartic acid protease

CDK2: cyclin-dependent kinase 2

CDK4: cyclin-dependent kinase 4

CDK4i: CDK4 inhibitor

CEP9: chromosome 9 centromeric probe

CLL: chronic lymphocytic leukemia

DAPI: 4'-6-diamidino-2-phenylindole

DMEM: Dulbecco's modified Eagle medium

DMSO: dimethyl sulfoxide

DTIC: dacarbazine

ERK: extracellular-signal-regulated kinase

FBS: fetal bovine serum

FDA: Food and Drug Administration

FGF: fibroblast growth factor

FISH: fluorescent *in situ* hybridization

FITC: fluorescein isothiocyanate

HGF: hepatocyte growth factor

IAP: inhibitor of apoptosis family

IHC: immunohistochemical staining

INK4A: inhibitor of cyclin-dependent kinase 4A; part of cyclin-dependent kinase inhibitor 2A gene (*CDKN2A*), also known as multiple tumor suppressor 1 (*MTS1*)

KIP1: kinase interacting protein 1

LOH: loss of heterozygosity

MEK: mitogen-activated protein kinase/ERK kinase

MEKi: MEK inhibitor

MST2: sterile 20- like-kinase 2

PAGE: polyacrylamide gel electrophoresis

PARP: poly (ADP-ribose) polymerase

PBS: phosphate buffered saline

PI3K: phosphatidylinositol 3-kinase

p-ERK: phopho-ERK

RAF: v-raf murine sarcoma viral oncogene homolog. Human has three RAF: CRAF, BRAF, and ARAF

RAS: rat sarcoma viral oncogene homolog. Human has three RAS: HRAS, NRAS, and KRAS (KRAS4A and KRAS4B proteins arise from alternative splicing)

RB: retinoblastoma proteins including pRB, p107, and p103

SDS: sodium dodecyl sulfate

siRNA: small interfering RNA

TdT: terminal deoxynucleotidyl transferase

TUNEL: terminal deoxynucleotidyl transferase-mediated dUTP nick end labeling

UV: ultra violate

WNT: wingless

http://dx.doi.org/10.5772/53620

Acknowledgments

We thank Dr. Stuart Aaronson for human melanoma cell lines. This work was supported by Bill Walter III Melanoma Research Fund, Harry J. Lloyd Charitable Trust, and Cancer and Leukemia Group B Foundation (to J.D.).

Author details

Jianli Dong*

Address all correspondence to: jidong@utmb.edu

Molecular Diagnostics Laboratory, University of Texas Medical Branch at Galveston, Galveston, USA

References

[1] Dong, J. and C.L. Schwab, Simultaneous knockdown of mutant BRAF and expression of INK4A in melanoma cells leads to potent growth inhibition and apoptosis. Treatment of Metastatic Melanoma, ed. R.M. R. 2011: InTech. 149-182.

[2] Li, J., et al., Simultaneous inhibition of MEK and CDK4 leads to potent apoptosis in human melanoma cells. Cancer Invest, 2010. 28(4): p. 350-6.

[3] Zhao, Y., et al., Simultaneous knockdown of BRAF and expression of INK4A in melanoma cells leads to potent growth inhibition and apoptosis. Biochem Biophys Res Commun, 2008. 370(3): p. 509-13.

[4] Davies, H., et al., Mutations of the BRAF gene in human cancer. Nature, 2002. 417(6892): p. 949-54.

[5] Peyssonnaux, C. and A. Eychene, The Raf/MEK/ERK pathway: new concepts of activation. Biol Cell, 2001. 93: p. 53-62.

[6] Flaherty, K.T., Next generation therapies change the landscape in melanoma. F1000 Med Rep, 2011. 3: p. 8.

[7] Flaherty, K.T., et al., Inhibition of mutated, activated BRAF in metastatic melanoma. N Engl J Med, 2010. 363(9): p. 809-19.

[8] Sherr, C.J., The INK4a/ARF network in tumour suppression. Nat Rev Mol Cell Biol, 2001. 2: p. 731-7.

[9] Flaherty, K., et al., Phase I/II expansion cohort of BRAF inhibitor GSK2118436 + MEK inhibitor GSK1120212 in patients with BRAF mutant metastatic melanoma who pro-

gressed on a prior BRAF inhibitor [abstract]. In: 8th International Congress of the Society for Melanoma Research. Tampa, FL, November 9–13, 2011. Abstract LBA 1-4. 2011.

[10] Bennett, D.C. and E.E. Medrano, Molecular regulation of melanocyte senescence. Pigment Cell Res, 2002. 15: p. 242-50.

[11] Kuilman, T., et al., The essence of senescence. Genes Dev, 2010. 24(22): p. 2463-79.

[12] Halaban, R., Melanoma cell autonomous growth: the Rb/E2F pathway. Cancer Metastasis Rev, 1999. 18(3): p. 333-43.

[13] Halaban, R., Rb/E2F: a two-edged sword in the melanocytic system. Cancer Metastasis Rev, 2005. 24(2): p. 339-56.

[14] Dent, P. and S. Grant, Pharmacologic interruption of the mitogen-activated extracellular-regulated kinase/mitogen-activated protein kinase signal transduction pathway: potential role in promoting cytotoxic drug action. Clin Cancer Res, 2001. 7: p. 775-83.

[15] English, J.M. and M.H. Cobb, Pharmacological inhibitors of MAPK pathways. Trends Pharmacol Sci, 2002. 23: p. 40-5.

[16] Halaban, R., The regulation of normal melanocyte proliferation. Pigment Cell Res, 2000. 13: p. 4-14.

[17] Busca, R., et al., Ras mediates the cAMP-dependent activation of extracellular signal-regulated kinases (ERKs) in melanocytes. Embo J, 2000. 19: p. 2900-10.

[18] Smalley, K.S., A pivotal role for ERK in the oncogenic behaviour of malignant melanoma? Int J Cancer, 2003. 104(5): p. 527-32.

[19] Hingorani, S.R., et al., Suppression of BRAF(V599E) in human melanoma abrogates transformation. Cancer Res, 2003. 63: p. 5198-202.

[20] Karasarides, M., et al., B-RAF is a therapeutic target in melanoma. Oncogene, 2004.

[21] Sumimoto, H., et al., Inhibition of growth and invasive ability of melanoma by inactivation of mutated BRAF with lentivirus-mediated RNA interference. Oncogene, 2004.

[22] Wojnowski, L., et al., Endothelial apoptosis in Braf-deficient mice. Nat Genet, 1997. 16: p. 293-7.

[23] Ivanov, V.N., A. Bhoumik, and Z. Ronai, Death receptors and melanoma resistance to apoptosis. Oncogene, 2003. 22(20): p. 3152-61.

[24] Soengas, M.S. and S.W. Lowe, Apoptosis and melanoma chemoresistance. Oncogene, 2003. 22: p. 3138-51.

[25] Johnstone, R.W., A.A. Ruefli, and S.W. Lowe, Apoptosis: a link between cancer genetics and chemotherapy. Cell, 2002. 108: p. 153-64.

[26] Schmitt, C.A., Senescence, apoptosis and therapy--cutting the lifelines of cancer. Nat Rev Cancer, 2003. 3: p. 286-95.

[27] Schmitt, C.A., et al., A senescence program controlled by p53 and p16INK4a contributes to the outcome of cancer therapy. Cell, 2002. 109: p. 335-46.

[28] Alavi, A., et al., Role of Raf in vascular protection from distinct apoptotic stimuli. Science, 2003. 301: p. 94-6.

[29] Erhardt, P., E.J. Schremser, and G.M. Cooper, B-Raf inhibits programmed cell death downstream of cytochrome c release from mitochondria by activating the MEK/Erk pathway. Mol Cell Biol, 1999. 19(8): p. 5308-15.

[30] Satyamoorthy, K., et al., Constitutive mitogen-activated protein kinase activation in melanoma is mediated by both BRAF mutations and autocrine growth factor stimulation. Cancer Res, 2003. 63(4): p. 756-9.

[31] Fan, M. and T.C. Chambers, Role of mitogen-activated protein kinases in the response of tumor cells to chemotherapy. Drug Resist Updat, 2001. 4: p. 253-67.

[32] Mandic, A., et al., The MEK1 inhibitor PD98059 sensitizes C8161 melanoma cells to cisplatin-induced apoptosis. Melanoma Res, 2001. 11: p. 11-9.

[33] Halaschek-Wiener, J., et al., Farnesyl thiosalicylic acid chemosensitizes human melanoma in vivo. J Invest Dermatol, 2003. 120: p. 109-15.

[34] Clark, W.H., Jr. and M.A. Tucker, Problems with lesions related to the development of malignant melanoma: common nevi, dysplastic nevi, malignant melanoma in situ, and radial growth phase malignant melanoma. Hum Pathol, 1998. 29: p. 8-14.

[35] Elder, D., Tumor progression, early diagnosis and prognosis of melanoma. Acta Oncol, 1999. 38: p. 535-47.

[36] Pollock, P.M., et al., High frequency of BRAF mutations in nevi. Nat Genet, 2003. 33: p. 19-20.

[37] Dong, J., et al., BRAF oncogenic mutations correlate with progression rather than initiation of human melanoma. Cancer Res, 2003. 63: p. 3883-5.

[38] Sherr, C.J. and F. McCormick, The RB and p53 pathways in cancer. Cancer Cell, 2002. 2: p. 103-12.

[39] Flores, J.F., et al., Loss of the p16INK4a and p15INK4b genes, as well as neighboring 9p21 markers, in sporadic melanoma. Cancer Res, 1996. 56(21): p. 5023-32.

[40] Tsao, H., et al., Melanoma: from mutations to medicine. Genes Dev, 2012. 26(11): p. 1131-55.

[41] Castellano, M., et al., CDKN2A/p16 is inactivated in most melanoma cell lines. Cancer Res, 1997. 57: p. 4868-75.

[42] Funk, J.O., et al., p16INK4a expression is frequently decreased and associated with 9p21 loss of heterozygosity in sporadic melanoma. J Cutan Pathol, 1998. 25: p. 291-6.

[43] von, E.F., et al., Analysis of the tumor suppressor gene p16(INK4A) in microdissected melanoma metastases by sequencing, and microsatellite and methylation screening. Arch Dermatol Res, 1999. 291: p. 474-7.

[44] Welch, J., et al., Lack of genetic and epigenetic changes in CDKN2A in melanocytic nevi. J Invest Dermatol, 2001. 117: p. 383-4.

[45] Zhang, H., J. Schneider, and I. Rosdahl, Expression of p16, p27, p53, p73 and Nup88 proteins in matched primary and metastatic melanoma cells. Int J Oncol, 2002. 21: p. 43-8.

[46] Bannert, N. and R. Kurth, The evolutionary dynamics of human endogenous retroviral families. Annu Rev Genomics Hum Genet, 2006. 7: p. 149-73.

[47] Bandyopadhyay, D., et al., Dynamic assembly of chromatin complexes during cellular senescence: implications for the growth arrest of human melanocytic nevi. Aging Cell, 2007. 6(4): p. 577-91.

[48] Daniotti, M., et al., BRAF alterations are associated with complex mutational profiles in malignant melanoma. Oncogene, 2004. 23(35): p. 5968-77.

[49] Chin, L., L.A. Garraway, and D.E. Fisher, Malignant melanoma: genetics and therapeutics in the genomic era. Genes Dev, 2006. 20(16): p. 2149-82.

[50] Flaherty, K.T., F.S. Hodi, and D.E. Fisher, From genes to drugs: targeted strategies for melanoma. Nat Rev Cancer, 2012. 12(5): p. 349-61.

[51] Johannessen, C.M., et al., COT drives resistance to RAF inhibition through MAP kinase pathway reactivation. Nature, 2011. 468(7326): p. 968-72.

[52] Nazarian, R., et al., Melanomas acquire resistance to B-RAF(V600E) inhibition by RTK or N-RAS upregulation. Nature, 2010. 468(7326): p. 973-7.

[53] Poulikakos, P.I., et al., RAF inhibitor resistance is mediated by dimerization of aberrantly spliced BRAF(V600E). Nature, 2011.

[54] Sondergaard, J.N., et al., Differential sensitivity of melanoma cell lines with BRAFV600E mutation to the specific Raf inhibitor PLX4032. J Transl Med, 2010. 8: p. 39.

[55] Villanueva, J., et al., Acquired resistance to BRAF inhibitors mediated by a RAF kinase switch in melanoma can be overcome by cotargeting MEK and IGF-1R/PI3K. Cancer Cell, 2010. 18(6): p. 683-95.

[56] Xing, F., et al., Concurrent loss of the PTEN and RB1 tumor suppressors attenuates RAF dependence in melanomas harboring (V600E)BRAF. Oncogene, 2011.

[57] Yang, G., A. Rajadurai, and H. Tsao, Recurrent patterns of dual RB and p53 pathway inactivation in melanoma. J Invest Dermatol, 2005. 125(6): p. 1242-51.

[58] Smalley, K.S., et al., Increased cyclin D1 expression can mediate BRAF inhibitor resistance in BRAF V600E-mutated melanomas. Mol Cancer Ther, 2008. 7(9): p. 2876-83.

[59] Dutton-Regester, K. and N.K. Hayward, Reviewing the somatic genetics of melanoma: from current to future analytical approaches. Pigment Cell Melanoma Res, 2012.

[60] Curtin, J.A., et al., Distinct sets of genetic alterations in melanoma. N Engl J Med, 2005. 353(20): p. 2135-47.

[61] Rotolo, S., et al., Effects on proliferation and melanogenesis by inhibition of mutant BRAF and expression of wild-type INK4A in melanoma cells. Int J Cancer, 2005. 115(1): p. 164-9.

[62] Serrano, M., G.J. Hannon, and D. Beach, A new regulatory motif in cell-cycle control causing specific inhibition of cyclin D/CDK4. Nature, 1993. 366(6456): p. 704-7.

[63] Lowe, S.W. and C.J. Sherr, Tumor suppression by Ink4a-Arf: progress and puzzles. Curr Opin Genet Dev, 2003. 13: p. 77-83.

[64] Su, F., et al., Resistance to Selective BRAF Inhibition Can Be Mediated by Modest Upstream Pathway Activation. Cancer Res, 2012.

[65] Recio, J.A. and G. Merlino, Hepatocyte growth factor/scatter factor activates proliferation in melanoma cells through p38 MAPK, ATF-2 and cyclin D1. Oncogene, 2002. 21(7): p. 1000-8.

[66] Spofford, L.S., et al., Cyclin D3 expression in melanoma cells is regulated by adhesion-dependent phosphatidylinositol 3-kinase signaling and contributes to G1-S progression. J Biol Chem, 2006. 281(35): p. 25644-51.

[67] Dong, J., et al., BRAF oncogenic mutations correlate with progression rather than initiation of human melanoma. Cancer Res, 2003. 63(14): p. 3883-5.

[68] Englaro, W., et al., Inhibition of the mitogen-activated protein kinase pathway triggers B16 melanoma cell differentiation. J Biol Chem, 1998. 273: p. 9966-70.

[69] Chin, L., et al., Cooperative effects of INK4a and ras in melanoma susceptibility in vivo. Genes Dev, 1997. 11: p. 2822-34.

[70] Sharpless, E. and L. Chin, The INK4a/ARF locus and melanoma. Oncogene, 2003. 22(20): p. 3092-8.

[71] O'Neill, E.E., D. Matallanas, and W. Kolch, Mammalian sterile 20-like kinases in tumor suppression: an emerging pathway. Cancer Res, 2005. 65(13): p. 5485-7.

[72] Delmas, V., et al., Beta-catenin induces immortalization of melanocytes by suppressing p16INK4a expression and cooperates with N-Ras in melanoma development. Genes Dev, 2007. 21(22): p. 2923-35.

[73] Schmidt, M., et al., Cell cycle inhibition by FoxO forkhead transcription factors involves downregulation of cyclin D. Mol Cell Biol, 2002. 22(22): p. 7842-52.

[74] Piras, F., et al., Nuclear survivin is associated with disease recurrence and poor survival in patients with cutaneous malignant melanoma. Histopathology, 2007. 50(7): p. 835-42.

[75] Zhuang, L., et al., Mcl-1, Bcl-XL and Stat3 expression are associated with progression of melanoma whereas Bcl-2, AP-2 and MITF levels decrease during progression of melanoma. Mod Pathol, 2007. 20(4): p. 416-26.

[76] Petitjean, A., et al., Impact of mutant p53 functional properties on TP53 mutation patterns and tumor phenotype: lessons from recent developments in the IARC TP53 database. Hum Mutat, 2007. 28(6): p. 622-9.

[77] Yu, B.D., et al., Distinct and nonoverlapping roles for pRB and cyclin D:cyclin-dependent kinases 4/6 activity in melanocyte survival. Proc Natl Acad Sci U S A, 2003. 100(25): p. 14881-6.

[78] Wang, X., et al., p27Kip1 overexpression causes apoptotic death of mammalian cells. Oncogene, 1997. 15(24): p. 2991-7.

[79] Engstrom, P.F., et al., NCCN molecular testing white paper: effectiveness, efficiency, and reimbursement. J Natl Compr Canc Netw, 2011. 9 Suppl 6: p. S1-16.

[80] Ong, F.S., et al., Personalized medicine and pharmacogenetic biomarkers: progress in molecular oncology testing. Expert Rev Mol Diagn, 2012. 12(6): p. 593-602.

[81] Grafstrom, E., et al., Biallelic deletions in INK4 in cutaneous melanoma are common and associated with decreased survival. Clin Cancer Res, 2005. 11(8): p. 2991-7.

[82] Jonsson, A., et al., High frequency of p16(INK4A) promoter methylation in NRAS-mutated cutaneous melanoma. J Invest Dermatol, 2010. 130(12): p. 2809-17.

[83] Miller, P.J., et al., Classifying variants of CDKN2A using computational and laboratory studies. Hum Mutat, 2011. 32(8): p. 900-11.

[84] Bennett, D.C., How to make a melanoma: what do we know of the primary clonal events? Pigment Cell Melanoma Res, 2008. 21: p. 27-38.

[85] Chung, C.T., et al., FISH assay development for the detection of p16/CDKN2A deletion in malignant pleural mesothelioma. J Clin Pathol, 2010. 63(7): p. 630-4.

[86] Gerami, P., et al., Fluorescence in situ hybridization (FISH) as an ancillary diagnostic tool in the diagnosis of melanoma. Am J Surg Pathol, 2009. 33(8): p. 1146-56.

[87] Straume, O., et al., Significant impact of promoter hypermethylation and the 540 C>T polymorphism of CDKN2A in cutaneous melanoma of the vertical growth phase. Am J Pathol, 2002. 161(1): p. 229-37.

[88] Tellez, C.S., et al., CpG island methylation profiling in human melanoma cell lines. Melanoma Res, 2009. 19(3): p. 146-55.

[89] Zainuddin, N., et al., Quantitative evaluation of p16(INK4a) promoter methylation using pyrosequencing in de novo diffuse large B-cell lymphoma. Leuk Res, 2011. 35(4): p. 438-43.

[90] Li, Z., et al., Expression of HERV-K correlates with status of MEK-ERK and p16INK4A-CDK4 pathways in melanoma cells. Cancer Invest, 2010. 28(10): p. 1031-7.

[91] Schlosshauer, P.W., et al., Loss of p16INK4A expression in low-grade ovarian serous carcinomas. Int J Gynecol Pathol, 2011. 30(1): p. 22-9.

[92] Middleton, L.P., et al., Implementation of American Society of Clinical Oncology/ College of American Pathologists HER2 Guideline Recommendations in a tertiary care facility increases HER2 immunohistochemistry and fluorescence in situ hybridization concordance and decreases the number of inconclusive cases. Arch Pathol Lab Med, 2009. 133(5): p. 775-80.

[93] Balch, C.M., et al., Final version of 2009 AJCC melanoma staging and classification. J Clin Oncol, 2009. 27(36): p. 6199-206.

[94] Alcala, A.M. and K.T. Flaherty, BRAF Inhibitors for the Treatment of Metastatic Melanoma: Clinical Trials and Mechanisms of Resistance. Clin Cancer Res, 2012. 18(1): p. 33-9.

[95] Patel, S.P. and S.E. Woodman, Profile of ipilimumab and its role in the treatment of metastatic melanoma. Drug Des Devel Ther, 2011. 5: p. 489-95.

[96] Ribas, A. and K.T. Flaherty, BRAF targeted therapy changes the treatment paradigm in melanoma. Nat Rev Clin Oncol, 2011. 8(7): p. 426-33.

[97] Jing, J., et al., Comprehensive predictive biomarker analysis for MEK inhibitor GSK1120212. Mol Cancer Ther, 2011. 11(3): p. 720-9.

[98] Noonan, D.M., et al., In vitro and in vivo tumor growth inhibition by a p16-mimicking peptide in p16INK4A-defective, pRb-positive human melanoma cells. J Cell Physiol, 2005. 202(3): p. 922-8.

[99] Robinson, W.A., et al., The effect of flavopiridol on the growth of p16+ and p16- melanoma cell lines. Melanoma Res, 2003. 13: p. 231-8.

Chapter 2

Targeted Therapies in Melanoma: Successes and Pitfalls

Giuseppe Palmieri, Maria Colombino,
Maria Cristina Sini, Paolo Antonio Ascierto,
Amelia Lissia and Antonio Cossu

Additional information is available at the end of the chapter

http://dx.doi.org/10.5772/53624

1. Introduction

Incidence of melanoma is steadily rising worldwide [1]. Lifetime risk of developing melanoma in Caucasians is estimated as 1 in 50 individuals [2-3]. The incidence of melanoma varies according to the geographical origins of the population and the extent of sun exposure. In Australia and United States, an incidence of melanoma higher than observed in the European countries (with the notable exception of Sweden) has been reported [4-5]. There is a gradient of melanoma incidence from north to south in Europe, with highest frequencies in the northern counties. This suggests that initiation and development of melanoma is due to a combination of the damaging effects of UV and a predisposing genetic background [5].

Melanoma arises from melanocytes, neural crest-derived cells that are located in the basal layer of the epidermis and skin appendages in humans. Melanocytes, by synthesizing melanin pigments and exporting them to adjacent keratonocytes play a key role in protecting the skin from the damaging effects of ultraviolet (UV) and other solar radiation [6]. Melanocytes can proliferate to form nevi (common moles), initially in the basal epidermis (junctional nevus) and later by limited local dermal infiltration (compound nevus). Nevi develop during embryonic life (congenital nevus) and in children and adults, (acquired nevus) partly as a result of solar exposure in the latter two populations. Further progression of melanocytic tumors relates to factors that include intermittent exposure to UV radiation (though a direct relationship between risk of melanoma and UV exposure remains somehow unclear), a history of sunburn and endogenous factors such as skin type and elevated numbers of nevi (especially dysplastic nevi, also known as atypical moles) [7-8].

Considering the growth patterns, four histological types of melanoma have been historically recognized: superficial spreading melanoma (SSM), lentigo maligna melanoma (LMM), nodular melanoma (NM), and acral lentiginous melanoma (ALM) [9]. Comparative genomic hybridization revealed that several genomic regions (mostly, 11q13, 22q11-13, and 5p15) were abnormally amplified in ALM [10]; such regions were different from those found altered in superficial SSM or NM (mainly, 9p21 and 1p22) [11]. Recently, a new classification of melanoma including the site of primary tumour and the degree of chronic sun-induced damage of the surrounding skin has been introduced [12]. Based on these criteria, melanomas are classified into four groups; melanoma on skin with chronic sun-damage (CSD melanoma), melanoma on skin without chronic sun-damage (non-CSD melanoma), melanoma on palms, soles and nail bed (acral melanoma), and melanoma on mucous membrane (mucosal melanoma) [12]. Non-CSD melanomas are characterized by high frequency of BRAF or NRAS mutations (which are mutually exclusive), while CSD, acral, and mucosal melanomas show a low frequency of BRAF/NRAS mutations but a high incidence of alterations in additional genes, such as mutations of receptor tyrosine kinase KIT gene, amplifications of cyclin D1 (CCND1) and cyclin-dependent kinase 4 (CDK4) genes [7, 12-13]. All genes affected into the different types of melanoma are involved in regulating cell-cycle progression and cell survival [12-13]. On the other hand, such a difference of genetic alterations indicates distinct genetic pathways in the pathogenesis of melanoma depending on the anatomical site of the primary lesion. Trying to merge the two classifications, it could be affirmed that non-CSD melanoma roughly corresponds to SSM, CSD melanoma to LMM, and acral melanoma to ALM. Since NM may arise at any anatomical site, this histological type can not be included in any of the subgroups of the latter classification (indeed, no distinct genetic pathway has been so far correlated with NM).

During recent past years, melanocytic transformation is being demonstrated to occur as a sequential accumulation of genetic and molecular alterations [13-14]. In this sense, it is becoming an unquestionable certainty that molecular classification of melanoma patients could be achieved through the assessment of the molecular profile of primary tumors and/or the correspondent metastases, by unveiling which gene or pathway is truly affected. Although pathogenetic mechanisms underlying melanoma development are still largely unknown, several genes and metabolic pathways have been shown to carry molecular alterations in melanoma.

2. Main genes and related pathways

2.1. *BRAF* and MAPK pathway

The *mitogen-activated protein kinase* (MAPK) signal transduction pathway regulates cell growth, survival, and invasion. MAPK signaling is initiated at the cell membrane, either by receptor tyrosine kinases (RTKs) binding ligand or integrin adhesion to extracellular matrix, which transmits activation signals via RAS on the cell membrane inner surface (Figure 1).

http://dx.doi.org/10.5772/53624

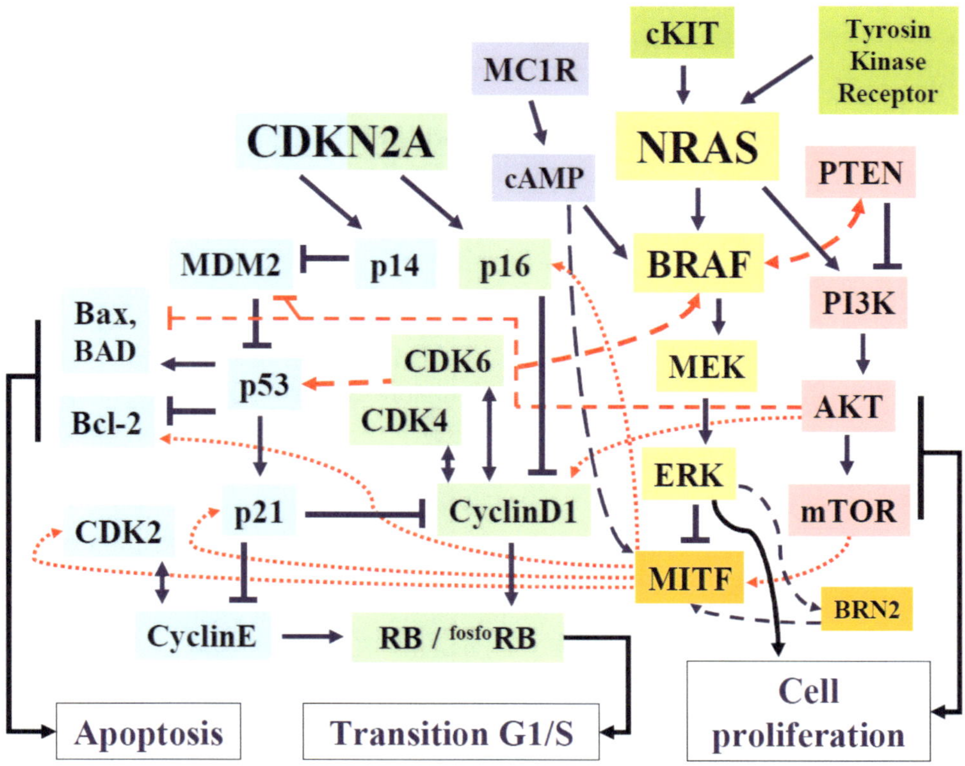

Figure 1. Main pathways involved in melanomagenesis. Arrows, activation signals. Interrupted lines, inhibition signals.

RAS proteins are small GTPases thatare activated by extracellular stimuli and regulate signal transduction of the BRAF-MEK1/2-ERK1/2 and AKT/PI3K pathways, controlling crucial cellular processes such as proliferation, differentiation, cell adhesion, apoptosis, and cell migration [14-16]. RAS gene is mutated in an estimated 20-30% of all cancers [17]. RAS proteins are constituted by three main isoforms - NRAS, KRAS, and HRAS, which present a similar function but a different specificity for tissue distribution [18]. On this regard, KRAS alterations mostly occur in gastrointestinal cancer [17-18], HRAS alterations are frequently observed in bladder cancer, and NRAS is mutated in 15-25% of melanomas [17-18]. Despite the huge amount of knowledge implicating RAS in tumour initiation and promotion, RAS itself has not become a successful target of therapy.

The RAF kinase family consists of three members - ARAF, BRAF, and CRAF, all of which can activate a series of protein kinases; such a signaling cascade culminate in the phosphorylation and activation of the extracellular signal-regulated kinase (ERK) downstream protein [19]. In melanoma, the most commonly mutated component of this pathway is the *BRAF* gene; the prevalent *BRAF* mutation (in nearly, 90% of cases) being a substitution of valine with glutamic acid at position 600 (V600E) [20]. Mutated *BRAF* induces constitutive ERK activation; activated ERK then translocates to the nucleus and initiates the transcription of a variety of growth-related genes, stimulating cell proliferation and survival [20]. Indeed, the increased activity of ERK seems to be implicated in rapid melanoma cell growth, enhanced cell survival and resistance to apoptosis [21]. High levels of activated ERK may further induce the metastatic potential of melanoma by increasing the expression of invasion-promoting integrins [22-23]. Presence of *BRAF* mutations in benign and dysplastic nevi supports the hypothesis that activation of the RAF/MEK/ERK pathway is an early event in melanoma progression [24-25]. In other words, *BRAF* activation is necessary but not sufficient for the development of melanoma and additional co-operating genetic events are required to achieve full malignancy.

In a study aimed to better define the role of BRAF in melanomagenesis, a transgenic zebra fish expressing ^{V600E}BRAF showed dramatic development of patches of ectopic melanocytes (designated as fish-nevi) [26]. Remarkably, activated *BRAF* in p53-deficient zebra fish induced the formation of melanocytic lesions that rapidly developed into invasive melanomas that resembled human melanomas in terms of their histology and biological behaviors [26]. These data provide direct evidence that the p53 and BRAF pathways interact functionally during melanomagenesis.

The *BRAF* gene also cooperates with the cyclin-dependent kinase inhibitor p16^{CDKN2A} (see below). Activating *BRAF* mutations have been reported to constitutively induce up-regulation of *p16*^{CDKN2A} and cell cycle arrest (this phenomenon appears to be a protective response to an inappropriate mitogenic signal). In particular, mutant BRAF protein induces cell senescence by increasing the expression levels of the p16^{CDKN2A} protein, which, in turn, may limit hyperplastic growth caused by *BRAF* mutations [25]. Therefore, inactivation of *p16*^{CDKN2A} gene may promote the melanocytic proliferation depending on oncogenic *BRAF*. In this sense, several factors seem to be able to induce the arrest of the cell cycle and cell senescence caused by *BRAF* activation [27-28].

Finally, it has been showed that primary melanomas arising from chronically sun-damages skin and from mucosal sites, which typically do not harbour *BRAF* and *NRAS* mutations, have increased copy number of the *CCND1/Cyclin D1* gene [12]. In contrast to primary melanomas, a subset (>15%) of metastatic melanoma samples with *BRAF* mutations also exhibit amplification of *CCND1/Cyclin D1*. These melanomas are resistant to BRAF inhibitors highlighting the need for combination therapy [29-30].

2.2. *CDKN2A* and senescence/apoptosis pathways

The cyclin-dependent kinase inhibitor 2 (*CDKN2A*; at chromosome 9p21) gene encodes two proteins, p16^{CDKN2A} and p14^{CDKN2A} (a product of an alternative splicing), that are known to function as tumor suppressors [31-33]. The cyclin proteins are regulatory effectors able to bind and activate the cyclin-dependent kinases (CDKs) that bear catalytic kinase activity. Several distinct cyclin/CDK complexes have been identified and functionally assigned to specific phases of the cell cycle: Cyclin D/CDK4 complex leads the passage from the pre-replicative (G1) to the DNA duplication (S) phase; the Cyclin E/CDK2 complex promotes the progression through the S phase and the Cyclin B/CDK1 complex induces cells to enter mitosis [31-32]. In such a functional network, proteins like p16^{CDKN2A} and p14^{CDKN2A} act as inhibitors of the cell cycle, negatively interfering with the activity of the cyclin/CDK complexes and, in this way, ensuring the control of the cell replication [33]. In particular, p16^{CDKN2A} is part of the G1–S cell cycle checkpoint mechanism that involves the retinoblastoma-susceptibility tumor suppressor protein (pRb). The p16^{CDKN2A} inhibits the Cyclin D/CDK4 complex, which, in turn, phosphorylates pRb and allows progression through the G1–S checkpoint (Figure 1) [33]. The *Cyclin D* (*CCND1*) and *CDK4* genes are found altered in less than 5% of total melanomas [12], though with an heterogeneous prevalence according to the distinct types of melanoma (see above). Somatic *CDK4* amplification is relatively common in acral and mucosal melanomas [12], whereas germline *CDK4* mutations are observed in a limited fraction of melanoma-prone families [34]. The *CCND1* gene amplifications is primarily found in ALM lesions (more than one third of cases) and to a lesser degree in other types (11% for LMM and 6% for SSM) [35]. Regarding the alternative *CDKN2A* gene product, p14^{CDKN2A} is an antagonist of the murine double minute 2 (MDM2) protein, which targets p53 to degradation by ubiquitination and proteasome processing, thus abrogating p53 control of cell growth (Figure 1) [32-33]. In particular, the p14^{CDKN2A} protein exerts a tumor suppressor effect by inhibiting the oncogenic actions of the downstream MDM2 protein, whose direct interaction with p53 blocks any p53-mediated activity and targets the p53 protein for rapid degradation [32-33]. The p53 is a transcription factor that functions as a major negative regulator of cell proliferation and survival, being activated by different adverse signals (i.e. growth factors withdrawal, DNA damage, oncogenic aberrations, hypoxia, etc.) and driving cells to either interrupt progression into the cell-cycle or enter apoptosis program, in order to avoid reproduction of altered cells [33, 36]. In normal conditions, expression levels of p53 within cells are low. In response to DNA damage, p53 accumulates and prevents cell division. Therefore, inactivation of the *TP53* gene results in an intracellular accumulation of genetic damage which promotes tumor formation [36]. In melanoma, such an inactivation is mostly due to functional gene silencing since the frequency of *TP53* mutations is low (less than 10% of cases) [37]. Impairment of the p14^{CDKN2A}-MDM2-p53 cascade, whose final effectors are the Bax/Bcl-2 proteins, has been implicated in defective apoptotic responses to genotoxic damage and, thus, to anticancer agents (in most cases, high expression levels of Bcl-2 protein have been demonstrated to reduce apoptosis and sensitivity of melanoma cells to proapoptotic stimuli, contributing to further increase tumor aggressiveness and refractoriness to therapy) [33].

More in general, genetic loss or rearrangement in the CDKN2A locus may result in impairing or silencing p16^{CDKN2A}, p14^{CDKN2A} or both genes, with the consequence of losing the mechanisms controlling cell proliferation and/or survival. In melanoma, the *CDKN2A* gene is somatically inactivated by genomic deletions (approximately 50% of cases) or point mutations (about 10% of cases); in addition, this gene is often transcriptionally silenced by promoter hypermethylation [38]. A reduced expression of the p16^{CDKN2A} protein seems to be strictly associated with malignant tumor invasion, varying from 5% to about 15% in benign melanocytic lesions, from 10% to about 50% in primary melanomas, and from 50% to about 60% in melanoma metastases [39]. The *CDKN2A* gene is frequently mutated at germline level in patients with a strong familial history of melanoma (three or more affected family members), indicating that it represents a key susceptibility gene for familial melanoma [40]. In melanoma, CDKN2A mutations typically occur in the $p16^{CDKN2A}$ gene, either alone or in combination with $p14^{CDKN2A}$ gene (some families harbor however mutations only in this latter gene) [33, 40].

A recent meta-analysis of studies conducted in independent populations indicated that multiple variants of the melanocortin-1 receptor (*MC1R*) gene increase the melanoma risk in *CDKN2A* mutation carriers [41]. The *MC1R* gene encodes a G-protein coupled receptor. In the skin, two types of melanin pigment, dark-protective eumelanin and red-photo reactive pheomelanin, are present [42]. MC1R plays an important role in determining the ratio of eumelanin and pheomelanin production. After stimulation by UV, keratinocytes produce alpha melanocyte stimulating hormone (MSH) that binds to the MC1R on melanocytes and shifts the balance of these two pigments in the direction of eumelanin [42]. In particular, stimulation of MC1R by MSH mediates activation of adenylate cyclase, subsequent elevation of cAMP levels, and activation of the microphthalmia transcription factor (MITF; see below). Activated MITF binds to a conserved region found in the promoters of the *tyrosinase* (*TYR*), *tyrosinase-related protein 1* (*TYRP1*), and *DOPAchrome tautomerase* (*DCT*) genes, stimulating the transcriptional up-regulation of these proteins and inducing maturation of the melanosomes [43]. This ultimately results in increased eumelanin production and darkening of the skin or hair.

New findings have shed light on the mechanisms by which MC1R contributes to melanoma risk. In vitro studies showed that acute UV irradiation of melanocytes with impaired MC1R results in an increased production of free radicals [44]. Melanomas that arise on body sites only intermittently exposed to sun, and which therefore lack marked signs of chronic solar damage, were found to have a high frequency of *BRAF* mutations [12]. One could speculate that induction of *BRAF* mutations may occur only when solar exposure is not sufficiently prolonged to induce the striking tissue changes that generate the hallmark signs of solar damage. Several *MC1R* variants, that impairing relevant protein function, have been associated with *BRAF* mutation in melanoma arising in Caucasian populations from United States and Europe [45-48]. On the basis of such indications, it is possible that increased production of free radicals following UV exposure is combination with impairment of *MC1R* may induce mutations in the *BRAF* gene.

Additional mechanisms promoting susceptibility to pathogenetic mutations of the *BRAF* gene may however exist since there is no demonstrable association between germ line *MC1R* status and the prevalence of somatic *BRAF* mutations in melanomas from Australian population, even after classifying the melanomas by their location relative to intermittent and chronic sun-exposure [49].

2.3. *PTEN* and mTORC pathways

Phosphatase and tensin homolog deleted in chromosome ten (PTEN) has a key role in cellular signal transduction by decreasing intracellular phosphatidylinositol [3,4-bisphosphate (PIP2) and 3,4,5-triphosphate (PIP3)] that are produced by the activation of phoshoinosite 3-kinase (PI3K) [50]. In the absence of extracellular growth stimuli mediated by cell surface receptors and G-proteins, PTEN dephosphorylates PIP3 generating the PIP2 phospholipid, unable to stimulate phosphorylation of the PI3K protein; this in turn maintains suppression of cell cycle progression and cell growth. In other words, there is a balance between PIP2 and PIP3 which is maintained by the opposite activities of PTEN and PI3K, which instead converts PIP2 into PIP3 [50]. Upon growth stimulation, mainly obtained by triggering the RAS kinase, PI3K is constitutively activated (Figure 1), resulting in an increase of intracellular levels of PIP3 and a consequent activation of AKT by phosphorylation [50-51]. Activated AKT in turn phosphorylates its substrate, the serine/threonine kinase mTOR, leading to increased synthesis of target proteins that promote cell division and survival as well as apoptotic escape [51]. The mechanisms associated with the ability of AKT to suppress apoptosis include the phosphorylation and inactivation of many pro-apoptotic proteins, such as BAD (Bcl-2 antagonist of cell death) and MDM2, as well as the activation of NF-kB [52] (Figure 1).

Three *AKT* genes have been described in humans: *AKT1*, which is involved in apoptosis and protein synthesis; *AKT2*, which is involved in controlling the glucose metabolism; and *AKT3*, whose increased activity (often associated with the amplification of the *AKT3* locus at chromosome 1q43-44) is mainly involved in stimulating cell growth and has been implicated in many cancers including melanoma [51-52]. More than two thirds of primary and metastatic melanomas exhibit higher levels of phosphorylated AKT [52], suggesting that such an alteration might be considered as an early event in melanoma pathogenesis.

Overall, PI3K expression is higher in malignant melanomas, as compared to nevi, and seems to correlate with a worse prognosis [53]. In primary melanomas, since activating mutations of PI3K are quite rare (about 1%), and comparative genomic hybridization did not reveal amplification at this gene locus [12, 37], activation of the PI3K pathway is mostly due to functional silencing of the tumour suppressor gene PTEN. Inactivation of *PTEN* gene is mainly due to hypermethylation-based epigenetic mechanisms, with a low incidence (less than 10%) of somatic mutations and/or allelic deletions; loss of (or reduced) PTEN protein is observed by immunohistochemistry in 20-40% of melanoma tissues [54-55]. Consistent with its role in the PI3K-AKT pathway, vast majority (more than 80%) of melanoma samples with loss of PTEN protein presents a significant increase in expression of phosphorylated AKT [37].

PTEN inactivation has been mostly observed as a late event in melanoma, although a dose-dependent down-regulation of PTEN expression has been implicated in early stages of tumorigenesis, often occurring in conjunction with mutations in *BRAF* gene (which have been demonstrated to indeed play a role in induction of the melanocytic proliferation and early steps of melanoma development) [50]. PTEN downregulation In addition, alterations of the BRAF-MAPK pathway are frequently associated with PTEN-AKT impairment [7, 56]. In summary, the combined effects of the inactivation of *PTEN* gene and activation of the PI3K-AKT effectors may result in aberrant cell growth, apoptosis escape, and abnormal cell spreading and migration [33, 50].

2.4. *MITF* and melanocytic differentiation

The microphthalmia-associated transcription factor (MITF) is a transcription factor that is involved in differentiation and maintenance of melanocytes, playing a role in melanoma development and pathogenesis [43, 57]. MITF is activated by the MAPK pathway as well as by the cAMP pathway (Figure 1), and leads to transcription of genes involved in pigmentation (TYR, TYRP1, and DCT; see above) as well as cell cycle progression and survival [43]. The *MITF* gene is amplified in melanoma (about 20% of cases); *MITF* amplification correlated with increased resistance to chemotherapy and decreased overall survival [57].

The connection between MITF and melanoma development is complex because it plays a double role of inducer/repressor of cellular proliferation. High levels of MITF expression lead to G1 cell-cycle arrest and differentiation, through induction of the cell cycle inhibitors $p16^{CDKN2A}$ and p21 [58-59] (Figure 1). Very low or null MITF expression levels predispose to apoptosis whereas inter-mediate MITF expression levels promote cell proliferation [57-59]. Therefore, it is thought that melanoma cells have developed strategies to maintain MITF levels in the range compatible with tumorigenesis. It has been shown that constitutive ERK activity, stimulated by ^{V600E}BRAF in melanoma cells, is associated with MITF ubiquitin-dependent degradation [60]. Nevertheless, continued expression of MITF is necessary for proliferation and survival of melanoma cells, because it also regulates CDK2 and Bcl-2 genes [61-62]. It has been recently shown that oncogenic BRAF may control intracellular levels of the MITF protein through a fine balance of two opposite mechanisms: a direct reduction of MITF levels, by inducing protein degradation, and an indirect increase of MITF levels, by stimulating transcription factors which increase protein expression levels [63]. Oncogenic *BRAF* mutations are associated with *MITF* amplification in a low fraction (10-15%) of melanomas [63], suggesting that other mechanisms are likely to be involved in ERK-dependent degradation of MITF.

2.5. *iNOS* and *NF-kB* pathways

Human melanoma cells are known to express the inducible nitric oxide synthase (iNOS) enzyme, which is responsible for synthesis of nitric oxide (NO), a free radical involved in several physiological processes such as neurotransmission, vasodilation, and regulation of immune responses [64]. The iNOS enzyme has been found to be frequently expressed in melanoma [65-66] and the subsequent increased concentrations of NO have been demonstrated to contribute to melanomagenesis through a sustained protection of the tumour from apoptosis [67]. However, the role of iNOS in melanoma progression remains controversial. Higher levels of iNOS have been found in subcutaneous and lymph node metastases of non-progressive melanoma as compared to metastases of progressive melanoma [68], however, iNOS was found to be expressed to a lesser extent in metastases as compared with nevi and primary melanomas [69]. Nevertheless, the expression of iNOS in patients with lymph nodes and in-transit metastases (stage III disease) has been proposed as an indicator of poor prognosis [70].

Recently, it has been reported that the constitutive iNOS expression in melanoma cells might be induced by activation of the MAPK pathway through stimulation of the activity of the Nuclear Factor-kB (NF-kB) [71-72]. NF-kB is a protein complex that acts as a transcriptional factor and regulates the transcription of several genes involved in many critical pathways [73]. In a quiescent status, proteins of the NF-kB complex are localized into the cytoplasm. NF-κB exists as cytoplasmic hetero- or homodimers associated with members of the inhibitor-of-kB (IkB) proteins (IkB*a*, Ik*Bb* and IkB*e*), which form complexes sequestering NF-kB into the cytoplasm [74]. Upon appropriate stimulation, the phosphorylation of IkB proteins is promoted, triggering their ubiquitination and degradation in the proteasome [74]. As a consequence, NF-kB may translocate to the nucleus where it binds to target DNA loci and induces transcription of several genes - including *iNOS* - associated with immune and inflammatory response, angiogenesis, cell proliferation, tumor promotion, and apoptosis [73-74].

Regarding the role of NF-kB in tumorigenesis, there are compelling evidence that activation of NF-kB controls multiple cellular processes in cancer due to its ability to promote cell proliferation, suppress apoptosis, promote cell migration, and suppress cell differentiation, opening the way for new therapeutic approaches against such a target [75-76]. In melanoma, NF-kB is constitutively activated since expression of the IkB proteins seems to be significantly reduced in comparison to nevi [77].

2.6. *cKIT* and tyrosinase kinase receptors

cKIT is a member of the transmenbrane receptor tyrosine kinase family that comprised five immunoglobin-like motifs, a single transmembrane region, an inhibitory cytoplasmic juxtamenbrane domain, and a split cytoplasmic kinase domain separated by a kinase insert segment [78]. Under physiological conditions, binding of the cKIT ligand stem-cell factor (SCF) to the extracellular domain of the receptor leads its dimerization, activation of the intracellular tyrosine kinase domain through autophosporylation of specific tyrosine residue [78]. The intracellular signaling through cKIT plays a critical role in the development of several mammalian cells, including growth, differentiation, migration, and proliferation of melanocytes [79]. It has been defined that cKIT recruits and activates a number of intracellular signaling pathways implicated in tumor progression, such as MAPK, PI3K/AKT, Src, activators of transcription (STAT), and phospholipase-C (PLC) [79-80].

Although the role of cKIT in melanomagenesis is still controversial, several studies have reported its downregulation during melanoma growth and invasion (in vertical growth phase of melanoma and metastatic lesions) [81-83]. Indeed, the majority of highly metastatic human melanomas do not express detectable levels of the cKIT receptor [83]. As a confirmation of this, over-expression of cKIT in metastatic melanoma cell lines led to important reduction in tumor growth, while cKIT activation through exposure to cKIT ligands induced apoptosis [83].

Specific mutations within the cKIT gene cause constitutive phosphorylation and activation of the kinase domain resulting in uncontrolled cell proliferation. [84]. Although such mutations seem to be more rare than *BRAF* and *NRAS* mutations, these may reflect the important role of cKIT tyrosine kinase in melanocyte development [84]. Sequencing of cKIT exons 11, 13, 17, and 18 revealed the most prevalent mutation to be K642, L576P, D816H-V, V559A [84]. The cKIT mutations are more common in mucosal and acral melanomas compared with cutaneous melanomas and are in most cases accompanied by an increase in gene copy number (40% mucosal or acral melanomas - frequently, associated with amplification of *cy-*

clin D1 - as well as 30% of melanomas on skin with chronic sun-induced damage) [84]. High expression levels of cKIT and CDK4 proteins have been identified in another subset of melanomas lacking *BRAF* mutations [85].

2.7. CTLA-4 and T-cell activation

The above-mentioned main intracellular molecular pathways are thus involved in tumor growth and survival, actively participating to the different phases of development and progression of melanoma. Additional extracellular factors, mainly represented by different components of the tumor microenvironment, have been implied to play a role in melanoma tissue invasion and metastatic dissemination. As an example, changes in the expression of adhesion molecules such as MCAM/MUC18, E-cadherin, and integrins occur in the transition from the radial growth phase (RGP) to the vertical growth phase (VGP) of melanoma; they are induced by both intracellular modifications [i.e., activation of the focal adhesion kinase (FAK) and integrin linked kinase (ILK) patways or high levels of activated ERK (phospoERK$_{1\text{-}2}$)] and biological signals directly generated by the extracellular matrix (ECM), which is composed of proteins, glycoproteins, proteoglycans, and glycosaminoglycans in complex arrangements [22-23].

Among others, a block of the anti-tumor immune response induced by changes in pericellular microenvironment has been demonstrated to contribute to melanoma progression [86]. In recent past years, research has tried to better define the molecular mechanisms underlying the downregulation of the immune system by such pericellular components, in order to develop new therapeutic targets [87]. Actually, two immunomodulant antibodies, such as anti-CTLA4 and anti-PD1, have been demonstrated to be effective in inhibiting some down-regulators of the anti-tumor immune response [30, 88]. Moreover, drugs able to interfere with the differentiation of the myeloid-derived suppressor cells (MDSC) and T regulatory cells (Treg), which are both physiologically involved in controlling an abnormal immune response during the inflammatory processes and pathologically favoring tumor progression through suppression of T-cell activation, represent additional therapeutic strategies to be exploited [89].

For T-cell activation, melanoma antigens that are bound to the major histocompatibility complex (MHC) on antigen-presenting cells (APCs) require the costimulation of CD28 receptor on T-cells by CD80 or CD86 ligands on APCs [90]. The cytotoxic T-lymphocyte antigen-4 (CTLA-4) can bind with greater affinity to CD80 and CD86, and thus disrupt the necessary costimulatory signal provided by APCs [88, 90]. This led to the hypothesis that blockade of CTLA-4 function may allow for optimal costimulation of CD28 receptors on T-cells by APC CD80/86, and enhanced T-cell activation [88, 90]. Ipilimumab (Yervoy™ Bristol-Myers Squibb, New York, NY) blocks the costimulatory signal required for T-cell activation [30, 88]. In particular, Ipilimumab is a recombinant human IgG1 monoclonal antibody that binds to CTLA-4 and blocks binding to CD80 or CD86 on APCs, thus increasing activation and proliferation of T cells [88]. Two randomized phase III trials have indicated a significant advantage in disease-free survival (DFS) and overall survival (OS) in either monotherapy or combination therapy [91-92]. The first trial compared monotherapy with Ipilimumab 3 mg/kg, combination of Ipilimumab with gp100 vaccine, and gp100 vaccine alone; the study demonstrated a significant advantage in OS for patients treated with Ipilimumab (regardless the addition off gp100) in comparison to those receiving the gp100 vaccine alone [median OS 10.0 vs 6.4 mesi; Hazard Ratio (HR) for death, 0.68; p<0,001) [91]. In the second study, Dacarbazine was administered as standard chemotherapeutic drug for melanoma patients, in association with Ipilimumab or placebo; the OS rate was significantly higher in the group of patients treated with Ipilimumab + Dacarbazine (11.2 *vs.* 9.1 months), with even more significant percentages of survival for such an association after one year (47.3% *vs.* 36.3%), two years (28.5% *vs.* 17.9%), or three years (20.8% *vs.* 12.2%) of follow-up [92]. The DFS and OS curves from the two studies have been indicated as largely overlapping, strongly demonstrating, for the first time in the history of medical treatments for the advanced disease, a clear survival benefit in metastatic (disease stage IV) melanoma. For these reasons, Ipilimumab has been recently approved by FDA and EMEA for the treatment of metastatic melanoma.

3. Melanoma subtypes and targeted therapeutic options

The different molecular *pathways* involved into the pathogenesis of melanoma are functionally linked each other (Figure 1). There is thus a need to consider such biological cascades as part of a functional web, and the alterations detected in distinct components of the various pathways must be globally considered for the effects determining in such a functional web. This new vision helps in clarifying the reasons by which some alterations may coexist or not in specific melanoma subtypes. As an example, *BRAF* mutations may be observed in conjunction with *PI3K* alterations, but none of them may coexist with *NRAS* mutations; since BRAF and PI3K kinases act downstream NRAS protein, occurrence of *NRAS* mutations activating both MAPK and PI3K-AKT pathways makes unnecessary the further activation of BRAF and PI3K (upstream effectors of the MAPK and PI3K-AKT pathways, respectively). Analogously, oncogenic *BRAF* mutations are able to more intensively activate ERK protein, main last effector downstream the MAPK pathway, when inactivation of the mechanisms controlling senescence and apoptosis concomitantly occurs.

In an attempt to simplify such complex processes underlying the different phases of development and progression of melanoma, the main pathogenetic molecular alterations may be grouped in the following way:

- oncogenic *BRAF* mutations, genomic rearrangements (mainly represented by allelic deletions) at the 9p21 chromosome, and increased expression levels of the AKT3 protein are the main alterations involved into the phase of stimulation of the proliferation for normal melanocytes (*initial preneoplastic phase*);
- impairments of the mechanisms controlling the cell senescence, apoptosis and cell survival (which particularly include alterations in the different components of *CDKN2A* pathways: functional deficit of $p16^{CDKN2A}$ gene, amplification of *CDK4-Cyclin D1/CCND1* loci, inattivation of *TP53* gene through a deregulation of the $p14^{CDKN2A}$-MDM2-p53 functional cascade), oncogenic mutations in *NRAS* gene, activating mutations and, to a lesser extent, gene amplifications of *cKIT* are the main alterations involved into the phase of acquisition of the malignant phenotype which underlay the development of melanoma (*intermediate neoplastic phase*);

- complete silencing of $p16^{CDKN2A}$ gene, functional loss of PTEN, activation of the PI3K-AKT pathway, and amplification of the *MITF* gene are the main alterations involved into the phase of acquisition of a more aggressive and invasive phenotype which underlay the progression and dissemination of melanoma (*final metasticase phase*).

All these findings clearly indicate the existence of a complex molecular machinery that provides checks and balances in normal melanocytes, allowing a physiologically controlled cell proliferation. Progression from normal melanocytes to malignant metastatic cell in melanoma patients is the result of a combination of down- or up-regulations of the various effectors acting into the different molecular pathways. According to this, it has been proposed a linear model of pathogenesis of melanoma based on the sequential accumulation of most of the previously-described molecular alterations (Figure 2A) [7, 13, 93]. In a limited fraction of cases, it has been recently hypothesized a second non-linear model of melanomagenesis based on accumulation of the same genetic alterations in tissue stem cells, with generation of malignant cells directly forming RGP or VGP or metastatic melanoma lesions (Figure 2B) [94]. This latter hypothesis has been derived by the evidence of some inconsistencies of the linear model in subgroups of melanomas (i.e., incidence of *BRAF* mutations higher in VGP lesions than that found in RGP lesions [94]).

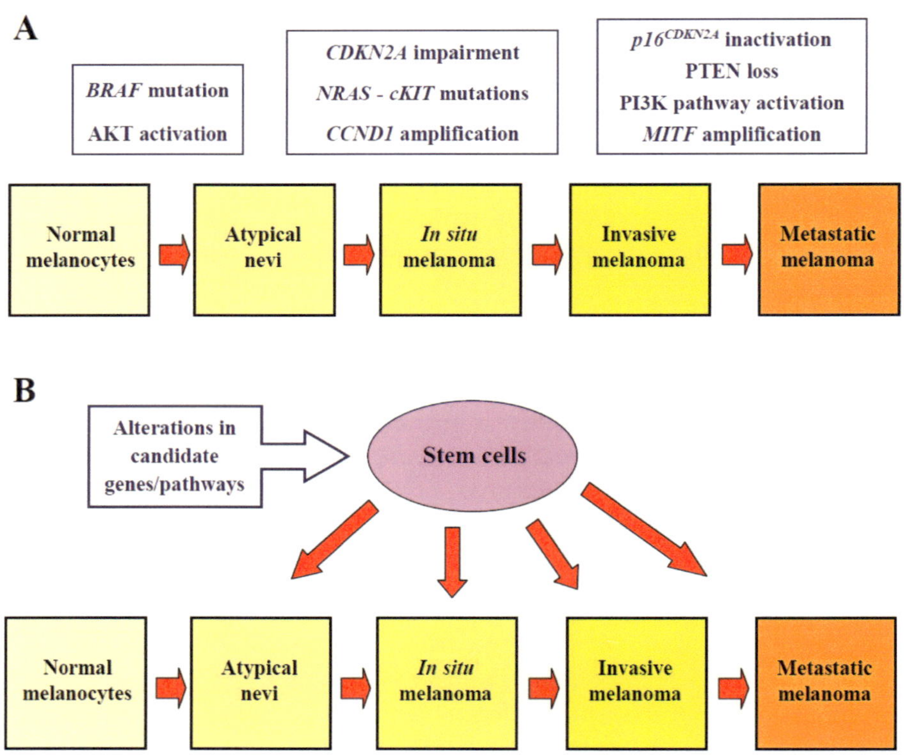

Figure 2. Models of development and progression for melanoma. A, sequential model. B, non-linear model.

Nevertheless, all these evidence represent a strong indication that the different molecular pathways associated with the melanomagenesis does correspond to different subsets of melanoma patients, with distinguished biological and clinical behavior of the disease. Identification of such different patients' subsets should be introduced in clinical trials, in order to better assess the classification of all predictive and prognostic factors associated with the disease as well as more accurately address patients to the most effective therapeutic intervention according to their biological and molecular status.

On the basis of the presence of the specific molecular features, a discrimination of the main subtypes of melanoma, along with the more appropriate therapeutic option for each subtype, could be schematically reported.

1. Subtype MAPK

Prevalence of *BRAF* mutations, with tendency to increased expression level of activated ERK (phospoERK$_{1\text{-}2}$) in melanoma tissues. This subtype benefits by the treatment with inhibitors of BRAF.

After failure of BAY 43-9006 (which is not specific for mutated BRAF, but suppresses activity of several different kinases [95]), a second generation BRAF inhibitor (Vemurafenib, also known as PLX4032 or RO5185426) was highly specific for ^{V600E}BRAF mutation and appeared very promising from the clinical point of view [96]. Very recently, results from a phase III study comparing the vemurafenib to dacarbazine have been indeed reported, indicating a relative reduction of 63% in the risk of death and of 74% in the risk of either death or disease progression, as compared with dacarbazine [97]. Preliminary data using an additional ^{V600E}BRAF inhibitor compound, Dabrafenib (previously known as GSK2118436), seemed to point out that this molecule is also active on ^{V600K}BRAF and ^{V600D}BRAF mutations [98]; actually, treatment with such a compound is under evaluation in a phase III study among BRAF mutation positive stage III-IV melanoma patients.

However, preliminary data seem to indicate that a large variety of induced alterations may drive resistance to BRAF inhibitors: upregulation of the receptor tyrosine kinase (RTK) effectors [99], mutation in *NRAS* gene and platelet-derived growth factor receptor β (PDGFRβ) [99], amplification of the *CCND1/Cyclin D1* gene or lack of phosphatase-and-tensin homologue (PTEN) function [100], mutations in downstream *MEK* gene [101], activation of MAPK pathway agonists such as COT kinase [102], or enhancement of the IGF-1R/PI3K signaling [103]. These findings highlight the need for combination therapy.

The MEK inhibitors (AS703026, E6201, GSK1120212, GDC0973, MEK162) as single agents have activity against melanoma, in patients either carrying BRAF mutations and unexposed to prior BRAF inhibitor therapy or presenting NRAS mutations [30]. A new combination of MEK and BRAF inhibitors as first line therapy for BRAF mutated melanoma patients naïve to prior anti-BRAF treatment is showing great promise [30].

The *BRAF* mutations may coexist with additional molecular alterations, with subsequent constitution of further biological and molecular subgroups of melanoma patients:

a. Impairment of the p16^{CDKN2A}-CDK4/CCND1-RB or p14^{CDKN2A}-MDM2-TP53 pathways, with reduced expression of the p16^{CDKN2A} protein and tendency to amplification of the *CDK4/CCND1* gene loci or inactivation of the TP53 gene (with consequent functional loss of the p53 protein), respectively. This subtype benefits by the treatment with inhibitors of the cyclin-dependent kinases.

Melanoma patients carrying genetic alterations affecting p16^{CDKN2A} could potentially be treated with inhibitors of CDK4/CDK6. There are currently no validated therapeutic options for melanoma with mutated p14^{CDKN2A}. Conversely, several CDK4 inhibitors (Alvocidib, AT-7519, P1446A-05, PD-0332991, Flavopiridol/alvocidib/HMR 1275, P276-00, R547, SNS-032/ BMS-387032, UCN-01, ZK 304709/MTGI) are currently under investigation for a variety of cancer types, including metastatic melanoma, and results are awaited. For p53, there are currently no drugs, approved or in trials, against such a target. Conversely, an anti-sense agent (Oblimersen) targeted at nuclear Bcl-2 has been evaluated in trials, failing to demonstrate a significant clinical benefit among patients with melanoma [104].

b. Amplification of *MITF* ± associated with reduction of the protein expression levels.

No drug targeting MITF has been developed; however, expression of MITF has been demonstrated to be reduced by compounds inhibiting the multiple histone deacetylase (HDAC) complex [105]. Ongoing trials based on HDAC-inhibitors [LBH589 (Panobinostat) or Valproic acid (Vorinostat)] will elucidate whether a clinical benefit could be obtained by down-regulating intracellular level of MITF protein.

c. Activation of NF-kB.

Proteasome inhibitors, such as Bortezomib (Velcade, previously known as PS-341), represent a new class of anticancer therapeutic agents which inhibit degradation of important cell cycle and/or regulatory proteins, including IkB [106-107]. Bortezomid has been demonstrated to contribute in maintaining integrity of the complexes sequestering NF-kB into the cytoplasm, thus reducing the NF-kB activity [106-107]. Phase 2 studies combinating Bortezomib with other chemotherapeutic agents, including paclitaxel, carboplatin, or temozolomide equally have been established [108-109]. A compound that more directly targets the NF-kB pathway is BMS-345541 (4(2'-aminoethyl) amino-1,8-dimethylimidazo(1,2-a)quinoxaline), identified as a selective inhibitor of the catalytic subunits of IKK that binds at an allosteric site of the enzyme [110].

Since mutational activation of BRAF in human melanomas has been demonstrated to contribute to constitutive induction of NF-kB activity through an increase of the IKK activity [111], inhibition of BRAF signaling using the above mentioned inhibitors may decrease the NF-kB transcriptional activity and sensitize melanoma cells to apoptosis.

2. Subtype NRAS

Prevalence of *NRAS* mutation, with markedly increased expression level of activated ERK (phospoERK$_{1-2}$) and eventual activation of AKT. This subtype benefits by the treatment with inhibitors of MEK or mTORC.

To date, two approaches have been considered in developing drugs against RAS. The first is based on the block of farnesylation. A small clinical trial using an inhibitor of the farnesyl transferase enzyme failed to be efficacious in a melanoma cohort; however, patients included into such a study were not selected on the basis of their *NRAS* mutation status [112-113]. In the light of recent successes of the target therapies based on anti-BRAF or anti-cKIT inhibitors, a more stringently selected cohort carrying alterations in *NRAS* gene would have increased responsiveness. On the other hand, a direct targeting of RAS has been demonstrated to be very difficult [114]; this is the reason why therapeutic strategies have focused on inhibiting downstream effectors into the pathways activated by RAS (i.e., MEK inhibitors for the MAPK pathway - see above - and mTORC inhibitors for the PI3K-AKT pathway - see below), which represent the second treatment approach against RAS.

3. Subtype cKIT

Prevalence of *cKIT* mutations ± gene amplification and/or increased protein expression levels. This subtype benefits by the treatment with inhibitors of cKIT (in particular, patients carrying gene mutations, with some sequence variants - such as K642E e L576P - which are highly responsive).

Activating cKIT mutations have been implicated in a variety of cancers, mainly represented by gastrointestinal stromal tumors (GIST) and chronic myelogenous leukemia (CML). This is the reason why several drugs targeting cKIT have been developed and tested in clinical trials, including Imatinib (approved for Philadelphia chromosome–positive CML and cKIT-positive GIST) and Sunitib (approved for advanced kidney cancer and Imatinib-resistant GIST) as well as Nilotinib and Dasatinib (approved for CML and Philadelphia chromosome-positive acute lymphoblastic leukemia).

The inhibitors of cKIT that may have a therapeutic benefit in melanoma, by inducing cell cycle arrest and apoptosis as well as significantly inhibiting cell migration and invasion of tumor cells, are:

Imatinib mesylate, formerly known as STI571, is designated chemically as 4-benzamide methanesulfonate. The efficacy of imatinib varies with the site of cKIT mutation; moreover, this drug can inhibit both the wild-type receptor activated by ligand and mutated receptor in the absence of ligand. However, imatinib is less effective at inhibiting the receptor with mutations in the enzymatic site (exon 17 mutations) [79];

Nilotinib (AMN107), which has been rationally designed based on the imatinib mesylate scaffold to have a more selective action. On this regard, Nilotinib inhibits both wild-type and cKIT mutants in exon 11 (V560del and V560G), exon 13 (K642E), double mutants involving exons 11, 13, and 17 as well as imatinib-resistant cKIT mutant (V560del/V654A) cells [115];

Dasatinib, which is a piperazinyl ethanol exhibiting increased potency but reduced selectivity compared with imatinib mesylate, has been demonstrated to inhibit both wild type and mutant cKIT in a dose-dependent manner, causing inhibition of cell migration and invasion through reduction of the phosphorylation of either Src kinase and FAK pathway [116-117].

4. Subtype mTORC

Prevalence of PTEN loss (± *PI3K* mutations, which are mostly infrequent) and phosphorylation of AKT, with absence of concurrent mutations in *BRAF* gene. This subtype mainly benefits by the treatment with inhibitors of mTOR.

In melanoma cells, three potential targets may be considered for therapeutic intervention against this pathway: AKT, PI3K and mTOR. Restoration of functional PTEN or interfering with AKT and PI3K activity would increase chemosensitivity to apoptotic agents and improve the efficacy of anti-tumor treatment. Several inhibitors of PI3K (BKM120, BEZ235, BGT226, GDC0941, PX-866, SF1126, and XL147) and AKT (GSK690693, MK2206, and VQD-002) have been developed; results of ongoing trials are thus awaited. To date, clinical trials using agents against the PI3K/AKT pathway have failed to demonstrate significant efficacy [118]. However, one therapeutic approach which seems to inhibit this pathway is based on the use of mTOR inhibitors [119]: rapamycin, Temsirolimus (CCI-779), Everolimus (RAD001), Sirolimus and AZD8055. While controversial data have been reported for rapamycin (suppressing disease progression in some patients with glioblastoma but ineffective in controlling the disease in others) [120], a limited advantage in response rates has been so far described for Temsirolimus [121]. It is to be underlined that none of the trials with mTOR inhibitors included patients specifically selected for alterations in the AKT/PI3K pathway. Several clinical trials are investigating specific combinations of mTOR inhibitors and chemotherapy drugs in the treatment of melanoma.

5. Subtype GNAQ/GNA11

Prevalence of *GNAQ/GNA11* mutations, with increased expression level of phosphoERK. This subtype benefits by the treatment with inhibitors of MEK.

The *GNAQ* and *GNA11* genes encodes specific GTP binding proteins that mediate signal transduction from the inner cell surface to the MAPK pathway through activation of the protein kinase C (PKC) enzyme [122]. Somatic mutations in *GNAQ* gene have been observed in about 90% of blue naevi, 50% of malignant blue naevi and 50% of primary uveal melanoma; conversely, the *GNA11* mutations have been found in less than 10% of blue nevi, about one third of primary uveal melanomas, and about 60% of metastatic uveal melanoma [122]. Since mutations in these two genes have non been detected among all the remaining types of melanoma (cutaneous, acral, mucosal), a clinical trial aimed at testing efficacy of a MEK inhibitor, Dabrafenib/GSK1120212, has been focused on patients with metastatic uveal melanoma carrying *GNAQ* and/or *GNA11* mutations [123].

4. Diagnostic panel of molecular alterations

The most prevalent molecular alterations within the heterogeneous patterns of biological features which characterize the distinct subtypes of melanoma are here summarized, according to the anatomical site of melanoma onset, the degree of exposure to the sun, and the histologic characteristics of the tumor lesions.

- Acral melanoma

Mutation ± amplification of *cKIT*; amplification of *CDK4* or *CCND1* (associated with increased expression levels of the related proteins); amplification of the 11q13, 22q11-13, and/or 5p15 genomic loci.

- Melanoma of the head and neck district and melanoma on skin with chronic sun-induced damage (CSD)

Amplification of *CDK4* and/or *CCND1*; increased expression levels of p53 protein; mutation ± amplification of *cKIT* (in about 5% of cases).

- Melanoma of the trunk and melanoma on skin without chronic sun-induced damage (non-CSD)

Mutation of *BRAF* or, alternatively, *NRAS* (with eventual coexistence of molecolar alterations which may ba associated with BRAF mutations; see above); tendency to reduced expression of the p53 protein; occurrence of specific polymorphisms in *MC1R* gene.

- Mucosal melanoma

Mutation ± amplification of *cKIT*; amplification of *CDK4* or *CCND1* (associated with increased expression levels of the related proteins); mutation of *BRAF* (in less than 10% of cases).

- Uveal melanoma

Mutation ± amplification of *cKIT*; mutation of *GNAQ* and/or *GNA11*.

Knowledge of the principal molecular alterations to be tested in patients with such distinct subtypes of melanoma will be of great clinical importance, because it is likely to result in separate targeted therapeutic approaches and prevention strategies. To date, it has been already developed a panel of molecular tests to be performed in patients with melanoma from different anatomical locations (Figure 3). This initial *"flow-chart"* will surely become more detailed and enriched on the basis of the progressive identification and validation of additional genetics and molecular alterations correlated with the disease.

Finally, recent meta-analyses tried to define the prognostic role of majority of molecular alterations previously described [124-125]:

- negative prognostic factors

loss of p53; over-expression of iNOS, AP-2, MMP-2 and metallothioneine; increased proliferation index (high expression levels of Ki-67);

- positive prognostic factors

reduced expression or loss of $p16^{CDKN2A}$; over-expression of Bcl-2 and ATF-2 (± associated with simultaneous increases expression of beta-catenin, fibronectin and p21 proteins).

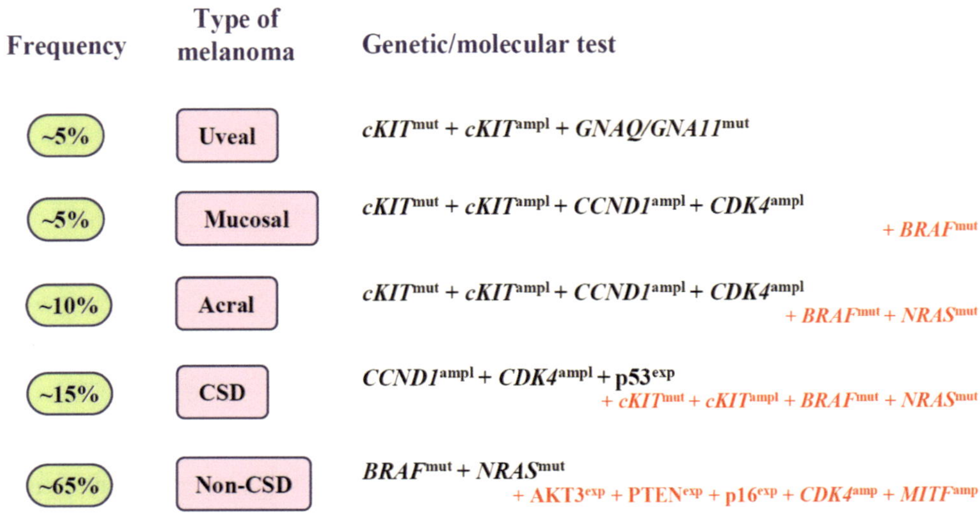

Figure 3. Principal genetic and molecular tests on tumor tissues for the different types of melanoma. Amp, gene amplification detected by *fluorescence in situ hybridization* (FISH) analysis. Exp, protein expression level detected by immunohistochemistry. Mut, gene sequence variation detected by mutation analysis. In red, tests for less prevalent alterations.

5. Conclusion

Taken together all the described molecular mechanisms involved in melanoma genesis and progression, data seem to emphasize the fact that in melanoma, but probably in all types of cancer, it is unlikely that targeting a single component in the signalling pathway will yield significant anti-tumour responses. For this purpose, molecular analyses could help clinicians to define the prognosis (prognostic value) as well as to make a prediction, identifying the subsets of patients who would be expected to be more or less likely to respond to specific therapeutic interventions (predictive value).

In other words, it is becoming evident that combination therapies targeting simultaneously several signaling pathways might be a winning therapeutic strategy to treat melanoma patients. Preclinical studies using combination of anti BRAF and AKT3 siRNA demonstrated a significantly higher reduction of tumor growth compared to single agent administration [126-127]. There is also evidence of synergism among MEK and PI3K inhibitors as well as promising results have been obtained by combinations of the mTOR inhibitors and sorafenib or MEK inhibitors [121, 128-129]. In contrast to single agent activity, these combinations of target drugs resulted in recovering of apoptosis by complete down-regulation of the anti-apoptotic proteins Bcl-2 and Mcl-1. Cooperation between BRAF and MEK inhibitors has also been demonstrated in preclinical studies with a consistent increase of apoptosis and abrogation of ERK activation compared to BRAF inhibitor alone [130]. Such cooperation was based on the observation that MEK activation was not abrogated in melanoma cells that develop resistance to BRAF inhibitors [131-134]. BRAF and MEK targeted synergic therapy is currently tested in a phase I clinical trial (NCT01072175) which combines the selective RAF inhibitor GSK2118436 with the MEK inhibitor GSK1120212 in patients with BRAF mutant tumors [135].

After decades without perspective, the history of medical treatment for the advanced melanoma is rapidly changing. Combined therapeutic approaches do represent the next challenge for treatment of patients with such a disease.

Acknowledgments

Authors are always grateful to patients for their cooperation into the various studies. Work was funded by Regione Autonoma della Sardegna and Ricerca Finalizzata Ministero della Salute.

Author details

Giuseppe Palmieri[1*], Maria Colombino[1], Maria Cristina Sini[1], Paolo Antonio Ascierto[2], Amelia Lissia[3] and Antonio Cossu[3]

*Address all correspondence to: gpalmieri@yahoo.com

1 Unit of Cancer Genetics, Institute of Biomolecular Chemistry (ICB), National Research Council (CNR), Traversa La Crucca, 3 - Baldinca Li Punti, Sassari, Italy

2 Unit of Medical Oncology and Innovative Therapy, Istituto Nazionale Tumori Fondazione "G. Pascale", Via Mariano Semmola, Napoli, Italy

3 University Hospital Health Unit - Azienda Ospedaliero Universitaria (AOU), Via Matteotti, Sassari, Italy

References

[1] Curado MP, Edwards B, Shin HR, Storm H, Ferlay J, Heanue M, Boyle P (eds). Cancer Incidence in Five Continents, Vol. IX, International Agency for Research on Cancer (IARC) Scientific Publications, No. 160, Lyon, IARC, 2007.

[2] Linos E, Swetter S, Cockburn MG, et al. Increasing burden of melanoma in the United States. J Invest Derm. 2009;129: 1666-74

[3] Rigel DS. Epidemiology of melanoma. Semin. Cutan. Med. Surg. 2010; 29: 204-209

[4] Welch HG, Woloshin S, Schwartz LM. Skin biopsy rates and incidence of melanoma: population based ecological study. BMJ 2005: 331: 481;

[5] de Vries E, Coebergh JW. Melanoma incidence has risen in Europe. BMJ. 2005: 331: 698

[6] Jhappan C, Noonan FP, Merlino G. Ultraviolet radiation and cutaneous malignant melanoma. Oncogene 2003: 22: 3099-3112

[7] Thompson JF, Scolyer RA, Kefford RF. Cutaneous melanoma. The Lancet 2005: 365: 687-701

[8] Cho E, Rosner BA, Feskanich D, Colditz GA. Risk factors and individual probabilities of melanoma for whites. J Clin Oncol. 2005: 23: 2669-2675

[9] Balch CM, Buzaid AC, Soong SJ, Atkins MB, Cascinelli N, Coit DG, Fleming ID, Gershenwald JE, Houghton A Jr, Kirkwood JM, McMasters KM, Mihm MF, Morton DL, Reintgen DS, Ross MI, Sober A, Thompson JA, Thompson JF. Final version of the American Joint Committee on Cancer Staging System for Cutaneous Melanoma. J Clin Oncol 2001; 19: 3635-48

[10] Bastian BC, Olshen AB, LeBoit PE, Pinkel D. Classifying melanocytic tumors based on DNA copy number changes. Am J Pathol 2003;163:1765-70

[11] Haluska FG, Tsao H, Wu H, Haluska FS, Lazar A, Goel V. Genetic alterations in signaling pathways in melanoma. Clin Cancer Res. 2006; 12: 2301-7

[12] Curtin JA, Fridlyand J, Kageshita T, Patel HN, Busam KJ, Kutzner H, Cho KH, Aiba S, Bröcker EB, LeBoit PE, Pinkel D, Bastian BC. Distinct sets of genetic alterations in melanoma. N Engl J Med. 2005; 353:2135-47

[13] Palmieri G, Capone ME, Ascierto ML, Gentilcore G, Stroncek DF, Casula M, Sini MC, Palla M, Mozzillo N, Ascierto PA. Main roads to melanoma. J Transl Med. 2009; 7: 86

[14] Miller AJ, Mihm MC. Melanoma. N Engl J Med 2006; 355, 51-65

[15] Giehl K. Oncogenic Ras in tumor progression and metastasis. Biol Chem. 2005;386:193–205

[16] Heidorn SJ, Milagre C, Whittaker S, et al. Kinase-dead BRAF and oncogenic RAS cooperate to drive tumor progression through CRAF. Cell. 2010 Jan 22;140:209-21

[17] Rajagopalan H, Bardelli A, Lengauer C, Kinzler KW, Vogelstein B, Velculescu VE. Tumorigenesis: RAF/RAS oncogenes and mismatch-repair status. Nature. 2002;418:934

[18] Quinlan MP, Settleman J. Isoform-specific ras functions in development and cancer. Future Oncol. 2009; 5:105-16

[19] Heidorn SJ, Milagre C, Whittaker S, et al. Kinase-dead BRAF and oncogenic RAS cooperate to drive tumor progression through CRAF. Cell. 2010; 140:209-21

[20] Davies H, Bignell GR, Cox C, Stephens P, Edkins S, Clegg S, Teague J, Woffendin H, Garnett MJ, Bottomley W, Davis N, Dicks E, Ewing R, Floyd Y, Gray K, Hall S, Hawes R, Hughes J, Kosmidou V, Menzies A, Mould C, Parker A, Stevens C, Watt S, Hooper S, Wilson R, Jayatilake H, Gusterson BA, Cooper C, Shipley J, Hargrave D, Pritchard-Jones K, Maitland N, Chenevix-Trench G, Riggins GJ, Bigner DD, Palmieri G, Cossu A, Flanagan A, Nicholson A, Ho JW, Leung SY, Yuen ST, Weber BL, Seigler HF, Darrow TL, Paterson H, Marais R, Marshall CJ, Wooster R, Stratton MR, Futreal PA. Mutations of the BRAF gene in human cancer. Nature. 2002; 417:949-54

[21] Smalley KSM. A pivotal role for ERK in the oncogenic behaviour of malignant melanoma? Int J Cancer 2003; 104:527-32

[22] McGary EC, Chelouche Lev D, Bar-Eli M. Cellular adhesion pathways and metastatic potential of human melanoma. Cancer Biol Ther 2002; 5: 459-465

[23] Kuphal S, Bauer R, Bosserhoff AK. Integrin signaling in malignant melanoma. Cancer Metastasis Reviews 24: 195–222, 2005

[24] Pollock PM, Harper UL, Hansen KS, Yudt LM, Stark M, Robbins CM, Moses TY, Hostetter G, Wagner U, Kakareka J, Salem G, Pohida T, Heenan P, Duray P, Kallioniemi O, Hayward NK, Trent JM, Meltzer PS. High frequency of BRAF mutations in nevi. Nat Genet. 2003, 33:19-20

[25] Michaloglou C, Vredeveld LC, Soengas MS, Denoyelle C, Kuilman T, van der Horst CM, Majoor DM, Shay JW, Mooi WJ, Peeper DS. BRAFE600-associated senescence-like cell cycle arrest of human naevi. Nature 2005; 436, 720–724

[26] Patton EE, Widlund HR, Kutok JL, Kopani KR, Amatruda JF, Murphey RD, Berghmans S, Mayhall EA, Traver D, Fletcher CD, Aster JC, Granter SR, Look AT, Lee C, Fisher DE, Zon LI. BRAF mutations are sufficient to promote nevi formation and cooperate with p53 in the genesis of melanoma. Curr Biol. 2005;15:249–54

[27] Wajapeyee N, Serra RW, Zhu X, et al. Oncogenic BRAF induces senescence and apoptosis through pathways mediated by the secreted protein IGFBP7. Cell. 2008;132:363–374

[28] Dhomen N, Reis-Filho JS, da Rocha Dias S, et al. Oncogenic Braf induces melanocyte senescence and melanoma in mice. Cancer Cell. 2009;15:294–303

[29] Smalley KS, Lioni M, Dalla Palma M, Xiao M, Desai B, Egyhazi S, Hansson J, Wu H, King AJ, Van Belle P, Elder DE, Flaherty KT, Herlyn M, Nathanson KL. Increased cyclin D1 expression can mediate BRAF inhibitor resistance in BRAF V600E-mutated melanomas. Mol Cancer Ther. 2008; 7: 2876-83

[30] Ascierto PA, Grimaldi AM, Curti B, Faries MB, Ferrone S, Flaherty K, Fox BA, Gajewski TF, Gershenwald JE, Gogas H, Grossmann K, Hauschild A, Hodi FS, Kefford R, Kirkwood JM, Leachmann S, Maio M, Marais R, Palmieri G, Morton DL, Ribas A, Stroncek DF, Stewart R, Wang E, Mozzillo N, Marincola FM. Future Perspectives in

melanoma research. Meeting report from the "Melanoma Research: a bridge from Naples to the World. Napoli, December 5th-6th 2011". J. Transl Med. 10: 83, 2012

[31] Pomerantz J, Schreiber-Agus N, Lie′ geois NJ. The Ink4a tumor suppressor gene product, 19Arf, interacts with MDM2 and neutralizes DM2's inhibition of p53. Cell 1998; 92: 713-23

[32] Zhang Y, Xiong Y, Yarbrough WG. ARF promotes MDM2 degradation and stabilizes p53: ARF-INK4a locus deletion impairs both the Rb and p53 tumor suppression pathways. Cell 1998: 92: 725–734

[33] Palmieri G, Capone ME, Ascierto ML, Gentilcore G, Stroncek DF, Casula M, Sini MC, Palla M, Mozzillo N, Ascierto PA. Main roads to melanoma. J Transl Med. 7: 86, 2009

[34] Soufir N, Avril MF, Chompret A, Demenais F, Bombled J, Spatz A, Stoppa-Lyonnet D, Bénard J, Bressac-de Paillerets B. Prevalence of p16 and CDK4 germline mutations in 48 melanoma-prone families in France. The French Familial Melanoma Study Group. Hum Mol Genet. 1998; 7: 209-16

[35] Sauter ER, Yeo UC, von Stemm A, Zhu W, Litwin S, Tichansky DS, Pistritto G, Nesbit M, Pinkel D, Herlyn M, Bastian BC. Cyclin D1 is a candidate oncogene in cutaneous melanoma. Cancer Res. 2002; 62:3200-6

[36] Box NF, Terzian T: The role of p53 in pigmentation, tanning and melanoma. Pigment Cell Melanoma Res 2008, 21:525-533

[37] Hocker TL, Singh MK, Tsao H. Melanoma genetics and therapeutic approaches in the 21st century: moving from the benchside to the bedside. J Invest Dermatol. 2008; 128:2575-95

[38] Bennett DC. How to make a melanoma: what do we know of the primary clonal events? Pigment Cell Melanoma Res. 2008; 21:27-38

[39] Sini MC, Manca A, Cossu A, Budroni M, Botti G, Ascierto PA, Cremona F, Muggiano A, D'Atri S, Casula M, Baldinu P, Palomba G, Lissia A, Tanda F, Palmieri G. Molecular alterations at chromosome 9p21 in melanocytic nevi and melanoma. Br. J. Dermatology 158: 243-250, 2008

[40] Meyle KD, Guldberg P. Genetic risk factors for melanoma. Hum Genet. 2009; 126: 499-510

[41] Fargnoli MC, Gandini S, Peris K, Maisonneuve P, Raimondi S. MC1R variants increase melanoma risk in famiglie with CDKN2A mutations: A meta-analysis. Eur J Cancer 2010; 46: 1413-20

[42] Scott MC, Wakamatsu K, Ito S, et al. Human melanocortin 1 receptor variants, receptor function and melanocyte response to UV radiation. J Cell Sci. 2002; 115: 2349-55

[43] Levy C, Khaled M, Fisher DE. MITF: master regulator of melanocyte development and melanoma oncogene. Trends Mol. Med. 2006;12, 406–414

[44] Hauser JE, Kadekaro AL, Kavanagh RJ, et al. Melanin content and MC1R function independently affect UVR-induced DNA damage in cultured human melanocytes. Pigment Cell Res. 2006; 19:303-14

[45] Landi MT, Bauer J, Pfeiffer RM, et al. MC1R germline variants confer risk for BRAF-mutant melanoma. Science 2006; 313:521-2

[46] Fargnoli MC, Pike K, Pfeiffer RM, et al. MC1R variants increase risk of melanomas harboring BRAF mutations. J Invest Dermatol. 2008; 128:2485-90

[47] Thomas NE, Kanetsky PA, Edmiston SN, et al. Relationship between germline MC1R variants and BRAF-mutant melanoma in a North Carolina population-based study. J Invest Dermatol. 2010; 130:1463-5

[48] Scherer D, Rachakonda PS, Angelini S, et al. Association between the germline MC1R variants and somatic BRAF/NRAS mutations in melanoma tumors. J Invest Dermatol. 2010; 130:2844-8

[49] Hacker E, Hayward NK, Dumenil T, et al. The association between MC1R genotype and BRAF mutation status in cutaneous melanoma: findings from an Australian population.J Invest Dermatol. 2010; 130:241-8

[50] Wu H, Goel V, Haluska FG. PTEN signaling pathways in melanoma. Oncogene. 2003; 22: 3113-22

[51] Vivanco I, Sawyers CL. The phosphatidylinositol 3-kinase AKT pathway in human cancer. Nat Rev Cancer. 2002;2:489-501

[52] Plas DR, Thompson CB. Akt-dependent transformation: there is more to growth than just surviving. Oncogene. 2005;24:7435–7442

[53] Aziz SA, Davies M, Pick E, Zito C, Jilaveanu L, Camp RL, Rimm DL, Kluger Y, Kluger HM. Phosphatidylinositol-3-kinase as a therapeutic target in melanoma. Clin Cancer Res. 2009; 15: 3029-36

[54] Mirmohammadsadegh A, Marini A, Nambiar S, et al. Epigenetic silencing of the PTEN gene in melanoma. Cancer Res. 2006; 66: 6546-52

[55] Goel VK, Lazar AJ, Warneke CL, Redston MS, Haluska FG. Examination of mutations in BRAF, NRAS, and PTEN in primary cutaneous melanoma. J Invest Dermatol. 2006; 126:154-60

[56] Tsao H, Goel V, Wu H, et al. Genetic interaction between NRAS and BRAF mutations and PTEN/MMAC1 inactivation in melanoma. J Invest Dermatol 2004; 122: 337–41

[57] Garraway LA, Widlund HR, Rubin MA, Getz G, Berger AJ, Ramaswamy S, Beroukhim R, Milner DA, Granter SR, Du J, Lee C, Wagner SN, Li C, Golub TR, Rimm DL, Meyerson ML, Fisher DE, Sellers WR. Integrative genomic analyses identify MITF as a lineage survival oncogene amplified in malignant melanoma. Nature. 2005; 436:117-22.

[58] Carreira S, Goodall J, Aksan I, et al. Mitf cooperates with Rb1 and activates p21Cip1 expression to regulate cell cycle progression. Nature 2005;433: 764-769

[59] Loercher AE, Tank EM, Delston RB, Harbour JW. MITF links differentiation with cell cycle arrest in melanocytes by transcriptional activation of INK4A. J Cell Biol 2005;168: 35-40

[60] Wellbrock C, Marais R: Elevated expression of MITF counteracts B-RAF stimulated melanocyte and melanoma cell proliferation. J Cell Biol 2005;170: 703-708

[61] McGill GG, Horstmann M, Widlund HR, et al. Bcl2 regulation by the melanocyte master regulator Mitf modulates lineage survival and melanoma cell viability. Cell 2002;109:707-718.

[62] Du J, Widlund HR, Horstmann MA, et al. Critical role of CDK2 for melanoma growth linked to its melanocyte-specific transcriptional regulation by MITF. Cancer Cell 2004;6: 565-576

[63] Wellbrock C, Rana S, Paterson H, et al. Oncogenic BRAF regulates melanoma proliferation through the lineage specific factor MITF. PLoS ONE 3:2734,2008

[64] Ekmekcioglu S, Tang CH, Grimm EA. NO news is not necessarily good news in cancer. Curr Cancer Drug Targets. 2005; 5:103-15

[65] Massi D, De Nisi MC, Franchi A, Mourmouras V, Baroni G, Panelos J, Santucci M, Miracco C. Inducible nitric oxide synthase expression in melanoma: implications in lymphangiogenesis. Mod Pathol. 2009; 22:21-30

[66] Grimm EA, Ellerhorst J, Tang CH, Ekmekcioglu S. Constitutive intracellular production of iNOS and NO in human melanoma: possible role in regulation of growth and resistance to apoptosis. Nitric Oxide. 2008; 19:133-7

[67] Sikora AG, Gelbard A, Davies MA, Sano D, Ekmekcioglu S, Kwon J, Hailemichael Y, Jayaraman P, Myers JN, Grimm EA, Overwijk WW. Targeted inhibition of inducible nitric oxide synthase inhibits growth of human melanoma in vivo and synergizes with chemotherapy. Clin Cancer Res. 2010; 16:1834-44

[68] Tschugguel W, Pustelnik T, Lass H, Mildner M, Weninger W, Schneeberger C, Jansen B, Tschachler E, Waldhör T, Huber JC, Pehamberger H: Inducible nitric oxide synthase (iNOS) expression may predict distant metastasis in human melanoma. Br J Cancer 1999, 79:1609-1612

[69] Ahmed B, Van den Oord JJ: Expression of the inducible isoform of nitric oxide synthase in pigment cell lesions of the skin. Br J Dermatol 2000, 142:432-40

[70] Ekmekcioglu S, Ellerhorst JA, Prieto VG, Johnson MM, Broemeling LD, Grimm EA. Tumor iNOS predicts poor survival for stage III melanoma patients. Int J Cancer. 2006; 119:861-6

[71] Dhawan P, Richmond A. A novel NF-kappa B-inducing kinase-MAPK signaling pathway up-regulates NF-kappa B activity in melanoma cells. J Biol Chem 2002; 277:7920-8

[72] Uffort DG, Grimm EA, Ellerhorst JA. NF-kappaB mediates mitogen-activated protein kinase pathway-dependent iNOS expression in human melanoma. J Invest Dermatol. 2009; 129:148-54

[73] Baldwin AS. Control of oncogenesis and cancer therapy resistance by the transcription factor NF-kB. J Clin Invest 2001;107:241–246

[74] Madonna G, Dansky Ullman C, Gentilcore G, Palmieri G, Ascierto PA. NF-kappaB as potential target in the treatment of melanoma. J. Transl Med. 2012; 10: 53

[75] Chaturvedi MM, Sung B, Yadav VR, Kannappan R, Aggarwal BB. NF-kB addiction and its role in cancer: 'one size does not fit all'. Oncogene. 2011; 30:1615-30.

[76] Kim HJ, Hawke N, Baldwin AS. NF-kappaB and IKK as therapeutic targets in cancer. Cell Death Differ. 2006; 13:738-47

[77] McNulty SE, del Rosario R, Cen D, et al. Comparative expression of NFkappaB proteins in melanocytes of normal skin vs. benign intradermal naevus and human metastatic melanoma biopsies. Pigment Cell Res. 2004; 17:173-80

[78] Clifford D, Mol, Kheng B. Lim. Structure of a c-Kit product complex reveals the basis for kinase transactivation. J. Biol Chem 2003; 278: 31461-64

[79] Smalley KS, Sondak VK, Weber JS. c-KIT signaling as the driving oncogenic event in sub-groups of melanomas. Histol Histopathol. 2009; 24:643-50.

[80] Alexeev V, Yoon K. Distinctive role of the cKit receptor tyrosine kinase signaling in mammalian melanocytes. J Invest Dermatol. 2006; 126: 1102-1110

[81] Shen SS, Zhang PS, Eton O, Prieto VG. Analysis of protein tyrosine kinase expression in melanocytic lesions by tissue array. J Cutan Pathol 2003; 30: 539-547

[82] Stefanou D, Batistatou A, Zioga A. Immunohistochemical expression of vascular endothelial growth factor (VEGF) and CKIT in cutaneous melanocytic lesions. Int J Surg Pathol 2004; 12: 133-138.

[83] Curtin JA, Busam K, Pinkel D, Bastian BC. Somatic activation of KIT in distinct subtypes of melanoma. J. Clin. Oncol. 2006; 24: 4340-43

[84] Beadling C, Jacobson-Dunlop E, Hodi FS, Le C, Warrick A, Patterson J, Town A, Harlow A, Cruz F 3rd, Azar S, Rubin BP, Muller S, West R, Heinrich MC, Corless CL. Kit gene mutations and copy numbering melanoma subtypes .Clin Cancer Res 2008; 14: 6821-6828

[85] Riviera RS, Nagatsuka H, Gunduz M, Cengiz B, Gunduz E, Siar CH, Tsujigiwa H, Tamamura R, Han K N, Nagai N. C-kit protein expression correlated with activating mutations in KIT gene in oral mucosal melanoma.Virchows Arch. 2008; 452: 27-32

[86] Postow MA, Harding J, Wolchok JD. Targeting immune checkpoints: releasing the restraints on anti-tumor immunity for patients with melanoma. Cancer J. 2012; 18:153-9

[87] Melero J, Hervas-Strubbs S, Glennie M et al. Immunostimulatory monoclonal antibodies for cancer therapy. Nat Rev Cancer 2007; 7:95-106

[88] Ascierto PA, Marincola FM, Ribas A. Anti-CTLA4 monoclonal antibodies: the past and the future in clinical application. J Transl Med. 2011 Nov 13;9:196

[89] Ozao-Choy J, Ma G, Kao J, Wang GX, Meseck M, Sung M, Schwartz M, Divino CM, Pan PY, Chen SH. The novel role of tyrosine kinase inhibitor in the reversal of immune suppression and modulation of tumor microenvironment for immune-based cancer therapies. Cancer Res. 2009 Mar 15;69(6):2514-22

[90] Lee KM, Chuang E, Griffin M, et al. Molecular basis of T cell inactivation by CTLA-4. Science. 1998; 282: 2263–2266

[91] Hodi FS, O'Day SJ, McDermott DF, Weber RW, Sosman JA, Haanen JB, Gonzalez R, Robert C, Schadendorf D, Hassel JC, Akerley W, van den Eertwegh AJ, Lutzky J, Lorigan P, Vaubel JM, Linette GP, Hogg D, Ottensmeier CH, Lebbé C, Peschel C, Quirt I, Clark JI, Wolchok JD, Weber JS, Tian J, Yellin MJ, Nichol GM, Hoos A, Urba WJ. Improved survival with ipilimumab in patients with metastatic melanoma. N Engl J Med. 2010; 363:711-23

[92] Robert C, Thomas L, Bondarenko I, O'Day S, M D JW, Garbe C, Lebbe C, Baurain JF, Testori A, Grob JJ, Davidson N, Richards J, Maio M, Hauschild A, Miller WH Jr, Gascon P, Lotem M, Harmankaya K, Ibrahim R, Francis S, Chen TT, Humphrey R, Hoos A, Wolchok JD. Ipilimumab plus dacarbazine for previously untreated metastatic melanoma. N Engl J Med. 2011; 364:2517-26

[93] Miller AJ, Mihm MC. Melanoma. N Engl J Med 2006; 355: 51-65

[94] Zabierowski SE, Herlyn M. Melanoma stem cells: the dark seed of melanoma. J Clin Oncol. 2008; 26: 2890-4

[95] Eisen T, Ahmad T, Flaherty KT, Gore M, Kaye S, Marais R, Gibbens I, Hackett S, James M, Schuchter LM, Nathanson KL, Xia C, Simantov R, Schwartz B, Poulin-Costello M, O'Dwyer PJ, Ratain MJ. Sorafenib in advanced melanoma: a phase II randomised discontinuation trial analysis. Br J Cancer 2006; 95: 581-86

[96] Flaherty KT, Puzanov I, Kim KB, Ribas A, McArthur GA, Sosman JA, O'Dwyer PJ, Lee RJ, Grippo JF, Nolop K, Chapman PB. Inhibition of mutated, activated BRAF in metastatic melanoma. N Engl J Med 2010; 363, 809-19

[97] Chapman PB, Hauschild A, Robert C, Haanen JB, Ascierto P, Larkin J, Dummer R, Garbe C, Testori A, Maio M, Hogg D, Lorigan P, Lebbe C, Jouary T, Schadendorf D, Ribas A, O'Day SJ, Sosman JA, Kirkwood JM, Eggermont AM, Dreno B, Nolop K, Li J, Nelson B, Hou J, Lee RJ, Flaherty KT, McArthur GA; BRIM-3 Study Group. Im-

proved survival with vemurafenib in melanoma with BRAF V600E mutation. N Engl J Med. 2011; 364:2507-16.

[98] Falchook GS, Long GV, Kurzrock R, Kim KB, Arkenau TH, Brown MP, Hamid O, Infante JR, Millward M, Pavlick AC, O'Day SJ, Blackman SC, Curtis CM, Lebowitz P, Ma B, Ouellet D, Kefford RF. Dabrafenib in patients with melanoma, untreated brain metastases, and other solid tumours: a phase 1 dose-escalation trial. Lancet. 2012; 379:1893-901

[99] Nazarian R, Shi H, Wang Q, Kong X, Koya RC, Lee H, Chen Z, Lee MK, Attar N, Sazegar H, Chodon T, Nelson SF, McArthur G, Sosman JA, Ribas A, Lo RS. Melanomas acquire resistance to B-RAF(V600E) inhibition by RTK or N-RAS upregulation. Nature 2010; 468: 973-77

[100] Smalley KS, Sondak VK. Melanoma--an unlikely poster child for personalized cancer therapy. N Engl J Med. 2010; 363:876-8

[101] Wagle N, Emery C, Berger MF, Davis MJ, Sawyer A, Pochanard P, Kehoe SM, Johannessen CM, Macconaill LE, Hahn WC, Meyerson M, Garraway LA. Dissecting therapeutic resistance to RAF inhibition in melanoma by tumor genomic profiling. J Clin Oncol. 2011; 29: 3085-96.

[102] Johannessen CM, Boehm JS, Kim SY, Thomas SR, Wardwell L, Johnson LA, Emery CM, Stransky N, Cogdill AP, Barretina J, Caponigro G, Hieronymus H, Murray RR, Salehi-Ashtiani K, Hill DE, Vidal M, Zhao JJ, Yang X, Alkan O, Kim S, Harris JL, Wilson CJ, Myer VE, Finan PM, Root DE, Roberts TM, Golub T, Flaherty KT, Dummer R, Weber BL, Sellers WR, Schlegel R, Wargo JA, Hahn WC, Garraway LA. COT drives resistance to RAF inhibition through MAP kinase pathway reactivation. Nature 2010; 468, 968-72

[103] Villanueva J, Vultur A, Lee JT, Somasundaram R, Fukunaga-Kalabis M, Cipolla AK, Wubbenhorst B, Xu X, Gimotty PA, Kee D, Santiago-Walker AE, Letrero R, D'Andrea K, Pushparajan A, Hayden JE, Brown KD, Laquerre S, McArthur GA, Sosman JA, Nathanson KL, Herlyn M. Acquired resistance to BRAF inhibitors mediated by a RAF kinase switch in melanoma can be overcome by cotargeting MEK and IGF-1R/PI3K. Cancer Cell 2010; 18, 683-95

[104] Bedikian AY, Millward M, Pehamberger H, Conry R, Gore M, Trefzer U, Pavlick AC, DeConti R, Hersh EM, Hersey P, Kirkwood JM, Haluska FG; Oblimersen Melanoma Study Group. Bcl-2 antisense (oblimersen sodium) plus dacarbazine in patients with advanced melanoma: the Oblimersen Melanoma Study Group. J Clin Oncol. 2006; 24:4738-45

[105] Yokoyama S, Feige E, Poling LL, Levy C, Widlund HR, Khaled M, Kung AL, Fisher DE. Pharmacologic suppression of MITF expression via HDAC inhibitors in the melanocyte lineage. Pigment Cell Melanoma Res. 2008; 21:457-63

[106] Adams J. The proteasome: a suitable antineoplastic target. Nat Rev Cancer 2004;4:349–60

[107] Amiri KI, Horton LW, LaFleur BJ, Sosman JA, Richmond A. Augmenting chemosensitivity of malignant melanoma tumors via proteasome inhibition: Implication for bortezomib (VELCADE, PS-341) as a therapeutic agent for malignant melanoma. Cancer Res 2004;64:4912–4918

[108] Su Y, Amiri KI, Horton LW, Yu Y, Ayers GD, Koehler E, Kelley MC, Puzanov I, Richmond A, Sosman JA. A phase I trial of bortezomib with temozolomide in patients with advanced melanoma: toxicities, antitumor effects, and modulation of therapeutic targets. Clin Cancer Res 2010;16:348-57

[109] Croghan GA, Suman VJ, Maples WJ, Albertini M, Linette G, Flaherty L, Eckardt J, Ma C, Markovic SN, Erlichman C. A Study of Paclitaxel, Carboplatin, and Bortezomib in the Treatment of Metastatic Malignant Melanoma. Cancer 2010;116:3463-8

[110] López-Guerra M, Roué G, Pérez-Galán P, Alonso R, Villamor N, Montserrat E, Campo E, Colomer D. p65 activity and ZAP-70 status predict the sensitivity of chronic lymphocytic leukemia cells to the selective IkappaB kinase inhibitor BMS-345541. Clin Cancer Res. 2009; 15:2767-76

[111] Liu J, Suresh Kumar KG, Yu D, Molton SA, McMahon M, Herlyn M, Thomas-Tikhonenko A, Fuchs SY. Oncogenic BRAF regulates β-Trcp expression and NF-kB activity in human melanoma cells. Oncogene 2007; 26:1954–1958

[112] Niessner H, Beck D, Sinnberg T, Lasithiotakis K, Maczey E, Gogel J, Venturelli S, Berger A, Mauthe M, Toulany M, Flaherty K, Schaller M, Schadendorf D, Proikas-Cezanne T, Schittek B, Garbe C, Kulms D, Meier F. The farnesyl transferase inhibitor lonafarnib inhibits mTOR signaling and enforces sorafenib-induced apoptosis in melanoma cells. J Invest Dermatol. 2011; 131:468-79

[113] Hong DS, Sebti SM, Newman RA, Blaskovich MA, Ye L, Gagel RF, Moulder S, Wheler JJ, Naing A, Tannir NM, Ng CS, Sherman SI, El Naggar AK, Khan R, Trent J, Wright JJ, Kurzrock R. Phase I trial of a combination of the multikinase inhibitor sorafenib and the farnesyltransferase inhibitor tipifarnib in advanced malignancies. Clin Cancer Res. 2009; 15:7061-8

[114] Konstantinopoulos PA, Karamouzis MV, Papavassiliou AG. Post-translational modifications and regulation of the RAS superfamily of GTPases as anticancer targets. Nat Rev Drug Discov. 2007; 6:541-55

[115] Tran A, Tawbi HA. A potential role for nilotinib in KIT-mutated melanoma. Expert Opin Investig Drugs. 2012; 21:861-9

[116] Serrels A, Macpherson IR, Evans TR, Lee FY, Clark EA, Sansom OJ, Ashton GH, Frame MC, Brunton VG. Identification of potential biomarkers for measuring inhibition of Src kinase activity in colon cancer cells following treatment with dasatinib. Mol Cancer Ther. 2006; 5: 3014–3022

[117] Gnoni A, Marech I, Silvestris N, Vacca A, Lorusso V. Dasatinib: an anti-tumour agent via Src inhibition. Curr Drug Targets. 2011; 12:563-78

[118] Courtney KD, Corcoran RB, Engelman JA. The PI3K pathway as drug target in human cancer.J Clin Oncol. 2010; 28:1075-83

[119] Abraham RT, Eng CH. Mammalian target of rapamycin as a therapeutic target in oncology.Expert Opin Ther Targets. 2008; 12:209-22

[120] Cloughesy TF, Yoshimoto K, Nghiemphu P, Brown K, Dang J, Zhu S, Hsueh T, Chen Y, Wang W, Youngkin D, Liau L, Martin N, Becker D, Bergsneider M, Lai A, Green R, Oglesby T, Koleto M, Trent J, Horvath S, Mischel PS, Mellinghoff IK, Sawyers CL. Antitumor activity of rapamycin in a Phase I trial for patients with recurrent PTEN-deficient glioblastoma. PLoS Med. 2008; 5:e8

[121] Margolin KA, Moon J, Flaherty LE, Lao CD, Akerley WL 3rd, Othus M, Sosman JA, Kirkwood JM, Sondak VK. Randomized phase II trial of sorafenib with temsirolimus or tipifarnib in untreated metastatic melanoma (S0438). Clin Cancer Res. 2012; 18:1129-37

[122] Van Raamsdonk CD, Griewank KG, Crosby MB, Garrido MC, Vemula S, Wiesner T, Obenauf AC, Wackernagel W, Green G, Bouvier N, Sozen MM, Baimukanova G, Roy R, Heguy A, Dolgalev I, Khanin R, Busam K, Speicher MR, O'Brien J, Bastian BC. Mutations in GNA11 in uveal melanoma. N Engl J Med. 2010; 363:2191-9

[123] Khalili JS, Yu X, Wang J, Hayes BC, Davies MA, Lizee G, Esmaeli B, Woodman SE. Combination Small Molecule MEK and PI3K Inhibition Enhances Uveal Melanoma Cell Death in a Mutant GNAQ- and GNA11-Dependent Manner. Clin Cancer Res. 2012 Jul 19

[124] Gould Rothberg BE, Bracken MB, Rimm DL. Tissue biomarkers for prognosis in cutaneous melanoma: a systematic review and meta-analysis. J Natl Cancer Inst. 2009; 101:452-74

[125] Gould Rothberg BE, Berger AJ, Molinaro AM, Subtil A, Krauthammer MO, Camp RL, Bradley WR, Ariyan S, Kluger HM, Rimm DL. Melanoma prognostic model using tissue microarrays and genetic algorithms. J Clin Oncol. 2009; 27:5772-80

[126] Cheung M, Sharma A, Madhunapantula SV, Robertson GP. Akt3 and mutant V600E B-Raf cooperate to promote early melanoma development. Cancer Res. 2008; 68, 3429–3439

[127] Tran MA, Gowda R, Sharma A, Park EJ, Adair J, Kester M, Smith NB, Robertson GP. Targeting V600EB-Raf and Akt3 using nanoliposomal small interfering RNA inhibits cutaneous melanocytic lesion development. Cancer Res. 2008; 68, 7638–7649

[128] Lasithiotakis KG, Sinnberg TW, Schittek B, Flaherty KT, Kulms D, Maczey E, Garbe C, Meier FE. Combined inhibition of MAPK and mTOR signaling inhibits growth, induces cell death, and abrogates invasive growth of melanoma cells. J Invest Dermatol. 2008;128:2013-23

[129] Davies MA, Fox PS, Papadopoulos NE, Bedikian AY, Hwu WJ, Lazar AJ, Prieto VG, Culotta KS, Madden TL, Xu Q, Huang S, Deng W, Ng CS, Gupta S, Liu W, Dancey

JE, Wright JJ, Bassett RL, Hwu P, Kim KB. Phase I study of the combination of sorafenib and temsirolimus in patients with metastatic melanoma. Clin Cancer Res. 2012;18:1120-8

[130] Paraiso KH, Fedorenko IV, Cantini LP, Munko AC, Hall M, Sondak VK, Messina JL, Flaherty KT, Smalley KS. Recovery of phospho-ERK activity allows melanoma cells to escape from BRAF inhibitor therapy. Br J Cancer. 2010; 102:1724-30

[131] Heidorn SJ, Milagre C, Whittaker S, Nourry A, Niculescu-Duvas I, Dhomen N, Hussain J, Reis-Filho JS, Springer CJ, Pritchard C, Marais R. Kinase-dead BRAF and oncogenic RAS cooperate to drive tumor progression through CRAF. Cell 2010;140:209-21

[132] Poulikakos PI, Zhang C, Bollag G, Shokat KM, Rosen N. RAF inhibitors transactivate RAF dimers and ERK signalling in cells with wild-type BRAF. Nature. 2010; 464:427-30

[133] Poulikakos PI, Persaud Y, Janakiraman M, Kong X, Ng C, Moriceau G, Shi H, Atefi M, Titz B, Gabay MT, Salton M, Dahlman KB, Tadi M, Wargo JA, Flaherty KT, Kelley MC, Misteli T, Chapman PB, Sosman JA, Graeber TG, Ribas A, Lo RS, Rosen N, Solit DB. RAF inhibitor resistance is mediated by dimerization of aberrantly spliced BRAF(V600E). Nature 2011; 480: 387-90

[134] Hatzivassiliou G, Song K, Yen I, Brandhuber BJ, Anderson DJ, Alvarado R, Ludlam MJ, Stokoe D, Gloor SL, Vigers G, Morales T, Aliagas I, Liu B, Sideris S, Hoeflich KP, Jaiswal BS, Seshagiri S, Koeppen H, Belvin M, Friedman LS, Malek S. RAF inhibitors prime wild-type RAF to activate the MAPK pathway and enhance growth. Nature 2010;464:431-5

[135] Arkenau H-T, Kefford R, Long GV. Targeting BRAF for patients with melanoma. Br J Cancer 2011; 104: 392-398

Chapter 3

Low-Penetrance Variants and Susceptibility to Sporadic Malignant Melanoma

G. Ribas, M. Ibarrola-Villava, M.C. Peña-Chilet,
L.P. Fernandez and C. Martinez-Cadenas

Additional information is available at the end of the chapter

http://dx.doi.org/10.5772/53097

1. Introduction

Although malignant melanoma (MM) is mainly a sporadic disease, about 3 to 15% of the cases may show familial aggregation [1, 2]. The diagnosis of melanoma in different members of the same families does indeed suggest there is a genetically-based hereditary predisposition in a significant percentage of the cases. However, this predisposition has proven to be genetically heterogeneous. Only two high-penetrance genes had been described so far: *CDKN2A* and *CDK4* [1]. Yet mutations in these genes are found in only 30–40% of melanoma kindreds, indicating the existence of additional genes involved in melanoma predisposition [1]. Also, common low-penetrance alleles of the human pigmentation *MC1R* gene have been implicated in melanoma predisposition as well [3-13]. More recently, several other pigmentation genes, such as *ASIP, TYR, TYRP1, SLC45A2* and *OCA2* have also emerged as being potentially important in both normal human pigmentation variation and in melanoma susceptibility [14-17].

Other putative low-penetrance genes involved in melanoma predisposition are DNA repair genes belonging to the base excision repair (BER) and the nucleotide excision repair (NER) mechanisms. BER and NER pathways eliminate a wide variety of DNA damage, including ultraviolet (UV) photoproducts. Therefore, the ability of each individual to repair DNA damage following different causes might explain at least in part the variability in melanoma susceptibility. Although several studies have investigated the association between polymorphisms in NER genes and risk of melanoma, most of the study sizes were relatively small, and the results were not consistent [18-24]. On the other hand, genetic polymorphisms have been identified in several BER genes and studies suggest that some of these polymorphisms may be associated with cancer risk [25-29].

Further candidate low-penetrance genes allegedly linked to melanoma predisposition are members of the glutathione S-transferase (*GST*) gene family. GSTs are multifunctional enzymes involved in the detoxification of a wide range of reactive oxygen species (ROS) which, together with inflammatory response to UV exposure, contribute to skin carcinogenesis by oxidative stress mechanisms [30-32]. Since UV radiation can also indirectly induce oxidative stress via ROS, several *GST* genes have been considered as possible low-penetrance melanoma predisposition genes. Among the *GST* genes, *GSTM1, GSTT1* and *GSTP1* commonly harbor functional polymorphisms in the general population [33]. The frequencies of variants in the *GSTM1* and *GSTT1* genes have been studied in relation to susceptibility to melanoma; however, conflicting results have been reported [34-39].

In recent years, several genome-wide association studies (GWAS) have identified novel genomic *loci* associated with pigmentation and skin cancer [40-44]. GWAS are the ideal strategy to identify common, low-penetrance susceptibility *loci* without prior hypothesis bias due to gene role knowledge. Some of the associations detected were already known, such as *MC1R* with pigmentation and skin cancer, *ASIP, TYR, OCA2,* etc. However, several novel chromosomal regions and genes have been revealed using large cohorts of samples, such as *IRF4, PARP1, CASP8, CCND1* and others.

What follows is a summary of the results obtained in our laboratory after the screening of genes belonging to three different genetic pathways: pigmentation, DNA repair and oxidative stress. For the past few years, our group has been studying melanoma candidate genes in Spain, a southern European population, displaying a considerably darker skin than most of the other well-studied Caucasian populations, including Australian, North American and Northern Europe populations.

2. Research methods

2.1. Study subjects and data collection

A case-control collection of 946 non-related MM cases from several Spanish Hospitals and 353 volunteer cancer-free controls were recruited from 1 September 2004 to January 2011. All participants were Caucasians of Spanish origin. A standardized questionnaire was used to collect information on pigmentation characteristics (eye, hair and skin color, number of nevi, presence of solar lentigines, sun exposure habits and presence of childhood sunburns), Fitzpatrick's classification of skin type (extracted from the medical record of cases only), tumor localization, Breslow index (depth index), and personal or family history of cancer. All study subjects gave informed consent and the study was approved by the Ethics Committee of Gregorio Marañón General University hospital and Clínico University Hospital.

Genomic DNA from cases and controls was isolated from peripheral blood lymphocytes and diluted to a final solution of 50ng/ml. MagNA Pure LC Instrument DNA extracción was used according to the manufacturer's protocol (Roche Applied Science, Mannheim, Germany); the DNAzol procedure (Invitrogen, Eugene, OR, USA) or traditional saline method was used. DNA concentration was quantified in samples prior to genotyping by using Quant-iT PicoGreen dsDNA Reagent (Invitrogen, Eugene, OR, USA).

2.2. SNP genotyping

2.2.1. MC1R sequencing

MC1R variants were detected by automated gene sequencing. The *MC1R* coding region was amplified by PCR using two overlapping pairs of primers previously described [9]. PCR products were 671 and 610 bp in length, respectively, and they overlapped by 104 bp. PCR amplification was performed according to Matichard and cols [9]. Sequence analysis was performed on the ABI Prism system (Life Technology, Foster city, CA) using the BigDye Terminator Cycle Sequencing kit and the ABI 3700 automated DNA sequencer according to the manufacturer's instructions. The sequence results were analyzed using Polyphred, Phred Phrap and Consed software [45-47] or SeqScape in order to detect all possible changes. All detected changes were confirmed manually.

2.2.2. Gene and SNP selection

The rest of the genes in the study were analyzed by genotyping selected SNPs. Public databases were used to collect information about single nucleotide polymorphisms (SNPs): NCBI (http://www.ncbi.nlm.nih.gov), Ensembl (http://www.ensembl.org/index.html) and HapMap (http://www.hapmap.org). SNPs selected were located in exons, in putative promoter regions or had been reported to be associated with cancer in previous studies. All SNPs had a minor allele frequency (MAF) greater than or equal to 5%. As a quality control measure we included two sample duplicates and a non-template sample per 96-well plate. For some high-throughput platforms three DNA duplicates (two intra-assays and one inter-assay) were added. For all the studies performed genotypes were scored by two different personnel in the laboratory and no discrepancies were observed.

2.2.3. Taqman and kaspar assays

The PCR primers and probes were designed by Life Technology (Foster City, CA) using their Custom Taqman SNP genotyping assays or KASPAR SNP Genotyping System KBiosciences (Hoddesdon, Herts UK). The primer and allele-specific probe sequences for Taqman as well as those used for Kaspar assays are detailed elsewhere [6, 7, 14, 16, 17, 27].

PCR conditions used were according to the manufacturer's protocol (Life technology, Foster City, CA). After PCR, the genotype of each sample was automatically determined by measuring allele-specific final fluorescence in the ABI Prism 7900HT Detection System, using the SDS 2.1 software for allele discrimination (Life technology, Foster City, CA).

2.2.4. Sequenom

Genotyping assays were designed according to the Sequenom MassARRAY Assay Design software (version 3.0.0; Sequenom Inc., San Diego, CA, USA). Assay primers are detailed elsewhere [15, 27]. One duplicate sample, one father–mother–child trio and two negative controls were included across the plates to assess the accuracy of genotyping. SNPs were genotyped using iPLEX™ chemistry on a MALDI-TOF Mass Spectrometer (Sequenom Inc, San Diego, CA, USA). PCR reactions were carried out according to their own instructions (Sequenom Inc.).

2.2.5. Illumina

A total of 384 SNPs were genotyped using the GoldenGate Genotyping Assay system according to the manufacturer's protocol (Illumina, San Diego, CA, USA) [16]. Genotyping was carried out using 350 ng of DNA per reaction. In addition, cases and control samples were always included in the same run. Genotypes were called using the proprietary software supplied by Illumina (BeadStudio, version 3.1.3.).

2.2.6. Taqman quantitative real-time PCR

The *GSTM1* and *GSTT1* copy number polymorphisms were determined using the TaqMan Quantitative real-time PCR. Assay designs were Hs02575461_cn *(GSTM1)* and Hs000100004_cn *(GSTT1)* and were used according to Life Technology instructions. After PCR, the genotype of each sample was automatically determined by measuring allele-specific final fluorescence in the ABI Prism 7900HT Detection System, using the SDS 2.3 software for allele discrimination (Life Technology, Foster City, Ca, USA). Analysis of PCR products was done using the COPY CALLER Software v1.0 (Life Technology, Foster City, USA) that allowed the classification of unambiguous homozygous (zero copies), heterozygous (one copy) and homozygous (two copies) *GSTM1* or *GSTT1* carrier individuals.

2.3. Statistical analysis

Associations between *MC1R* variants and melanoma risk were initially assessed individually using Fisher's exact test. Associations with melanoma were assessed using logistic regression. Estimating odds ratios (ORs), their associated 95% confidence intervals (CIs) and P-values were obtained using SPSS v19. Multivariate logistic regression was also applied, including age, sex, hair color, skin color, solar lentigines and childhood sunburn as covariates. Associations between the number of variants carried and various individual and tumor characteristics were assessed via logistic regression.

To study the effect of combined protective and risk genotypes, we reduced the sample set to 528 samples successfully genotyped for all the associated SNPs. We used a 2x2 contingency table and a t-student test between *SLC45A2* (rs35414) and both *SILV* (rs2069398) and *NOS1* (rs2682826), as well as with all three genes together. In addition, we studied the results between the risk alleles, *TYR* (rs17793678), *ADAMTS20* (rs1510521), *GSTP1* (rs1695) and *OCA2/HERC2* (rs12913832). Finally, we analyzed possible interactions between *MC1R* (0, 1 or 2 variants) and all previous risk and protective alleles

http://dx.doi.org/10.5772/53097

3. Results

3.1. MC1R

Of the 946 individuals studied, 559 (59.15%) carried at least one *MC1R* variant, including 388 (65.43%) of 593 cases and 171 (48.4%) of the 353 controls. A total of 36 *MC1R* variants were identified.

Among these, 25 variants were non-synonymous changes, 20 of which had been described previously [5] and 5 were identified for the first time: S41F, M128T, P268R, A285V and N281S. Six variants of the receptor have been traditionally associated with red hair color (RHC): D84E, R142H, R151C, R160W, I155T and D294H.

Similarly, another three variants have not been associated with RHC phenotype and have been designated as NRHC (V60L, V92M and R163Q). These amino acid changes have been studied in different populations because their frequency is greater than 1%.

The other variants detected in the *MC1R* gene have frequencies lower than 1% in control samples and included C35Y, F45L, a trinucleotide deletion that results in a new amino acid in position 54 (c.161delTGG, V54E), S83P, G89R, V92L, T95M, a nonsense change (Y152X), two nucleotide insertions (c.537insC, p.ins179C; and c.537insT, p.ins179T), R213W, R272M, K278E, and T308M, plus all novel ones described before. These rare variants have been designated as "ns_rare SNPs" in Figure 1. The synonymous variants included the most common change, T314T (A>G), and the rare changes I63I, Q233Q, I264I, F300F as well as I180I and S316S, the last two described for the first time. These synonymous variants are called "s_rare" with or without T314T in Figure 1. The estimated frequency of common *MC1R* variants and some combinations such as all synonymous changes with and without the common T314T and all non-synonymous rare variants, as well as the corresponding estimated OR for MM and associated P-values are shown in Figure 1.

Among the 36 changes detected, five were individually associated with melanoma risk: V60L, R151C, I155T, R160W and D294H ($P< 0.05$). The highest OR was estimated for I155T (OR 3.65, 95% CI: 1.40–9.52; $P=0.006$). The estimated OR associated with carrying one non-synonymous variant was 1.58 (95% CI: 1.19–2.097; $P=0.0013$); however, the OR for carrying two non-synonymous variants was 4.38 (95% CI: 2.72–7.05; $P=1.33\times 10^{-9}$). The MM associated OR among those Spanish patients carrying one RHC variant was 2.36 (95% CI: 1.71–3.26; $P=1.86\times 10^{-7}$). However if we consider individuals homozygous or compound heterozygous for two RHC variants, the OR increased to 12.76 (95% CI: 3.06–53.29; $P=1.9\times 10^{-5}$).

We considered blue /green eye color, blond /red hair color, solar lentigines and childhood sunburns as confounders in a multivariate model. *MC1R* variant analysis retained statistically significant results when adjusted for all potential confounders (OR: 1.77, 95% CI: 1.37–2.27; $P=9.57\times 10^{-6}$). Hair color, solar lentigines and childhood sunburns were independently associated with MM (OR: 2.11, 95% CI: 1.22–3.66, $P=0.008$; OR: 2.28 95% CI: 1.61–3.23, $P=3.54\times 10^{-6}$; OR: 4.77, 95% CI: 3.37–6.77, $P=9.57\times 10^{-6}$, respectively).

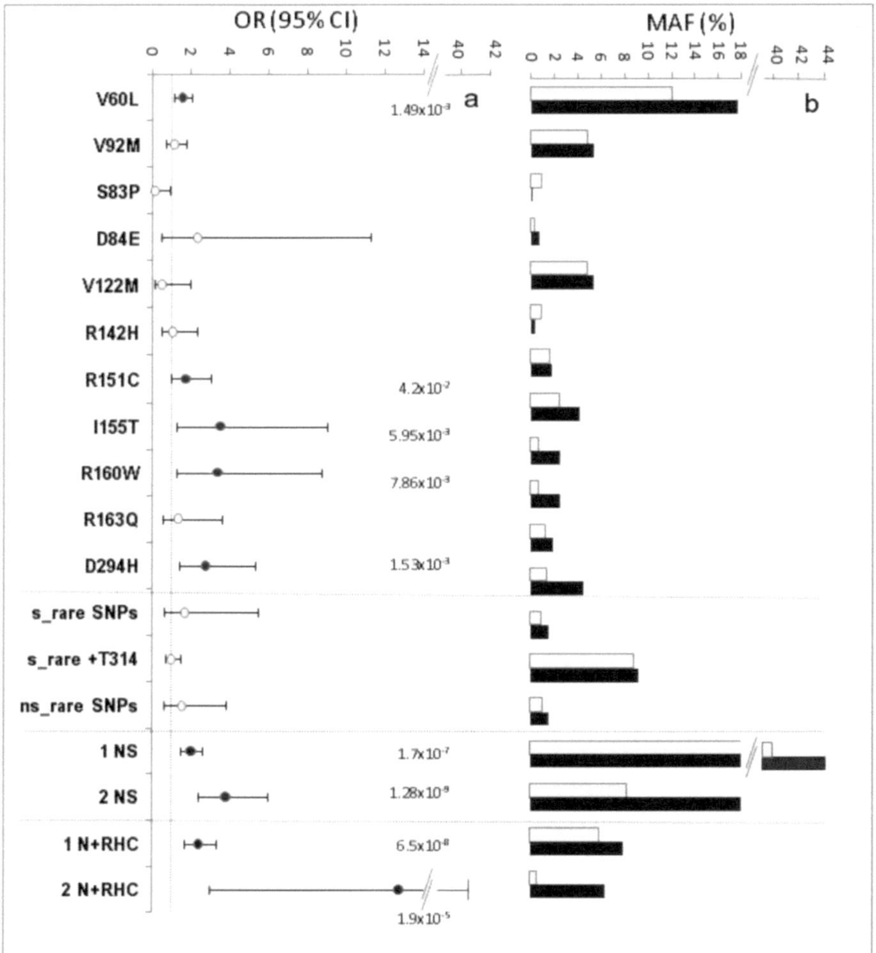

Figure 1. a) Summary of all *MC1R* variants associated with MM. Odds Ratios (OR), 95% confidence interval (95% CI) and P-values. b) Minor Allele Frequencies (MAF) of *MC1R* genetic variants. ns: non-synonymous variants :V60L, V92M, S83P, D84E,V122M, R142H, R151C, I155T R160W, R163Q and D294H; s_rare SNPs: synonymous variants with MAFs in controls lower than 1%: I63I, I180I, Q233Q, I264I, F300F and S316S; s_rare +T314T: same variants as before plus the addition of T314T; ns_rare SNPs: non-synonymous variants with less than 1% frequency in controls: C35Y;S41F, F45L, 54delTGG, G89R, V92L,T95M, M128T, Y152X, 179insTor C, R213W, P268R, T272M, K278E, N281S, A285V and T308M. Grey squares represent control data whereas black bars represent MM cases. Dark circles denote statistically significant values.

3.2. Other genes from pathways associated to melanoma

Several studies have been performed in order to evaluate other pigmentation-related genes and their relationship to MM susceptibility. The first results generated by Fernandez and cols. [4] analyzed the oculocutaneous albinism (OCA) genes: *TYR* (MIM#606933), *OCA2* (MIM#611409), *TYRP1* (MIM#115501) and *SLC45A2* (MIM#606202); the melanocyte protein *SILV* (MIM#155550) and *MC1R* inverse agonist *ASP* (MIM#600201).

Allele frequencies for each SNP and the P-value for their comparisons between case and control subjects are detailed in Figure 2. After discarding two of the selected SNPs, one in the *OCA2* gene due to its monomorphic nature in our sample collection, and one in the *SLC45A2* gene due to its departure from HWE, we observed evidence of differences in allele frequency for one SNP in the *SLC45A2* gene, corresponding to F374L (NCBI dbSNP rs16891982). The estimated OR per minor allele copy was 0.41 (95% CI, 0.24–0.70; P =0.001) with the minor allele being more frequent in controls than cases (16% vs. 7%; adjusted P=0.001).

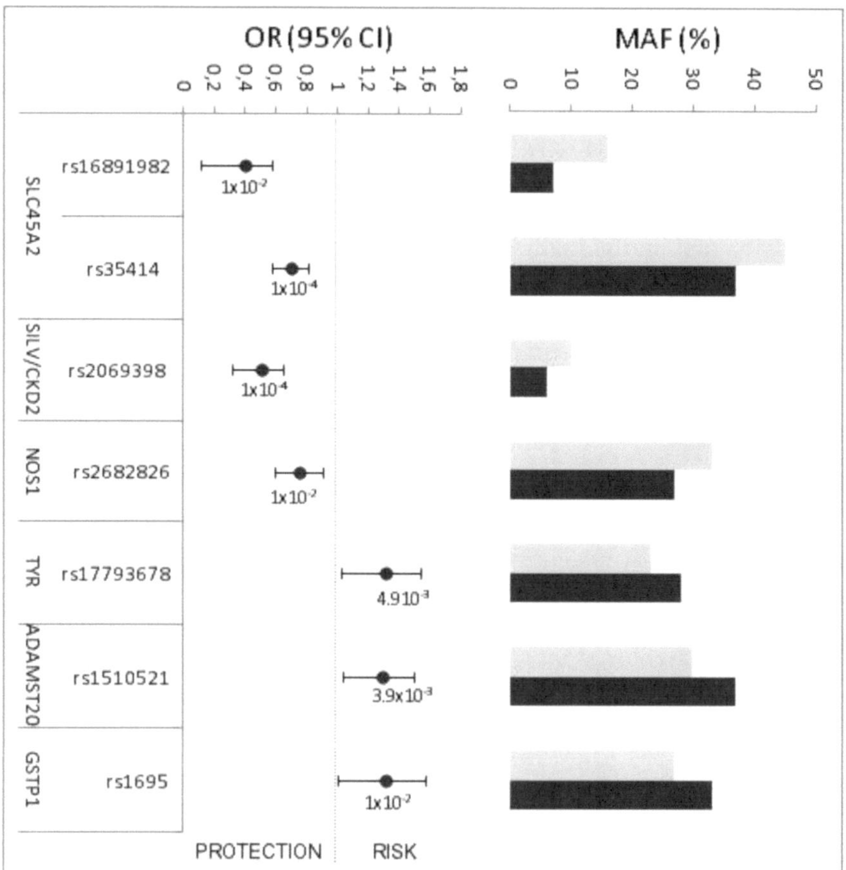

Figure 2. Odds ratios (OR), 95% confidence interval (95% CI), P-values and Minor Allele Frequency (MAF) for the best seven genetic variants in genes belonging to pigmentation, DNA repair and oxidative stress pathways. Grey bars represent control data while black bars represent MM cases. Dark circles denote statistically significant values. Exact P-values are indicated in number.

In a second study we genotyped 384 SNPs from 65 genes belonging mainly to the pigmentation pathway [16]. Ten SNPs located on six individual chromosomes (one in each of *ADAMTS20*, *TYR* and *SILV/CDK2*; two in each of *KIT* and *MYO7A*; and three in *SLC45A2*) constituted the top ten MM phase I associated SNPs in our sample after establishing a restrictive P-value threshold of 0.01. A phase II validation study was conducted to analyze the most significant SNP of each of the 6 candidate genes. One SNP, rs35414 in the *SLC45A2* gene, had an unadjusted P=0.002 in this phase II and overall OR of 0.75 (95% CI 0.67–0.84, P=0.0001) (Figure 2). None of the other five SNPs tested in phase II reached statistical significance at this stage. However, three of them, located in *TYR*, *SILV/CDK2* and *ADAMTS20* had an overall P<0.05 when phase I and II were considered together.

After analysis of genes in the pigmentation pathway, we conducted two studies where 16 genes belonging to both base excision repair (BER) and nucleotide excision repair (NER) pathways, as well as 14 genes involved in oxidative stress, including *GSTT1* and *GSTM1*, were screened for copy number variation [17, 27]. Two statistically significant results suggested a putative role of oxidative stress processes in the genetic predisposition to melanoma.

First of all, a novel variant in the *NOS1* oxidative stress gene (rs2682826) was detected (P=0.01). A second association pointed to *GSTP1* polymorphism rs1695, encoding the amino acid change I105V, and individually associated with MM (OR: 1.32, 95%CI: 1.06–1.63, P=0.01) found associated with melanoma for the first time. The best seven SNPs associated with MM in our population are shown in Figure 2. We could not detect any association between *GSTM1* or *GSTT1* deletions and MM risk.

3.3. Phenotypic characteristics

If we take into account *MC1R* and the associated phenotypic characteristics we detect the estimated ORs for melanoma associated with various phenotypic characteristics based on univariate analyses. MM risk was associated with the presence of blond or RHC (OR: 4.86, 95% CI: 2.35–10.03, P=$2x10^{-5}$), solar lentigines (OR: 1.71, 95% CI: 1.04–2.81, P =0.032) and childhood sunburn (OR: 10.41, 95%CI: 5.81–18.65, P=$3x10^{-13}$). No association with melanoma risk was observed for eye color, skin color or number of nevi.

The number of *MC1R* variants was statistically significantly associated with blond or RHC (OR: 1.80, 95% CI: 1.26–2.58, P=0.001), fair skin (OR: 1.42, 95% CI: 1.06–1.89, P=0.018) and with the presence of childhood sunburn (OR: 1.71, 95% CI: 1.28–2.27, P= $2x10^{-4}$). The corresponding ORs for the number of functional *MC1R* variants were 2.32 (95% CI: 1.42–3.78, P=0.001) for blond or RHC, 1.58 (95% CI: 1.09–2.3, P= 0.014) for fair skin and 2.35 (95% CI: 1.6–3.45, P=5 $x10^{-5}$) for the presence of childhood sunburn.

We assessed whether *SLC45A2* polymorphisms were associated with various phenotypic characteristics. The F374L variant allele was associated with dark eye color, dark hair color, darker skin and absence of both solar lentigines and childhood sunburns. Finally, we tested for associations between *SLC45A2* SNPs and phototype, tumor location, and tumor depth among cases only (Table 5). The minor (G) allele of the F374L variant was found to be associated with phototypes III/IV (per allele OR, 3.25; 95% CI, 1.05–10.03; P=0.04). Additionally, *SLC45A2* SNPs rs35414 and rs35415 were also associated with dark skin color (P=0.028 and P=0.0485) and only rs35414 with dark hair color (P=0.0183).

Evidence of association with phenotypic characteristics for two *KIT* SNPs, rs759083 and rs13135792, were also present. Both SNPs appeared to be associated with both light hair color (P=0.0021 and P=0.0072) and childhood sunburns (P=0.0112 and P=0.0167).

Two different SNPs in *MYO7A* were associated with dark hair color (rs948970, P=0.04), and childhood sunburn (rs3758708, P=0.0474). One SNP in the *TYR* gene (rs17793678) was associated with light eye color (P=0.0239). Likewise, the *ADAMTS20* gene was associated with light eye color (P=0.0339), blond or red hair color (P=0.0353) and with number of nevi (rs1510521; P=0.0338). Finally, *SILV/CDK2* SNP rs2069398 was associated with absence of childhood sunburns (P=0.0353).

3.4. Gene-gene interactions

We explored the combined effects of the individually associated SNPs located in the six relevant genes studied: *SLC45A2*, *SILV*, *NOS1* (protective associated genes) and *TYR*, *ADAMTS20* and *GSTP1* (risk associated genes). Although in our series it does not show individual association with MM, we added rs12913832 from the *OCA2/HERC2* gene due to its strong association with eye color [6, 48] and the fact that it has been demonstrated to have epistatic effects with the *MC1R* gene [49].

3.4.1. Interaction between protective alleles

Two SNPs, rs16891982 and rs35414, located in the *SLC45A2* gene were associated with MM. Both of them could have been used to perform the interaction analyses; however, rs35414 was chosen due to its higher MAF. SNPs rs2069398, located in the *SILV/CDK2* gene region, and rs2682826 in *NOS1* were also included in the analyses. Interaction results are shown in Figure 3.

We observed some degree of epistatic protective interaction between rs35414 (*SLC45A2* gene) and rs2069398 (*SILV/CDK2* gene region) when considering rare allele carriers at both *loci*. A significant decrease in MM associated OR was observed when two (heterozygotes for both *SLC45A2* and *SILV*) or three (heterozygous for *SLC45A2* and minor homozygotes for *SILV*) rare alleles were present at both *loci* (OR: 0.54, 95% CI: 0.39–0.75, P=0.0003). Similarly, when three (minor homozygotes for *SLC45A2* and heterozygous for *SILV*) or four (minor homozygous for both *SLC45A2* and *SILV*) rare alleles were carried, a greater decrease in MM risk was observed (OR: 0.31, 95% CI: 0.18–0.55, P=0.0001). Results including joint genotypes for rs35414 and rs2069398 SNPs, individual status (heterozygous or minor homozygous), ORs with their corresponding 95% CIs and P-values are shown in Figure 3a.

In addition, we observed some degree of epistatic protective interaction between rs35414 (*SLC45A2*) and rs2682826 (*NOS1*) when considering heterozygote alleles at both *loci* (OR 0.23, 95% CI 0.16–0.55, P=0.0001). However, a trend toward protective effect was detected when both homozygous rare alleles were compared (OR: 0.50, 95% CI 0.18–1.20; P=0.1). This lack of statistically significant results is most probably due to the reduced number of samples in this category (21 MM cases vs. 17 controls). Results are shown in Figure 3b.

The interaction analyses between *NOS1* rs2682826 SNP and *SILV* rs20693989 SNP revealed a trend toward significance when both rare alleles are considered (OR: 0.19, 95% CI: 0.03–1.07, P=0.055). Results are shown in Figure 3c.

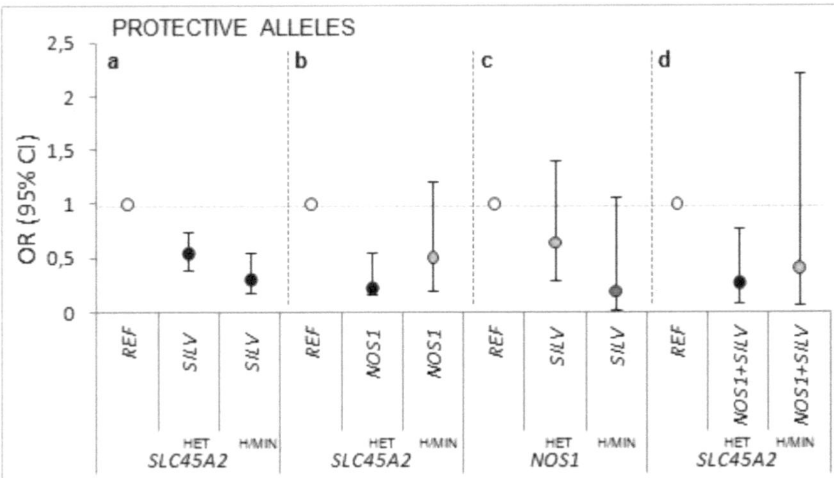

Figure 3. Interaction between protective allele variants and their effect on MM susceptibility. a) *SLC45A2* and *SILV*, b) *SLC45A2* and *NOS1*, c) *NOS1* and *SILV* and d) *SLC45A2*, *NOS1* and *SILV* all together. OR: odds ratios per minor allele; 95% CI: 95% confidence intervals; REF: reference value; HET: heterozygotes; and HMIN: minor homozygotes. For the genes labeled in vertical, we joined heterozygotes and minor homozygotes. Dark circles denote statistically significant results.

Finally, when the effect of the interaction between the three *loci* protectively associated with MM, rs35414 (*SLC45A2*), rs2682826 (*NOS1*) and rs2069398 (*SILV*) were analyzed, statistically significant results were observed. Individuals heterozygous for the three genes were more common in controls than in MM cases (OR: 0.09, 95% CI: 0.022–0.316, P=0.0001), showing a cumulative protective effect. The comparison with rare homozygous alleles in all three *loci* was statistically not relevant due to the small number of samples found (Figure 3d).

3.4.2. Interaction between risk alleles

In order to show the distinct combinations of MM risk alleles we performed two different analyses. The first comparison studied the effect in MM susceptibility by taking together four genotypes: rs17793678 (*TYR*), rs1510521 (*ADAMTS20]*; rs1695 (*GSTP1*), and rs12913832 (*OCA2/HERC2*). Results are shown in Figure 4a-d.

Some degree of epistatic risk interaction was seen between rs17793678 (*TYR*) and rs1510521 (*ADAMTS20*) when considering either heterozygous or rare alleles at both *loci*. We observed an increased risk effect when two or three rare alleles were present at both *loci* (rs17793678 heterozygotes and rs1510521 heterozygous, and minor homozygous carriers; OR: 1.41, 95% CI: 1.12–1.78, P=0.004). When three or four rare alleles (rs17793678 minor homozygotes and rs1510521 heterozygotes, and minor homozygous carriers) were analyzed together, we obtained an OR of 1.54 (95% CI 0.96–2.48) with a trend toward significance (P=0.088). Results are shown in Figure 4a.

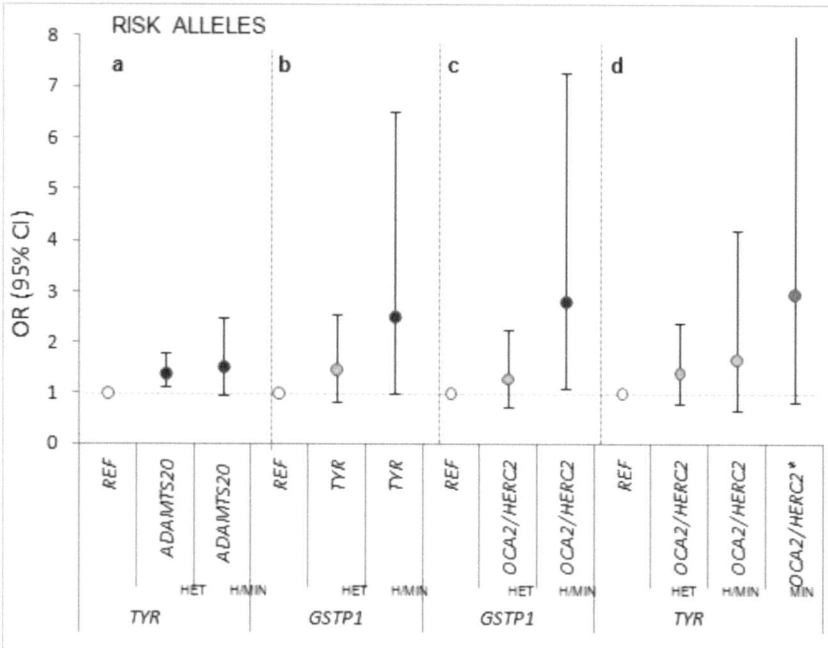

Figure 4. Interactions between risk allele variants and their effect on MM susceptibility. a) *TYR* and *ADAMTS20*, b) *GSTP1* and *TYR*, c) *GSTP1* and *OCA2/HERC2* and d) *TYR* and *OCA2/HERC2*. OR: odds ratios per minor allele; 95% CI: 95% confidence intervals; REF: reference value; HET: heterozygotes; H MIN: minor allele homozygotes; and MIN: only minor homozygotes for *TYR* and *GSTP1* respectively. For genes labeled in vertical we joined heterozygous and minor homozygous status. Dark circles denote statistically significant results.

A similar effect was observed when we compared rs1695 (*GSTP1*) with both rs1510521 (*ADAMTS20*) and rs12913832 (*OCA2/HERC2*) polymorphisms. We detected some degree of epistatic risk interaction when considering homozygous rare alleles at both *loci*. Results for rs1695 and rs1510521 showed an OR of 2.53 (95% CI 1.005–6.49, P=0.04, data shown in Figure 4b), while the interaction between rs1695 and rs12913832 had an OR of 2.81 (95% CI 1.11–7.27, P=0.018, see Figure 4c).

An additional comparison with rs17793678 (*TYR*) and rs12913832 (*HERC2/OCA2)* showed increasing epistasis as the number of risk alleles augmented, showing a trend toward significance only when homozygous minor alleles were considered at both *loci*, OR=2.95 (95% CI 0.84–11.326] (p=0.077). See Figure 4d. All other complex comparisons did not add further information.

For the second type of analyses we included the *MC1R locus* together with the previous four polymorphisms. As *MC1R* had already been associated with MM, it seemed biologically plausible that genetic interactions would be detected between risk variants within *MC1R* and other associated genes. Indeed, increased risks appeared when heterozygotes or rare alleles at *MC1R* were combined with heterozygotes plus rare homozygous at *GSTP1* (OR: 5.3, 95% CI: 2.80–417.42; P =1x10^{-4}, see Figure 5a), at *TYR* (OR: 6.42; 95% CI 2.32–18.64; P=0.0001, see Figure 5b), and at *OCA2/HERC2* (OR: 7.163; 95% CI 2.659–20.05; P=0.0001, see Figure 5c).

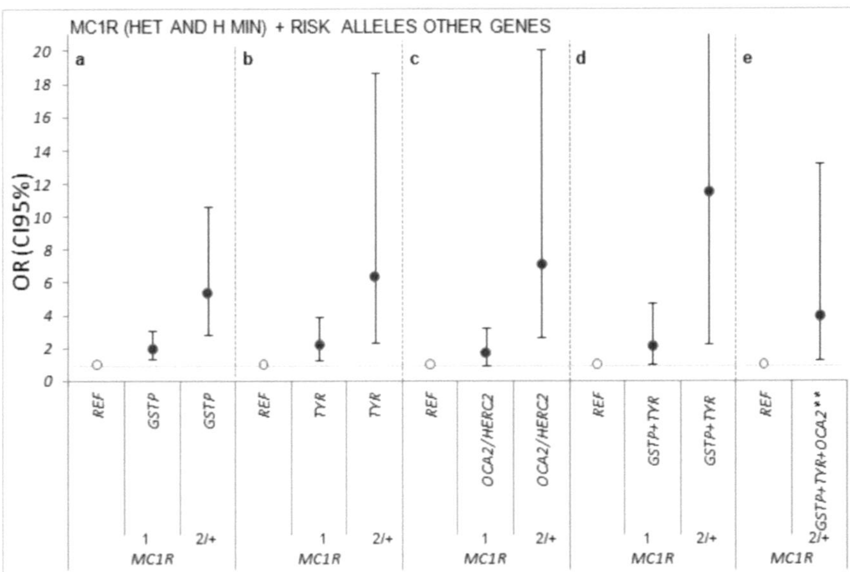

Figure 5. Interactions between risk allele variants on *MC1R* together with other risk associated genes alone or in multiple combinations, and their effect on MM susceptibility. a) *MC1R* and *GSTP1*, b) *MC1R* and *TYR*, c) *MC1R* and *OCA2/HERC2* and d) *MC1R, TYR* and *OCA2/HERC2*, e) *MC1R, GSTP1, TYR* and *OCA2/HERC2.* OR: odds ratios per minor allele; 95% CI: 95% confidence intervals; REF: reference value; HET: heterozygotes; H MIN: minor allele homozygotes. For the genes labeled in vertical we joined heterozygotes and minor homozygotes. Dark circles denote statistically significant results.

The last group of comparisons was done taking into consideration three and four genes at the same time. Firstly, we showed that combining *MC1R* genotypes with both *TYR* and *GSTP1* resulted in the highest MM associated risk (OR: 11.56, 95% CI 2.25–79.54, P=0.0001; data shown in Figure 5d). Secondly, we performed a final analysis taking into account only rare homozygotes of the four risk alleles and compared them, for MM association, with wild type genotype individuals. We obtained an OR of 4.008 (95% CI 1.25–13.2) with a P-value of 0.016 (see Figure 5e). There is not enough power to consider any other comparison with statistical significance.

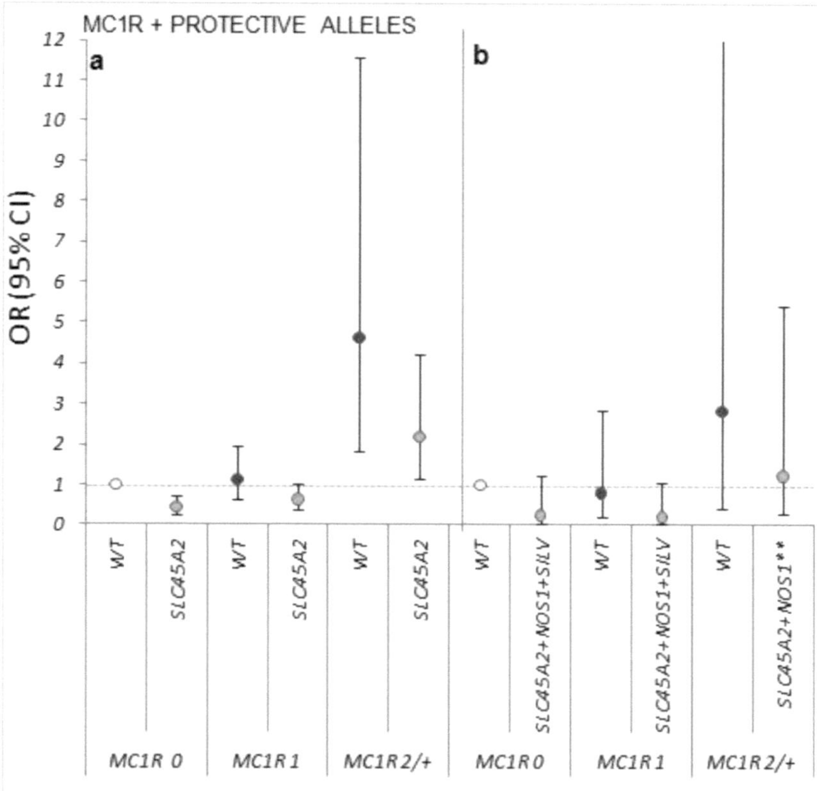

Figure 6. Interactions between risk variants on *MC1R* compared with protective alleles in a) *SLC45A2*, b) *SLC45A2*, *NOS1* and *SILV*, and their effect on MM susceptibility. OR: odds ratios per minor allele; 95% CI: 95% confidence intervals; WT: wild type alleles; *MC1R* 0: normal sequence in the *MC1R* gene; *MC1R* 1: carriers of 1 non-synonymous variant in *MC1R*; *MC1R* 2/+: carriers of two or more non-synonymous variants in the *MC1R* gene. For the genes labeled in vertical we have joined heterozygotes and minor homozygotes. Red circles represent carriers of risk alleles in *MC1R* whereas green circles correspond to carriers of risk alleles in *MC1R* and protective alleles either in *SLC45A2* alone or in combination.

3.4.3. Complex interactions

The role of *SLC45A2* and the other protective genes (*NOS1* and *SILV*) in melanoma predisposition was further analyzed in relation to *MC1R*, the main low-penetrance gene associated to melanoma. Since all these genes have been studied by our group, we analyzed the interaction effects between both *MC1R* and *SLC45A2 loci* (see Figure 6a) and between *MC1R* and all the protective alleles (see Figure 6b).

A great reduction of risk was detected when the rare protective alleles at *SLC45A2* were carried in individuals with two *MC1R* variants (OR: 2.20, 95% CI 1.14–4.23, P=0.02), in comparison to individuals carrying only two *MC1R* variants (OR: 4.64; 95% CI 1.85–11.58, P=0.001). Individuals having only one *MC1R* mutation plus the rare protective *SLC45A2* allele also showed a reduction in MM risk, although this decline does not seem to reach significant values (data shown in Figure 6a). These results confirmed the protective role of the rs35414 variant in *SLC45A2* regarding MM risk. Similar effects are observed when we included in the calculations the protective SNPs located in *NOS1* and *SILV*, however less statistically significant results were obtained due to the small number of samples in each class.

4. Discussion

Since *MC1R* genetic variability is strongly associated with the RHC phenotype [12], a large number of studies have investigated the involvement of this gene in MM susceptibility. *MC1R* is highly polymorphic, with more than 100 variants described in Caucasian populations [13]. Despite of its high variability, the synonymous changes are greatly reduced, with only three described in the literature: T314T (A>G), F300F (C>T) and C273C (C>T) [50, 51]. Results obtained from our laboratory confirmed the association between five *MC1R* polymorphic variants and MM risk in the Spanish population. We found 36 *MC1R* variants, this number being quite similar to the number found in other Mediterranean population studies (16 in France, 26–29 in Italy and 18 in Greece) [9, 11]. The most frequent Spanish variant is V60L with a frequency of 12.03%. This value is close to that reported in other populations (15.7% among Northern Italians, 12.4% among fair-skinned Australians and 15.0% among Northern Europeans) [52]. The RHC phenotype-associated variants (R151C, R160W and D294H) were present at frequencies of 0,71, 0.71 and 1.42%, respectively, in our population, compared to 9.9, 8.7 and 3.6%, respectively, reported in Northern European populations [52]. There were very few red-haired individuals among the control sample, and only 36 (6%) of MM cases had red hair. This finding is consistent with other results from Mediterranean populations and is at odds with red hair frequencies found in Northern European populations [12]. Red-haired subjects with no *MC1R* variants are not uncommon and have been seen in a Northern European population as well [53].

RHC variants have been consistently associated with MM in Northern European populations [3, 10, 12] and also in the Northern French population [9]. In Spain, we detected statistically significant individual associations for R151C, R160W and D294H. These three variants have been detected in the Northern French and Central Italian populations [9, 54]. We did not observe any MM risk associated with the rare RHC variant D84E (OR: 1.63, 95% CI: 0.02–128, P= 0.99), as detected in Northern Europeans [32, 55, 56], probably due to its low prevalence in Spain (0.28% in controls). The I155T variant has not been associated with MM in other populations to date, but this may also be due to its low frequency. However, our results clearly suggest that this rare variant increases risk of MM, at least in the Spanish population (OR: 3.51, 95% CI: 1.35–9.12, P= 0.006). While the associations of RHC with MM were expected, the case of V60L (an NRHC variant) was more intriguing, since its involvement in MM pathology has been generally unclear in Caucasian populations. However, V60L could play a role in MM susceptibility only in darker skinned populations since it has been found associated with MM in other Mediterranean populations such as France and Greece [9, 11]. The fact that NRHC variants could be important in MM risk is also supported by our finding that risk increased with the number of non-synonymous changes carried, regardless of whether they were RHC or NRHC. The presence of two non-synonymous changes implies that both copies of the MC1R protein are compromised. In addition, the presence of two NRHC increases by more than five times the risk of only one non-synonymous variant ($P=1.9x10^{-5}$). All these results taken together strongly support the role of the *MC1R* gene as highly linked to the susceptibility of developing MM in Mediterranean countries such as Spain [3, 5, 10, 52].

In recent years, *SLC45A2* has joined the group of genes (including *MC1R*, *OCA2*, and *ASP*) identified as being related to pigmentation, and it is now considered integral to pigmentation variation. Mutations in the *SLC45A2* or *MATP* gene (MIM #606202), which encodes the membrane-associated transporter, have recently been associated with the *OCA4* albinism subtype [57]. The non-synonymous variant F374L (rs16891982) has been reported to have a strong association with dark hair, skin and eye color in Europeans [58]. These phenotypic correlations were replicated in our analysis on the Spanish population and we also established for the first time its role in MM susceptibility [14]. We also found that other polymorphisms on *SLC45A2* other than rs16891982 were also associated with dark phenotypic characteristics [16], confirming the role of *SLC45A2* in pigmentation. A parallel work by Guedj and cols. [59] also detected association of this variant with melanoma in a French population, supporting our previous results. It has been proposed that the F374 allele causes a reduction of protein function that alters the intracellular trafficking of melanosomal proteins, creating an environment for decreased melanin production [58]. More than 90% of European genes carry the F374 allele, which is rare or absent in Africans. The remaining 10% of people of European descent with the Leucine ancestral allele (the most common in Africans) appear to have significantly more pigmented skin. There is a clear evidence of selective sweep of the chromosomal segment around the *SLC45A2* gene in the European population, which is consistent with our data [60]. The derived L374 allele shows unusually large allele frequency differences between Europeans and other populations, and has reduced haplotype diversity. These patterns are consistent with the action of recent natural selection on these genes in Europeans.

The *NOS1* gene is located on chromosome 12q24.2 and consists of 29 exons, encompassing more than 160kb of genomic DNA [61] and it is the main NO synthesizing enzyme in the central nervous system [62, 63]. The rs2682826 SNP is located in the 3' UTR of exon 29 of the *NOS1* gene and was selected as the tag SNP of one of the most frequent haplotypes. However, rs2682826 seems to be the most likely functional SNP due to its location close to several miRNAs binding sites in 3'UTR region. Possibly, differences in protein translation might be elicited depending on the allele present in the mRNA of this gene. No other regulatory element close to this region seems to modulate this gene. We propose this SNP as a novel variant related to melanoma (P=0.01).

Despite not being able to detect association between MM and the absence of either *GSTM1* or *GSTT1* copies, minor homozygotes for rs1695 in the *GSTP1* gene appeared to be strongly associated with MM. The latter SNP encodes an amino acid change, I105V, that was described for the first time associated with MM (P =0.01) in our population. This finding is consistent with the hypothesis that patients with the *GSTP1* V105 variant enzyme have a reduced ability to detoxify compounds, which results in lower clearance and reduced efficacy. The *GSTP1* V105 variant is associated with a lower thermal stability and altered catalytic activity to a variety of substrates compared with those for *GSTP1* I105 [34].

It seemed biologically plausible that genetic interactions would be detected between several of the SNPs identified in our studies, and for that reason we grouped protective alleles located in the genes *SLC45A2, SILV/CDK2* and *NOS1*. On one hand, a great reduction of risk was detected when rare alleles at these *loci* were combined. The strongest protective combination was between *SLC45A2* and *SILV/CDK2*, followed by the combination of heterozygote samples at *SLC45A2* and *NOS1*. Other protective effects were seen, although they did not reach statistical significance due to the low number of samples in the analyzed categories.

In order to determine possible genetic interactions between *MC1R* and the rest of the genes studied, we compared individuals carrying risk variants in *TYR, ADAMTS20* or *OCA2/HERC2* with the *MC1R locus*. Indeed, increasing risk effects were observed in all comparisons when as more risk alleles accumulated in the same individuals. However, when *MC1R* was taken into consideration, the epistatic effect was far stronger, increasing from an OR of 4.38 when combined with *GSTP1* up to an OR of 11.56 when *MC1R, TYR* and *GSTP1* heterozygotes and homozygotes are considered together, and achieving risk effect values similar to having two *MC1R* RHC alleles. It is worth mentioning here that some genetic interactions, for instance between *MC1R* and *OCA2,* have already been described among pigmentation genes [49, 64].

Finally, we tried to see whether protective alleles were going to be able to reduce the risk induced by the accumulation of risk alleles. Some comparisons were not possible due to the absence of individuals in some of the categories. Therefore, we present only the results between *MC1R* risk alleles and the more robust protective gene, *SLC45A2,* alone or in combination with *NOS1* and *SILV*. We could indeed observe a great reduction in risk in individuals carrying two risk alleles in *MC1R* when simultaneously carrying protective alleles in the other genes. These results are important because the overall risk for an individual does not rely in only one gene but in the interaction of all his/hers genetic background and this should be considered in the future.

In summary, we found that five *MC1R* variants (V60L, R151C, I155T, R160W and D294H) are individually associated with MM risk in the Spanish population. Carrying two non-synonymous *MC1R* variants was associated with even higher risk, more than doubling the risk of carrying a single variant and having a five time higher risk than when carrying an NRHC variant. We described for the first time an association with the F374L variant, located on the *SLC45A2* gene, which appears to be a novel protective low-penetrance melanoma susceptibility gene. We therefore propose an integral study when trying to assert the MM risk of an individual, because the combination of rare alleles at several *loci* modulates the final risk/protective value that predisposes him/her to MM.

http://dx.doi.org/10.5772/53097

Acknowledgements

All these works were supported by several grants from the Ministerio de Educación y Ciencia (MEC) (SAF2007-65542-C02-01), Fundación Mutua Madrileña (FMMA 2009), and Ministerio Salud Carlos III (CP08/00069 and FI10_0405). LPF was funded by the Ministerio de Ciencia y Tecnología (MCT) and a grant from the Fondo de Investigación Sanitaria (FIS) FI05/00918; MI-V and MP-Ch were funded by the Spanish Ministerio de Educación y Ciencia under a grant FPI (BES-2008-009234) and by Generalitat Valenciana ValI+D under a grant (ACIF[2011/207) respectively. GR is funded by Ministerio de Salud Carlos III (MS08/00069). We thank the staff at the Spanish National Genotyping Centre in Santiago de Compostela and Madrid for their expert technical support with Sequenom and Illumina. Quantitative real-time PCR and Taqman was performed at the Unidad Central de Investigacion Medica (UCIM) of the Faculty of Medicine at the University of Valencia. Sequencing was done at the Sequencing Unit at CNIO and the Diagnostic and Genotyping Unit at UCIM, Faculty of Medicine at the University of Valencia.

Author details

G. Ribas[1], M. Ibarrola-Villava[1], M.C. Peña-Chilet[1], L.P. Fernandez[2] and C. Martinez-Cadenas[3]

1 Health Research Institute-INCLIVA, Av. Blasco Ibañez, Valencia, Spain

2 IIB Instituto de Investigaciones Biomédicas "Alberto Sols", Madrid, Spain

3 Department of Medicine, University of Castellon Jaume I, Castellon, Spain

References

[1] Bataille, V. Genetic epidemiology of melanoma. Eur J Cancer, 39: 1341-7, 2003

[2] Ferlay, J., Autier, P., Boniol, M., Heanue, M., Colombet, M., and Boyle, P. Estimates of the cancer incidence and mortality in Europe in 2006. Ann Oncol, 18: 581-92, 2007.

[3] Bastiaens, M. T., ter Huurne, J. A., Kielich, C., Gruis, N. A., Westendorp, R. G., Vermeer, B. J., and Bavinck, J. N. Melanocortin-1 receptor gene variants determine the risk of nonmelanoma skin cancer independently of fair skin and red hair. Am J Hum Genet, 68: 884-94, 2001

[4] Fernandez, L., Milne, R., Bravo, J., Lopez, J., Aviles, J., Longo, M., Benitez, J., Lazaro, P., and Ribas, G. MC1R: three novel variants identified in a malignant melanoma association study in the Spanish population. Carcinogenesis, 28: 1659-64, 2007

[5] Han, J., Kraft, P., Colditz, G. A., Wong, J., and Hunter, D. J. Melanocortin 1 receptor variants and skin cancer risk. Int J Cancer, 119: 1976-84, 2006.

[6] barrola-Villava, M., Fernandez, L. P., Pita, G., Bravo, J., Floristan, U., Sendagorta, E., Feito, M., Aviles, J. A., Martin-Gonzalez, M., Lazaro, P., Benitez, J., and Ribas, G. Genetic analysis of three important genes in pigmentation and melanoma susceptibility: CDKN2A, MC1R and HERC2/OCA2. Exp Dermatol, 19: 836-44, 2010

[7] Ibarrola-Villava, M., Hu, H. H., Guedj, M., Fernandez, L. P., Descamps, V., Basset-Seguin, N., Bagot, M., Benssussan, A., Saiag, P., Fargnoli, M. C., Peris, K., Aviles, J. A., Lluch, A., Ribas, G., and Soufir, N. MC1R, SLC45A2 and TYR genetic variants involved in melanoma susceptibility in Southern European populations: Results from a Meta-analysis. Eur J Cancer, 2012

[8] Kanetsky, P. A., Ge, F., Najarian, D., Swoyer, J., Panossian, S., Schuchter, L., Holmes, R., Guerry, D., and Rebbeck, T. R. Assessment of polymorphic variants in the melanocortin-1 receptor gene with cutaneous pigmentation using an evolutionary approach. Cancer Epidemiol Biomarkers Prev, 13: 808-19, 2004

[9] Matichard, E., Verpillat, P., Meziani, R., Gerard, B., Descamps, V., Legroux, E., Burnouf, M., Bertrand, G., Bouscarat, F., Archimbaud, A., Picard, C., Ollivaud, L., Basset-Seguin, N., Kerob, D., Lanternier, G., Lebbe, C., Crickx, B., Grandchamp, B., and Soufir, N. Melanocortin 1 receptor (MC1R) gene variants may increase the risk of melanoma in France independently of clinical risk factors and UV exposure. J Med Genet, 41: e13, 2004.

[10] Smith, R., Healy, E., Siddiqui, S., Flanagan, N., Steijlen, P. M., Rosdahl, I., Jacques, J. P., Rogers, S., Turner, R., Jackson, I. J., Birch-Machin, M. A., and Rees, J. L. Melanocortin 1 receptor variants in an Irish population. J Invest Dermatol, 111: 119-22, 1998.

[11] Stratigos, A. J., Dimisianos, G., Nikolaou, V., Poulou, M., Sypsa, V., Stefanaki, I., Papadopoulos, O., Polydorou, D., Plaka, M., Christofidou, E., Gogas, H., Tsoutsos, D., Kastana, O., Antoniou, C., Hatzakis, A., Kanavakis, E., and Katsambas, A. D. Melanocortin receptor-1 gene polymorphisms and the risk of cutaneous melanoma in a low-risk southern European population. J Invest Dermatol, 126: 1842-9, 2006

[12] Valverde, P., Healy, E., Jackson, I., Rees, J. L., and Thody, A. J. Variants of the melanocyte-stimulating hormone receptor gene are associated with red hair and fair skin in humans. Nat Genet, 11: 328-30, 1995.

[13] Wong, T. H., and Rees, J. L. The relation between melanocortin 1 receptor (MC1R) variation and the generation of phenotypic diversity in the cutaneous response to ultraviolet radiation. Peptides, 26: 1965-71, 2005

[14] Fernandez, L. P., Milne, R. L., Pita, G., Aviles, J. A., Lazaro, P., Benitez, J., and Ribas, G. SLC45A2: a novel malignant melanoma-associated gene. Hum Mutat, 29: 1161-7, 2008.

[15] Fernandez, L. P., Milne, R. L., Pita, G., Floristan, U., Sendagorta, E., Feito, M., Aviles, J. A., Martin-Gonzalez, M., Lazaro, P., Benitez, J., and Ribas, G. Pigmentation-related genes and their implication in malignant melanoma susceptibility. Exp Dermatol, 18: 634-42, 2009

[16] Ibarrola-Villava, M., Fernandez, L. P., Alonso, S., Boyano, M. D., Pena-Chilet, M., Pita, G., Aviles, J. A., Mayor, M., Gomez-Fernandez, C., Casado, B., Martin-Gonzalez, M., Izagirre, N., De la Rua, C., Asumendi, A., Perez-Yarza, G., Arroyo-Berdugo, Y., Boldo, E., Lozoya, R., Torrijos-Aguilar, A., Pitarch, A., Pitarch, G., Sanchez-Motilla, J. M., Valcuende-Cavero, F., Tomas-Cabedo, G., Perez-Pastor, G., Diaz-Perez, J. L., Gardeazabal, J., Martinez de Lizarduy, I., Sanchez-Diez, A., Valdes, C., Pizarro, A., Casado, M., Carretero, G., Botella-Estrada, R., Nagore, E., Lazaro, P., Lluch, A., Benitez, J., Martinez-Cadenas, C., and Ribas, G. A customized pigmentation SNP array identifies a novel SNP associated with melanoma predisposition in the SLC45A2 gene. PLoS One, 6: e19271, 2011.

[17] Ibarrola-Villava, M., Martin-Gonzalez, M., Lazaro, P., Pizarro, A., Lluch, A., and Ribas, G. Role of glutathione S-transferases in melanoma susceptibility: association with GSTP1 rs1695 polymorphism. Br J Dermatol, 166: 1176-83, 2012

[18] Baccarelli, A., Calista, D., Minghetti, P., Marinelli, B., Albetti, B., Tseng, T., Hedayati, M., Grossman, L., Landi, G., Struewing, J. P., and Landi, M. T. XPD gene polymorphism and host characteristics in the association with cutaneous malignant melanoma risk. Br J Cancer, 90: 497-502, 2004.

[19] Blankenburg, S., Konig, I. R., Moessner, R., Laspe, P., Thoms, K. M., Krueger, U., Khan, S. G., Westphal, G., Berking, C., Volkenandt, M., Reich, K., Neumann, C., Ziegler, A., Kraemer, K. H., and Emmert, S. Assessment of 3 xeroderma pigmentosum group C gene polymorphisms and risk of cutaneous melanoma: a case-control study. Carcinogenesis, 26: 1085-90, 2005

[20] Han, J., Colditz, G. A., Liu, J. S., and Hunter, D. J. Genetic variation in XPD, sun exposure, and risk of skin cancer. Cancer Epidemiol Biomarkers Prev, 14: 1539-44, 2005.

[21] Liu, D., O'Day, S. J., Yang, D., Boasberg, P., Milford, R., Kristedja, T., Groshen, S., and Weber, J. Impact of gene polymorphisms on clinical outcome for stage IV melanoma patients treated with biochemotherapy: an exploratory study. Clin Cancer Res, 11: 1237-46, 2005.

[22] Millikan, R. C., Hummer, A., Begg, C., Player, J., de Cotret, A. R., Winkel, S., Mohrenweiser, H., Thomas, N., Armstrong, B., Kricker, A., Marrett, L. D., Gruber, S. B., Culver, H. A., Zanetti, R., Gallagher, R. P., Dwyer, T., Rebbeck, T. R., Busam, K., From, L., Mujumdar, U., and Berwick, M. Polymorphisms in nucleotide excision repair genes and risk of multiple primary melanoma: the Genes Environment and Melanoma Study. Carcinogenesis, 27: 610-8, 2006.

[23] Tomescu, D., Kavanagh, G., Ha, T., Campbell, H., and Melton, D. W. Nucleotide excision repair gene XPD polymorphisms and genetic predisposition to melanoma. Carcinogenesis, 22: 403-8, 2001

[24] Wei, Q., Lee, J. E., Gershenwald, J. E., Ross, M. I., Mansfield, P. F., Strom, S. S., Wang, L. E., Guo, Z., Qiao, Y., Amos, C. I., Spitz, M. R., and Duvic, M. Repair of UV light-induced DNA damage and risk of cutaneous malignant melanoma. J Natl Cancer Inst, 95: 308-15, 2003

[25] Hu, Z., Ma, H., Chen, F., Wei, Q., and Shen, H. XRCC1 polymorphisms and cancer risk: a meta-analysis of 38 case-control studies. Cancer Epidemiol Biomarkers Prev, 14: 1810-8, 2005.

[26] Hung, R. J., Hall, J., Brennan, P., and Boffetta, P. Genetic polymorphisms in the base excision repair pathway and cancer risk: a HuGE review. Am J Epidemiol, 162: 925-42, 2005.

[27] Ibarrola-Villava, M., Pena-Chilet, M., Fernandez, L. P., Aviles, J. A., Mayor, M., Martin-Gonzalez, M., Gomez-Fernandez, C., Casado, B., Lazaro, P., Lluch, A., Benitez, J., Lozoya, R., Boldo, E., Pizarro, A., Martinez-Cadenas, C., and Ribas, G. Genetic polymorphisms in DNA repair and oxidative stress pathways associated with malignant melanoma susceptibility. Eur J Cancer, 47: 2618-25, 2011.

[28] Lockett, K. L., Hall, M. C., Xu, J., Zheng, S. L., Berwick, M., Chuang, S. C., Clark, P. E., Cramer, S. D., Lohman, K., and Hu, J. J. The ADPRT V762A genetic variant contributes to prostate cancer susceptibility and deficient enzyme function. Cancer Res, 64: 6344-8, 2004.

[29] Wilson, D. M., 3rd, and Bohr, V. A. The mechanics of base excision repair, and its relationship to aging and disease. DNA Repair (Amst), 6: 544-59, 2007.

[30] Baars, A. J., and Breimer, D. D. The glutathione S-transferases: their role in detoxification and toxification of xenobiotics. Ann Biol Clin (Paris), 38: 49-56, 1980.

[31] Lusini, L., Tripodi, S. A., Rossi, R., Giannerini, F., Giustarini, D., del Vecchio, M. T., Barbanti, G., Cintorino, M., Tosi, P., and Di Simplicio, P. Altered glutathione anti-oxidant metabolism during tumor progression in human renal-cell carcinoma. Int J Cancer, 91: 55-9, 2001

[32] Mossner, R., Anders, N., Konig, I. R., Kruger, U., Schmidt, D., Berking, C., Ziegler, A., Brockmoller, J., Kaiser, R., Volkenandt, M., Westphal, G. A., and Reich, K. Variations of the melanocortin-1 receptor and the glutathione-S transferase T1 and M1 genes in cutaneous malignant melanoma. Arch Dermatol Res, 298: 371-9, 2007

[33] Nebert, D. W., and Vasiliou, V. Analysis of the glutathione S-transferase (GST) gene family. Hum Genomics, 1: 460-4, 2004

[34] Bu, H., Rosdahl, I., Holmdahl-Kallen, K., Sun, X. F., and Zhang, H. Significance of glutathione S-transferases M1, T1 and P1 polymorphisms in Swedish melanoma patients. Oncol Rep, 17: 859-64, 2007.

[35] Dolzan, V., Rudolf, Z., and Breskvar, K. Genetic susceptibility to environmental carcinogenesis in Slovenian melanoma patients. Acta Dermatovenerol Alp Panonica Adriat, 15: 69-78, 2006.

[36] Heagerty, A. H., Fitzgerald, D., Smith, A., Bowers, B., Jones, P., Fryer, A. A., Zhao, L., Alldersea, J., and Strange, R. C. Glutathione S-transferase GSTM1 phenotypes and protection against cutaneous tumors. Lancet, 343: 266-8, 1994

[37] Kanetsky, P. A., Holmes, R., Walker, A., Najarian, D., Swoyer, J., Guerry, D., Halpern, A., and Rebbeck, T. R. Interaction of glutathione S-transferase M1 and T1 genotypes and malignant melanoma. Cancer Epidemiol Biomarkers Prev, 10: 509-13, 2001

[38] Lafuente, A., Molina, R., Palou, J., Castel, T., Moral, A., and Trias, M. Phenotype of glutathione S-transferase Mu (GSTM1] and susceptibility to malignant melanoma. MMM group. Multidisciplinary Malignant Melanoma Group. Br J Cancer, 72: 324-6, 1995.

[39] Shanley, S. M., Chenevix-Trench, G., Palmer, J., and Hayward, N. Glutathione S-transferase GSTM1 null genotype is not overrepresented in Australian patients with nevoid basal cell carcinoma syndrome or sporadic melanoma. Carcinogenesis, 16: 2003-4, 1995

[40] Amos, C. I., Wang, L. E., Lee, J. E., Gershenwald, J. E., Chen, W. V., Fang, S., Kosoy, R., Zhang, M., Qureshi, A. A., Vattathil, S., Schacherer, C. W., Gardner, J. M., Wang, Y., Bishop, D. T., Barrett, J. H., MacGregor, S., Hayward, N. K., Martin, N. G., Duffy, D. L., Mann, G. J., Cust, A., Hopper, J., Brown, K. M., Grimm, E. A., Xu, Y., Han, Y., Jing, K., McHugh, C., Laurie, C. C., Doheny, K. F., Pugh, E. W., Seldin, M. F., Han, J., and Wei, Q. Genome-wide association study identifies novel loci predisposing to cutaneous melanoma. Hum Mol Genet, 20: 5012-23, 2011.

[41] Barrett, J. H., Iles, M. M., Harland, M., Taylor, J. C., Aitken, J. F., Andresen, P. A., Akslen, L. A., Armstrong, B. K., Avril, M. F., Azizi, E., Bakker, B., Bergman, W., Bianchi-Scarra, G., Bressac-de Paillerets, B., Calista, D., Cannon-Albright, L. A., Corda, E., Cust, A. E., Debniak, T., Duffy, D., Dunning, A. M., Easton, D. F., Friedman, E., Galan, P., Ghiorzo, P., Giles, G. G., Hansson, J., Hocevar, M., Hoiom, V., Hopper, J. L., Ingvar, C., Janssen, B., Jenkins, M. A., Jonsson, G., Kefford, R. F., Landi, G., Landi, M. T., Lang, J., Lubinski, J., Mackie, R., Malvehy, J., Martin, N. G., Molven, A., Montgomery, G. W., van Nieuwpoort, F. A., Novakovic, S., Olsson, H., Pastorino, L., Puig, S., Puig-Butille, J. A., Randerson-Moor, J., Snowden, H., Tuominen, R., Van Belle, P., van der Stoep, N., Whiteman, D. C., Zelenika, D., Han, J., Fang, S., Lee, J. E., Wei, Q., Lathrop, G. M., Gillanders, E. M., Brown, K. M., Goldstein, A. M., Kanetsky, P. A., Mann, G. J., Macgregor, S., Elder, D. E., Amos, C. I., Hayward, N. K., Gruis, N. A., Demenais, F., Bishop, J. A., and Bishop, D. T. Genome-wide association study identifies three new melanoma susceptibility loci. Nat Genet, 43: 1108-13, 2011.

[42] Bishop, D. T., Demenais, F., Iles, M. M., Harland, M., Taylor, J. C., Corda, E., Randerson-Moor, J., Aitken, J. F., Avril, M. F., Azizi, E., Bakker, B., Bianchi-Scarra, G., Bres-

sac-de Paillerets, B., Calista, D., Cannon-Albright, L. A., Chin, A. W. T., Debniak, T., Galore-Haskel, G., Ghiorzo, P., Gut, I., Hansson, J., Hocevar, M., Hoiom, V., Hopper, J. L., Ingvar, C., Kanetsky, P. A., Kefford, R. F., Landi, M. T., Lang, J., Lubinski, J., Mackie, R., Malvehy, J., Mann, G. J., Martin, N. G., Montgomery, G. W., van Nieuwpoort, F. A., Novakovic, S., Olsson, H., Puig, S., Weiss, M., van Workum, W., Zelenika, D., Brown, K. M., Goldstein, A. M., Gillanders, E. M., Boland, A., Galan, P., Elder, D. E., Gruis, N. A., Hayward, N. K., Lathrop, G. M., Barrett, J. H., and Bishop, J. A. Genome-wide association study identifies three loci associated with melanoma risk. Nat Genet, 41: 920-5, 2009.

[43] Han, J., Kraft, P., Nan, H., Guo, Q., Chen, C., Qureshi, A., Hankinson, S. E., Hu, F. B., Duffy, D. L., Zhao, Z. Z., Martin, N. G., Montgomery, G. W., Hayward, N. K., Thomas, G., Hoover, R. N., Chanock, S., and Hunter, D. J. A genome-wide association study identifies novel alleles associated with hair color and skin pigmentation. PLoS Genet, 4: e1000074, 2008

[44] Macgregor, S., Montgomery, G. W., Liu, J. Z., Zhao, Z. Z., Henders, A. K., Stark, M., Schmid, H., Holland, E. A., Duffy, D. L., Zhang, M., Painter, J. N., Nyholt, D. R., Maskiell, J. A., Jetann, J., Ferguson, M., Cust, A. E., Jenkins, M. A., Whiteman, D. C., Olsson, H., Puig, S., Bianchi-Scarra, G., Hansson, J., Demenais, F., Landi, M. T., Debniak, T., Mackie, R., Azizi, E., Bressac-de Paillerets, B., Goldstein, A. M., Kanetsky, P. A., Gruis, N. A., Elder, D. E., Newton-Bishop, J. A., Bishop, D. T., Iles, M. M., Helsing, P., Amos, C. I., Wei, Q., Wang, L. E., Lee, J. E., Qureshi, A. A., Kefford, R. F., Giles, G. G., Armstrong, B. K., Aitken, J. F., Han, J., Hopper, J. L., Trent, J. M., Brown, K. M., Martin, N. G., Mann, G. J., and Hayward, N. K. Genome-wide association study identifies a new melanoma susceptibility locus at 1q21.3. Nat Genet, 43: 1114-8, 2011.

[45] Ewing, B., and Green, P. Base-calling of automated sequencer traces using phred. II. Error probabilities. Genome Res, 8: 186-94, 1998.

[46] Gordon, D., Abajian, C., and Green, P. Consed: a graphical tool for sequence finishing. Genome Res, 8: 195-202, 1998.

[47] Nickerson, D. A., Tobe, V. O., and Taylor, S. L. PolyPhred: automating the detection and genotyping of single nucleotide substitutions using fluorescence-based resequencing. Nucleic Acids Res, 25: 2745-51, 1997.

[48] Jannot, A. S., Meziani, R., Bertrand, G., Gerard, B., Descamps, V., Archimbaud, A., Picard, C., Ollivaud, L., Basset-Seguin, N., Kerob, D., Lanternier, G., Lebbe, C., Saiag, P., Crickx, B., Clerget-Darpoux, F., Grandchamp, B., Soufir, N., and Melan, C. Allele variations in the OCA2 gene (pink-eyed-dilution locus) are associated with genetic susceptibility to melanoma. Eur J Hum Genet, 13: 913-20, 2005.

[49] Duffy, D. L., Box, N. F., Chen, W., Palmer, J. S., Montgomery, G. W., James, M. R., Hayward, N. K., Martin, N. G., and Sturm, R. A. Interactive effects of MC1R and OCA2 on melanoma risk phenotypes. Hum Mol Genet, 13: 447-61, 2004.

[50] Harding, R. M., Healy, E., Ray, A. J., Ellis, N. S., Flanagan, N., Todd, C., Dixon, C., Sajantila, A., Jackson, I. J., Birch-Machin, M. A., and Rees, J. L. Evidence for variable selective pressures at MC1R. Am J Hum Genet, 66: 1351-61, 2000.

[51] Rana, B. K., Hewett-Emmett, D., Jin, L., Chang, B. H., Sambuughin, N., Lin, M., Watkins, S., Bamshad, M., Jorde, L. B., Ramsay, M., Jenkins, T., and Li, W. H. High polymorphism at the human melanocortin 1 receptor locus. Genetics, 151: 1547-57, 1999.

[52] Sturm, R. A., Teasdale, R. D., and Box, N. F. Human pigmentation genes: identification, structure and consequences of polymorphic variation. Gene, 277: 49-62, 2001.

[53] Sturm, R. A., Box, N. F., and Ramsay, M. Human pigmentation genetics: the difference is only skin deep. Bioessays, 20: 712-21, 1998.

[54] Fargnoli, M. C., Chimenti, S., Keller, G., Hofler, H., and Peris, K. Identification of four novel melanocortin 1 receptor (MC1R) gene variants in a Mediterranean population. Hum Mutat, 21: 655, 2003.

[55] Palmer, J. S., Duffy, D. L., Box, N. F., Aitken, J. F., O'Gorman, L. E., Green, A. C., Hayward, N. K., Martin, N. G., and Sturm, R. A. Melanocortin-1 receptor polymorphisms and risk of melanoma: is the association explained solely by pigmentation phenotype? Am J Hum Genet, 66: 176-86, 2000.

[56] Valverde, P., Healy, E., Sikkink, S., Haldane, F., Thody, A. J., Carothers, A., Jackson, I. J., and Rees, J. L. The Asp84Glu variant of the melanocortin 1 receptor (MC1R) is associated with melanoma. Hum Mol Genet, 5: 1663-6, 1996

[57] Sturm, R. A., and Frudakis, T. N. Eye color: portals into pigmentation genes and ancestry. Trends Genet, 20: 327-32, 2004.

[58] Graf, J., Hodgson, R., and van Daal, A. Single nucleotide polymorphisms in the MATP gene are associated with normal human pigmentation variation. Hum Mutat, 25: 278-84, 2005.

[59] Guedj, M., Bourillon, A., Combadieres, C., Rodero, M., Dieude, P., Descamps, V., Dupin, N., Wolkenstein, P., Aegerter, P., Lebbe, C., Basset-Seguin, N., Prum, B., Saiag, P., Grandchamp, B., and Soufir, N. Variants of the MATP/SLC45A2 gene are protective for melanoma in the French population. Hum Mutat, 29: 1154-60, 2008.

[60] Jackson, I. J. Identifying the genes causing human diversity. Eur J Hum Genet, 14: 979-80, 2006.

[61] Hall, A. V., Antoniou, H., Wang, Y., Cheung, A. H., Arbus, A. M., Olson, S. L., Lu, W. C., Kau, C. L., and Marsden, P. A. Structural organization of the human neuronal nitric oxide synthase gene (NOS1]. J Biol Chem, 269: 33082-90, 1994.

[62] Baranano, D. E., Ferris, C. D., and Snyder, S. H. Atypical neural messengers. Trends Neurosci, 24: 99-106, 2001

[63] Snyder, S. H., and Ferris, C. D. Novel neurotransmitters and their neuropsychiatric relevance. Am J Psychiatry, 157: 1738-51, 2000.

[64] Duffy, D. L., Zhao, Z. Z., Sturm, R. A., Hayward, N. K., Martin, N. G., and Montgomery, G. W. Multiple pigmentation gene polymorphisms account for a substantial proportion of risk of cutaneous malignant melanoma. J Invest Dermatol, 130: 520-8, 2010.

Chapter 4

Melanoma Genetics: From Susceptibility to Progression

Guilherme Francisco, Priscila Daniele Ramos Cirilo,
Fernanda Toledo Gonçalves,
Tharcísio Citrângulo Tortelli Junior and
Roger Chammas

Additional information is available at the end of the chapter

http://dx.doi.org/10.5772/54143

1. Introduction

Melanoma genetics has been for a long time a great challenge to cancer biologists, in part due to a complete lack of a single candidate gene to melanoma development. Different from breast and colorectal cancers, where BRCA-1/2 and *APC*/mismatch repair genes, respectively, characterize familial clusters of cancer susceptibility (reaching penetrance rates as high as 90% in some cases), in melanomas, the mutation rate of the most commonly altered genes associated with disease progression do not exceed 60% of the cases in familial clusters. Among the "classical melanoma genes" are those coded at the *CDKN2A locus* (coding for p14 and p16, both related to cell cycle arrest), BRAF (specially the V600E mutation), a downstream transducer of the RAS signaling pathway and critical for the cellular response to growth signals, and mutations in NRAS, somewhat related to initiation and progression of melanoma.

However, alterations in those genes, either by mutations or by epigenetic alterations do not account for all melanoma cases. Moreover, the mutations found in the classical melanoma genes are not typical UV signature mutations (such as C to T transitions). This observation poses an interesting problem in melanoma biology. Extensive epidemiological data indicates that intermittent exposure to UV radiation, mainly UVB is a major etiologic factor for melanoma development. On the other hand, genes commonly mutated in melanomas lack UV signature mutations. Thus, evidence so far for the presence of UVB-generated signature mutations in melanoma that could be defined as driver mutations has been less than compelling. Two critical questions need therefore to be answered; (1) If the classical melanoma genes do not account for the majority of cases, what other genes are involved in melanomagenesis? And, (2) what is the real relationship between the mutagenic potential of UV radiation and melanoma genetics?

In the following pages, we will discuss the new findings about the biology of this neoplasia, besides discussing the known genes involved in melanomagenesis. A systematic review of to date GWAS data, deep-sequencing data and functional genomics will serve as the background for this discussion. As examples, GWAS studies have identified genetic variations in genes related to pigmentation that confer susceptibility to melanomas. The importance of these studies resides in the identification of new variants that can represent low penetrance susceptibility genes. Other classes of genes that have emerged as critical genes to melanoma are DNA repair genes, especially NER genes (Nucleotide Excision Repair – a pathway that repair typical UV DNA damages). New studies have identified polymorphisms in those genes that confer higher risk to melanoma development. This susceptibility, in an interesting manner, seems to be influenced by the UV index of a certain region. On the other hand, microarray studies have suggested that DNA repair genes may be critical to metastasis sucess of melanomas, through stabilization of a "metastatic genome". Deep-sequencing studies of melanoma cells have also identified genes and patterns of mutational status that correlate with UV signatures, bringing new clues to melanoma genetics. Are these driver or passenger mutations? The importance of other genes and pathways is also highlighted. One good example of a gene involved with melanoma progression is the *Microphthalmia*-associated *transcription factor* (*MITF*). *MITF* has been found to be expressed in several melanomas and its function is related to a diversity of cell processes, contributing to melanoma progression. The importance of *TP53* gene and its pathways in melanocyte/melanoma biology is also discussed. The *TP53* gene has intrigued biologists for a long time, since its mutational frequency is very low in melanomas, differently from other skin cancers, which harbor a high frequency of p53 mutations, which in turn are UV-type mutations. Functional data indicate however that the p53 pathway is dysfunctional in melanomas. What are the bases for this malfunction in this critical pathway for genome stability?

Thus, in this chapter we discuss both the "old" and the "new" genetics of melanoma susceptibility and progression. A discussion that will allow for the readers a systematic overview of what is known about the classical melanoma genetics, at the same time that may provide the basis to explore the new concepts that are emerging in this field.

2. UV exposure, deep-sequencing and melanomas – Understanding the melanoma development in depth

Skin constitutes the first defense barrier in protection of internal environment and it is therefore subjected to several aggressions by pathogenic microorganisms or by chemical or physical damaging agents. Among these several agents, sunlight ultraviolet radiation (UV) is considered the most potent carcinogenic factor for skin cancers, although the precise relationship between dose, time and nature of sunlight exposure to skin cancer development remains controversial [1]. Ultraviolet radiation can be classified according to its wavelength in UVA

(320-400 nm), UVB (280-320 nm) and UVC (200-280 nm). Despite the fact that UVA is more abundant in sunlight (90 %), UVB is about 1000-fold more efficient to cause sunburns and DNA damage than UVA [2]. Skin exposure to UV light affects epidermal and dermal cell survival and proliferation, besides other cutaneous functions [3]. Acute effects of UV exposure are usually the most harmful, including DNA damage, apoptosis, erythema, immunosuppression, all factors contributing to aging and skin cancer [4].

One of the main effects of UV exposure on cancer development is direct damages to DNA. Photoreactions due to absorption of UV (mainly UVB) by DNA lead to the establishment of covalent linkages of adjacent pyrimidine bases (cytosine or thymine) thus forming cyclobutane pyrimidine dimers (CPD) and 6-4 photoproducts. CPDs are constituted by the ligation of C-4 and C-5 carbons in both pyrimidines, whereas 6-4 photoproducts are produced between C-6 and C-4 carbons of two adjacent pyrimidines, more frequently between TC and CC residues. CPDs are also considered more carcinogenic than 6-4 photoproducts, the frequency of CPD formation is three times higher and are less efficiently repaired [5]. If not repaired, both photoproducts lead to genetic mutations such as C→T and CC→TT transitions, besides single and double strand breaks on DNA [6]. Other genotoxic agents associated with excessive exposure to UV are reactive oxygen species (ROS), characterizing an indirect effect of radiation [7]. ROS can promote deanimation and adduct formation, leading to errors in base pairing and, thus, mutations and chromosomal reorganization, contributing to carcinogenic process.

Epidemiologic studies have indicated that a pattern of intense and intermittent exposure to sunlight is a major risk factor for developing melanoma [8]. History of skin sunburns have been frequently used as measure to intermittent exposure and can be a marker for high risk of melanoma development. One or more severe sunburns on younger ages increase the risk of melanoma [9-11]. Besides the clear risk attributed to sunlight and thus UV exposure in melanomagenesis, the lack of a typical signature of UV mutation in genes classically related to melanoma development and progression had intrigued researchers for years. First, *CDKN2A* and *CDK4* genes had inheritable mutations and thus not showed typical UV mutations. Even somatic alterations in *CDKN2A* show very low levels of UV mutations and the majority of *CDKN2A* alterations in melanomas are epigenetic silencing and homozygous deletions [12]. Regarding *NRAS*, another "old gene" involved with melanoma progression, the most commonly described mutation lies in codon 61 and does not correspond to typical UV mutations (CAA(Gln) to AAA(Lys) or CAA(Gln) to CGA(Arg)) and can be found in about 10% of somatic melanomas [13]. Regarding *BRAF* mutation, the most prevalent V600E (found in about 40% of melanomas – [14]), shows a transversion of thymine substituted by adenine. Finally, regarding the *PTEN* gene, increased allelic loss can be detected ranging to 40 to 60% of melanoma cases; less than 10% of melanoma samples show mutations in *PTEN*, the extensive majority consisting of frameshift mutations [15]. All those cited reports are the opposite to the high frequency of typical UV mutations in critical genes related to the other two skin cancers, namely basal cell carcinomas and squamous cell carcinomas, such as *TP53* [16].

In a seminal study, a comparison of four distinct sets of melanomas at the genomic level gave important clues about the role of UV in melanomagenesis [17]. The authors compared the number of copies of DNA and the mutational status of two critical genes to melanoma development, *BRAF* and *NRAS* in a panel consisting of 126 melanomas from four groups differing among them according the degree of exposure to ultraviolet light: 30 melanomas from skin with chronic sun-induced damage; 40 melanomas from skin without such damage; 36 melanomas from palms, soles, and subungual (acral) sites; and 20 mucosal melanomas. The results indicated that melanomas from sun-protected areas (acral and mucosal) had more frequent chromosomal aberrations including amplifications and losses compared to sun-exposed melanomas. Frequent amplification was identified in *CCND1* gene (cyclin D1 gene) and *CDK4* gene (more frequent in acral and mucosal melanomas). Moreover, deletions of the *CDKN2A* locus in were found in 50 percent of all melanomas, making it the most commonly lost genomic region, being also more frequent in acral and mucosal melanomas). Mutations in *BRAF* gene were significantly more common in the group of melanomas that were on skin without chronic sun-induced damage than in the other three groups. Therefore, there are distinct patterns of genetic alterations in the four groups of primary melanomas. The differences in both chromosomal aberrations and the frequency of mutations of specific genes suggest that these tumors develop through different mechanistic routes, and likely respond to different selective influences.

The unanswered question about the real impact of UV light on melanoma genetics began to be solved with the development of new technologies in DNA sequencing, the so called "deep-sequencing method". With this technology, the researchers could perform large-scale sequencing, covering the whole genome. In one of the first studies using deep-sequencing methods, the authors reported more than 1000 mutations using 210 diverse human cancers, including melanomas [18]. This study covered 274 megabases (Mb) and was restricted to 518 protein kinase genes. The results showed that melanomas (in that case, melanoma cell lines), had a high prevalence of mutations showing a mean number of 18.54 mutations per Mb of DNA. The main result from this first study was that of 144 mutations in melanomas, more than 90% was C to T mutations, the typical transition of UV-related mutations. Most somatic mutations found were classified as "passengers" mutations, i.e. those which do not contribute directly to carcinogenesis. "Driver" mutations, those mutations that contribute to carcinogenesis, were found in approximately 120 genes.

A second study, in this time a comprehensive catalogue of the whole genome of a melanoma cell line and a lymphoblastoid cell line from the same person, provided the first catalogue of somatic mutations from an individual cancer [19]. The numbers generated by the deep-sequencing are impressive. The study identified 33345 somatic mutations, where 32325 were single base mutations and 510 were double-base mutations. A total of 292 somatic base substitutions were in protein-coding sequences and of these, 187 were non-synonymous mutations leading to amino acid changes, including 172 missense mutations and 15 nonsense. Several individual substitutions highlighted novel candidate cancer genes such as mutations in *SPDEF* gene, which codes to an ETS transcription factor family, described as associated with some cancers types [20]. Moreover, mutations in *MMP28* gene (a member of matrix metalloproteinases) and in *UVRAG* (a putative tumor suppressor gene – [21]) were found. In addition, a 12-kilobase internal homozygous deletion was found in PTEN gene.

Of the total number of mutations found (33345), almost 25000 were C to T mutations, and of the 510 dinucleotide substitutions, 360 were CC to TT changes [19]. The mutational spectrum observed is consistent with UV-associated mutations, fact that denotes the influence of UV on melanoma development. C to T and CC to TT changes were significantly more frequent in CpG dinucleotides than the expected by chance. The mutational pattern also indicated a strong relation of UV mutations with the nucleotide excision DNA repair pathway (NER) due to the high frequency of mutations in non-transcribed strands when compared to mutational frequency in transcribed strands. The transcription-coupled repair (a sub-pathway of NER system), which operates in transcribed strands, is credited to be more efficiently in repair UV lesions when compared to NER system that operates in non-transcribed strands. Finally, besides the majority of C to T mutations, the second commonest mutation frequency was substitution of G to T. High production of ROS can lead to oxidized guanines and in turn causes G to T changes. As UV exposure can also lead to ROS production, is tempting to suggest that besides the direct DNA damage caused by UV, contributing to C to T changes, indirect effects such as ROS production also may contribute to melanoma carcinogenesis. Thus, this first entire catalogue of mutations in melanoma by whole genome sequencing supports the notion that UV exposure plays a critical role in melanoma development.

A third whole genome sequencing study also confirmed the elevated mutational rate in melanomas, that in mean was about 30 mutations per Mb, and the C to T mutations were the most frequent, once again reinforcing the role of UV irradiation in melanomas [22]. However, the great advantage of the study was using metastatic melanoma samples and also including melanomas from different body areas. Thus, the authors could present an interesting panel of mutational rate across the different melanoma subtypes. As example, acral melanomas showed mutational rates comparable to other solid tumor types (3 mutations per Mb), whereas melanomas from the trunk showed higher mutational rates. The sequencing of a melanoma from an individual with history of chronic sun exposure exhibited the higher mutational rate across the samples analyzed (111 somatic mutations per Mb). Moreover, that melanoma with the higher mutational rate showed 93% of C to T substitutions, while acral melanomas showed only 36% of such mutations. These data strongly support the contribution of sun exposure in melanoma etiology. From the most significantly genes, the authors identified frequent mutations in *PREX2* gene, mutated in 11 of the 25 melanomas samples. PREX2 is involved with PTEN pathway modulating its function [23]. Functional analysis by expressing the mutant forms of PREX2 in melanocytes injected in immunodeficient significantly accelerated *in vivo* tumorigenesis, suggesting that PREX2 mutations contribute to melanoma progression. Whole genome sequence of acral melanomas also identified low frequency of mutations (2.16 per Mb in the primary tumor and 1.95 per Mb in metastasis sample) [24].

Additional studies from exome sequencing have identified new genes related to melanoma development and also chemoresistance. From exome sequencing study performed in seven melanomas the authors found a total of 4933 somatic mutations, 3611 of which were located in protein-coding regions in 2586 genes [25]. Confirming previous results, C to T transitions were the most representative mutations (ranging from 73 to 87% of all mutations). In order to get a more comprehensive view of melanoma genome, the authors looked to genes involved with MAPK pathway, which includes NRAS and BRAF. Two of seven melanomas analyzed showed a somatic G to A transition at homologous site in the *MAP2K1* and *MAP2K2* genes, kinases that are downstream targets of BRAF. In an independent set of 127 melanomas, 8% confirmed the existence of damaging mutations in either gene. Following functional studies with either gene demonstrated a constitutive activation and resulted in ERK1/2 phosphorylation and the oncogenic activity of such mutations was also evaluated in transformation assays. Moreover, in four of the seven melanomas, mutations were found in *FAT4, DSC1* and *LRP1B* genes, which might be candidate genes, as suggested by the authors [25].

In an independent study [26], other melanoma exome sequencing also identified mutations in genes participating of MAPK pathway, more precisely *MAP3K5* and *MAP3K9*. Validation of such data indicated mutations in *MAP3K5* in 8 of 85 melanoma cell lines and mutation in 13 of 85 cell lines to *MAP3K9*. Functional analysis of such mutations indicated a significantly reduction in kinase activity of both proteins. Moreover, such mutations in both genes resulted in decreased levels of phosphorylated MEK-ERK and JNK, pathways involved with apoptosis, differentiation, survival and senescence. Interestingly, decreased expression of MAP3K5 and MAP3K9 by siRNA method led to chemoresistance to temozolomide [26]. A third exome sequencing study, using a large sample size (147 melanomas from sun-exposed areas), identified a recurrent UV-signature in *RAC1* gene in 9.2% of cases. Biochemical and functional analysis of mutated RAC1 showed that such alteration promotes melanocyte proliferation and migration [27].

All of these genome sequence studies identified a great number of mutations, however most mutations are passenger mutations. In order to differentiate passenger from driver mutations, Linda Chin coordinated an effort to sequence exons and introns of melanoma samples, comparing their frequency in order to identify positively selected genes, based on enrichment of mutations in exons [28]. The authors identified positive selection in melanoma genes including well-know genes such as *BRAF, NRAS, PTEN, TP53, p16* and also indentify new candidate genes, such as *PPP6C, RAC1* (previously described in [26]), *SNX31, TACC1* and *STK19*. Noteworthy, to *PPP6C* (a subunit of PP6C protein phosphatase), a candidate to tumor suppressor gene, showed 60% of mutations clustered within a 12 amino acid region flanking an arginine at codon 264. Regarding *RAC1*, the mutant forms also indicated gain-of-function. The study also indicated the role of UV in the advent of melanoma driver mutations. Of 262 driver mutations found in 21 genes identified by the study, 46% were caused by C to T mutations (37%) or G to T (9%), alterations characteristics of UVB/UVA-induced mutations. These numbers increased to 67% by excluding mutations in *BRAF* or *NRAS* genes.

Innovative strategies exploiting deep sequencing will contribute to the understanding of the diversity of pathways involved with melanoma. We anticipate that studies of melanomas arising in different ethnic groups, and mainly from individuals who migrated from low-UV index regions to high-UV index regions in the globe will help us understanding more about the genes involved in melanomagenesis.

3. Melanoma genetics: Susceptibility genes

When we talk about susceptibility genes to diseases, especially to cancer, we are talking about inheritable genetic alterations. Such alterations in critical genes related to tumor suppression contribute to modulate the susceptibility to certain tumors. Inheritable alterations can be classified as mutations or polymorphisms (also known as single nucleotide polymorphism – SNP). Both genetic alterations have different features such as: (i) related to population allelic frequency (mutations < 1% and polymorphisms > 1%); (ii) related to its impact to gene functionality, where mutations cause deleterious alterations to the function while polymorphisms may modify the function, however not in a deleterious manner; (iii) related to penetrance, where mutations exerts its deleterious function in a high penetrance to development of the disease. Conversely, polymorphisms exert its function in a low penetrance to disease and may be more susceptible to environmental influence; (iv) age of tumor onset, where high penetrance mutated genes contribute to disease development in younger ages while polymorphisms are related to older ages to cancer development. Temporally, high susceptibility genes to melanoma were well established through the years, however low susceptibility genes have been identified recently. Appreciation of high penetrance genes came from multiple studies of melanoma-predisposed families studies; in which linkage analysis, cytogenetic and candidate gene studies helped to identify those genes. However, the high-penetrance genes account for 5 to 10% melanoma cases, indicating that other genes, including low penetrance genes may modulate the susceptibility. The development of new technologies has contributed to identify new susceptible genes and understand their roles to melanoma. In this section we discuss the "old" and the "new" genetics for melanoma susceptibility.

3.1. High penetrance genes: "The old genetics" for melanoma

3.1.1. CDKN2A – The classical susceptibility gene

The best-established gene for melanoma susceptibility is the *CDKN2A* (cyclin-dependent kinase inhibitor 2A gene) locus, which is located in chromosome 9p21. Involvement of a 9p locus in melanomas was first indicated by cytogenetically detectable loss or translocation of this region. Subsequent loss of heterozigosity (LOH) studies and later studies indicated the existence of a tumor suppressor gene in this region. Germline mutations in this locus have been described among melanoma-predisposed families since 1995, and approximately 40% of familial melanomas cases harbor *CDKN2A* mutations [29]. The *CDKN2A* locus encodes for two different proteins, which are related to cell cycle control and tumor suppression. The two proteins are produced by alternative reading frame of four exons [30]. The proteins produced by *CDKN2A* locus, p16/Ink4a and p14/Arf, are involved with regulation of cell cycle from G1 to S phase, besides the ability of p14/Arf to induce apoptosis [30]. Regarding p16/Ink4a, its main function is to bind to CDK4 and to inhibit its kinase activity. By inhibiting CDK4 activity, p16/Ink4a avoids the phosphorylation of retinoblastoma (*Rb*) tumor suppressor gene, acting therefore as a negative regulator of E2F function. Thus, loss-of-function mutations or loss of p16/Ink4a expression, allow for CDK4 to phosphorylate Rb, thereby releasing E2F activity in the transition of G1 to S phase.

The role of p14/Arf in tumor suppression is related to regulation of p53 pathway. Its function is related to binding to HDM-2 protein and inhibition of its activity. The MDM-2 protein is a key regulator of p53 protein due to its ability to ubiquitinate p53, leading to p53 degradation. Thus, by p14/Arf function, MDM-2 is depleted and p53 is stabilized. Inactivation of p14/Arf functions is associated with MDM-2 accumulation, which in turn leads to p53 degradation and consequently loss of its tumor suppressor function. In summary, loss-of-function alterations in *CDKN2A* simultaneously impair two of the most critical pathways in tumor suppression, the Rb and p53 pathways. Most germline mutations in *CDKN2A* locus are missense mutations, usually found in exons 1α and exon 2, although mutations in 5′ UTR and intron regions are also found, affecting thus translation initiation and splicing events [31]. Overall, *CDKN2A* mutations have been found in 20 – 40% of families with 3 or more affected members and in 10% of families with 2 melanoma cases. However the frequency can vary according to different populations, fact that can be explained by different founder mutations in some of those populations. The low mutation detection rate has suggested that other susceptibility genes exist in melanomas. Moreover, the penetrance of mutations in *CDKN2A* shows geographical variations [32].

Some studies have suggested that the penetrance of the *CDKN2A* mutations may be modulated by other genetic risk modifiers. Certain MC1R variants (discussed below) increase melanoma risk in familial melanomas harboring mutations in *CDKN2A* [33]. As MC1R, a gene strongly related to skin color, plays a role as a modifier gene, it seems logical that other pigmentation genes might similarly act as genetic modifiers to *CDKN2A* penetrance. Environmental factors, such as relative exposure to UV radiation may contribute to the variability in penetrance of *CDKN2A* mutations according to geographical reasons, as suggested by previous studies [32].

3.1.2. CDK4 – The second line in melanoma susceptibility

Another well known gene associated with melanoma susceptibility is the *CDK4* gene. The gene is located in chromosome 12q13 and codes for cyclin-dependent kinase. Mutations in the *CDK4* gene were just described in 15 families with melanoma predisposition [34], where just two known mutations are described and located in codon, Arg24Cys e Arg24His. Curiously, these mutations can be also found in sporadic melanomas. Although less frequent than the inheritable mutations in *CDKN2A* locus, patients harboring mutations in *CDK4* usually show the same clinical characteristics as patients with mutations in *CDKN2A* such as mean age at diagnostics, mean number of melanomas and mean number of nevi [35]. These clinical similarities (phenocopies) shown by mutations in different genes may be explained by the same pathway that *CDK4* and p16 protein share together the Rb (retinoblastoma) tumor suppressor pathway. Both CDK4 mutant variants described above are unable to bind p16, and therefore CDK4 activity is not inhibited. The functional consequence is then phosphorylation of Rb, leading to Rb inactivity and thus allowing the cell to progress on cell cycle. Only in a few reports the whole *CDK4* gene was sequenced. Expansion of *CDK4* sequencing, including the whole gene, instead of only codon 2, might help to identify new mutations in non-9p-linked melanoma families.

3.1.3. Evidence of new susceptibility locus and other critical genes that confer risk to melanoma

Different from other familial cancer, such as breast and HNPCC colon cancers, a unique candidate gene seems not responsible to all familial cases of melanoma. As cited above, up to 40% of familial melanomas could be attributed to *CDKN2A* mutations. This fact opens the possibility to other susceptibility genes with high penetrance. A study performed in families with no *CDKN2A* and *CDK4* mutations identified a possible candidate locus in 1p22 chromosome [36]. Subsequent analysis of this locus in additional pedigrees supported this previous evidence. Moreover, LOH studies also indicated a putative tumor suppressor gene is this region, however, sequence analysis has not identified any mutations [37].

Other germline mutations in critical genes responsible for cancer susceptibility, which melanoma is not a clinically feature, also increase the risk for melanoma, where some melanoma cases have been reported. Individuals harboring germline mutations in *RB1* gene (Retinoblastoma); *TP53* and *CHEK2* genes (Li-Fraumeni and Li-Fraumeni Like syndrome respectively); *NF1* gene (Neurofibromatosis type 1); *Xeroderma Pigmentosum* genes (XP) and *BRCA2* were also associated with melanoma. Even melanomas cases were reported in such syndromes. The absolute low number of melanomas reported in these syndromes, especially in Li-Fraumeni syndrome, creates a debate regarding whether melanomas could be a rare manifestation of these cancer syndromes. A detailed discussion on the role of these genes and melanoma was published elsewhere [38].

3.2. Low penetrance genes: The "new genetics" of melanoma

The great development in low penetrance genes search for melanoma risk came with the development of genome-wide association studies (GWAS). With GWAS, several hundreds of thousands DNA variants can be detected and larger samples sizes can be used, thus increasing the power of analysis. A great advantage of using GWAS is the possibility to identify variants that are not located in protein coding regions. Coupled with the development of GWAS, the use of meta-analysis has also contributed to identify new low penetrance genes. Meta-analysis is a widely accepted method that summarizes the results from multiple published studies, then producing results with larger sample size and increasing statistical power. We discuss below the main findings regarding low-penetrance genes and melanoma of GWAS and meta-analysis studies in melanoma.

3.2.1. MC1R gene – Coloring the knowledge of melanoma susceptibility

The *MC1R* (melanocortin 1 receptor) is a critical gene related to human skin pigmentation. *MC1R* codes for a transmembrane protein receptor that binds to α-melanocyte stimulating hormone (α-MSH), upon binding the activation of adenylate cyclase is triggered and consequently intracellular cAMP levels increases, then leading to a switch in melanin production from pheomelanin pigments to eumelanin (a photoprotective pigment). The activation of MC1R is an integral part of the tanning response following UV irradiation.

The *MC1R* gene is highly polymorphic, a fact that denotes the huge variation in pigmentation phenotypes and skin colors in humans. This huge variation can create different haplotypes (many of them with amino acid substitutions) which have been show to modify the receptor functions altering the ratios of pheomelanin and eumelanin. The high levels of pheomelanin associated with some *MC1R* variants cause the red hair and fair skin phenotype. In European and Asian populations, there is considerable diversity of *MC1R* haplotypes, while in African populations the variation is less common, indicating an evolutional pressure to keep the high levels of eumelanin [39]. Germline variants that compromise the signaling of MC1R are present in about 80% of red hair and fair skin individuals; about 20% in individuals with brown or black hair and less than 4% in persons with a robust tanning response [40].

Epidemiological studies have indicated that red hair and fair skin are host characteristics predisposing to melanoma [11]. This phenotype is known to be more sensitive to harmful effects of UV exposure, mainly because the low capacity of tanning in red hair and fair skin individuals. As certain *MC1R* variants are strongly associated with skin color, and the type of skin color is associated with melanoma risk, it is not surprising therefore than some *MC1R* polymorphisms could influence susceptibility to melanoma development. Molecular epidemiology studies have reported melanoma patients as significantly harboring some *MC1R* variants more than control healthy subjects. Individuals that carry *MC1R* variants present a 2.2-to-3.9 fold risk to develop melanomas. Notably, there is an additive effect on having multiple variants, for example carriers of two *MC1R* variants have a 4.1-to-4.8 fold risk of developing melanoma [41-44].

In a recent meta-analysis, of 9 *MC1R* variants analyzed (V60L, D84E, V92M, R142H, R151C, I155T, R160W, R163Q, D294H), all variants were associated with melanoma risk. The odds ratio (OR) and the 95% confidence interval (95% CI), ranged from 1.18 (95% CI 1.04 – 1.35) to V60L to 2.40 (95% CI 1.64 – 3.51) to R142H [45]. Besides the risk values, the study showed a critical variation of a certain polymorphism among control and case populations. As example, to V60L variant, the frequency ranged from 5% in controls to 19.75 in cases, while to R160W, this variation was from 3.95% in controls to 11.64% in cases. The meta-analysis also validated the risk of melanoma associated with the so-called RHC and NRHC phenotypes [45]. The RHC phenotype (from red hair color) is defined by a nonfunctional melanocortin receptor, which leads to accumulation of pheomelanin, phenotype associated with fair skin, red hair, freckles and poor tanning ability [46]. Conversely, variants giving rise to receptors with a weak or without loss of function are called NRHC (from nonred hair color) convert pheomelanin into eumelanin less efficiently than control individuals. The RHC is composed by the variants R151C, R160W and D294H, a dominant effect of these variants is observed and the odds ratio to development of melanoma is 2.44 (95% CI 1.72 – 3.45) while to NRHC variants, the attributed odds ratio is 1.29 (95% CI 1.10 – 1.51) [45].

3.2.2. *MITF*

As it is well established, melanin is one of the major protective factors against ultraviolet radiation DNA damage that results in melanoma development. The formation of this pigment is triggered by melanocyte-stimulating hormone, a peptide hormone coded by the the proopiomelancortin gene (*POMC*). Melanocyte-stimulating hormone binding to *MC1R* also results in the induction of microphthalmia-associated transcription factor (MITF) [47;48]. This transcription factor is coded by *MITF* gene located in chromosome 3 (3p14.2-p14.1) and it regulates a suite of genes involved in cell cycle control and melanogenesis [49]. These functions allow MITF to mediate differentiation and survival of melanocytes while limiting their uncontrolled progression. It was observed by Cheli et al. (2010) [49] that loss of *MITF* in the germline abolishes melanocyte formation in mice, whereas its loss in established melanocyte gives rise to their expansion [49]. MITF achieves this partly via inducing senescence through expression of p16INK4a, p21, and anti-apoptosis genes such as B-cell lymphoma 2 (*BCL2*) and apex nuclease 1 (*APEX1*) [49]. Recently, two independent groups identified a rare functional non-synonymous SNP (E318K) in *MITF* gene that alters MITF transcriptional activity, and it is associated with a large population-wide melanoma risk estimated between odds ratio 2.19 (95% CI 1.41, 3.45) and 4.78 (95% CI 2.05, 11.75) ([50],[51]; respectively). *MITF* gene is also associated with increased nevus count and non-blue eye color, consistent with its enhanced transcriptional ability. Adjusting for these traits reduced (odds ratio 1.82, 95% CI 0.85, 3.92) but did not abolish E318K association with melanoma [50].

There is a positive feedback loop in melanocytes caused by UV radiation damage, which increases melanin production and blocks cell cycle progression via MITF until DNA damage is no longer detected [48]. Given its protective nature, melanoma researchers have spent significant effort testing skin coloration genes derived from animal studies or genetic association studies identified as targets of *MITF*, or highlighted by human pigmentation GWAS [52;53].

3.2.3. *Other pigmentation genes*

SLC45A2

Genetic epidemiological studies have recently identified a subset of other pigmentation genes that are associated with risk for melanoma and other cutaneous malignancies as well as photosensitivity for MITF-regulated solute carrier family 45 member 2 gene - *SLC45A2* [54;55]. This gene is located in chromosome 5p, comprised of seven exons spanning 40 kb, and encodes a 530 amino acid protein presumably located in the melanosome membrane [56-57]. The protein SLC45A2 probably directs the traffic of melanosomal proteins and other substances to the melanosomes [57]. The mutation 1122C>G in *SLC45A2*gene, which results in non-synonymous amino acid change (Phe374Leu) has been related with pigmentation variation and ethnic ancestry in different populations [58]. However, according to meta-analysis that summarize some association studies [54;55], this mutation confers protection from cutaneous melanoma in individuals with a fair phenotype in populations from South European regions (France, Italy and Spain) – OR =0.41 (95% CI: 0.33–0.50). This meta-analysis may explain the incidence of melanoma in cases with skin phototypes III–IV, dark eye and hair color, absence of ephelides, lentigines and with a low number of nevi [57].

ASIP

Another pigmentation gene extensively studied in melanoma is *ASIP*, located in chromosome 20q11.22, which encodes agouti signaling protein. Agouti signalling protein (ASIP) was first described to inhibit eumelanogenesis in human melanocytes [59]. The protein ASIP is a MC1R ligand of 132 amino acids that antagonises the function of the transmembrane receptor [60]. According with a recent review [34], in a large study of European population descendants, a significant association was found between two SNP haplotype (rs1015362 and rs4911414), at the *ASIP* locus and cutaneous melanoma, with a modest OR =1.45 [61]. In another study [62], the haplotype near *ASIP* with same SNPs was associated with fair skin color (OR, 2.28; 95% CI, 1.46-3.57) as well as the risks of melanoma (OR 1.68; 95% CI 1.18-2.39). Similar results were described [63] in a German population study with increased risk to melanoma development in carriers of the rs4911414 variant (OR 1.27; 95% CI 1.03–1.57). An Australian genome-wide association study [64] also indicated the presence of a melanoma susceptibility locus on chromosome 20q11.22, with an OR of 1.72 for *ASIP* SNPs, (rs910873 and rs1885120). As the *ASIP* gene encodes the antagonist melanocortin receptor, polymorphisms of this gene can alter the protein conformation or decreased level of ASIP mRNA in melanocytes. As a consequence of low ASIP protein levels, its inhibiting effect is diminished, while eumelanogenesis is increased. If there are some altered ratio of pheomelanin and eumelanin caused by huge variation in *MC1R* gene, the high level of pheomelanin synthesis will increase, resulting in phenotypes with increased risk of cutaneous melanoma (red hair and fair skin phenotype).

TYR

The gene *TYR*, located in 11q14-q21, coded tyrosinase, which is a copper-dependent enzyme that catalyzes the first two steps during melanogenesis. The protein is required for the synthesis of both types of melanin, eumelanin and pheomelanin. While a basal activity of the enzyme leads to pheomelanin synthesis, a switch to eumelanogensis occurs upon increased protein activity. It has been reported that TYR presents higher enzymatic activity in a neutral environment than in acidic conditions. This formed the basis for the assumption that a neutral environment is required for the formation of eumelanosomes instead of pheomelanosomes and that the pH value is a control mechanism for melanin synthesis [65]. In a recent review of the literature [34] polymorphisms in *TYR* gene has also been implicated in cutaneous malignant melanoma susceptibility, where variants in coding region (rs1126809) of the gene increased melanoma risk (OR 1.27; 95% CI 1.16: 1.40 and OR 1.22 ; 95% CI 1.14 : 1.31) ([66] [67]; respectively).

Genome-wide association studies (GWAS) have unveiled single nucleotide polymorphisms (SNPs) or genetic variants in other genes involved with pigmentation pathways that can contribute to melanoma susceptibility. Examples follow; two pore segment channel 2 (*TPCN2*), KIT ligand (*KITLG*), solute carrier family 24, member 5 (*SLC24A5*), interferon regulatory factor 4 (*IRF4*), oculocutaneous albinism II (*OCA2*), HECT and RLD domain containing E3 ubiquitin protein ligase 2 (*HERC2*) and tyrosinase-related protein 1 (*TYRP1*) pigmentation genes. These findings emphasize the contribution of pigmentation pathways to melanoma predisposition and tumorigenesis through gene-environment interactions. Since pigmentation genes in the melanin synthesis pathway also confer risk for cutaneous malignancy, a better understanding of the operative molecular mechanisms involved in this relationship has the potential to impact individual risk assessment for cutaneous malignant melanoma in the future [68].

3.2.4. DNA repair genes – Polymorphisms contributing to a mutator phenotype?

Epidemiological and experimental data suggest that UV radiation is the main carcinogenic agent responsible for melanoma development. While UV-B radiation (290–320 nm) induces critical damage to DNA in the form of cyclobutane pyrimidine dimers (CPD) and pyrimidine photoproducts, UV-A radiation (320–400 nm) induces single strand breaks and generates free radicals that cause oxidative damage [69]. While UV-induced DNA damage often activates distinct DNA repair pathways that maintain genome integrity, the main processes involve the Base Excision Repair (BER), which operates mainly to repair damage caused by oxidative stress and single strand breaks and Nucleotide Excision Repair (NER) that acts to neutralize photoproducts such as CPD and 6–4 dimers [2].

The differences in DNA repair capacity among individuals are genetically determined in function of mutations and polymorphisms in many genes implicated in these pathways and it has been examined in relation to cutaneous malignant melanoma. According with a recent review [34], some studies found significant association between variations in DNA repair genes and melanoma. The gene *XPD*, located in 19q13.3, codes a protein that is involved in transcription-coupled nucleotide excision repair and is an integral member of the basal transcription factor BTF2/TFIIH complex. The SNP 13181 A>C in exon 23 of the gene, with amino acid change in protein (Lys751Gln) was described as a risk factor for cutaneous melanoma susceptibility, with an OR of 1.12 (95% CI, 1.03-1.21) [70]. Other polymorphisms in members of XP family genes involved with NER pathway were also described. Another recent study found melanoma protection for the *XPG* (13q33) 1104 His/His genotype (OR 0.32; 95% CI 0.13-0.75), and increased risk for three polymorphisms in chromosome 3p25 at *XPC* gene (OR 3.64; 95% CI 1.77-7.48) (PAT+; IV-6A and 939Gln), which represent a haplotype for *XPC* [71].

In other repair pathways significant association has been described, for example variants in exon 7 of *XRCC3* (14q32.3). This gene encodes a member of the RecA/Rad51-related protein family that participates in homologous recombination to maintain chromosome stability and repair DNA damage. T241M *XRCC3* was associated with an increased risk for cutaneous melanoma [72]. Individuals who carry variant alleles had a decreased risk of cutaneous melanoma (OR 0.83, 95% CI, 0.79-0.98) [72]. Same results were found in a previous study [73]. An additional study reported a significant association between *MGMT* haplotypes and cutaneous melanoma risk, with a greater risk observed among 84Phe or 143Val carriers, who have a lower alkylation-damage repair capacity due to the variant alleles [74].

A summary of the main founds regarding low penetrance genes and melanoma risk can be found in Table 1.

Gene/ Polymorphism	rs	OR (95% CI)	References
MC1R - V60L	1805005	1.10 (1.04-1.35)	[45]
MC1R - D84E	1805006	1.67 (1.21-2.30)	[45]
MC1R - V92M	2228479	1.32 (1.04-1.68)	[45]
MC1R - R142H	11547464	2.40 (1.64-3.51)	[45]
MC1R - R151C	1805007	1.93 (1.54-2.41)	[45]
MC1R - I155T	1110400	1.39 (1.05-1.83)	[45]
MC1R - R160W	1805008	1.55 (1.21-1.97)	[45]
MC1R - R163Q	885479	1.21 (1.02-1.42)	[45]
MC1R - D294H	1805009	1.89 (1.39-2.56)	[45]
MITF - E318K	149617956	2.19 (1.41-3.45) 4.78 (2.05-11.75)	[50] [51]
SLC45A2 - F374L	16891982	0.41 (0.33-0.50)	[57]
ASIP - haplotype G;T	1015362/ 4911414	1.45 ($P = 1.2 \times 10^{-9}$) 1.68 (1.18-2.39) 1.27 (1.03-1.57)	[61] [62] [63]
ASIP - haplotype G;G	910873/ 1885120	1.72 (1.53, 2.01)	[64]
TYR - R402Q	1126809	1.27 (1.16-1.40) 1.22 (1.14-1.31)	[66] [67]
XPD - K751Q	1052559	1.12 (1.03-1.21)	[70]
XPG - D1104H	17655	0.32 (0.13-0.75)	[71]
XPC - IV11-6C/A		3.10 (1.65–5.83)	[71]
XPC - K939Q	2228001	2.89 (1.52–5.50)	[71]
XPC - PAT(-/+)		3.27 (1.75–6.12)	[71]
XPC haplotype PAT+; 6A,Gln allele		3.64 (1.77–7.48)	[71]
XRCC3 - T241M	861539	0.83 (0.79-0.98) 2.36 (1.44–3.86)	[72] [73]
MGMT haplotype L84F/ I143V	12917/ 2308321	1.75 (1.11-2.76)	[74]

Table 1. Summary of low-penetrance candidate melanoma susceptibility genes

4. Melanoma genetics: Progression genes

4.1. "Old genetics" of melanoma progression

The here called "old-genetics" of melanoma progression consist of known genes which its functions are well described and are also related to several other cancer types, mainly due to its function in controlling survival and proliferation pathways. An overview of such "old-genetics" of melanoma is shown in Figure 1.

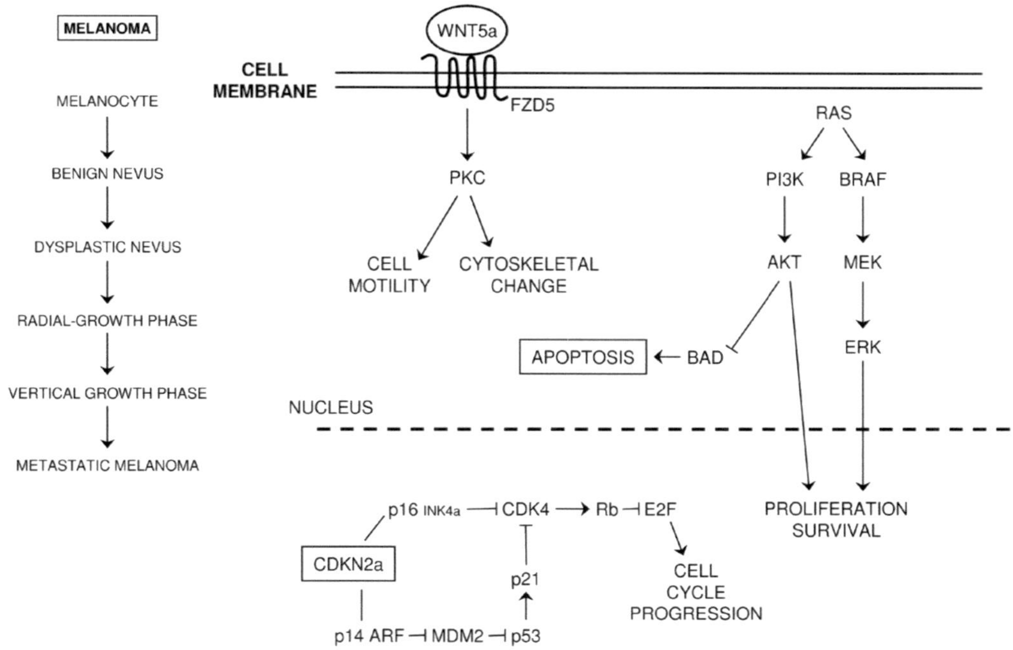

Figure 1. A schematic view of the main genes and pathways related to melanoma progression. The genes and pathways described are the here called "old genetics" of melanoma progression. Arrows indicate activation and blunt arrows indicate inhibition.

4.1.1. Mitogen-Activated Protein Kinases (MAPK) pathway – MAPing the first melanoma progression pathway

Several molecular pathways are activated/deactivated during tumor formation and some of them are responsible for the development of specific phases of tumor progression. Among them, is the Mitogen-activated protein kinases (MAPK) pathway. The pathway consists in a chain-like activation cascade of serine/threonine-specific protein kinases, where one protein must be phosphorylated to activate another. The proteins involved in this pathway are the RAS oncogene, discovered in the early 80s, with three known isoforms (H-Ras, K-RAS and N-RAS); RAF kinase, with also three isoforms (A-RAF, B-RAF and C-RAF or RAF-1); MEK kinase and ERK kinase, which have cytoplasmic targets or can phosphorylate transcription factors in the nucleus. The MAPK pathway is one of the most well-known pathways involved not only in melanoma formation, but probably in most types of tumors. The pathway is responsible to conduct an extracellular signal, like growth signal, from receptors in cell surface towards cell nucleus. After activation of RAS, the first protein of the cascade, a multitude of cellular responses, like protein synthesis, regulation of cell survival, differentiation and proliferation can be observed, showing the importance of this pathway for melanoma progression. Mutations in MAPK pathway are necessary for the development of early stages melanomas, as the transfection of constitutively activated MEK into immortalized melanocytes is sufficient to induce tumorigenesis in nude mice, activation of the angiogenic switch, and increased production of the pro-angiogenic factor, vascular endothelial growth factor (VEGF), and matrix metalloproteinases (MMPs) [75].

The most common mutations found in MAPK proteins in melanomas are in RAS protein, more specific in N-RAS and in RAF proteins, in B-RAF. The RAS proteins are members of a large superfamily of low molecular-weight GTP-binding proteins. The activation state of RAS proteins depends on whether they are bound to GTP (in which case, they are active and are able to engage downstream target enzyme) or GDP (in which case, they are inactive and fail to interact with these effectors). In normal cells, the activity of RAS proteins is controlled by the ratio of bound GTP to GDP [76]. N-RAS mutations can be found in over 15% of all melanoma cases and are most commonly the result of the substitution from leucine to glutamine at position 61 [77]. It is correlated to the vertical growth phase of melanoma progression. Although initially thought to occur mainly at the plasma membrane, there is increasing evidence that isoform-specific RAS signaling can take place at different cellular compartments and within different regions of the plasma membrane. Such compartmentalization and trafficking of endogenous RAS oncogenes is likely to play an important role in regulating downstream signaling processes involved in tumorigenesis [78]. For its activation and function as a signal transducer, N-RAS needs to be modified by a farnesylation near its C-terminal domain. Several farnesylation inhibitors were tested in the clinics and all results were disappointing [79]. In part, the failure of the clinical trials can be explained due to the fact that the farnesylation inhibitors may work in Rho (a subfamily of RAS superfamily) rather than RAS, or the fact that the inhibitors works on normal and mutated RAS.

Other important component of MAPK pathway that is mutated in melanomas is the RAF kinase B-RAF, the primer mediator of RAS protein. Some reports have shown that over 60% of all melanoma cases have mutation in B-RAF [80]. RAF mutations occur in the kinase domains and the most common mutation found in melanomas, approximately 80%, is the substitution of valine at position 600 with glutamic acid also called B-RAF^{V600E} mutation. This mutation creates a constitutively active status for B-RAF, independently of a previous activation by RAS oncogene and extracellular stimulus and it is more frequently found in skin of individuals with intermittent sun exposure than unexposed or chronically sun-damaged skin. Interestingly, B-RAF mutation frequency in benign melanocytic nevi seems to be equal or even higher than in that for melanomas. The frequency also varies, like melanomas, from 0% in Spitz nevi up to 90% in intradermal nevi. These differences, between B-RAF mutation in nevi and melanomas make the assessment of the impact of these mutations on prognosis difficult to determine [38]. B-RAF mutation in nevi might be a critical step in melanoma development, suggesting its importance in early stages of the disease.

Melanomas usually do not have B-Raf^{V600E} mutation at the same time they have mutations in any RAS isotype. However, some small proportions of cases carry mutation in both B-RAF and any RAS isoform, but in these cases, B-RAF mutation almost never is in V600E locus [81]. Recently, a link between B-RAF and the cell cycle controller E2F has been shown. B-RAF is able to phosphorylate the retinoblastoma (Rb) protein and release E2F transcription factor family to work [82]. E2F family is a classic cell cycle controller, but can also induce DNA repair, regulates autophagy and MMPs expression. The link between MAPK pathway and E2F transcription factor family may provide new strategies for melanoma treatment. New drugs using the B-Raf^{V600E} mutation as a target is currently being used in the clinics. Vemurafenib (PLX-4032) is a novel treatment for metastatic disease for melanomas with the V600E mutation. Vemurafenib treatment has demonstrated improved progression-free and prolonging overall survival in three months, compared with chemotherapy in a randomized trial, and represents a new standard of care in patients with advanced melanoma harboring a BRAF-V600 mutation [83]. However, Vemurafenib treatment induces several resistance pathways in B-Raf^{V600E} cells and is expected to failure after a few months, but it is the best treatment for melanoma disease so far. Among the resistance pathway induced by the drug are MEK activation by MAP3K8 [84], up regulation of N-RAS [85] and activation of fibroblast growth factor receptor 3 (FGFR3) [86].

4.1.2. PI3K pathway – Supporting MAPK pathway to melanoma progression

RAS can also activate other effectors pathways rather than RAF. RAS can interact directly with phosphatidylinositol 3-kinases (PI3Ks), activating other molecular pathways. One of the pathways activated by PI3Ks is the AKT/PKB pathway, which has a strong anti-apoptotic function by phosphorylating various targets and seems to be an important part of the survival signal that is generated by RAS activation.

MAPK activation is necessary for early stages melanomas, but is not sufficient for the development of advanced disease. Other molecular mechanisms are necessary for melanoma invade other tissues and survive in different microenvironments. AKT/PKB seems to be important for the development of radial growth melanomas, from cell lines which are characterized as radial growth melanomas. In this model, AKT overexpression induced VEGF expression and switched to a more glycolytic metabolism [87]. The AKT family consists of three members, AKT1–3 and 43–50% of melanomas have a selective constitutively active AKT3. AKT3 overexpression may occur as a result of copy number increases in the long arm of chromosome 1. Another mechanism for PI3K/AKT pathway activation in melanoma is through the acquisition of activating E17K mutations in AKT3. AKT has a critical role in cancer development through its ability to block apoptosis through the direct phosphorylation of BAD as well as through its effects in many other pathways, including the inhibition of forkhead signaling and the inhibition of glycogen synthase kinase-3. One of the most critical regulators of AKT is the phosphatase and tensin homolog (PTEN), which degrades the products of PI3K, preventing AKT activation. The mechanism by which the PI3K/AKT pathway is activated in melanoma may involve the loss of expression or functional inactivation of PTEN [88]. However, PI3K pathway mutations, though more heterogeneous, were present in 41% of the melanoma, with PTEN being the highest mutated gene of the PI3K pathway in melanomas (22%) [89].

PTEN is a tumor suppressor gene located in chromosome 10q23.3 and is a dual specificity phosphatase capable of dephosphorylating both tyrosine phosphate and serine/threonine phosphate residues in proteins. It also functions as a major lipid phosphatase, counteracting PI3K by dephosphorylating the second messengers phosphatidylinositol-3,4,5-triphosphate

(PIP3) and phosphatidylinositol-3,4-diphosphate (PIP2), which are required for the activation of AKT/PKB [17]. PTEN can work in other pathways than AKT/PKB. PTEN is involved in cell migration, spreading, and focal adhesion formation through direct dephosphorylation and inactivation of focal adhesion kinase (FAK). Also, PTEN inhibits Shc phosphorylation, preventing the association of Shc with Grb2/Sos and activation of the Ras/Raf/MEK1/MAPK pathway. PTEN suppresses the stabilization of hypoxia-mediated HIF-1α, which when stabilized through the PI3K/AKT pathway, upregulates VEGF expression suggesting a possible role for PTEN in angiogenesis [88]. An interesting study sequenced the PTEN gene from melanomas from patients harboring the *Xeroderma Pigmentosum* syndrome [90]. A total of 59 melanomas from 8 XP patients showed a mutation rate of 56% in *PTEN* gene. A detailed look for the mutational spectrum revealed that 91% of the melanomas with mutations had 1 to 4 UV type mutations (C to T changes) occurring at adjacent pyrimidines. Functional analyses also indicated impared PTEN function caused by the mutations. The study showed critical data to the understanding of melanoma progression in XP patients.

4.1.3. WNT5A – Progression to the edges, leading to melanoma metastasis

The metastatic disease does not have fixed histopathological subclasses. That is why there is a need to look for genetic profiles that could predict a behavior in advanced stages. WNT5A, a protein of Wnt family, was identified as the gene that best defined the new subclasses of tumors. The Wnt family of proteins has over 19 members, all of which are secreted, that are very closely structurally related. The activation of Wnt signaling can have very different results depending on which members of the family are involved. Wnt proteins work through three different pathways: the β-catenin pathway, the Wnt/Ca2+ pathway and the planar cell polarity pathway. The activation of WNT5A in melanomas uses the non-canonical pathway Wnt/Ca2+ together with Frizzled receptors, activating phospholipase C, which translocate to the membrane and hydrolyzes membrane phospholipids, initiating phosphatidylinositol signaling [91]. *In vitro* analysis of melanoma cell lines differing in WNT5A expression levels showed that WNT5A overexpression is correlated with increased motility and invasiveness of the cell [91]. WNT5A correlates with high aggressive metastatic disease and its activation is mediated through PKC pathways which are associated to cytoskeletal organization and invasion. WNT5A protein expression in human melanoma biopsies directly correlates with increasing tumor grade while inversely correlating with patient survival [92]. Members of the Wnt pathways have been identified in melanoma. WNT5A and others members like Rho pathway and frizzled 7 may play an important role in transition of melanoma from VGP to metastases. It is very likely that the temporal activation of Wnt pathways is very important for melanoma development and progression. It would not be surprising if β-catenin expression was an early event, and metastatic cells need to down regulate expression of this protein prior to invading, and escaping the immune system. WNT5A may provide a survival advantage to melanoma cells, despite the fact that in others tumor it may act as a tumor suppressor. Thus, its early expression may result in suppression of tumorigenesis, whereas if it is expressed at a later stage, it becomes a potent inducer of migration and motility. Wnt signaling and its effects on melanoma establishment and progression are complex, and surely temporal and context dependent [92].

4.2. "New genetics" of melanoma progression

Melanoma is a complex genetic disease. Recent studies have begun to characterize the mechanisms underlying melanoma plasticity, relating to intratumoral switching between varying malignant capacities, such as proliferation, invasion, or tumorigenesis. The rate at which somatic and germline genetic alterations have been cataloged in melanoma has accelerated greatly in recent years. The ability to modulate genes and proteins of interest, even when pharmacologic agents are not available, has provided preclinical evidence that many putative oncogenes represent potential therapeutic targets [93]. At the same time, the notorious resistance of melanoma to treatments with its strong potential to metastasize represents the major clinical obstacle in the treatment of these tumors. These observations allow the scientists to improve staging and subtype classification and lead them to design better therapeutic agents and approaches. New insights about genetics of melanoma, including high-throughput strategies such as gene expression microarrays, comparative genomic hybridization, mutation analysis by deep sequencing and microRNAs gene regulation have helped researchers to elucidate the crucial cell-signaling pathways or validate the already postulated pathways as modified in melanomas. The genes and pathways discussed below for the "new genetics" of melanoma progression are represented in Figure 2.

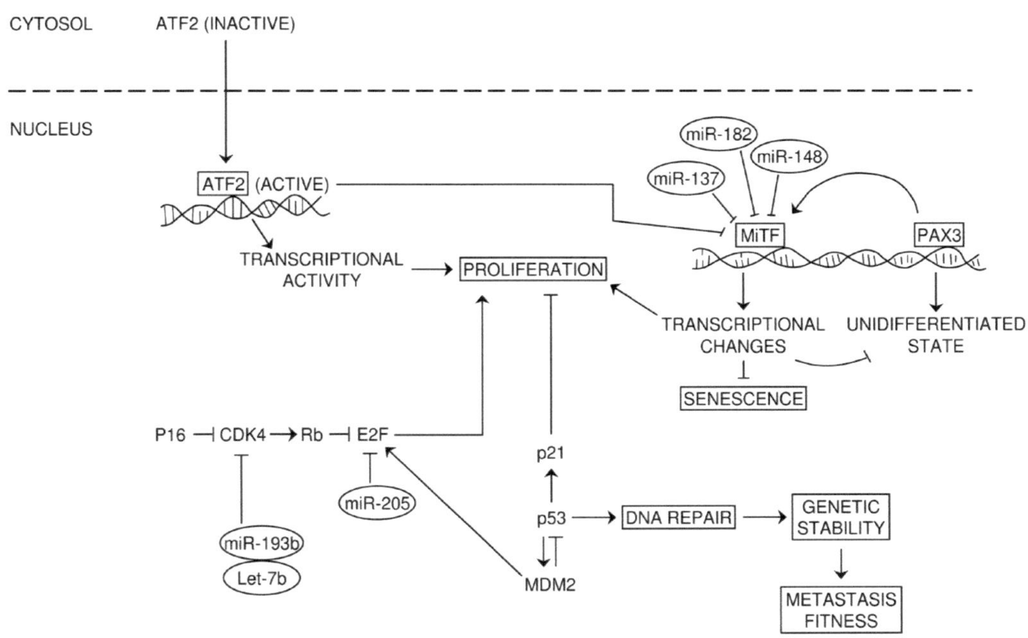

Figure 2. A schematic view of the main genes and pathways related to melanoma progression. The genes and pathways described are the here called "new genetics" of melanoma progression. Arrows indicate activation and blunt arrows indicate inhibition.

4.2.1. Activating Transcription Factor 2 (ATF2) – Helping melanoma progression activation

The ATF2 (Activating Transcription Factor-2 or cAMP response element [CRE]) it was first identified as an inducible enhancer of genes that can be transcribed in response to increased cAMP levels and mediates various transcriptional regulatory effects, for example, ATF2/Jun complex is implicated in multiple cellular processes [94,95]. The ATF2 transcriptional targets genes is divided into (a) regulation of transcription factors and proteins engaged in stress and DNA damage response (b) regulation of genes associated with growth and tumorigenesis (c) regulation of genes important for maintenance and physiological homeostasis [94]. In addition to its function as a transcription factor, ATF2 was found to play an important role in DNA damage response. After damage occurs, ATF2 is phosphorylated by ATM and its results in rapid localization of ATF2 to ionizing radiation (IR) induced foci (IRIF), which contain DNA repair proteins and chromatin-modifying enzymes. Furthermore, ATF2 phosphorylated is required for an intact intra-S-phase checkpoint response necessary to stop DNA replication [96]. In recent years, the study of ATF2 activity in melanoma cells has revealed a probably oncogenic function. In the early '90s, Ronai and Weinstein [97] elucidated the cellular response to UV irradiation. The authors characterized a UV-responsive element (URE;TGACAACA) and soon after, its binding proteins, AP1 and ATF family members [98]. Interesting, the URE was found within the promoter sequences of stress-responsive genes, including c-jun, DNA polymerase B, and cyclin A, as well as on regulatory regions of viruses that respond to UV irradiation [99]. Differences in transcriptional activities of URE-bound proteins were found after UV-irradiation of keratinocytes, melanocytes and melanoma, and also in repair deficient cells of patients with *Xeroderma pigmentosum*, or Cockayne syndrome [for review 9]. In 1998, the Ronai´s group investigated which of the CREB-associated proteins is directly involved in modifying specific characteristics of melanoma phenotypes. They demonstrate that ATF2 is the primary binding protein and regulator of URE-mediated transcription and it contributes specifically to radiation resistance of human melanoma cells.

An approach to selectively inhibit ATF2 activity in human melanoma was designed, based on peptides derived from ATF2 trans-activating domain which affect ATF2 transcriptional activity. In an attempt to sensitize melanoma cells to UV irradiation, Ronai *et al*. investigated the ability of cells to enter in apoptosis competing by endogenous ATF2 expression with ATF2-derived peptide(s) alone and/or combined with inhibition of p38 activity (one Mitogen-activated Protein Kinases that is responsive to stress stimuli) via its pharmacological inhibitor (SB203580) [100]. The expression of a 50-amino acid peptide derived from the NH2-terminal domain of ATF2 ($ATF2^{50-100}$) was sufficient to sensitize melanoma cells to radiation. Combination of this peptide with SB203580 induced programmed cell death in late stage melanoma cells via Fas signaling, whereas Fas ligand/receptor interactions play an important role in the progression of cancer. In 2002, experimental mouse models validated the expression of this peptide. The $ATF2^{50-100}$ not only sensitized melanoma cells to apoptosis but efficiently inhibited tumor growth and metastasis [101]. Analysis of mouse cell lines derived from melanomas formed in the HGF/SF (Hepatocyte Growth Factor/Scatter Factor) transgenic mouse, revealed that the proliferation rate in culture increased with increased ATF-2 activity [102], confirming the role of ATF2 in melanoma development. Along these lines, B16 mouse melanoma cells exhibit higher levels of phosphorylated ATF2 compared to immortalized non-malignant mouse melanocytes. Following treatment with retinoic acid, ATF2 phosphorylation was reduced, resulting in c-Jun dimerization with c-Fos and promoting a shift from proliferation towards differentiation [103]. Additional experiments showed that delivery of ATF2 inhibitory peptides elicited efficient inhibition of melanoma tumor growth [104].

Even with these encouraging results, one question remains unanswered: how ATF2 inhibition induces apoptosis in melanoma cells? It was demonstrated that $ATF2^{50-100}$ induced apoptosis by sequestering ATF2 to the cytoplasm, thereby inhibiting its transcriptional activities [105]. In addition, mutations within the c-Jun N-terminal kinases (JNK) binding region of $ATF2^{50-100}$ or expression of TAM67, a dominant negative of the Jun family of transcription factors, or JunD-RNA interference attenuate inhibition of melanoma tumorigenicity by $ATF2^{50-100}$. The JNKs are kinases responsive to stress stimuli, such as ultraviolet irradiation used in this study. These results were crucial to show that inhibition of ATF2 in concert with increased JNK/Jun activities is central for the sensitization of melanoma cells to apoptosis and inhibition of their tumorigenicity. Furthermore, $ATF2^{50-100}$ increases ATF2 localization within the cytoplasm. Indeed, one study evaluating the ATF2 as a prognostic marker among patients with melanomas validated this result. A study to determine the prognostic value of ATF2 evaluating the pattern and level of its expression in a tissue microarray was conducted [106]. Cytoplasmic ATF2 expression was associated with primary tumor rather than metastases and with better patient survival whereas nuclear ATF2 expression was associated with metastatic tumor and with poor survival. Nuclear ATF2 seems to be transcriptionally active while cytoplasmic ATF2 probably represents an inactive form. These findings support one preclinical finding in which transcriptionally active ATF2 is involved in tumor progression-proliferation in melanoma, suggesting that ATF2 might be a useful prognostic marker in early-stage melanoma. Although the use peptide $ATF2^{50-100}$ have shown good results to sensitize melanoma cells to treatments, Ronai group´s continued investigating peptides with smaller size but producing the same effect. In 2004, Bhoumik *et al.* [107] presented one peptide with only 10aa - $ATF2^{51-60}$. This peptide sensitizes melanoma cells to spontaneous apoptosis and inhibits the *in vivo* growth. Furthermore, the $ATF2^{51-60}$ expression coincides with activation of caspase 9, an important molecule activated during apoptosis. This study points to mechanisms underlying the activities of the ATF2 peptide while highlighting its possible use in drug design.

Based on these findings, ATF2 present oncogenic action, but could it act as one tumor suppressor molecule? Although genetic changes in ATF2 have not been identified in human tumors, many data sustain the notion that ATF2 is not only oncogenic, whereas its altered expression and sub cellular localization is associated with tumor stage and prognosis in melanomas, but it also acts as a tumor suppressor molecule, under specific conditions. This hypothesis arose from independent studies with skin and mammary tumors. Studies from a mouse mammary tumor model revealed that loss of ATF2 *per se,* does not promote mammary tumor formation, but heterozygous mouse *ATF2* mutants developed mammary tumors when crossed with p53 mutant mice, indicating that ATF2 may have a suppressor function only when combined with a p53 mutant background [108]. Likewise, loss of ATF2 transcriptional activities in keratinocytes promotes faster development of skin papillomas. Deletion of functional *ATF2* in keratinocytes was achieved using a K14-cre mouse which was crossed with mutant ATF2 mice. Exposure of K14-ATF2 mutant mice to DMBA (a carcinogen that causes Ras mutation) followed by application of TPA (a tumor promoter) resulted in faster formation of papillomas which were bigger, compared with mice bearing wild-type (WT) *ATF2* in their keratinocytes [109]. Importantly, mice in which *ATF2* was deleted only in keratinocytes did not develop papillomas, differently from WT mice when treated with the carcinogens DMBA or TPA alone. Therefore, ATF2 can limit tumor development by cooperating with existing oncogenes and inactivated tumor suppressor genes.

Present knowledge positions ATF2 as important transcription factor and DNA damage response protein, which is also implicated in the regulation of cellular growth control. Along the growing complexity of understanding ATF2 regulation and function are the observations that point to its ability to elicit oncogenes or tumor suppressor functions, depending on the tissue type. Based on these findings, it was proposed one model for ATF2 oncogenic *versus* tumor suppressor functions. Future studies will reveal the nature of these major differences, and further delineate the important role ATF2 plays in cellular growth control prior and following DNA damage, as in transformation and cancer development. In addition, the ATF2 function findings highlight the importance of transcriptional regulation, which enables the sensitization of melanoma to treatment and inhibits their growth and metastasis *in vivo*.

4.2.2. Microphthalmia-associated Transcription Factor (MITF) the conductor of melanoma players

Microphthalmia locus displays important roles for biology and pathology of pigmentation of the skin, as well as eye development and degeneration. Ever since, many other mutant alleles of the locus have been found in mice and other vertebrates [for review 110].The human *MITF* gene (3p14.2-p14.1) was cloned in 1994 [111] and so far, *MITF-A*, *MITF-B*, *MITF-H*, and *MITF-M* splice variants were described [112;113]. MITF contains a basic DNA binding domain and binds to DNA sequences primarily consisting of a 5′-CATGTG-3′ or 5′-CACGTG-3′ motif [114-116]. Ten isoforms of MITF have been described [117], but the m-MITF isoform is exclusively expressed in melanocytes. All MITF isoforms have a central transcriptional activation domain. MITF acts as a transcription factor which controls proliferation and apoptosis and plays a central role in the differentiation, growth, and survival of cells of the melanocytic lineage [118]. MITF is the main transcription activator for key genes involved in melanogenesis (*TYR*, *TYRP1*, *MLANA*, *SILV*), but its function can switch, in balance with *POU3F2*, to activate proliferation and inhibit invasion [119].

Recent observations of reversible phenotypic heterogeneity in melanoma have proposed a novel "phenotypic plasticity model" of cancer, whereas MITF seems to be one of the central players in melanoma phenotypic plasticity. The "dynamic epigenetic model" or rheostat model proposes that variations in the tumor microenvironment result in epigenetic lesions, leading to alterations observed in melanomas [for review 120]. In this model, high expression levels of MITF regulate genes involved with differentiation and cell cycle arrest. When MITF is expressed at average levels, melanoma cells proceed through cell cycle, while reduction of MITF to low levels switches off the cell proliferation program, inducing cell cycle arrest, and promotes invasion and metastasis. For example, prolonged MITF depletion leads melanomas to either quiescence or senescence [121]. So, MITF regulates distinct functions in melanocytic cells at different levels of expression. While MITF lower levels are commonly observed in melanoma cells rather than in melanocytes, high levels of MITF activate the expression of differentiation-associated genes implicated on melanosome function and promote a differentiation-associated cell cycle arrest via up regulation of the p16 (*CDKN2A*) and p21 (*CDKN1A*) cyclin-dependent kinase inhibitors ([122-124]. Chromatin immunoprecipitation of MITF from 501 melanoma cell line followed by high-throughput deep sequencing and RNA sequencing from MITF-depleted cells, showed *TYROSINASE, MET, LIG1, BRCA1, CCND1,* and *CCNB1* genes transcriptionally-regulated by *MITF*. Thus, MITF-depleted cells exhibit diminished capacity to passage through S-phase and repair DNA damage. These data highlight the multitasking role of MITF that, in addition to differentiation, survival, and its anti-proliferative roles, also includes a role in the S phase, controling mitosis and suppressing senescence. In an opposite way, increased MITF levels reduce melanoma cell proliferation even in the presence of oncogenic BRAF [124]. MITF can cooperate with $BRaf^{V600E}$ to transform immortalized melanocytes by expression of telomerase (TERT), dominant-negative p53 and activated Cdk4 [121]. These data indicates that, although MITF alone cannot transform normal human melanocytes, it can cooperate with $BRaf^{V600E}$ to contribute to the transformation process, functioning as a "lineage-specific oncogene", because it provides essential survival functions and contributes to proliferation. In this context, and bearing in mind that ERK is hyperactivated in melanoma and required for proliferation and survival, it is striking that MITF is targeted for degradation after its phosphorylation by ERK [125]. Indeed, constitutive activation of ERK by $BRaf^{V600E}$ in melanocytes results in constant down regulation of MITF [for review 126].

One interesting example from different levels of MITF action came from an elegant translational study [127]. The authors demonstrated that the transcription factor ATF2 negatively regulates *MITF* transcription in melanocytes and around 50% of melanoma cells. Increased MITF expression (upon inhibition of ATF2), effectively attenuated the ability of $BRaf^{V600E}$-melanocytes to exhibit a transformed phenotype. This effect was partially rescued when MITF expression was also blocked. The development of melanoma in mice carrying genetic changes seen in human tumors was inhibited upon inactivation of ATF2 in melanocytes. Melanocytes from mice lacking active ATF2 increased levels of MITF, confirming that ATF2 negatively regulates MITF and implicating this newly discovered regulatory link in melanomagenesis. Additionally, primary melanoma specimens that exhibit a high nuclear ATF2-to-MITF ratio were found to be associated with metastatic disease and poor prognosis, substantiating the significance of MITF control by ATF2. Taken together, these findings provide a genetic evidence for the role of ATF2 in melanoma development and indicate an ATF2 function as a regulator of MITF expression, which is central to understanding MITF control at the early phases of melanocyte transformation.

Another possible mechanism that could explain the different levels of expression of *MITF* observed in melanoma cells is DNA copy number alterations (CNAs). Copy number alterations involving "driver genes" can modulate substantially their expression

[128]. Melanoma genomes frequently contain somatic copy number alterations that can significantly perturb the expression level of affected genes. Recently, accurate strategies have been used to identify new genes and/or focus on molecular pathways already described as affected in melanomas (*BRAF, PTEN* and *MITF* alterations) [129]. By using integrative strategy of SNP (Single Nucleotide Polymorphism) array-based genetic, which has higher genomic resolution than CGH arrays, with gene expression signatures derived from NCI60 cell lines identified *MITF* as the target of novel melanoma amplification [121]. *MITF* amplification was more prevalent in metastatic disease and correlated with decreased overall patient survival. *BRAF* mutation and p16 inactivation was accompanied by *MITF* amplification in melanoma cell lines. Moreover, it was described that ectopic MITF expression in conjunction with the $BRAF^{V600E}$ mutant transformed primary human melanocytes, reinforcing the MITF as a melanoma oncogene. Although *MITF* amplification (10–100-fold) is observed around 10–16% of metastatic melanomas (in which *BRAF* is mutated), *MITF* levels are only increased about 1.5-fold compared with cells without amplification [121], again suggesting that MITF levels must be maintained within narrow limits. However, because only 10–16% of *BRAF*-mutated melanomas have *MITF* amplification, this raises the crucial question of how the remaining 84–90% counteracts MITF degradation mediated by hyperactivated ERK. One mechanism could involve β-catenin (molecule which regulates cell growth and adhesion between cells). β-catenin can induce MITF expression through a LEF-1/TCF binding site in the MITF promoter [130]. Although mutations in β-catenin are rare in melanoma [131], nuclear and/or cytoplasmic localization of β-catenin was found in 28% of metastatic melanoma [132]. Therefore, regardless the mechanism of activation, MITF was shown to be a key mediator of switching between the slow-growing invasive phenotype and the proliferative phenotype in melanoma cells.

Recent studies have shown the role of germline mutations associated with MITF function. Evidence for germline mutations in melanomas comes from studies with relatives of patients with melanoma with increased risk of melanoma development, indicating the presence of mutations in genes with high penetrance [for review 133]. A study conducted by Bertolotto et al. involving patients with melanoma and renal cell carcinoma (RCC) supports the hypothesis of genetic predisposition for both cancers [51]. MITF stimulates the transcription of HIF1A, the pathway of which is targeted by kidney cancer susceptibility genes, indicating that MITF might have a role in conferring a genetic predisposition to co-occurring melanoma and RCC. A germline missense substitution in *MITF* (Mi-E318K) was identified occurring at a significantly higher frequency in genetically enriched patients affected with melanoma, RCC or both cancers. Overall, patients bearing the Mi-E318K genotype had more than fivefold increased risk of developing melanoma, RCC or both cancers. The E318K variant was significantly associated with melanoma in a large case–control sample. The variant allele was significantly over-represented in cases with a family history of melanoma, multiple primary melanomas, or both. The variant allele was also associated with increased nevus count and no blue eye colour. In addition, Mi-E318K enhanced MITF protein binding to the HIF1A promoter and increased its transcriptional activity. Gene expression profiling from RCC cell line identified a Mi-E318K signature related to cell growth, proliferation and inflammation. Therefore, the mutant MITF present all features of a gain-of-function variant associated with tumorigenesis.

4.2.3. MITF as therapeutic strategy?

The understanding of the tumor stage, microenvironment, and mechanisms employed in phenotype switching have significant implications for clinical strategies in melanoma management. The description of *BRAF* and *KIT* mutations provided the first basis for a molecular classification of cutaneous melanoma and brought up insights about therapeutic approaches. Therapies based on BRAF moves on direction of regulatory approval and incorporation as standard therapy for patients with metastatic disease, as well as targeting mutated *KIT* has also been established for melanoma patients. *NRAS* mutations have been known to be present in a subset of melanomas and represent a complicated subgroup for targeted therapies. Matching patient subgroups defined by genetic aberrations in the phosphoinositide 3-kinase (PI3K) and p16/cyclin dependent kinase 4 (CDK4) pathways with appropriate targeted therapies has not yet been realized. So, an increasing understanding of lineage-specific transcriptional regulators, as MITF, and how they could play a role in melanoma pathophysiology provided other clues to therapies. Modulating MITF in a direct way with pharmacologic inhibitors would be challenging, particularly if the interaction of MITF with certain promoter regions on specific genes is desired. Reduction of MITF activity sensitizes melanoma cells to different chemotherapeutic agents [for review 121]. Targeting MITF combined with BRAF or cyclin-dependent kinase inhibitors is an exciting therapeutic strategy for melanoma patients.

One therapeutic strategy is target one or more of the post-translational processes that determine MITF activity, stability, or degradation. Another approach is targeting the melanocyte-specific mechanisms controlling MITF expression. Nonspecific histone deacetylases seem to function in such a manner [134]. Furthermore, MITF and its target genes have been used as diagnostic markers for melanoma [135]. As cited above, MITF-M isoform is involved in the *in vivo* growth control and contribute to the phenotype of human melanoma whereas MITF-M may qualify as a marker capable of identifying subgroups of melanoma patients with different tumor biology and prognosis [136]. Many MITF transcriptional targets are emerging, and it is likely that their identification may bring therapeutic strategies based on lineage-specific conditions. One candidate is cyclin dependent kinase 2 (CDK2). This molecule seems to contribute to deregulate cell cycle control via its transcriptional control by MITF, which is unique in the melanocyte lineage due to its genomic location adjacent to a *MITF*. Another molecule that seems to be regulated by MITF is BCL2 and it may contribute to resistance to apoptosis in melanomas [134].

4.2.4 DNA repair genes – Dual effect of DNA repair genes in melanoma progression

Exposure to UV radiation from sunlight induces DNA damage, which can lead to melanocyte carcinogenesis when not efficiently corrected. UV radiation may induce direct alterations through formation of pyrimidine dimmers, indirect alterations through formation of reactive oxygen species that may oxidize DNA bases and also induce DNA breaks. In a scenario where such alterations may facilitate the carcinogenic process, DNA repair systems are critical to suppress malignant transformation. There are different DNA repair systems inside the cells, which may repair a variety of DNA lesions, since mismatch base pairing formation during replication process, oxidized DNA bases, bulky addictions, intra and interstrand damages and single and double strand breaks. The main DNA repair systems are: Base excision repair (BER), Nucleotide Excision Repair (NER), Mismatch Repair (MMR), Homologous Repair (HR) and Non-Homologous End-Joinning Repair (NHEJ) [137].

The critical role of DNA repair systems in cancer suppression is observed in a diversity of cancer predisposition syndromes which the main cause is due to mutations in DNA repair genes. Mutations in genes of nucleotide excision repair (NER), which preferentially corrects UV damages, caused the so-called *Xeroderma Pigmentosum* syndrome. The affected individuals have a one thousand fold greater chances of developing skin cancer under the age of 20 years [138], including melanomas, compared to DNA repair proficient individuals.

As discussed above, genetic variants that may alter the functionality of DNA repair genes, mainly genes from NER repair systems, may also modulate the susceptibility for melanoma. DNA repair systems were pointed as a functional network that could contribute to melanocyte carcinogenesis process by complete inactivating (such as in XP patients) or by differential functionality due to genetic variants associated with environmental factors such as UV exposure. However, this intuitive thought regarding the role of DNA repair systems restrict to the initials steps of melanoma development has changed in the last years. A study published in 2008 [139] has suggested a new role of DNA repair systems in melanoma progression and metastasis. Aiming at the better understanding of primary melanoma to metastasis progression, the authors used a collection of frozen primary melanomas to study their gene expression by microarray. Those patients that had primary melanomas included in the study had a follow up for four years. After that, 26 of 60 patients showed metastasis while the other 34 patients did not. Gene expression of primary melanomas that originated metastasis (called M+ by the authors) was compared with the gene expression of primary melanomas that did not originate metastasis (M-). The results indicated a high and robust significant expression of genes involved with DNA replication (p = 4.02 x 10^{-14}) and DNA repair genes (p = 1.4 x 10^{-16}) in those M+ primary melanomas. Besides the high expression of such class of genes, a strong correlation with Breslow index was also observed. To certain genes, its high expression was positively correlated to tumor thickness. To genes with low expression in M+ primary melanomas compared to M- melanomas, a negative correlation with tumor thickness was observed.

The study indentified a total of 48 genes with higher expression in M+, which are related to DNA repair genes and genes related to maintenance of genetic stability in replication process [139]. Among those genes, genes from the BER repair systems (a repair system strongly related to repair oxidized bases and single strand breaks) such as *OGG1* and *EXO1* were high expressed. A possible biological interpretation is that the high expression of these genes could facilitate tumor growth and invasiveness, since base oxidation is the most frequent spontaneous and deleterious lesions observed in actively replicating cells. Overexpression of genes of

MMR repair systems was also observed. Since the inactivation of the MMR system leads to DNA damage hypersensitivity, it is likely that over-expression of the MMR system could improve the cellular resistance to DNA lesions. However, the main results indicate an over-expression of genes related to rescue of stalled DNA replication forks, DNA double strand breaks and interstrand crosslink repair. These processes, acting on the S-phase checkpoint and post-replicative repair mechanisms, are essential for cell proliferation and survival by correcting eventual damages and replicative stress, such as cancer cells may exhibit higher rate of DNA synthesis. Thus, by maintaining an elevate activity of such DNA repair systems and checkpoints in S-phase during replicative stress, metastatic cancer cells can grow and survive, and further be resistant to chemotherapy.

As example, a gene overexpressed in M+ melanomas was *TOP2A*, an enzyme that plays a role in replication and chromosome segregation by solving torsional stress [140]. Moreover, cells over-expressing *TOP2A* were more resistant to chemotherapeutic drugs such as alkylating agents [141]. Finally, over-expression of genes related to FANC-BRCA pathways (genes acting in double strand breaks repair and rescue of blocked replication forks) in melanomas M+ suggest the critical role that these process exerts on keeping the genetic stability in cancer cells with metastatic fitness. These findings demonstrate an important duality of DNA repair genes in tumor progression. First, the development of malignant cells from normal cells has been credited to a reduction or lack of DNA repair genes, thereby allowing the accumulation of mutations and subsequent transformation of the cells. This concept is well documented, since the relationship of individuals with genetic predisposition to certain tumors, where such predisposition may be is attributed to genes related to DNA repair or pathways that do support to DNA repair pathways [142]. However, at some point in the progression of melanoma, genetic stability appears to be a crucial factor to ensure that the tumor cells maintain the genetic repertoire that guarantees the ability of invasion and metastasis. Thus, melanoma cells with higher expression of DNA repair genes, would have greater capacity for metastasis due to maintenance of genetic capability. The genetic stability suggested [139] is not limited to the repair genes. Genes linked to telomere stability, as well as genes that ensure proper chromosome separations were also highly expressed in melanomas M+. Another important implication based on the results is that high expression of repair gene may be responsible for the characteristic low response of metastatic melanoma to chemotherapy, since many of the chemotherapeutic agents used to treat melanoma act causing DNA damage. It was also observed a higher expression of genes correlated to resistance to chemotherapeutic agents such as cisplatin and dacarbazine (e.g., *BRCA1, XRCC5, XRCC6*). In addition, other genes related to the maintenance of DNA replication machinery were also highly expressed, leading to translesion replication, thereby preventing the apoptosis signal being secondary to the arrest of DNA/RNA polymerase.

Following studies, confirmed the high expression of FANC DNA repair genes in melanoma samples when compared to normal skin and non-melanoma skin cancers [143]. Moreover, there is a positive correlation regarding FANC genes and melanoma thickness by Breslow index. Conversely, NER genes were significantly decreased in melanomas, albeit its expression was not correlated with melanoma thickness. Immunohistochemistry of independent melanoma and non-melanoma skin cancers, confirmed the results previous discovered in gene expression regarding FANC genes and melanomas. Interestingly, down regulation of NER genes may have contributed to initial steps of melanomagenesis, however, the high expression of gene products of DNA repair pathways, mainly those regarding to solve double strand breaks, may be related to melanoma progression.

In another study, expression of DNA repair genes was associated with prognosis, disease relapse, tumor thickness and response to chemotherapy in melanomas [144]. In that study, high expression of genes *RAD51, RAD52 and TOP2A* was significantly associated to poor relapse-free survival. Expression of *RAD51* was 1.22 times greater in tumors from patients who relapsed versus those who did not; the fold changes between tumors from relapsers and non-relapsers for *RAD52* and *TOP2A* were 1.16 and 1.12 respectively. *RAD54B, RAD52, TOP2A* and *RAD51* were also overexpressed in tumours from patients who died versus surviving patients. As reported by the studies cited above [139;143], expression of DNA repair genes was also correlated with tumor thickness and to mitotic rate. Finally, when the chemotherapy response was analyzed, *RAD51* and *TOP2A* had significantly higher expression in tumors from non-responders compared to responders [144]. Finally, the results described point to new methods for melanoma treatment, where in addition to chemotherapy and radiotherapy for melanoma cells, the development of new drugs capable to modify the activity of proteins related to DNA repair, may increase the efficiency of treatment.

4.2.5. PAX3 – Back to stemness?

The *PAX* family genes (from Paired Box) consist of transcriptional factors highly conserved and also essential to development of different tissues during embryogenesis as well as essential to maintenance of stem cells in the adult organism. Indeed, *PAX* genes are related to regulation of several processes such as proliferation, migration, avoiding apoptosis and sustaining stemness phenotype in undifferentiated cells. There are nine PAX proteins, of which PAX3 is a particularly interesting protein for its function in regulating the development of melanocytes and other cell types.

Together with SOX10, PAX3 regulate transcription of MITF [145] and c-RET [146] in melanocytes. PAX3 is a key transcription factor during the development of the neural crest and its derivatives in the embryo. The neural crest cells detach from the dorsal neural epithelium and give origin to a diverse set of cells, including melanocytes. PAX3 starts its expression in neural crest precursors that are further committed with melanocytic cells lineage, such as melanoblasts [147]. PAX3 exerts its activity by expressing MITF and repressing Dct (Dopachrome-tautomerase), thus leading to an undifferentiated cell state [148]. When MITF levels reach a threshold, a complex consisting of MITF and β-catenin binds to Dct promoter, abolishing PAX3 inhibition, which leads to Dct expression and melanocyte differentiation. It is thought that upon terminal differentiation, the expression of PAX3 is reduced as suggested by initial studies that reported no expression of PAX3 in normal skin melanocytes [148;149] PAX3 expression has been described in nevi, in most primary melanoma tumors, melanoma cell lines [150-152]. The first study described the expression of PAX3 in 8/8 melanoma cell lines [150]. The study also showed that PAX3 was commonly expressed in primary melanoma samples (21/58) but significantly less frequently in benign pigmented lesions (9/75). However, the following studies found PAX3 expression in melanoblasts localized in hair follicles and also in mature melanocytes in hair follicles, in 100% of the nevi examined, 94% of primary melanomas and in 90% of metastatic melanomas examined [151;152].

A most complete study performed in melanocytic lesions [152], analyzed PAX3 expression in normal skin, nevi, primary melanoma and melanoma metastases by immunohistochemistry. PAX3 was expressed in all samples and in normal cells. PAX3 expression showed a pattern of distribution characteristic of melanocytes (at epidermal-dermal boundary and along the hair follicle). Moreover, PAX3-positive cells were fewer and had a weaker staining in normal skin, as compared to nevi and melanomas. Co-expression of PAX3 with MITF was also observed in all samples, however, in normal skin some cells expressed only MITF, highlighting the differences in melanocyte phenotype. PAX3-positive cells were also co-stained with markers of less or more melanocyte differentiation, such as HES1 and Melan-A respectively. The samples indicated PAX3-positive cells co-stained with either markers, showing then a variable differentiation status of epidermal and follicular melanocytes, however a higher proportion of PAX3 and Melan-A positive cells. Finally, to further describe the phenotype of PAX3-positive melanocytes and melanoma cells, antiapoptotic factor BCL2L1 and melanoma progression marker MCAM were also analyzed in those cells. Regarding BCL2L1, a high similar proportion of PAX3-positive cells were also BCL2L1 positive cells, in all samples, with exception of melanoma metastases. These results suggest a role for PAX3 in regulation of survival of melanocytes and melanomas. Regarding MCAM, all melanocytic lesions showed its expression. Co-staining of MCAM and PAX3 increased in proportion from nevi to primary melanoma to melanomas metastases. As suggested above, PAX3 also plays a role in regulating genes involved in protecting cancer cells from apoptosis, as indicated by studies where the down-regulation of PAX3 increased the levels of apoptosis [153;154]. One of the mechanisms by which PAX3 may be involved with resistance to apoptosis resides in the fact that PAX3 interacts with the enhancer element of Bcl-XL gene, triggering its activation [155]. Another mechanism described for the anti-apoptotic role of PAX3 is via the regulation of tumor supressor PTEN [156]. In melanoma cells, the down regulation of PAX3 showed a dose-dependent reduction of proliferation and induction of apoptosis when cells were treated with cisplatin [157]. Indeed, PAX3 down-regulation lead to increase in p53 protein and also caspase3 (a critical protein involved with apoptosis).

Functional studies have clarified the PAX3 function on melanocytes/melanomas [158]. PAX3, acting synergistically with SOX10, play a role in the regulation of MET expression. MET is a transmembrane receptor tyrosine kinase activated by Hepatocyte Growth Factor (HGF) and plays a role in normal development and in cell migration, growth, survival, differentiation, angiogenesis [159]. The HGF-MET pathway is involved in melanocyte biology acting on survival and maintenance of specific genes. MET is commonly over-expressed in melanoma and is associated with a more aggressive phenotype in terms of invasion and metastasis [160;161]. A strong correlation of expression of MET with PAX3 and SOX10 in primary melanomas was observed [158]. Thus, the expression of PAX3 may facilitate melanoma progression and metastasis through the expression of MET, a classical proto-oncogene involved in invasion, metastasis, resistance of apoptosis, and tumor cell expansion.

PAX3 activities as a transcription factor were also analyzed by comparing melanocytic and melanoma cell lines [162]. Initially, PAX3 binding to promoter regions of specific genes was analyzed and a enrichment of binding in melanoma cells was observed in genes such as HES1, SOX9 and NES (genes related to maintenance of stemness phenotype), CCNA2 and TPD52 (genes related to proliferation), BCL2L1, PTEN and TGFB1 (genes related to survival) and MCAM, CSPG4 and CXCR4 (genes related to migration). Conversely, in melanocytic cell lines, enrichment of PAX3 binding was just observed in HES1, SOX9, MCAM, TGFB1 and CSPG4, however quantitative analysis indicated lower PAX3 binding activity in melanocyte promoters, as compared to melanomas. Finally, a correlation of PAX3 promoter binding levels in melanocyte/melanoma cell line with gene expression of those genes indicated up-regulation of SOX9, NES, CCNA2, TPD52, TGFB1, MCAM, CSPG4 and CXCR4 in melanoma. Regarding BCL2L1 and PTEN, lower levels were observed in melanoma. In general, the study described a correlation between PAX3 binding to the target gene and its expression level, identified possible PAX3-regulated genes and also suggested the differential activity of PAX3 in transcriptional activity in melanocytes and melanoma cells. The interpretation of the results indicates critical features of the PAX3 function. Those genes up-regulated are genes related to cancer progression (SOX9 and NES), genes involved with cell motility, spread and metastatic potential (MCAM, CSPG4 and CXCR4) and with proliferation (TPD52). Moreover, down regulation of PTEN also contributes to melanoma progression due to tumor suppression activity of PTEN. Decreased of CDK2, BCL2 and MelanA (a melanocyte differentiation marker) gene expression and inhibition of cell growth was observed with PAX3 knock-down in melanoma cell lines, although the results were strongly cell line dependent [157]. Moreover, an induced cell cycle arrest in S and G2/M phases and increase in apoptosis was also observed in PAX3 knock-down melanoma cells, and in one cell line. Silencing of PAX3 induced terminal differentiation.

In general, there is convincing evidence that PAX3 is expressed in melanomas and in melanocytic lesions, such as nevi. Indeed, PAX3 expression in melanomas may play a role in progression regulating processes such as survival, proliferation, metastases and participating in the maintenance of stemness. However, PAX3 seems expressed in a subset of differentiated melanocytes. Further clarification of PAX3 function in these cells is necessary. Environmental stimuli may be related to PAX3 expression in melanocytic lesions, as reported by up-regulation of PAX3 under UV-induced loss of TFG-β signaling from keratinocytes [163]. Thus, PAX3 may be a good target gene to understanding the melanomagenesis process and more studies regarding its function are required.

4.2.6 TP53 gene and melanoma – What is its function?

The *TP53* gene is thought to be the “guardian of the genome” due to its pleiotropic function in protecting cells from genotoxic events, acting on cell cycle control, DNA repair and also triggering apoptosis. In general, *TP53* is frequently mutated in a diversity of cancer types and its inactivation confers advantage to tumor initiation and progression. Regarding the sources of mutagenic agents to TP53, sun exposure is a potent mechanism of induction of *TP53* mutations as suggested by the frequent occurrence of such mutations in skin cancers such as basal cell carcinomas (BCC) and squamous cell carcinomas (SCC). In such skin cancers, UV-related mutations (C to T and CC to TT transitions) are frequently described in *TP53* and in other genes, confirming then the role of UV exposure in skin cancers. As melanocytes from exposed skin areas have UV-exposure as the major environmental factor to its tumorigenesis, one could expect a high frequency of UV-related mutations in *TP53* in melanomas, as those found in the melanoma genome [19] and *PTEN* gene [90].

However, the proportion of primary melanomas harboring *TP53* mutations is frequently low, around 7% of melanoma samples, although ranging from 0 to 24% between individual studies [38]. Data from meta-analysis of 645 melanoma specimens showed that only 13.2% were *TP53* mutants, and more than half were UV signature changes [164]. Curiously, *TP53* mutations have been described in some nevi and in melanomas from XP patients [165]. In fact, on one hand *TP53* inactivating mutations play a role in cancer progression, however, on the other hand, TP53 mutations in melanomas are frequently low. With this duality in mind, interesting question arises: What is the function of *TP53* in melanoma initiation and progression? Moreover, is there a positive pressure to keep wild-type *TP53* in melanomas? Recent functional studies start to address these questions. Indeed, inactivation of p53 pathway may be relevant for melanocyte transformation [166]. Study from melanocytes indicated that murine cells engineered to have high levels of p53 developed less pigmented lesions, primary melanomas and metastases [167]. Besides this feature, melanomas from elevated p53 levels had lower size and growth rate, indicating a role for p53 as a suppressor of tumor development. Regarding human melanocytes and melanoma cells, pharmacological activation of p53 by a specific inhibitor of HDM-2, led cells to cell cycle arrest in low doses and to apoptosis in high doses. In addition, chemical activation of p53 in primary human melanocytes and melanoma cells demonstrated that these cells were far more sensitive to cell cycle arrest than to apoptosis. Moreover, *CDKN1A* (also known as p21) was identified as the predominant network operating in such tumor suppressor activity in melanocytes and melanomas [167]. In summary, such study indicated an anti-proliferative role of p53, both *in vivo* and *in vitro*, as the preferential mode for tumor suppression in melanocytes, indicating then the "need" for p53 supression to allow melanomagenesis. However, as mutations are infrequent in *TP53* from melanomas, a possible way to inactivate p53 pathway is by regulating its activity. One possible mechanism for the inactivation of the p53 pathway in melanoma may be attributed to mutations in the *CDKN2A* locus. As discussed above, *CDKN2A* is frequently mutated, lost or even epigenetically silenced in melanomas. Besides p16 protein, the locus also codes for p14ARF protein, which is regulates HDM-2 protein, the classical negative regulator of p53. Thus, one manner to contribute to melanoma progression through inactivation of p53-dependent pathways is by inactivation of p14 protein, or even by amplification of *HDM-2* gene. Under both circumstances, abundance of p53 protein decreases. However, p14 mutations are frequently associated with familial melanomas, which does not explain the somatic cases, *HDM-2* amplification in melanomas occurs in a very low frequency (ranging 3 to 5% - [168]) and high-level expression of wild-type p53 can be found in melanoma tissues and cell lines [169].

Some reports have indicated that high expression of p53 can be found in both melanoma samples and melanoma cell lines. In addition, others reports have also indicated that this high expression does not correlate with p53 functionality. Melanoma cell lines harboring wild-type p53 showed transcriptional inactivity [169], a feature of melanoma cell lines that corroborates with data showing different gene expression of p53 targets in melanomas compared with nevi, strongly suggesting a dysfunctional p53 [166]. Moreover, melanoma cell lines with wild-type p53 shows an absent p53 DNA-binding activity [170]. All these reports indicate that downstream mechanisms could be operating to down-regulate p53 pathway in melanomas. One of the challenges of melanoma genetics in the coming years is to identify and characterize those downstream mechanisms, which certainly will improve our knowledge about p53 dysfunction in melanoma biology as well as identifying possible windows for melanoma treatment. There are at this moment critical candidates genes to act as negative regulator of p53 activity. Proteins such as iASPP (Inhibitor of apoptosis-stimulating protein of p53) [171], delta Np73 [172], YB-1 [173] and Parc protein [174] has been described as p53 inhibitors. Alternatively, posttranslational modifications may also be responsible to p53 transcriptional silencing, such as phosphorylation, acetylation, methylation, sumoylation and neddlyation. Some findings have suggested that accumulation and increase in wild type p53 expression during melanoma progression may be indicative of dysfunctional p53 activity, reflecting posttranslational p53 modifications. Cytoplasmatic functions of transcriptionally inactive p53 have also emerged as a good hypothesis to a new p53 activity in either limit or promote tumor growth [175].

Additional reports have also confirmed the p53 transcriptional inability in melanomas [176]. The results from such study showed that p53 downstream genes involved in apoptosis have low expression in melanoma metastases and melanoma cell lines. Conversely, genes involved with cell cycle were over-expressed in melanoma cell lines. Curiously, little difference between melanomas with wild-type p53 and mutant p53 could be observed regarding expression of p53 target genes, which confirm the notion that possible negative regulators are involved in the suppression of the p53 pathway. Even with down-regulation of p53 by using short-harpin method, there was limited effect on p53 target genes in p53 wild-type melanomas, however to melanocytes, p53 inhibition leads to alteration of several p53-dependent transcripts. An interesting feature observed was related to the proliferative capacity in melanocytes and melanomas, down regulation of p53 in melanocytes resulted in a gene expression similar to melanomas and increased proliferation rates while in melanomas, down regulation of p53 contributed to decreased proliferation, corroborating the results described by an independent study [177] (discussed below).

Although melanomas may have an inability to exert p53 full transcriptional capability, the p53 accumulation observed in such melanomas may still have basal activity. A central question is to understand the role of this basal p53 transcriptional activity in progression of melanomas. Recent functional studies start to address this interesting question. Melanoma cells are described as largely adapted to certain stress such as endoplasmic reticulum (ER) stress [178], a situation where melanomas acquire resistance to ER stress-induced apoptosis as well as resistance to chemotherapy [179]. This adaptative response may be attributed to expression of Mcl-1 protein, which acts antagonizing the pro-apoptotic proteins PUMA and NOXA. Under ER stress, melanoma cells accumulate p53, which in turn (even in basal activity) induces the transcription of the microRNA miR149* [180]. The p53-dependent expression of miR149* decrease the activity of GSK3α, resulting in Mcl-1 increase and consequent resistance to apoptosis. Moreover, decrease of miR149* elevated the rate of cell death in these melanoma cells and inhibited melanoma growth in a xenograft model. Finally, elevated expression of miR149 was found in melanoma samples, associated with decrease of GSK3α and increase of Mcl-1.

Other elegant functional study indicated critical features of p53 role in melanocytes and melanoma cells [177]. First, the study indicated that p53 may be dispensable for melanoma cells due to lack of increase in DNA damage and enhanced proliferative potential in p53 depleted cells. Conversely, depletion of p53 in melanocytes increased mitotic defects. This last result is consistent with animal models in which genetic depletion of p53 cooperates with cell transformation [167]. Indeed, in melanoma cells p53 is kept in a basal state of functionality. This basal activity showed to be critical to melanoma growth, as: (i) basal p53 activity leads to HDM-2 expression, which in turn keeps the basal levels of p53; (ii) this basal level of p53 avoids the activation of a p53-dependent pro-senescence program; (iii) in a basal state, p53 does not induce expression of p21, which in turn does not inhibits E2F1. The following E2F1 activation contributes to melanoma cell proliferation; (iv) expression of HMD-2 leads to activation of E2F1 in a p53-independet manner, contributing to melanoma cell proliferation. Instead, the "so-called" HDM-2 addiction in melanoma cells seems not to be related to melanocytes due to maintenance of viability and absence of senescence when p53 is activated by MDM-2 depletion. In summary, this study [177] elucidates new functions of the p53-HDM-2 axis in melanomas. Besides, the p53-HDM-2 axis in melanomas is now suggested as a promising target for melanoma treatment, since the use of specific HDM-2 antagonist rescues the p53 activity, leading to melanoma growth suppression and melanoma cell death [181].

The identification of negative p53 regulators that keep p53 pathway dysfunctional seems critical for a better understanding of the involvement of p53-dependent pathways in melanomagenesis and progression. Further functional studies will elucidate the intriguing questions regarding the real function of p53 to melanoma biology: Why has TP53 low frequency of mutations? How is p53 basal state maintained? What are p53 functions in melanomas?

4.2.7. MicroRNAs and melanoma – Another level of gene expression in melanomas

MicroRNAs (miRNAs) are small non-coding RNAs (21–23 nucleotides) encoded in the genome of plants, invertebrates, and vertebrates. These small molecules bind imperfectly to the 3′ untranslated (3′UTR) regions of target messenger RNAs (mRNAs) thus, miRNAs are central regulators of gene expression and can act both in a positive and a negative way to control protein levels in the cell. More than a thousand miRNAs exist in the human genome and each one can potentially regulate hundreds of mRNAs. Target prediction algorithms can be helpful in identifying potential mRNA targets of the miRNA of interest and further they should be validated by functional studies [182]. MicroRNAs play an important role in many cellular processes, such as differentiation, proliferation, apoptosis, and stress response. Additionally, they are key regulators in many diseases, including cancer [183]. These molecules regulate pathways in cancer by targeting various oncogenes and tumor suppressors and there is an increasing body of evidence suggesting that genomic instability regions harbor miRNA genes [184]. The first study to associate genomic instability regions, miRNAs and cancer was published in 2002 [185]. The authors found frequent deletions at 13q14 involving miR-15 and miR-16 genes in B-cell from chronic lymphocytic leukaemia. Since then, hundreds miRNAs have been reported acting as oncogenes or tumour suppressor genes in a wide variety of cancers [for review 183]. The first miRNAs described as involved in cancer formation was miR-let-7 [186] and further the family of miRs let 7a and let 7b were reported to play a role in melanomas [for review 187]. For example, miR-let 7-b acts as a negative regulator of melanoma cell proliferation via regulation of cyclin D1, whereas miR-let-7a was demonstrated to regulate the expression of integrin-β3 and the Ras [188]. So, modulation of miRNA expression is increasingly thought to be an important mechanism by which tumour suppressor proteins and oncoproteins exert some of their effects. Studies assessing the role of miRNAs in melanomas are still very recent and many efforts have been made to identify the 'melano-miRs'. Despite the increasing number of studies (NCBI searching in September 2012 retrieved 162 results) a small number of miRNAs were identified to regulate genes involved specifically in melanomagenesis and some of them will be discussed here.

The linking between expression of miR-137 and *MITF* expression, a crucial gene involved in melanomas and already presented above have been described [189]. However, *MITF* seems to be also regulated by miR-182, miR-148, and miR-340, respectively [190;191]. Additionally, melanoma tumors preferentially express *MITF* mRNA isoforms with shorter 3′UTR, "to avoid" miRNA post-transcriptional regulation. Although the translation of the transcripts can be regulated by miRNAs the transcriptional regulation of miRNAs is still poorly known [192]. Some studies have searched for miRNA promoters that are specific to melanoma progression [193]. In an opposite way, the authors identified miRNAs that are specifically regulated by *MITF* transcription factor/oncoprotein and identified miR-146a, miR-221/222 and miR-363 as MITF-regulated. This high-throughput identification of miRNA promoters and enhancer regulatory elements sheds light on evolution of miRNA transcription and permits rapid identification of transcriptional networks of miRNAs, inclusive in melanomas. Moreover, expression of *MITF* has been recently shown to be involved in the regulation of DICER, the central regulator of miRNA maturation and key enzyme involved in the formation of the RNA-induced silencing complex. MITF binds and activates a conserved regulatory element upstream of DICER's transcriptional start site upon melanocyte differentiation [194]. Moreover, when DICER was knocked out, melanocytes failed to survive [194].

Besides miRNAs "*MITF* regulators" or miRNAs "regulated by MITF", other molecules with known target genes in melanoma are also regulated by miRNAs. Recently an interesting review focusing on miRNAs that act in major pathways of formation of melanomas: RAS-RAF-MEK-ERK, $p16^{INK4A}$-CDK4-RB, PIK3-AKT and the MITF pathway was published [195]. As cited, mutation $BRaf^{V600E}$ occurs in 50–70% of sporadic melanomas which active constitutively the MEK/ERK signaling pathway, promoting tumor progression and metastasis through enhanced cell proliferation, survival, motility and invasion. Two studies have investigated the correlation between B-Raf mutational status and miRNA expression in melanomas and only one study linking three miRNAs to $BRaf^{V600E}$ [196]. Recently, [197] a network of 420 miRNAs deregulated in B-Raf/MKK/ERK pathway in melanoma cells whereas majority of which modulate the expression of key cancer regulatory genes and functions was identified. In addition to MEK/ERK pathway, new insights about miRNAs and $p16^{INK4A}$-CDK4-RB pathway have been described. The mains senescence pathway associated with miRNAs are p53/p21 and p16/Rb pathways [for review 198]. Several miRNAs have been shown to be involved in the regulation of pathways involved in cellular senescence exerting negative effects on cell cycle progression, such as E2F family of transcription factors acting in cell cycle [198-200]. Recent studies reported that E2F1 to E2F3 are targets of several miRNAs, such as miR-34a [201]. In addition, miR-205 in human melanoma cells induces senescence by targeting E2F1 [202] and miR-203 also induces senescence by targeting E2F3 in melanoma cells [203]. Therefore, miRNA/E2F interaction is an important mechanism that leads melanomas cells to senescence.

Other studies have identified a cluster of miRNAs that are either involved in melanomagenesis or predictors of survival. A study has identified the miR-506–514 cluster as a transforming oncogene that regulates melanoma progression and melanocyte transformation [204]. Moreover, the authors showed that ectopic expression of this cluster in melanocytes was sufficient to transform them, activating cell growth, cell proliferation and migration/invasion along with inhibiting apoptosis. Although this study did not identify any direct gene targets of the miRNAs, further investigation is necessary because this cluster may reveal pathways that contribute to both the initiation and the maintenance of melanoma. As presented above, studies showed the increased expression of the miR-221/222 cluster associated with melanoma progression [for review 205]. A cascade involving *PLZF* transcription factor as a repressor of miR-221 and miR-222 by direct binding to their putative regulatory region was described [206]. These miRNAs regulate directly *KIT* and *CDKN1B*, respectively resulting in cell cycle inhibition and differentiation. Thus, over-expression of these miRNAs cluster increases proliferation and tumourigenesis and activates invasion/migration in melanomas.

Approaches investigating miRNAs expression are also based on gene silencing by CpG methylation. Since miRNAs precursor genes are usually within regions of coding genes (intron sequences, for example), dysfunction of these protein-coding genes by epigenetic mechanisms may also be expected to cause aberrant regulation of the miRNA target genes [207]. For example, miRNA-34a is highly methylated in melanoma cell lines and primary tumors and additionally, it was described that *MET* transcript is miRNA-34a target [for review 188]. Besides miR-34a, the miR-34b, belonging to the same family, seems to have an important effect on melanomas. A group of epigenetically regulated miRNA genes in melanoma cells, and confirmed the upstream hypermethylated CpG island sequences of several miRNAs genes in cell lines derived from different stages of melanoma, but not in melanocytes and keratinocytes was identifies [208]. Among them, miR-34b expression reduced cell invasion and motility rates of melanoma cell lines. After deep sequencing, the authors identified network modules that are potentially regulated by miR-34b, and which suggest a mechanism for the role of miR-34b in regulating normal cell motility and cytokinesis. Additionally, this same group identified the epigenetic regulation of miR-375 in human melanomas. Melanoma cells were treated with one demethylating agent (5-aza-2'-deoxycytidine) and it was identified the miR-375 highly methylated. Ectopic expression of miR-375 inhibited melanoma cell proliferation, invasion, and cell motility, and induced cell shape changes, suggesting that miR-375 may have an important function in the development and progression of human melanomas [209].

All of these studies investigated the biological functions of miRNAs and their contribution to melanomagenesis. Other studies have attempted to identify miRNAs signatures for diagnostic and prognostic, melanoma progression by comparing the expression profiles in different stages of transformation, and others focused on specific pathways. Some of these studies will be presented here. In 2007, assays were performed using the well established NCI-60 cancer cell line panel and normal tissue [210]. The study was able to discriminate between the malignancies, including melanomas cell lines whereas miR-146, miR-204 and miR-211 miRNAs shown to be highly expressed in melanomas. Large cohorts of miRNAs associated with malignant transformation as well as with the progression and with metastatic colonization in melanocytes and subsets of melanoma cell lines also was identified [211]. Subsequently, down regulation of miRNA-200c in melanocytes, melanoma cell lines, and patient samples could be reported, whereas miRNA-205 and miRNA-23b were markedly reduced among patient samples [212]. In contrast, miR-146a and miR-155 were upregulated in all analyzed patients but none of the cell lines. Using deep sequencing approach of a diverse set of melanoma and pigment cell libraries it was identified 539 known mature sequences along with the prediction of 279 novel miRNAs candidates [213]. Some of these novel candidate miRNAs may be specific to the melanocytic lineage and as such could be used as biomarkers in the early detection of distant metastases by measuring the circulating levels in blood. The expression of 611 miRNAs in 59 metastatic specimens was profiled and the authors were able to identify a "miRNA classifier" consisting of miR-150, miR-342-3p, miR-455-3p, miR-145, miR-155 and miR-497 that were considered predictors of post-recurrence survival [214]. Similarly the analyses of the miRNA expression profiling from melanoma lymph node metastases reported a unique signature consisting of down regulation of miR-191, combined with up regulation of miR-193a, miR-193b, miR-365, miR-338 and let-7. Together, this miRNAs also serves as predictors of short-term survival in melanoma patients [215]. These findings indicate that miRNAs are differentially expressed in melanoma subtypes and that their dysfunction can be impacted by inherited gene variants, supporting the hypothesis that miRNA dysfunction reflects biological differences in melanoma. Recently, the use of microarray analysis of formalin-fixed and paraffin-embedded samples from different stages of melanomagenesis identified differentially expressed microRNAs [216]. The miR-203 and miR-205 were differentially expressed between primary and metastatic melanomas and functional *in vitro* assays validated this found. So, these results indicated that differentially expressed miRNAs that could be useful as diagnostic or prognostic markers for melanoma.

As such, miRNAs represent a new class of molecules that might prove to be powerful cancer biomarkers useful in future staging systems and used as stratification criteria in clinical trials as well as treatment of patients with disseminated disease. It was demonstrated that miR-214 is over-expressed in metastatic melanoma cell lines as well as tumor specimens. MiR-214 regulates the expression of two transcription factors, AP-2c and AP-2a [217]. These molecules have been previously shown to play major roles in melanoma metastasis via regulation of genes involved in invasion and angiogenesis. Histological examination of skin biopsies remains the standard method for melanoma diagnosis and prognosis. Significant morphological overlap between benign and malignant lesions complicates diagnosis, and tumour thickness is not always an accurate predictor of prognosis. For purpose of clinical management, the microRNA profiling of clinical melanoma subtypes samples considering the somatic and inherited mutations associated with melanomas, including the presence of one variant in a miRNA binding site in the 3'UTR of the *KRAS* oncogene has been evaluated [218]. The authors showed that miR-142-3p, miR-486, miR-214, miR-218, miR-362, miR-650 and miR-31 were significantly correlated with acral as compared to non-acral melanomas. In addition, the *KRAS*-variant was enriched in non-acral melanoma and that miR-137 under expression was significantly associated with melanomas with the *KRAS*-variant. Recently, it was develop one *in situ* measurement methodology to evaluate the miR-205 in a cohort of human melanomas [219]. Based on previous findings, the authors hypothesized that decreased miR-205 would be associated with more aggressive tumors. So, multiplexing miR-205 qISH (quantitative *in situ* hybridization) with immunofluorescent assessment of S100/GP100 (melanocytic markers), the authors evaluated quantitatively the miR-205 expression. Outcome was assessed on the Yale Melanoma Discovery Cohort consisting of 105 primary melanoma specimens and then, validated the results on an independent set of 206 primary melanomas. Measurement of melanoma cell miR-205 levels shows a significantly shorter melanoma-specific survival in patients with their low expression and it was significantly independent of stage, age, gender, and Breslow depth. Low levels of miR-205 expression in melanoma cell quantified by ISH show worse outcome, supporting the role of miR-205 as a tumor suppressor miRNA. This promising result indicates that the quantification of miR-205 *in situ* suggests its potential use for future prognostic or predictive models. Studies investigating the various roles of miRNAs in melanocytes and melanoma are gaining momentum and should continue to provide fertile ground for both clinical and basic research.

5. Conclusions

In this chapter we proposed to discuss the melanoma genetics, starting from the genes that may confer susceptibility to the genes that may be involved with progression. Moreover, we addressed the already known genes (here called as "old genetics") as well as new genes that have been discovered as involved in melanoma (here called as "new genetics). It is noteworthy that the new technologies such as GWAS and deep-sequencing have improved our knowledge about melanoma genetics. Nowadays we have critical information about the disease, such as the clear involvement of UV in carcinogenic process and the many pathways that contribute significantly to it. As could be observed, conversely to other cancer types where single genes has great impact on susceptibility and progression, such as BRCA in breast and ovarian, mismatch repair pathways and colorectal cancer or *TP53* to Li-Fraumeni syndrome, a single gene cannot be pointed as "the melanoma gene". Huge amplitude of genetic pathways may be related to melanoma progression and this same amplitude may be responsible for melanoma metastasis and chemoresistance, making this neoplasia of complex management. However, in a biologist point of view such huge amplitude makes this neoplasia fascinating to understand, challenging researchers to approach the problem in creative ways.

It is tempting to assume that the more we know about melanoma biology, including melanoma genetics, much more efficacious melanoma prevention and treatment will be. Heterogeneity within the very same tumor will certainly hamper treatment. We will need to take it in account in the days of personalized medicine. To this, improvement of technologies, coordinated studies of gene-environment interactions, allied to functional studies and critical clinical trials, will be necessary for the adequate translation of this body of information into patient benefit.

Acknowledgements

The authors thank Cristina Grandal for helping with figures editing.

Author details

Guilherme Francisco[1,2], Priscila Daniele Ramos Cirilo[1,2], Fernanda Toledo Gonçalves[3], Tharcísio Citrângulo Tortelli Junior[1,2] and Roger Chammas[1,2]

*Address all correspondence to: guilherme@lim24.fm.usp.br

*Address all correspondence to: rchammas@usp.br

1 Department of Radiology and Oncology, School of Medicine, University of São Paulo, Brazil

2 Center of Translational Research in Oncology, São Paulo State Cancer Institute (ICESP), São Paulo, Brazil

3 Department of Ethical and Legal Medicine, School of Medicine, University of São Paulo, Brazil

References

[1] Jhappan C, Noonan FP, Merlino G. Ultraviolet radiation and cutaneous malignant melanoma. Oncogene 2003; 22:3099-112.

[2] Costa RM, Chiganças V, Galhardo R da S, Carvalho H, Menck CF. The eukaryotic nucleotide excision repair pathway. Biochimie 2003;85(11):1083-99.

[3] Kadekaro AL, Kavanagh RJ, Wakamatsu K, Ito S, Pipitone MA, Abdel-Malek ZA. Cutaneous photobiology. The melanocyte vs. the sun: who will win the final round? Pigment Cell Res 2003; 16:434-47.

[4] Brash DE, Ziegler A, Jonason AS, Simon JA, Kunala S, Leffell DJ. Sunlight and sunburn in human skin cancer: p53, apoptosis, and tumor promotion. J Investig Dermatol Symp Proc 1996; 1:136-42.

[5] You YH, Lee DH, Yoon JH, Nakajima S, Yasui A, Pfeifer GP. Cyclobutane pyrimidine dimers are responsible for the vast majority of mutations induced by UVB irradiation in mammalian cells. J Biol Chem 2001; 276:44688-94.

[6] Cleaver JE, Crowley E. UV damage, DNA repair and skin carcinogenesis. Front Biosci 2002; 7:1024-43.

[7] Sander CS, Chang H, Hamm F, Elsner P, Thiele JJ. Role of oxidative stress and the antioxidant network in cutaneous carcinogenesis. Int J Dermatol 2004; 43:326-35.

[8] Nelemans PJ, Groenendal H, Kiemeney LA, Rampen FH, Ruiter DJ, Verbeek AL. Effect of intermittent exposure to sunlight on melanoma risk among indoor workers and sun-sensitive individuals. Environ Health Perspect 1993; 101:252-5.

[9] Weinstock MA, Colditz GA, Willett WC, Stampfer MJ, Bronstein BR, Mihm MC Jr, Speizer FE. Nonfamilial cutaneous melanoma incidence in women associated with sun exposure before 20 years of age. Pediatrics 1989; 84:199-204.

[10] Elwood JM. Melanoma and sun exposure: contrasts between intermittent and chronic exposure. World J Surg 1992; 16:157-65.

[11] Luiz OC, Gianini RJ, Gonçalves FT, Francisco G, Festa-Neto C, Sanches JA, et al. Ethnicity and cutaneous melanoma in the city of Sao Paulo, Brazil: a case-control study. PLoS One 2012;7(4):e36348.

[12] Law MH, Macgregor S, Hayward NK. Melanoma genetics: recent findings take us beyond well-traveled pathways. J Invest Dermatol 2012;132(7):1763-74.

[13] Eskandarpour M, Hashemi J, Kanter L, Ringborg U, Platz A, Hansson J. Frequency of UV-inducible NRAS mutations in melanomas of patients with germline CDKN2A mutations. J Natl Cancer Inst 2003;95(11):790-8.

[14] Mann GJ, Pupo GM, Campain AE, Carter CD, Schramm SJ, Pianova S, et al. BRAF Mutation, NRAS Mutation, and the Absence of an Immune-Related Expressed Gene Profile Predict Poor Outcome in Patients with Stage III Melanoma. J Invest Dermatol 2012 Aug 30. doi: 10.1038/jid.2012.283.

[15] Birck A, Ahrenkiel V, Zeuthen J, Hou-Jensen K, Guldberg P. Mutation and allelic loss of the PTEN/MMAC1 gene in primary and metastatic melanoma biopsies. J Invest Dermatol 2000;114(2):277-80.

[16] Giglia-Mari G, Sarasin A. TP53 mutations in human skin cancers. Hum Mutat 2003;21(3):217-28.

[17] Curtin JA, Fridlyand J, Kageshita T, Patel HN, Busam KJ, Kutzner H, et al. Distinct sets of genetic alterations in melanoma. N Engl J Med 2005;353(20):2135-47.

[18] Greenman C, Stephens P, Smith R, Dalgliesh GL, Hunter C, Bignell G, et al. Patterns of somatic mutation in human cancer genomes. Nature 2007;446(7132):153-8.

[19] Pleasance ED, Cheetham RK, Stephens PJ, McBride DJ, Humphray SJ, Greenman CD, et al. A comprehensive catalogue of somatic mutations from a human cancer genome. Nature 2010;463(7278):191-6.

[20] Sood AK, Saxena R, Groth J, Desouki MM, Cheewakriangkrai C, Rodabaugh KJ, et al. Expression characteristics of prostate-derived Ets factor support a role in breast and prostate cancer progression. Hum Pathol 2007;38(11):1628-38.

[21] Liang C, Feng P, Ku B, Dotan I, Canaani D, Oh BH, Jung JU. Autophagic and tumour suppressor activity of a novel Beclin1-binding protein UVRAG. Nat Cell Biol 2006;8(7): 688-99.

[22] Berger MF, Hodis E, Heffernan TP, Deribe YL, Lawrence MS, Protopopov A, et al. Melanoma genome sequencing reveals frequent PREX2 mutations. Nature 2012;485(7399):502-6.

[23] Fine B, Hodakoski C, Koujak S, Su T, Saal LH, Maurer M, et al. Activation of the PI3K pathway in cancer through inhibition of PTEN by exchange factor P-REX2a. Science 2009;325(5945):1261-5.

[24] Turajlic S, Furney SJ, Lambros MB, Mitsopoulos C, Kozarewa I, Geyer FC, et al. Whole genome sequencing of matched primary and metastatic acral melanomas. Genome Res 2012;22(2):196-207.

[25] Nikolaev SI, Rimoldi D, Iseli C, Valsesia A, Robyr D, Gehrig C, et al. Exome sequencing identifies recurrent somatic MAP2K1 and MAP2K2 mutations in melanoma. Nat Genet 2011;44(2):133-9.

[26] Stark MS, Woods SL, Gartside MG, Bonazzi VF, Dutton-Regester K, Aoude LG, et al. Frequent somatic mutations in MAP3K5 and MAP3K9 in metastatic melanoma identified by exome sequencing. Nat Genet 2011;44(2):165-9.

[27] Krauthammer M, Kong Y, Ha BH, Evans P, Bacchiocchi A, McCusker JP, et al. Exome sequencing identifies recurrent somatic RAC1 mutations in melanoma. Nat Genet 2012;44(9):1006-14. doi: 10.1038/ng.2359.

[28] Hodis E, Watson IR, Kryukov GV, Arold ST, Imielinski M, Theurillat JP, et al. A landscape of driver mutations in melanoma. Cell 2012;150(2):251-63.

[29] Hansson J. Familial cutaneous melanoma. Adv Exp Med Biol 2010;685:134-45.

[30] Hayward NK. Genetics of melanoma predisposition. Oncogene 2003;22(20):3053-62.

[31] Maubec E, Chaudru V, Mohamdi H, Blondel C, Margaritte-Jeannin P, Forget S, et al. Familial melanoma: Clinical factors associated with germline CDKN2A mutations according to the number of patients affected by melanoma in a family. J Am Acad Dermatol 2012.

[32] Bishop DT, Demenais F, Goldstein AM, Bergman W, Bishop JN, Bressac-de Paillerets B, et al. Geographical variation in the penetrance of CDKN2A mutations for melanoma. J Natl Cancer Inst 2002;94(12):894-903.

[33] Box NF, Duffy DL, Chen W, Stark M, Martin NG, et al. MC1R genotype modifies risk of melanoma in families segregating CDKN2A mutations. Am J Hum Genet 2001;69(4): 765-73.

[34] Ward KA, Lazovich D, Hordinsky MK. Germline melanoma susceptibility and prognostic genes: A review of the literature. J Am Acad Dermatol 2012.

[35] Goldstein AM, Struewing JP, Chidambaram A, Fraser MC, Tucker MA. Genotype-phenotype relationships in U.S. melanoma-prone families with CDKN2A and CDK4 mutations. J Natl Cancer Inst 2000;92(12):1006-10.

[36] Gillanders E, Juo SH, Holland EA, Jones M, Nancarrow D, Freas-Lutz D, et al. Localization of a novel melanoma susceptibility locus to 1p22. Am J Hum Genet 2003;73(2): 301-13.

[37] Walker GJ, Indsto JO, Sood R, Faruque MU, Hu P, Pollock PM, et al. Deletion mapping suggests that the 1p22 melanoma susceptibility gene is a tumor suppressor localized to a 9-Mb interval. Genes Chromosomes Cancer 2004;41(1):56-64.

[38] de Snoo FA, Hayward NK. Cutaneous melanoma susceptibility and progression genes. Cancer Lett 2005;230(2):153-86.

[39] Harding RM, Healy E, Ray AJ, Ellis NS, Flanagan N, Todd C, et al. Evidence for variable selective pressures at MC1R. Am J Hum Genet 2000;66(4):1351-61.

[40] Valverde P, Healy E, Jackson I, Rees JL, Thody AJ. Variants of the melanocyte-stimulating hormone receptor gene are associated with red hair and fair skin in humans. Nat Genet 1995;11(3):328-30.

[41] Valverde P, Healy E, Sikkink S, Haldane F, Thody AJ, Carothers A, et al. The Asp84Glu variant of the melanocortin 1 receptor (MC1R) is associated with melanoma. Hum Mol Genet 1996;5(10):1663-6.

[42] Ichii-Jones F, Lear JT, Heagerty AH, Smith AG, Hutchinson PE, Osborne J, et al. Susceptibility to melanoma: influence of skin type and polymorphism in the melanocyte stimulating hormone receptor gene. J Invest Dermatol 1998;111(2):218-21.

[43] Palmer JS, Duffy DL, Box NF, Aitken JF, O'Gorman LE, Green AC, et al. Melanocortin-1 receptor polymorphisms and risk of melanoma: is the association explained solely by pigmentation phenotype? Am J Hum Genet 2000;66(1):176-86.

[44] Kennedy C, ter Huurne J, Berkhout M, Gruis N, Bastiaens M, Bergman W, et al. Melanocortin 1 receptor (MC1R) gene variants are associated with an increased risk for cutaneous melanoma which is largely independent of skin type and hair color. J Invest Dermatol 2001;117(2):294-300.

[45] Williams PF, Olsen CM, Hayward NK, Whiteman DC. Melanocortin 1 receptor and risk of cutaneous melanoma: a meta-analysis and estimates of population burden. Int J Cancer 2011;129(7):1730-40.

[46] Smith R, Healy E, Siddiqui S, Flanagan N, Steijlen PM, Rosdahl I, et al. Melanocortin 1 receptor variants in an Irish population. J Invest Dermatol 1998;111(1):119-22.

[47] Buscà R, Ballotti R. Cyclic AMP a key messenger in the regulation of skin pigmentation. Pigment Cell Res. 2000;13(2):60-9.

[48] Law MH, Macgregor S, Hayward NK. Melanoma genetics: recent findings take us beyond well-traveled pathways. J Invest Dermatol. 2012;132(7):1763-74.

[49] Cheli Y, Ohanna M, Ballotti R, Bertolotto C. Fifteen-year quest for microphthalmia-associated transcription factor target genes. Pigment Cell Melanoma Res 2010;23(1): 27-40.

[50] Yokoyama S, Woods SL, Boyle GM, Aoude LG, MacGregor S, Zismann V, et al. A novel recurrent mutation in MITF predisposes to familial and sporadic melanoma. Nature 2011;480(7375):99-103.

[51] Bertolotto C, Lesueur F, Giuliano S, Strub T, de Lichy M, Bille K, et al. A SUMOylation-defective MITF Germline Mutation Predisposes to Melanoma and Renal Carcinoma. Nature 2011;480(7375):94-98.

[52] Sulem P, Gudbjartsson DF, Stacey SN, Helgason A, Rafnar T, et al. Two newly identified genetic determinants of pigmentation in Europeans. Nat Genet 2008;40(7):835-7.

[53] Meng S, Zhang M, Liang L, Han J. Current opportunities and challenges: genome-wide association studies on pigmentation and skin cancer. Pigment Cell Melanoma Res 2012;25(5):612-7.

[54] Fernandez LP, Milne RL, Pita G, Avilés JA, Lázaro P, Benítez J, et al. SLC45A2: a novel malignant melanoma-associated gene. Hum Mutat 2008;29(9):1161-7.

[55] Guedj M, Bourillon A, Combadières C, Rodero M, Dieudé P, Descamps V, et al. Variants of the MATP/SLC45A2 gene are protective for melanoma in the French population. Hum Mutat 2008;29(9):1154-60.

[56] Newton JM, Cohen-Barak O, Hagiwara N, Gardner JM, Davisson MT, King RA, et al. Mutations in the human orthologue of the mouse underwhite gene (uw) underlie a new form of oculocutaneous albinism, OCA4. Am J Hum Genet 2001;69(5):981-8.

[57] Ibarrola-Villava M, Hu HH, Guedj M, Fernandez LP, Descamps V, Basset-Seguin N, et al. MC1R, SLC45A2 and TYR genetic variants involved in melanoma susceptibility in Southern European populations: Results from a Meta-analysis. Eur J Cancer 2012;48(14):2183-91.

[58] Graf J, Hodgson R, van Daal A. Single nucleotide polymorphisms in the MATP gene are associated with normal human pigmentation variation. Hum Mutat 2005;25(3): 278-84.

[59] Suzuki I, Tada A, Ollmann MM, Barsh GS, Im S, Lamoreux ML, et al. Agouti signaling protein inhibits melanogenesis and the response of human melanocytes to alpha-melanotropin. J Invest Dermatol 1997;108(6):838-42.

[60] Scherer D, Rachakonda PS, Angelini S, Mehnert F, Sucker A, Egberts F, et al. Association between the germline MC1R variants and somatic BRAF/NRAS mutations in melanoma tumors. J Invest Dermatol. 2010 Dec;130(12):2844-8.

[61] Gudbjartsson DF, Sulem P, Stacey SN, Goldstein AM, Rafnar T, Sigurgeirsson B, et al., ASIP and TYR pigmentation variants associate with cutaneous melanoma and basal cell carcinoma. Nat Genet 2008;40(7):886-91.

[62] Nan H, Kraft P, Hunter DJ, Han J. Genetic variants in pigmentation genes, pigmentary phenotypes, and risk of skin cancer in Caucasians. Int J Cancer 2009;125(4):909-17.

[63] Maccioni L, Rachakonda PS, Scherer D, Bermejo JL, Planelles D, Requena C, et al. Variants at chromosome 20 (ASIP locus) and melanoma risk. Int J Cancer 2012. doi: 10.1002/ijc.27648.

[64] Brown KM, Macgregor S, Montgomery GW, Craig DW, Zhao ZZ, Iyadurai K, et al. Common sequence variants on 20q11.22 confer melanoma susceptibility. Nat Genet 2008;40(7):838-40.

[65] Ancans J, Tobin DJ, Hoogduijn MJ, Smit NP, Wakamatsu K, Thody AJ. Melanosomal pH controls rate of melanogenesis, eumelanin/phaeomelanin ratio and melanosome maturation in melanocytes and melanoma cells. Exp Cell Res 2001;268(1):26-35.

[66] Bishop DT, Demenais F, Iles MM, Harland M, Taylor JC, Corda E, et al. Genome-wide association study identifies three loci associated with melanoma risk. Nat Genet 2009;41(8):920-5.

[67] Chatzinasiou F, Lill CM, Kypreou K, Stefanaki I, Nicolaou V, Spyrou G, et al. Comprehensive field synopsis and systematic meta-analyses of genetic association studies in cutaneous melanoma. J Natl Cancer Inst 2011;103(16):1227-35.

[68] Pho LN, Leachman SA. Genetics of pigmentation and melanoma predisposition. G Ital Dermatol Venereol 2010;145(1):37-45.

[69] Schuch AP, Menck CF. The genotoxic effects of DNA lesions induced by artificial UV-radiation and sunlight. J Photochem Photobiol B 2010;99(3):111-6.

[70] Mocellin S, Verdi D, Nitti D. DNA repair gene polymorphisms and risk of cutaneous melanoma: a systematic review and meta-analysis. Carcinogenesis 2009;30(10):1735-43.

[71] Gonçalves FT, Francisco G, de Souza SP, Luiz OC, Festa-Neto C, Sanches JA, et al., European ancestry and polymorphisms in DNA repair genes modify the risk of melanoma: a case-control study in a high UV index region in Brazil. J Dermatol Sci 2011;64(1):59-66.

[72] Figl A, Scherer D, Nagore E, Bermejo JL, Botella-Estrada R, Gast A, et al. Single-nucleotide polymorphisms in DNA-repair genes and cutaneous melanoma. Mutat Res 2010;702(1):8-16.

[73] Winsey SL, Haldar NA, Marsh HP, Bunce M, Marshall SE, Harris AL, et al. A variant within the DNA repair gene XRCC3 is associated with the development of melanoma skin cancer. Cancer Res 2000;60(20):5612-6.

[74] Gu F, Qureshi AA, Kraft P, Guo Q, Hunter DJ, Han J. Polymorphisms in genes involved in DNA repair, cell growth, oxidative stress and inflammatory response, and melanoma risk. Br J Dermatol 2009;161(1):209-12.

[75] Govindarajan B, Bai X, Cohen C, Zhong H, Kilroy S, Louis G, et al. Malignant transformation of melanocytes to melanoma by constitutive activation of mitogen-activated protein kinase kinase (MAPKK) signaling. J Biol Chem 2003;278(11):9790-9795.

[76] Downward J. Targeting RAS signalling pathways in cancer therapy. Nat Rev Cancer 2003;3(1):11-22.

[77] Brose MS, Volpe P, Feldman M, Kumar M, Rishi I, Gerrero R, et al. BRAF and RAS mutations in human lung cancer and melanoma. Cancer Res 2002;62(23):6997-7000.

[78] Dhillon AS, Hagan S, Rath O, Kolch W. MAP kinase signalling pathways in cancer. Oncogene 2007;26(22):3279-90.

[79] Beeram M, Patnaik A, Rowinsky EK. Regulation of c-Raf-1: therapeutic implications. Clin Adv Hematol Oncol 2003;1:476–481.

[80] Davies H, Bignell GR, Cox C, Stephens P, Edkins S, Clegg S, et al., Mutations of the BRAF gene in human cancer. Nature 2002;417:949–954.

[81] R. Kumar, S. Angelini, K. Hemminki, Activating BRAF and N-Ras mutations in sporadic primary melanomas: an inverse association with allelic loss on chromosome 9, Oncogene 22 2003 9217–9224.

[82] Singh S, Davis R, Alamanda V, Pireddu R, Pernazza D, Sebti S, et al. Rb-Raf-1 interaction disruptor RRD-251 induces apoptosis in metastatic melanoma cells and synergizes with dacarbazine. Mol Cancer Ther 2010;9(12):3330-41.

[83] Fisher R, Larkin J. Vemurafenib: a new treatment for BRAF-V600 mutated advanced melanoma. Cancer Manag Res 2012;4:243-52.

[84] Johannessen CM, Boehm JS. COT drives resistance to RAF inhibition through MAP kinase pathway reactivation. Nature 2010;468(7326):968-72.

[85] Nazarian R, Shi H. Melanomas acquire resistance to B-RAF(V600E) inhibition by RTK or N-RAS upregulation. Nature 2010;468(7326):973-7.

[86] Yadav V, Zhang X. Reactivation of Mitogen-activated Protein Kinase (MAPK) Pathway by FGF Receptor 3 (FGFR3)/Ras Mediates Resistance to Vemurafenib in Human B-RAF V600E Mutant Melanoma. J Biol Chem 2012;287(33):28087-98.

[87] Govindarajan B, Sligh JE, Vincent BJ, Li M, Canter JA, Nickoloff BJ, et al. Overexpression of Akt converts radial growth melanoma to vertical growth melanoma. J Clin Invest 2007;117(3):719-29.

[88] Bogenrieder T, Herlyn M. The molecular pathology of cutaneous melanoma. Cancer Biomark 2010;9(1-6):267-86.

[89] Shull AY, Latham-Schwark A, Ramasamy P, Leskoske K, Oroian D, Birtwistle MR, et al., Novel Somatic Mutations to PI3K Pathway Genes in Metastatic Melanoma. PLoS One 2012;7(8):e43369.

[90] Wang Y, Digiovanna JJ, Stern JB, Hornyak TJ, Raffeld M, Khan SG, et al. Evidence of ultraviolet type mutations in xeroderma pigmentosum melanomas. Proc Natl Acad Sci U S A 2009;106(15):6279-84.

[91] Weeraratna AT. A Wnt-er wonderland--the complexity of Wnt signaling in melanoma. Cancer Metastasis Rev 2005;24(2):237-50.

[92] Bittner M, Meltzer P. Molecular classification of cutaneous malignant melanoma by gene expression profiling. Nature 2000;406(6795):536-40.

[93] Flaherty KT, Fisher DE. New Strategies in Metastatic Melanoma: Oncogene-Defined Taxonomy Leads to Therapeutic Advances. Clinical Cancer Research 2011;17(15): 4922-4928.

[94] Bhoumik A, Lopez-Bergami P, Ronai Z. ATF2 on the Double—Activating Transcription Factor and DNA Damage Response Protein. Pigment Cell Research 2007;20(6):498-506.

[95] Hai T, Curran T. Cross-Family Dimerization of Transcription Factors Fos/Jun and ATF/ CREB Alters DNA Binding Specificity. Proceedings of the National Academy of Sciences of the United States of America 1991;88(9):3720-3724.

[96] Bhoumik A, Ronai Z. ATF2: A Transcription Factor that Elicits Oncogenic or Tumor Suppressor Activities. Cell Cycle 2008;7(15):2341-2345.

[97] Ronai ZA, Weinstein IB. Identification of Ultraviolet-Inducible Proteins that Bind to a TGACAACA Sequence in the Polyoma Virus Regulatory Region. Cancer Research 1990;50(17):5374-5381.

[98] Rutberg SE, Goldstein IM, Yang YM, Stackpole CE ,Ronai Z. Expression and Transcriptional Activity of AP-1, CRE, and URE Binding Proteins in B16 Mouse Melanoma Subclones. Molecular Carcinogenesis 1994;10(2) 82-87.

[99] Ronai Z, Yang Y, Fuchs SY, Adler V, Sardana M, Herlyn M. ATF2 Confers Radiation Resistance To Human Melanoma Cells. Oncogene 1998;16(4) 523-531.

[100] Bhoumik A, Ivanov V, Ronai Z. Activating Transcription Factor 2-derived Peptides Alter Resistance of Human Tumor Cell Lines to Ultraviolet Irradiation and Chemical Treatment. Clinical Cancer Research 2001;7(2):331-342.

[101] Bhoumik A, Huang TG, Ivanov V, Gangi L, Qiao RF, Woo SL, et al. An ATF2-Derived Peptide Sensitizes Melanomas to Apoptosis and Inhibits their Growth and Metastasis. The Journal of Clinical Investigation 2002;110(5): 643-650.

[102] Recio JA, Merlino G. Hepatocyte Growth Factor/Scatter Factor Activates Proliferation in Melanoma Cells through p38 MAPK, ATF-2 and Cyclin D1. Oncogene 2002;21(7): 1000-1008.

[103] Huang Y, Minigh J, Miles S, Niles RM. Retinoic Acid Decreases ATF-2 Phosphorylation and Sensitizes Melanoma Cells to Taxol-Mediated Growth Inhibition. Journal of Molecular Signaling 2008;3(3):1-11.

[104] Bhoumik A, Gangi L, Ronai Z. Inhibition of Melanoma Growth and Metastasis by ATF2-Derived Peptides. Cancer Research 2004;64(22):8222–8230.

[105] Bhoumik A, Jones N, Ronai Z. Transcriptional Switch by Activating Transcription Factor 2-Derived Peptide Sensitizes Melanoma Cells to Apoptosis and Inhibits their Tumorigenicity. Proceedings of the National Academy of Sciences of the United States of America 2004 23;101(12):4222-4227.

[106] Berger AJ, Kluger HM, Li N, Kielhorn E, Halaban R, Ronai Z, Rimm DL. Subcellular Localization of Activating Transcription Factor 2 in Melanoma Specimens Predicts Patient Survival. Cancer Research 2003;63(23): 8103-8107.

[107] Bhoumik A, Gangi L, Ronai Z. Inhibition of Melanoma Growth and Metastasis by ATF2-Derived Peptides. Cancer Research 2004;64(22):8222-8230.

[108] Maekawa T, Shinagawa T, Sano Y, Sakuma T, Nomura S, Nagasaki K, et al. Reduced Levels of ATF-2 Predispose Mice to Mammary Tumors. Molecular and Cellular Biology 2007;27(5):1730-1744.

[109] Bhoumik A, Fichtman B, Derossi C, Breitwieser W, Kluger HM, Davis S, et al. Suppressor role of activating transcription factor 2 (ATF2) in skin cancer. Proceedings of the National Academy of Sciences of the United States of America 2008;105(5): 1674-1679.

[110] Steingrimsson E, Copeland NG, Jenkins NA. Melanocytes and the Microphthalmia Transcription Factor Network. Annual Review of Genetics 2004;38:365–411.

[111] Tachibana M, Perez-Jurado LA, Nakayama A, Hodgkinson CA, Li X, Schneider M, Miki T, et al. Cloning of MITF, The Human Homolog of the Mouse Microphthalmia Gene and Assignment to Chromosome 3p14.1-p12.3. Human Molecular Genetics 1994;3(4): 553-557.

[112] Fuse N, Yasumoto K, Takeda K, Amae S, Yoshizawa M, Udono T, Takahashi K, et al. Molecular Cloning of cDNA Encoding a Novel Microphthalmia-Associated Transcription Factor Isoform with a Distinct Amino-Terminus. Journal of Biochemistry 1999;126(6):1043-1051.

[113] Udono T, Yasumoto K, Takeda K, Amae S, Watanabe K, Saito H, et al. Structural Organization of the Human Microphthalmia-Associated Transcription Factor Gene

Containing Four Alternative Promoters. Biochimica et Biophysica Acta 2000;1491(1-3): 205-219.

[114] Lowings P, Yavuzer U, Goding CR. Positive and Negative Elements Regulate a Melanocyte-Specific Promoter. Molecular and Cellular Biology 1992;12(8):3653–3662.

[115] Yasumoto KI, Mahalingam H, Suzuki H, Yoshizawa M, Yokoyama K, Shibahara S. Transcriptional Activation of the Melanocyte-Specific Genes by the Human Homolog of the Mouse Microphthalmia Protein. Journal of Biochemistry 1995;118(5):874–881.

[116] Cheli Y, Ohanna M, Ballotti R, Bertolotto C. Fifteen-Year Quest for Microphthalmia-Associated Transcription Factor Target Genes. Pigment Cell and Melanoma Research 2010;23(1):27–40.

[117] Boeckmann B, Blatter MC, Famiglietti L, Hinz U, Lane L, Roechert B, Bairoch A. Protein Variety And Functional Diversity: Swiss-Prot Annotation in its Biological Context. Comptes Rendus Biologies 2005;328(10-11):882–899.

[118] Goding CR. Mitf from Neural Crest to Melanoma: Signal Transduction and Transcription in the Melanocyte Lineage. Genes and Development 2000;14(14):1712–1728.

[119] Hoek KS, Goding CR. Cancer Stem Cells versus Phenotype-Switching in Melanoma. Pigment Cell and Melanoma Research 2010;23(6):746–759.

[120] Bell RE, Levy C. The three M's: Melanoma, Microphthalmia-Associated Transcription Factor and microRNA. Pigment Cell and Melanoma Research 2011;24(6):1088-1106.

[121] Garraway LA, Widlund HR, Rubin MA, Getz G, Berger AJ, Ramaswamy S Beroukhim R, et al. Integrative Genomic Analyses Identify MITF as a Lineage Survival Oncogene Amplified in Malignant Melanoma. Nature 2005;436(7047):117–122.

[122] Carreira S, Goodall J, Denat L, Rodriguez M, Nuciforo P, Hoek KS Testori A, Larue L, Goding CR. Mitf Regulation of Dia1 Controls Melanoma Proliferation and Invasiveness. Genes and Development 2006;20(24):3426–3439.

[123] Goding CR. A Picture of Mitf in Melanoma Immortality. Oncogene 2011;30(20): 2304-2306.

[124] Wellbrock C, Marais R. Elevated Expression Of MITF Counteracts B-RAF-Stimulated Melanocyte And Melanoma Cell Proliferation. The Journal of Cell Biology 2005;170(5): 703–708.

[125] Wu M, Hemesath TJ, Takemoto CM, Horstmann MA, Wells AG, Price ER, Fisher DZ, Fisher DE. c-Kit Triggers Dual Phosphorylations, Which Couple Activation and Degradation of the Essential Melanocyte Factor Mi. Genes and Development 2000;14(3):301–312.

[126] Gray-Schopfer V, Wellbrock C, Marais R. Melanoma Biology and New Targeted Therapy. Nature 2007;22 445(7130):851-857.

[127] Shah M, Bhoumik A, Goel V, Dewing A, Breitwieser W, Kluger H, et al. A role for ATF2 in regulating MITF and melanoma development. PLoS Genetics 2010;6(12):e1001258.

[128] Akavia UD, Litvin O, Kim J, Sanchez-Garcia F, Kotliar D, Causton HC, Pochanard P, Mozes E, Garraway LA, Pe'er D. An integrated approach to uncover drivers of cancer. Cell 2010;143(6):1005-1017.

[129] Valsesia A, Rimoldi D, Martinet D, Ibberson M, Benaglio P, Quadroni M, et al. Network-guided analysis of genes with altered somatic copy number and gene expression reveals pathways commonly perturbed in metastatic melanoma. PLoS One 2011;6(4):e18369.

[130] Takeda K, Yasumoto K, Takada R, Takada S, Watanabe K, Udono T, et al. Induction of Melanocyte-Specific Microphthalmia-Associated Transcription Factor by Wnt-3a. The Journal of Biological Chemistry 2000;275(19):14013–14016.

[131] Omholt K, Platz A, Ringborg U, Hansson, J. Cytoplasmic and Nuclear Accumulation of b-Catenin is Rarely Caused by CTNNB1 Exon 3 Mutations in Cutaneous Malignant Melanoma. International Journal of Cancer 2001;92(6):839–842.

[132] Rimm DL, Caca K., Hu, G., Harrison, F. B. & Fearon, E. R. Frequent Nuclear/Cytoplasmic Localization of b-Catenin without Exon 3 Mutations in Malignant Melanoma. The American Journal of Pathology 1999;154(2):325–329.

[133] Bishop JN, Harland M, Randerson-Moor J, Bishop DT. Management of Familial Melanoma. The Lancet Oncology 2007;8(1):46-54.

[134] Flaherty KT, Fisher DE. New Strategies in Metastatic Melanoma: Oncogene-defined Taxonomy Leads to Therapeutic Advances. Clinical Cancer Research 2011;17(15): 4922-4928.

[135] Levy C, Khaled M, Fisher DE. MITF: Master Regulator Of Melanocyte Development And Melanoma Oncogene. Trends in Molecular Medicine 2006;12(9):406-414.

[136] Selzer E, Wacheck V, Lucas T, Heere-Ress E, Wu M, Weilbaecher KN, Schlegel W, Valent P, Wrba F, Pehamberger H, Fisher D, Jansen B. The Melanocyte-Specific Isoform of the Microphthalmia Transcription Factor Affects the Phenotype of Human Melanoma. Cancer Research 2002;62(7):2098-2103.

[137] Sancar A, Lindsey-Boltz LA, Unsal-Kaçmaz K, Linn S. Molecular mechanisms of mammalian DNA repair and the DNA damage checkpoints. Annu Rev Biochem 2004;73:39-85.

[138] DiGiovanna JJ, Kraemer KH. Shining a light on xeroderma pigmentosum. J Invest Dermatol 2012;132(3 Pt 2):785-96.

[139] Kauffmann A, Rosselli F, Lazar V, Winnepenninckx V, Mansuet-Lupo A, Dessen P, et al. High expression of DNA repair pathways is associated with metastasis in melanoma patients. Oncogene 2008;27(5):565-73.

[140] Wang L, Eastmond DA. Catalytic inhibitors of topoisomerase II are DNA-damaging agents: induction of chromosomal damage by merbarone and ICRF-187. Environ Mol Mutagen 2002;39(4):348-56.

[141] Eder JP Jr, Chan VT, Ng SW, Rizvi NA, Zacharoulis S, Teicher BA, et al. DNA topoisomerase II alpha expression is associated with alkylating agent resistance. Cancer Res 1995 Dec 15;55(24):6109-16.

[142] Sarasin A. An overview of the mechanisms of mutagenesis and carcinogenesis. Mutat Res 2003;544(2-3):99-106.

[143] Kao WH, Riker AI, Kushwaha DS, Ng K, Enkemann SA, Jove R, et al., Upregulation of Fanconi anemia DNA repair genes in melanoma compared with non-melanoma skin cancer. J Invest Dermatol 2011;131(10):2139-42.

[144] Jewell R, Conway C, Mitra A, Randerson-Moor J, Lobo S, Nsengimana J, et al. Patterns of expression of DNA repair genes and relapse from melanoma. Clin Cancer Res 2010;16(21):5211-21.

[145] Bondurand N, Pingault V, Goerich DE, Lemort N, Sock E, Le Caignec C, et al., Interaction among SOX10, PAX3 and MITF, three genes altered in Waardenburg syndrome. Hum Mol Genet 2000;9(13):1907-17.

[146] Lang D, Epstein JA. Sox10 and Pax3 physically interact to mediate activation of a conserved c-RET enhancer. Hum Mol Genet 2003;12(8):937-45.

[147] Medic S, Ziman M. PAX3 across the spectrum: from melanoblast to melanoma. Crit Rev Biochem Mol Biol 2009;44(2-3):85-97.

[148] Lang D, Lu MM, Huang L, Engleka KA, Zhang M, et al. Pax3 functions at a nodal point in melanocyte stem cell differentiation. Nature 2005;433(7028):884-7.

[149] Scholl FA, Kamarashev J, Murmann OV, Geertsen R, Dummer R, Schäfer BW. PAX3 is expressed in human melanomas and contributes to tumor cell survival. Cancer Res 2001;61(3):823-6.

[150] Plummer RS, Shea CR, Nelson M, Powell SK, Freeman DM, Dan CP, Lang D. PAX3 expression in primary melanomas and nevi. Mod Pathol 2008;21(5):525-30.

[151] He S, Yoon HS, Suh BJ, Eccles MR. PAX3 Is extensively expressed in benign and malignant tissues of the melanocytic lineage in humans. J Invest Dermatol 2010;130(5): 1465-8.

[152] Medic S, Ziman M. PAX3 expression in normal skin melanocytes and melanocytic lesions (naevi and melanomas). PLoS One 2010;5(4):e9977.

[153] Bernasconi M, Remppis A, Fredericks WJ, Rauscher FJ 3rd, Schäfer BW. Induction of apoptosis in rhabdomyosarcoma cells through down-regulation of PAX proteins. Proc Natl Acad Sci U S A 1996;93(23):13164-9.

[154] Borycki AG, Li J, Jin F, Emerson CP, Epstein JA. Pax3 functions in cell survival and in pax7 regulation. Development 1999;126(8):1665-74.

[155] Margue CM, Bernasconi M, Barr FG, Schäfer BW. Transcriptional modulation of the anti-apoptotic protein BCL-XL by the paired box transcription factors PAX3 and PAX3/FKHR. Oncogene 2000;19(25):2921-9.

[156] Kubic JD, Mascarenhas JB, Iizuka T, Wolfgeher D, Lang D. GSK-3 Promotes Cell Survival, Growth, and PAX3 Levels in Human Melanoma Cells. Mol Cancer Res 2012;10(8):1065-76.

[157] He SJ, Stevens G, Braithwaite AW, Eccles MR. Transfection of melanoma cells with antisense PAX3 oligonucleotides additively complements cisplatin-induced cytotoxicity. Mol Cancer Ther 2005;4(6):996-1003.

[158] Mascarenhas JB, Littlejohn EL, Wolsky RJ, Young KP, Nelson M, Salgia R, Lang D. PAX3 and SOX10 activate MET receptor expression in melanoma. Pigment Cell Melanoma Res 2010;23(2):225-37.

[159] Gentile A, D'Alessandro L, Lazzari L, Martinoglio B, Bertotti A, Mira A, et al. Met-driven invasive growth involves transcriptional regulation of Arhgap12. Oncogene 2008;27(42):5590-8.

[160] Cruz J, Reis-Filho JS, Silva P, Lopes JM. Expression of c-met tyrosine kinase receptor is biologically and prognostically relevant for primary cutaneous malignant melanomas. Oncology 2003;65(1):72-82.

[161] Puri N, Ahmed S, Janamanchi V, Tretiakova M, Zumba O, Krausz T, et al. c-Met is a potentially new therapeutic target for treatment of human melanoma. Clin Cancer Res 2007;13(7):2246-53.

[162] Medic S, Rizos H, Ziman M. Differential PAX3 functions in normal skin melanocytes and melanoma cells. Biochem Biophys Res Commun 2011;411(4):832-7.

[163] Yang G, Li Y, Nishimura EK, Xin H, Zhou A, Guo Y, et al. Inhibition of PAX3 by TGF-beta modulates melanocyte viability. Mol Cell 2008;32(4):554-63.

[164] Hocker T, Tsao H. Ultraviolet radiation and melanoma: a systematic review and analysis of reported sequence variants. Hum Mutat 2007;28(6):578-88.

[165] Ragnarsson-Olding BK, Karsberg S, Platz A, Ringborg UK. Mutations in the TP53 gene in human malignant melanomas derived from sun-exposed skin and unexposed mucosal membranes. Melanoma Res 2002;12(5):453-63.

[166] Yu H, McDaid R, Lee J, Possik P, Li L, Kumar SM, et al. The role of BRAF mutation and p53 inactivation during transformation of a subpopulation of primary human melanocytes. Am J Pathol 2009;174(6):2367-77.

[167] Terzian T, Torchia EC, Dai D, Robinson SE, Murao K, Stiegmann RA, et al. p53 prevents progression of nevi to melanoma predominantly through cell cycle regulation. Pigment Cell Melanoma Res 2010;23(6):781-94.

[168] Muthusamy V, Hobbs C, Nogueira C, Cordon-Cardo C, McKee PH, Chin L, Bosenberg MW, et al. Amplification of CDK4 and MDM2 in malignant melanoma. Genes Chromosomes Cancer 2006;45(5):447-54.

[169] Houben R, Hesbacher S, Schmid CP, Kauczok CS, Flohr U, Haferkamp S, et al. High-level expression of wild-type p53 in melanoma cells is frequently associated with inactivity in p53 reporter gene assays. PLoS One 2011;6(7):e22096.

[170] Haapajärvi T, Pitkänen K, Laiho M. Human melanoma cell line UV responses show independency of p53 function. Cell Growth Differ 1999;10(3):163-71.

[171] Bergamaschi D, Samuels Y, Sullivan A, Zvelebil M, Breyssens H, Bisso A, et al. iASPP preferentially binds p53 proline-rich region and modulates apoptotic function of codon 72-polymorphic p53. Nat Genet 2006;38(10):1133-41.

[172] Grob TJ, Novak U, Maisse C, Barcaroli D, Lüthi AU, Pirnia F, et al. Human delta Np73 regulates a dominant negative feedback loop for TAp73 and p53. Cell Death Differ 2001;8(12):1213-23.

[173] Homer C, Knight DA, Hananeia L, Sheard P, Risk J, Lasham A, et al. Y-box factor YB1 controls p53 apoptotic function. Oncogene 2005;24(56):8314-25.

[174] Nikolaev AY, Li M, Puskas N, Qin J, Gu W. Parc: a cytoplasmic anchor for p53. Cell 2003;112(1):29-40.

[175] Kastan MB, Berkovich E. p53: a two-faced cancer gene. Nat Cell Biol 2007;9(5):489-91.

[176] Avery-Kiejda KA, Bowden NA, Croft AJ, Scurr LL, Kairupan CF, Ashton KA, et al. P53 in human melanoma fails to regulate target genes associated with apoptosis and the cell cycle and may contribute to proliferation. BMC Cancer 2011;11:203.

[177] Verhaegen M, Checinska A, Riblett MB, Wang S, Soengas MS. E2F1-dependent oncogenic addiction of melanoma cells to MDM2. Oncogene 2012;31(7):828-41.

[178] Hersey P, Zhang XD. Adaptation to ER stress as a driver of malignancy and resistance to therapy in human melanoma. Pigment Cell Melanoma Res 2008;21(3):358-67.

[179] Griffith TS, Chin WA, Jackson GC, Lynch DH, Kubin MZ. Intracellular regulation of TRAIL-induced apoptosis in human melanoma cells. J Immunol 1998;161(6):2833-40.

[180] Jin L, Hu WL, Jiang CC, Wang JX, Han CC, Chu P, et al. MicroRNA-149*, a p53-responsive microRNA, functions as an oncogenic regulator in human melanoma. Proc Natl Acad Sci U S A 2011;108(38):15840-5.

[181] Ji Z, Njauw CN, Taylor M, Neel V, Flaherty KT, Tsao H. p53 rescue through HDM2 antagonism suppresses melanoma growth and potentiates MEK inhibition. J Invest Dermatol 2012;132(2):356-64.

[182] Glud M, Gniadecki R. MicroRNAs in the Pathogenesis of Malignant Melanoma. Journal of the European Academy of Dermatology and Venereology 2012, doi: 10.1111/j. 1468-3083.2012.04579.x.

[183] Kong YW, Ferland-McCollough D, Jackson TJ, Bushell M. MicroRNAs in Cancer Management. The Lancet Oncology 2012;13(6):249-258.

[184] Zhang L, Huang J, Yang N, Greshock J, Megraw MS, Giannakakis A, et al.. MicroRNAs Exhibit High Frequency Genomic Alterations in Human Cancer. Proceedings of the National Academy of Sciences of the United States of America 2006;103(24):9136-9141.

[185] Calin GA, Dumitru CD, Shimizu M, Bichi R, Zupo S, Noch E, et al. Frequent Deletions and Down-Regulation of Micro-RNA Genes miR-15 and miR-16 at 13q14 in Chronic Lymphocytic Leukemia. Proceedings of the National Academy of Sciences of the United States of America 2002;99(24):15524–15529.

[186] Johnson SM, Grosshans H, Shingara J, Byrom M, Jarvis R, Cheng A, et al. RAS is Regulated by the let-7 microRNA Family. Cell 2005;120(5):635–647.

[187] Mueller DW, Bosserhoff AK. Role of miRNAs in the Progression of Malignant Melanoma. British Journal of Cancer 2009;101(4):551–556.

[188] Bar-Eli M. Searching for the 'melano-miRs': miR-214 Drives Melanoma Metastasis. The EMBO Journal 2011;30(10):1880-1881.

[189] Bemis LT, Chen R, Amato CM, Classen EH, Robinson SE, Coffey DG, et al. MicrorRNA-137 Targets Microphtalmia-Associated Transcription Factor in Melanoma Cell Lines. Cancer Research 2008;68(5):1362–1368.

[190] Segura MF, Hanniford D, Menedez S, Reavie L, Zou X, Alvarez-Diaz S, et al. Aberrant miR-182 Expression Promote Melanoma Metastasis by Repressing FOX03 and Microphtalmia-Associated Transcription Factor. Proceedings of the National Academy of Sciences of the United States of America 2009;106(6):1814–1819.

[191] Haflidadóttir BS, Bergsteinsdóttir K, Praetorius C, Steingrímsson E. miR-148 regulates Mitf in Melanoma Cells. PLoS One 2010;5(7):e11574.

[192] Goswami S, Tarapore RS, Teslaa JJ, Grinblat Y, Setaluri V, Spiegelman VS. MicroRNA-340-mediated Degradation of Microphthalmia-Associated Transcription Factor mRNA is Inhibited by the Coding Region Determinant-Binding Protein. The Journal of Biological Chemistry 2010;285(27):20532-20540.

[193] Ozsolak F, Poling LL, Wang Z, Liu H, Liu XS, Roeder RG, et al. Chromatin structure analyses identify miRNA promoters. Genes and Development 2008;22(22):3172–3183.

[194] Levy C, Khaled M, Robinson KC, Veguilla RA, Chen PH, Yokoyama S, et al. Lineage-Specific Transcriptional Regulation of DICER by MITF in Melanocytes. Cell 2010;141(6): 994–1005.

[195] Glud M, Gniadecki R. MicroRNAs in the pathogenesis of malignant melanoma. J Eur Acad Dermatol Venereol. 2012 May 23. doi: 10.1111/j.1468-3083.2012.04579.x

[196] Chan E, Patel R, Nallur S, Ratner E, Bacchiocchi A, Hoyt K, et al. MicroRNA Signatures Differentiate Melanoma Subtypes. Cell Cycle 2011;10(11):1845–1852.

[197] Couts KL, Anderson EM, Gross MM, Sullivan K, Ahn NG. Oncogenic B-Raf Signaling in Melanoma Cells Controls a Network of microRNAs with Combinatorial Functions. Oncogene 2012, doi: 10.1038/onc.2012.209.

[198] Liu FJ, Wen T, Liu L. MicroRNAs as a Novel Cellular Senescence Regulator. Ageing Research Review 2012;11(1):41–50.

[199] Gorospe M, Abdelmohsen K. MicroRegulators Come of Age in Aenescence. Trends in Genetics 2011;27(6):233–241.

[200] Bueno MJ, Malumbres M. MicroRNAs and the Cell Cycle. Biochimica et Biophysica Acta 2011;1812(2):592–601.

[201] Tazawa H, Tsuchiya N, Izumiya M, Nakagama H. Tumor-suppressive miR-34a induces senescence-like growth arrest through modulation of the E2F pathway in human colon cancer cells. Proceedings of the National Academy of Sciences of the United States of America 2007;104(39):15472-15427.

[202] Dar AA, Majid S, de Semir D, Nosrati M, Bezrookove V, Kashani-Sabet M. miRNA-205 Suppresses Melanoma Cell Proliferation and Induces Senescence Via Regulation of E2F1 Protein. The Journal of Biological Chemistry 2011;286(19):16606-16614.

[203] Noguchi S, Mori T, Otsuka Y, Yamada N, Yasui Y, Iwasaki J, et al. Anti-oncogenic microRNA-203 induces senescence by targeting E2F3 protein in human melanoma cells. The Journal of Biological Chemistry 2012;287(15):11769-11777.

[204] Streicher KL, Zhu W, Lehmann KP, Georgantas RW, Morehouse CA, Brohawn P, et al. A novel oncogenic role for the miRNA-506-514 cluster in initiating melanocyte transformation and promoting melanoma growth. Oncogene 2012;31(12):1558-1570.

[205] Bonazzi VF, Stark MS, Hayward NK. MicroRNA Regulation of Melanoma Progression. Melanoma Research 2012;22(2):101-113.

[206] Felicetti F, Errico MC, Bottero L, Segnalini P, Stoppacciaro A, Biffoni M, et al. The Promyelocytic Leukemia Zinc Finger-microrna-221/-222 Pathway Controls Melanoma Progression Through Multiple Oncogenic Mechanisms. Cancer Research 2008;68(8): 2745-2754.

[207] Lujambio A, Ropero S, Ballestar E, Fraga MF, Cerrato C, Setién F, et al. Genetic Unmasking of an Epigenetically Silenced microRNA in Human Cancer Cells. Cancer Research 2007;67(4):1424–1429.

[208] Mazar J, Khaitan D, DeBlasio D, Zhong C, Govindarajan SS, Kopanathi S, et al.. Epigenetic Regulation of microRNA Genes and the Role of miR-34b in Cell Invasion and Motility in Human Melanoma. PLoS One 2011;6(9):e24922.

[209] Mazar J, DeBlasio D, Govindarajan SS, Zhang S, Perera RJ. Epigenetic Regulation of microRNA-375 and its Role in Melanoma Development in Humans. FEBS Letters 2011;585(15):2467-2476.

[210] Gaur A, Jewell DA, Liang Y, Ridzon D, Moore JH, Chen C, et al. Characterization of microRNA Expression Levels and Their Biological Correlates in Human Cancer Cell Lines. Cancer Research 2007;67(6):2456-2468.

[211] Mueller DW, Rehli M, Bosserhoff AK. miRNA Expression Profiling in Melanocytes and Melanoma Cell Lines Reveals miRNAs Associated with Formation and Progression of Malignant Melanoma. The Journal of Investigative Dermatology 2009;129(7) 1740–1751.

[212] Philippidou D, Schmitt M, Moser D, Margue C, Nazarov PV, Muller A, et al. Signatures of microRNAs and selected microRNA target genes in human melanoma. Cancer Research 2010;70(10):4163–4173.

[213] Stark MS, Tyagi S, Nancarrow DJ, Boyle GM, Cook AL, Whiteman DC, et al. Characterization of the Melanoma miRNAome by Deep Sequencing. PLoS One 2010;12(5):e9685.

[214] Segura MF, Belitskaya-Lévy I, Rose AE, Zakrzewski J, Gaziel A, Hanniford D, et al. Melanoma MicroRNA Signature Predicts Post-Recurrence Survival. Clinical Cancer Research 2010;16(5):1577-1586.

[215] Caramuta S, Egyházi S, Rodolfo M, Witten D, Hansson J, Larsson C, Lui WO. MicroRNA expression profiles associated with mutational status and survival in malignant melanoma. The Journal of Investigative Dermatology 2010;130(8):2062-2070.

[216] Xu Y, Brenn T, Brown ER, Doherty V, Melton DW. Differential expression of microRNAs during melanoma progression: miR-200c, miR-205 and miR-211 are downregulated in melanoma and act as tumour suppressors. Britsh Journal of Cancer 2012;106(3) 553-561.

[217] Penna E, Orso F, Cimino D, Tenaglia E, Lembo A, Quaglino E, et al. microRNA-214 Contributes to Melanoma Tumour Progression Through Suppression of TFAP2C. The EMBO Journal 2011;30(10):1990-2007.

[218] Chan E, Patel R, Nallur S, Ratner E, Bacchiocchi A, Hoyt K, et al. MicroRNA Signatures Differentiate Melanoma Subtypes. Cell Cycle 2011;10(11):1845-1852.

[219] Hanna JA, Hahn L, Agarwal S, Rimm DL. In Situ Measurement of miR-205 in Malignant Melanoma Tissue Supports its Role as a Tumor Suppressor microRNA. Laboratory Investigation 2012, doi: 10.1038/labinvest.2012.119.

Chapter 5

Diagnosis, Histopathologic and Genetic Classification of Uveal Melanoma

J.G.M. van Beek, A.E. Koopmans, R.M. Verdijk,
N.C. Naus, A. de Klein and E. Kilic

Additional information is available at the end of the chapter

http://dx.doi.org/10.5772/53631

1. Introduction

Uveal melanoma (UM) is the most common cause of primary eye cancer in the western world. During embryogenesis neural crest cells migrate to the neural tract where they develop into melanocytes. Melanomas of the uvea are derived from these melanocytes. UM may arise in the iris (5%), ciliary body (23%) or choroid (72%). Choroidal melanomas are the most common and usually display a discoid, dome-shaped or mushroom shaped growth pattern. Approximately 80% of the primary intraocular tumours are diagnosed as UM in patients above the age of 20 years, with a mean age of 60 years (Singh & Topham, 2003). Despite a shift towards more conservative eye treatments, survival has not improved during 1973 to 2008 (Singh et al, 2011). Growth of the primary tumour is related with histopathological features, as well as the genetic changes within these tumours. In this chapter we will not discuss iris melanoma, as this shows a different clinical and genetic behaviour, compared to ciliary body and choroidal melanoma. The clinical features, histopathological profile and genetic alterations of UM, as well as therapeutic options for primary tumours and metastases will be discussed.

2. Epidemiology

The incidence of UM ranges from 4.3 to 10.9 per million (Singh et al, 2009). For the past fifty years, the incidence has remained stable, unlike trends indicating a higher incidence of cutaneous melanoma. The incidence in Europe and United States is comparable to that in Australia and New Zealand. In Europe, a lower incidence is reported in Spain and the south of

Italy, about 2 per million, whereas registries in France, the Netherlands, Switzerland and Germany has intermediate values around 4 to 5 per million. The United Kingdom registered over 6 per million, and the highest incidence is up to > 8 per million in Norway and Denmark (Virgili et al, 2007).

3. Predisposing factors

Men and women with UM are more or less affected equally (Damato & Coupland, 2012; Singh et al, 2011). Iris melanoma is more common in women than in men (Damato & Coupland, 2012). Several phenotypes, like blue or grey eyes and fair skin have been suggested to predispose for UM (Schmidt-Pokrzywniak et al, 2009). This might explain why Caucasians are approximately 150 times more frequently affected than Africans (Margo et al, 1998; Singh et al, 2005a). In Asians UM is less common (Biswas et al, 2002).

From all the parts of the uvea the iris is most exposed to ultraviolet light, because of filtering effects of the lens and retinal pigment epithelium (RPE), the choroid receives less light (Singh et al, 2004). Although several epidemiologic and case control studies have been performed to investigate the influence of sunlight exposure on UM, the results are not conclusive (Guenel et al, 2001; Holly et al, 1990; Pane & Hirst, 2000; Shah et al, 2005; Vajdic et al, 2002). UM may occur as a part of familial syndromes, like xeroderma pigmentosa, Li-Fraumeni syndrome and familial breast and ovarian cancer. Of all UM 0.6% is considered to be familial (Singh et al, 1996). In a retrospective study 0.0017% of the primary UM patients were in the setting of familial atypical mole and melanoma syndrome (FAMM). These patients were relatively young with a mean age of 40 years (Singh et al, 1995). Furthermore, an association of neurofibromatosis type 1 and UM has been suggested, since both are of neural crest origin, however this association remains unclear (Honavar et al, 2000). Ocular and oculodermal melanocytosis (Nevus of Ota), dysplastic nevi and cutaneous melanoma are correlated with an increased risk of UM development (Carreno et al, 2012; Gonder et al, 1982; Hammer et al, 1995; Richtig et al, 2004; Singh et al, 1998; Toth-Molnar et al, 2000; van Hees et al, 1994). Additionally, in UM patients ocular and oculodermal melanocytosis are about 35 to 70 times more common (Carreno et al, 2012; Singh et al, 1998).

4. Clinical presentation

Depending on de location and size of the tumour, patients can present with visual complaints. Most UMs are detected during a routine ophthalmic examination. Approximately 30% of the patients have no symptoms at time of diagnosis, and if there are any complaints these consist mostly of blurred vision, floaters, photopsias and visual field loss (Damato, 2010) (figure 1). Usually patients do not present with severe ocular pain, however, this can occur secondary to inflammation or neovascular glaucoma.

http://dx.doi.org/10.5772/53631

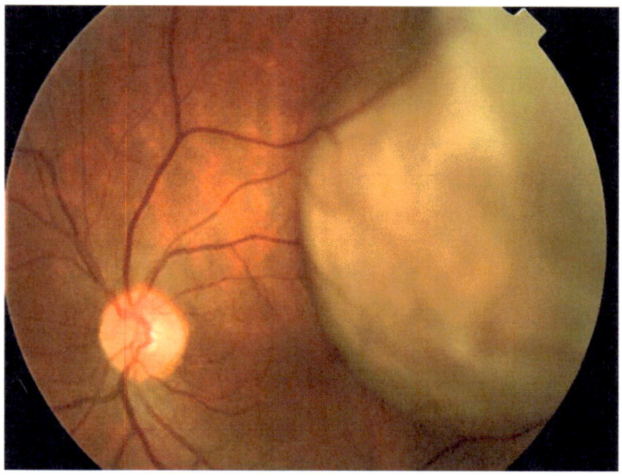

Figure 1. A large amelanotic uveal melanoma leads to a visual field defect.

5. Diagnosis

Diagnosis of UM is based on a combination of clinical examination with slit lamp biomicroscopy, indirect ophthalmoscopy (figure 1, 2a, 3a) and ultrasonography (US) (figure 2b, 3b). Iris melanomas are readily detectable by slit lamp biomicroscopy, whereas ciliary body tumours are hidden behind the iris and can be visualized by US. Choroidal tumours, depending on their location, are diagnosed by dilated indirect ophthalmoscopy and US. In suspect cases of intravenous fluorescein angiography can be helpful in differentiating melanomas from other diagnoses. Also optical coherence tomography (OCT) and autofluorescence can provide additional information (Lavinsky et al, 2007; Shields et al, 2008). In selected cases, when in doubt, an intraocular biopsy is taken of the tumour.

Indirect ophthalmoscopy through a dilated pupil provides a correct diagnosis in more than 95% of the cases (Char et al, 1980). Accuracy of the right diagnosis is established to be over 99% by experienced clinicians with US, ophthalmoscopy, and fluorescein angiography and confirmed by histopathology (Collaborative Ocular Melanoma Study Group, 1990). The ability to differentiate melanoma from other lesions has improved over the last decades. When comparing studies of 1964 and 1973, in 19% of the enucleated patients with the clinical diagnosis melanoma no histopathological evidence of a melanoma was found (Ferry, 1964; Shields, 1973). The accuracy in diagnosing medium to small sized tumours is quite challenging. Nine percent of presumed melanomas are found to have another diagnosis by fine needle aspiration biopsy (Char & Miller, 1995). Most important is to minimise the delay in referring patients with melanoma to a specialised centre. It is reported that in 29% of the patients a melanoma is missed during the first visit by an ophthalmologist, and that 31.5% of the patients referred to an oncology centre with the diagnosis of melanoma actually had a mimicking lesion (Eskelin & Kivelä, 2002; Khan & Damato, 2007).

5.1. Characteristics

Melanoma are generally pigmented, but one fourth are relatively non-pigmented or amelanotic (figure 1). Melanoma can develop into two different directions: towards the vitreous and outwards, through the underlying sclera. Having broken through Bruch's membrane, into the vitreous, UMs achieve a characteristic shape, even pathognomonic, like a 'collar button' or 'mushroom'. Small melanomas can appear flat or dome shaped.

5.2. Clinical prognostic factor

Well-known clinical prognostic factors are age and location of the tumour. Older patients tend to have a worse prognosis (Shields et al, 2012). One study found that UMs were located predominantly posterior and temporal or had a preference for macular zone, while others found a more equal distribution of melanoma (Krohn et al, 2008; Li et al, 2000; Shields et al, 2009b). Patients with larger tumours, tumours that ruptured through Bruch membrane and in patients who have developed metastasis, the tumours were significantly more often located anterior to the equator (Krohn et al, 2008).

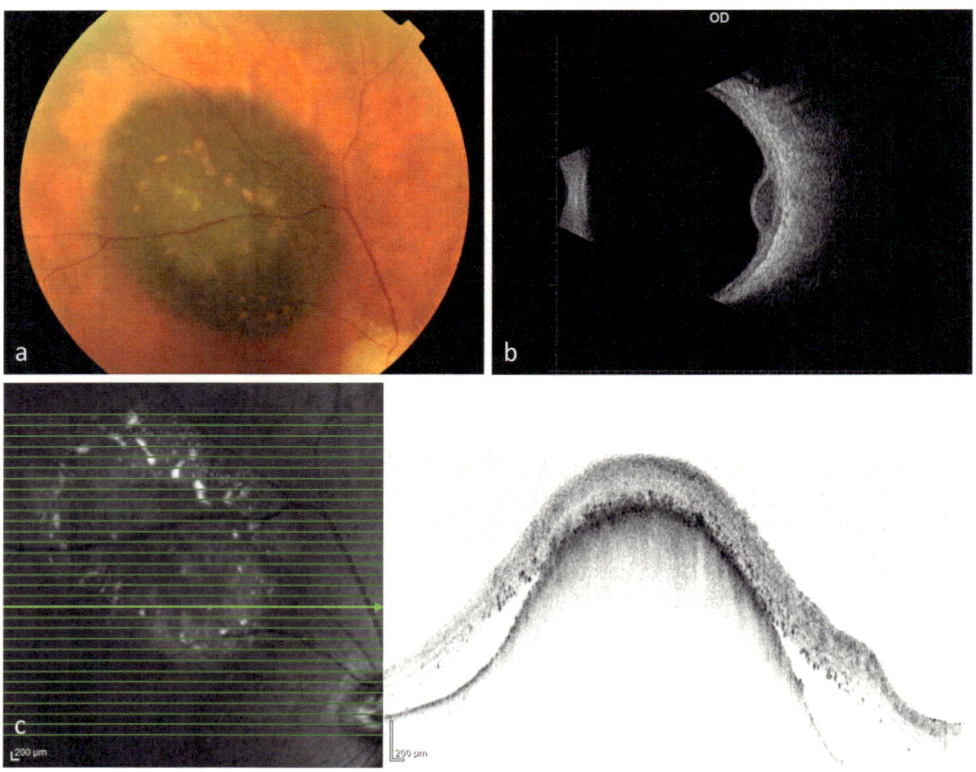

Figure 2. a: A dark pigmented uveal melanoma with orange pigment; 2b: On B-scan ultrasonography acoustic hollowing and choroidal excavation is present, 2c: Subretinal fluid and retinal pigment epithelial alterations are visible on optical coherence tomography scan at the top of the tumour.

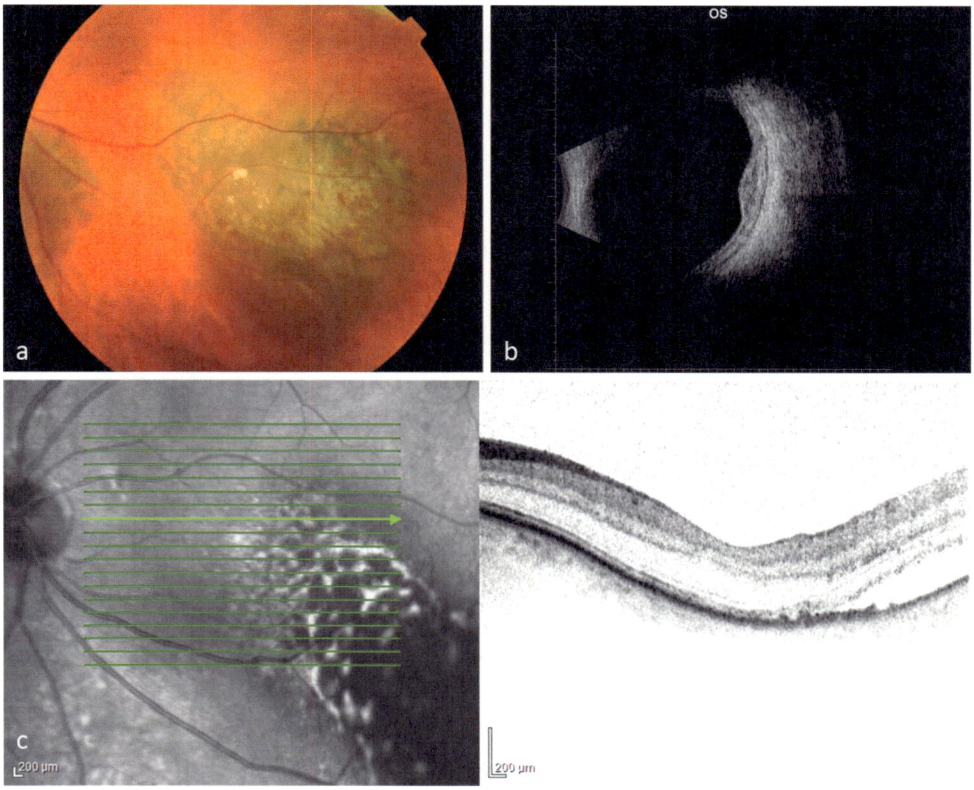

Figure 3. a: Pigmented uveal melanoma with orange pigment (lipofuscin); 3b: A homogeneous grey scale in the tumour and choroidal excavation on B-scan ultrasonography; 3c: Optical coherence tomography of the same tumour with subretinal fluid.

The most important clinical prognostic factor is tumour size, and is often used for selection of the treatment. There are several treatment options, which will be discussed later in this chapter. UM are subdivided into different categories depending on the apical size and diameter, however, many centres use their own definition. Most widely used definition is suggested by the COMS study. Small melanomas are 1.0 - 2.5 mm in apical height and > 5.0 mm in largest basal dimension (Collaborative Ocular Melanoma Study Group, 1997). Medium tumours are defined as tumours 2.5 to 10 mm in apical height and ≤ 16 mm in largest basal diameter. Large tumours are ≥ 2 mm in apical height and > 16 mm in maximal basal diameter, or a melanoma > 10 mm in apical height, regardless of the basal diameter (Collaborative Ocular Melanoma Study Group, 2003). One large study described that each increase in millimeter of tumour thickness increased the risk for metastasis by 5% (Shields et al, 2009b). The mortality rate for small (< 2 - 3 mm height), medium (3 - 8 mm height) and large (> 8 mm height) melanoma was 16%, 32% and 53% in 5 years, respectively, and has not changed in recent years (Diener-West et al, 1992). This supports the model of tumour doubling time of melanoma and its' related metastasis. The model suggests that micrometastasis already exist several years before diagnosis of the primary tumour (Eskelin et al, 2000). This emphasizes the importance of identifying small melanoma and reducing the risk of metastases.

5.3. Clinical predictive factors of small melanoma

In general, choroidal nevi have a less than 5 mm basal diameter and are minimal in height (< 2 mm), although several definitions of nevi have been proposed. Due to different examination methods and definitions, the prevalence of nevi is between 0.2% and 30% (Gass, 1977; Wilder, 1946). Overall in a Caucasian population the incidence is 6.5% (Sumich et al, 1998). Whenever, growth of a nevus is measured on US in a short time a transformation into a small melanoma is suspected. On the other hand benign nevi can also grow slowly. Mashayekhi *et al* observed in 31% of nevi a slight growth, without evidence of development into a melanoma over a mean follow up of 15 years (Mashayekhi et al, 2011). As described by Singh and co-workers, assuming that all melanoma result from nevi, 1 out of 8845 choroidal nevi can undergo malignant transformation into melanoma in the Caucasian population in the USA (Singh et al, 2005b). In Australia this is estimated 1 out of 4300 nevi (Sumich et al, 1998).

It is important to differentiate melanoma form other choroidal pathologies, such as choroidal nevi, by identifying indicators of potential malignancy which may differentiate nevi from small UM. Shields *et al* constructed a mnemonic "TFSOM", i.e. "to find small ocular melanoma" to assist in identifying small choroidal melanoma at risk for growth (Shields et al, 1995). The letters of the mnemonic indicate: Thickness > 2 mm, subretinal Fluid, Symptoms, Orange pigment and Margin to the optic disc. Tumours with no, one or more than two factors have 4%, 36% or > 45% chance of growth, respectively (Shields et al, 2000). A tumour with a thickness of more than 2 mm is considered suspect of being a melanoma rather than a nevus. Subretinal fluid is the strongest indicator of malignancy. Exudative retinal detachment, overlying or adjacent to the tumour, is associated with tumour growth (Augsburger et al, 1989). Presence of symptoms, as mentioned earlier or a change in symptoms is a risk factor for malignancy. Orange pigment is formed on melanomas of the posterior pole, although this can also be seen on the surface of presumed benign nevi and haemangioma. Orange pigment is an accumulation of lipofuscin within the RPE. In amelanotic tumours it appears brown-black of colour. Besides orange pigment as a risk factor, a tumour margin within 3 mm of the optic disc is also suspect for malignant potential (figure 4a).

Later "Using Helpful Hints Daily" was added to "TFSOM" mnemonic (Shields et al, 2009a). These features indicate a low acoustic profile or Ultrasound Hollowness, absence of a Halo around the tumour and absence of Drusen over the tumour. US hollowness is shown in 25% of nevi that transformed into melanoma, compared to the 4% with growth without US hollowness (Shields et al, 2009a). A halo around a tumour is a pigmented lesion with a surrounding depigmentation, as can also be noticed in dysplastic nevi. Drusen suggest a chronic lesion and usually indicate that the tumour is benign, however this is not conclusive.

http://dx.doi.org/10.5772/53631

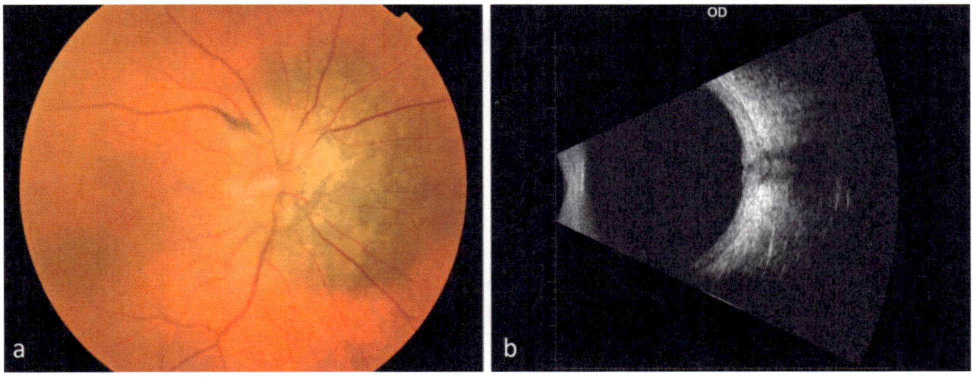

Figure 4. a: Peripapillary nevus, barely elevated, with margin located < 3 mm to the optic disc in the right eye of a 72 year-old man; 4b: High reflectivity on B-scan ultrasonography.

5.4. Ancillary testing

5.4.1. Ultrasonography

US is a non-invasive tool and helps to establish the diagnosis of UM, despite media opacities or whether the tumour is located far peripherally. UM shows characteristic low to medium internal reflectivity on A-scan. B-scan US is primarily used to plan therapy based on the first measurement, and to periodically measure tumour prominence (height) and basal diameter for follow-up. The B-scan can identify possible extraocular extension as an empty area behind the sclera. On B-scan US the internal structure of the tumour is typically seen as a relative homogeneous grey scale, although this pattern is not specifically diagnostic (figure 3b). At the base of the tumour an acoustically silent zone (called acoustic hollowing) is seen, as well as choroidal excavation and shadowing in the orbit (figure 2b). Eighty-eight percent of the UM show US hollowness or low acoustic reflectivity (Boldt et al, 2008). Choroidal excavation is not observed in all melanomas and varies from 42% to 70% (Coleman et al, 1974; Sobottka et al, 1998; Verbeek, 1985). US provides accurate measurements with an interobserver variability of 0.5 mm (Char et al, 1990).

5.4.2. Fluorescein angiography

The diagnostic value of fluorescein angiography in UM is limited. Fluorescein angiography does not show pathognomonic patterns and is especially helpful in differentiating lesions, which simulate melanoma. The pigmentation, size and effect on the RPE of the tumour influence the fluorescein angiogram. It is of little help in some medium to large melanomas that have an intrinsic tumour circulation. This 'double circulation' (simultaneous visualization of retinal and choroidal circulation) consists of late staining of the lesion and multiple pin-point leaks at the level of the RPE, which is evident in the early phase of the angiogram. Blockage of background fluorescence and late staining, when fluorescein leaks from the vessels can be seen on an angiogram as well (Atmaca et al, 1999). Characteristic signs are hypofluorescence in the early phase followed by diffuse hyperfluorescence and hyperfluorescent spots (due to changes in RPE). In the late phase the dye accumulates in the tumour tissue and hyperfluorescents (figure 5b). Hypofluorescent spots correspond with deposits of orange pigment on the surface of the tumour.

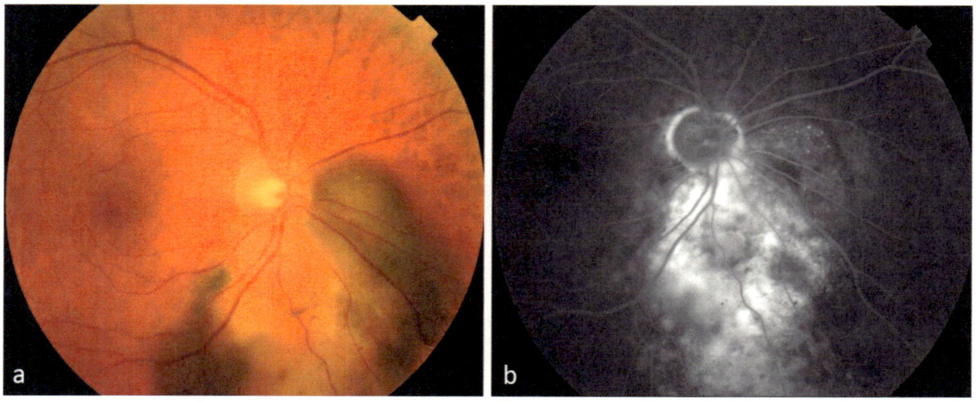

Figure 5. a: A partly pigmented and non-pigmented uveal melanoma; 5b: Fluorescein angiogram with blockage of the background and fluorescein leaking from the vessels.

5.4.3. Indocyanine green angiography

Indocyanine green angiography is designed to visualize the choroidal vessels and provides more information than fluorescein angiography. Whether an evident pattern can be seen on an angiogram depends on the pigmentation, thickness, disruption through Bruch's membrane and vascularisation of the tumour (Atmaca et al, 1999). More fluorescence is seen in less pigmented and larger tumours. The choroidal vasculature can be better visualised with indocyanine green than fluorescein. On indocyanine green late staining is observed, because of the leaking of indocyanine green in the extracellular space of the tumour (Frenkel et al, 2008; Guyer et al, 1993; Stanga et al, 2003).

5.4.4. Optical coherence tomography and fundus autofluorescence

OCT and fundus autofluorescence imaging have limited use in detecting changes in the choroid, however, both techniques are non-invasive and of help in identifying subtle changes in the RPE, retina and vitreoretinal interface. By means of an OCT subretinal fluid can be visualized and quantified, small tumours can be measured, whereas with fundus autofluorescence orange pigment can be shown. Spectral domain OCT can be useful in the detection of subretinal deposits, vitreous seeding and transretinal tumour extension (Heindl et al, 2009).

Although OCT itself is not useful in diagnosing uveal melanoma, it aids in differentiating other pigmented lesions from melanomas (Schaudig et al, 1998). For example, melanocytoma tend to have a high reflective signal anteriorly, corresponding with the nerve fibre layer, and an optical shadowing posteriorly (Muscat et al, 2001). In most choroidal nevi no charac-

http://dx.doi.org/10.5772/53631

teristic or subtle patterns of autofluorescence were observed (Lavinsky et al, 2007; Shields et al, 2008). Choroidal melanoma and related retinal and RPE changes, show different autofluorescence patterns, and secondary changes, such as subclinical retinal detachments associated with presence of small amounts of subretinal fluid can discriminate small choroidal melanoma and nevi at risk for growth (Muscat et al, 2004). Like some nevi UM show brighter hyperautofluorescence in overlying orange pigment, RPE detachment and subsequently decreased brightness in subretinal fluid and drusen (Shields et al, 2008) (figures 2c and 3c).

5.4.5. Magnetic resonance imaging and computed tomography

Magnetic resonance imaging (MRI) and computed tomography (CT) can be of additional value in the differential diagnosis of UM. On CT an UM appears as a hyperdense lesion with moderate contrast enhancement. Tumours thinner than 2 mm are not detectable on CT. Besides that, CT is less accurate than US in differentiating melanoma and is more expensive (Mafee et al, 1986; Peyster et al, 1985). For extrascleral extension CT is inferior to US (Scott et al, 1998). On the other hand, MRI seems more sensitive and more specific than US for detection of extraocular extension of UM (Hosten et al, 1997). A choroidal melanoma appears hyperintense on a T1 and hypointense on a T2 weighted scan. As this can also be the appearance of a melanocytoma, MRI is not specific for uveal melanoma. Due to the higher expenses of CT and MRI and the superiority of US, both techniques are not routinely used for diagnostic evaluation.

5.5. Differential diagnosis

About 54 different conditions are able to simulate UM. The most frequent diagnosis is choroidal nevus, accounting for 49% of the approximately 1739 presumed melanoma patients referred to a large tertiary Oncology Department in the USA (Shields et al, 2005b). The differentiation between small melanomas and choroidal nevi remains a clinical challenge. Clinical features that are more prevalent in *choroidal nevi* than in melanomas are drusen and RPE changes, whereas retinal detachment, choroidal neovascularisation or haemorrhagic retinal detachment can occur in both. On B-scan US, nevi have a high internal reflectivity (figure 4b). Also orange pigment and subretinal fluid, which are features of potential malignancy as mentioned previously, can be present in nevi. Ten percent of the nevi have orange pigment and 18% have subretinal fluid.

Congenital hypertrophy of the retinal pigment epithelium (CHRPE) has sharper edges than melanoma and usually sharply bordered nonpigmented areas (lacunae), or a depigmentated or pigmented halo within. The lesions might be slightly elevated and are black or grey of colour. CHRPE is a benign lesion and is typically located in the peripheral fundus. On the other hand, adenocarcinomas arising from a CHRPE have been reported (Shields et al, 2009e).

Optic disc melanocytoma is a heavily pigmented benign lesion with a fibrillated or feathery margin. Although it can occur anywhere in the uveal tract, the tumour is most often located unilateral and on or nearby the optic disc. Optic disc melanocytoma is a variant of melanocytic nevus. Most patients (75%) have no visual complaints, whereas patients with visual loss were related to neuroretinitis from tumour necrosis and secondary subretinal fluid of the fovea (Shields et al, 2006; Shields et al, 2004). In addition, visual field defects have been described (Meyer et al, 1999; Shields et al, 2006). Ocular melanocytosis is associated with melanocytoma in 8% of cases, and melanocytoma enlargement is noticed in 57% within 8 years (Lee et al, 2010) and 32% within 10 years (Shields et al, 2004). Although malignant transformation is extremely rare, it has been reported (Meyer et al, 1999; Shields et al, 2004).

Hyperplasia of the RPE is a common ocular finding, which is idiopathic or develops in response to trauma, inflammation, haemorrhage and retinal detachment. It is characterised as a black irregular usually small retinal lesion consisting of proliferated RPE cells. Intraretinal pigmented spicules can be seen, and when it manifests as a subretinal localized mass, a melanoma can be suspected.

Choroidal haemangioma is a benign tumour consisting of blood vessels with a typical red to orange colour. Some areas of increased pigmentation can be observed, which makes it difficult to differentiate from melanoma. On angiography typical early hyperfluorescence is shown and on US a characteristic high internal reflectivity is present.

Choroidal metastases are the most common intraocular malignancies. The prevalence of uveal metastases from all forms of carcinoma is between 2% and 9%, with a mean of 7% for breast cancer and 5% for lung cancer (Kanthan et al, 2007). The origin of choroidal metastases is predominantly breast cancer in woman and lung cancer in man. Less frequently patients are diagnosed with other primary tumours, such as gastrointestinal tract, kidney, skin and prostate carcinoma (Shields et al, 1997). Choroidal metastases typically develop after the diagnosis of breast cancer and in some cases systemic metastases have already been detected. In 66% to 97% of lung cancer patients, choroidal metastases are detected after the primary tumour has been diagnosed (Kanthan et al, 2007). In conclusion, uveal metastases can also be observed before the diagnosis of breast or lung cancer (Demirci et al, 2003; Singh et al, 2012). The median interval between diagnosis of the primary tumour and uveal metastasis is 1 - 4.5 years (Amer et al, 2004; Ratanatharathorn et al, 1991; Rosset et al, 1998; Rottinger et al, 1976; Tsina et al, 2005). Choroidal metastases are creamy yellow, flat or elevated and often multilobulated lesions that can occur bilateral. More than half of the patients may develop subretinal fluid (Demirci et al, 2003). The lesion can show clumps of brown pigmentation, known as leopard spots and RPE alterations. Metastases grow in a different fashion than primary UMs, they infiltrate and replace the normal choroidal architecture more diffusely. On US metastases from breast carcinoma show a higher internal reflectivity than UM (Sobottka et al, 1998).

Choroidal osteoma is a rare ossifying benign lesion of the choroid that appears as a yellowish to orange well-defined, juxtapapillary or macular choroidal tumour. These lesions mostly occur in young women with a mean age of 26 years; usually it occurs unilateral, although in 20-30% of cases it appears to be bilateral. Over time an osteoma may enlarge and decalcify partially or totally (Ross & Kemp, 2009; Shields et al, 2005a). There is a 31% chance of developing choroidal neovascularisation after 10 years (Shields et al, 2005a). On B-scan US a highly reflective lesion that shadows the orbit can be seen.

http://dx.doi.org/10.5772/53631

Peripheral exudative hemorrhagic chorioretinopathy (PEHC) lesions, unilateral and often bilateral, have peripheral (> 3 mm outside the fovea) subretinal or sub-RPE haemorrhage that arises from choroidal neovascularisation. In the periphery signs of macular degeneration, such as lipid exudation, subretinal fluid and fibrosis can be observed (Mantel et al, 2009; Shields et al, 2009c). Also in the macula drusen, RPE alterations or choroidal neovascularisation can be present, which is then consistent with macular degeneration (Shields et al, 2009c). On B-scan internal lesion characteristics show a solid or hollow acoustic quality and no choroidal excavation (Mantel et al, 2009; Shields et al, 2009d). The majority of the peripheral lesions resolve spontaneously over time, leaving a scar.

Hemorrhagic detachment of the retina and RPE may also simulate melanoma.

Choroidal haemorrhage may be distinguished from UM by partially or totally resorption of the haemorrhage over a few weeks, and on US an after-movement can be noticed by kinetic evaluation. Key features are elevated eye pressure, forward movement of diaphragm combined with severe pain (Yang et al, 2003).

Posterior nodular scleritis is rare, but often underdiagnosed. It is twice as common in women as in men, and in 35% of the patients it occurs in both eyes. The most common symptoms are periocular pain, pain with eye movement and decreased vision. The differentiation between scleritis and melanoma can be made by US. On B-scan echogenic scleral nodules, fluid in Tenon's capsule, swelling of the optic disc and serous retinal detachment are found (McCluskey et al, 1999).

Intraocular leiomyoma is a rare benign amelanotic tumour of the uvea and mimics an UM. It presents as a dome-shaped lesion, showing light translucency and often contains dilated episcleral vessels, with a predilection in young females (Shields et al, 1994). Sometimes the diagnosis cannot be made by non-invasive examination and intraocular biopsy is necessary (Richter et al, 2003).

Adenoma of the RPE is infrequently diagnosed before enucleation. RPE adenoma is dome-shaped and has in contrast to melanoma a higher internal reflectivity on A-scan US (Nakamura et al, 2012). Compared to UM, RPE adenoma has more frequently retinal feeder vessels, retinal or subretinal exudates and exudative retinal detachment (Wei et al, 2010).

6. Classification and histopathologic features

UMs develop from melanocytes of the uvea that are derived from neural crest cells. Initially Callender and colleagues described several melanoma cell types, (Callender, 1931) currently three histopathological uveal melanoma categories are being recognised: spindle, epithelioid and mixed cell type (Campbell et al, 1998). Haematoxylin and eosin (H&E) staining is used to differentiate between cell types. Spindle cells exhibit elongated nuclei that may contain eosinophilic nucleoli. In general, Ums containing spindle cells grow slowly and might be associated with better prognosis. On the other hand, UMs consisting of faster growing epithelioid cells, have a more aggressive behaviour, and are therefore associated with poor clinical outcome. Epithelioid cells have more polygonal cytoplasm and contain eccentric placed large pleomorphic nuclei and prominent eosinophilic nucleoli (figure 6). The mixed-cell type melanoma has variable proportion of spindle and epithelioid cells with a minimum of 10% of any one type (Edge & American Joint Committee on Cancer, 2010). Other inter-tumour factors, like the presence of certain extracellular matrix patterns (three closed loops located back to back identified by Periodic-acid Schiff (PAS) staining) and increased mitotic figures (number of mitoses per 50 high-power fields equal to 8mm2) can both provide additional adverse prognostic information (Folberg et al, 1993; Mooy et al, 1995). Other histological features associated with mortality and metastases are mean diameter of ten largest nucleoli, degree of pigmentation, presence of inflammation and tumour necrosis (Gill & Char, 2012). Extrascleral extension by perineural, perivascular, intravascular or direct scleral invasion is correlated with a worse prognosis, especially when the orbital fat resection margin is positive (Collaborative Ocular Melanoma Study Group, 1998).

Immunohistochemistry may be of diagnostic value. S-100 is expressed by cells of neuroectodermal origin. HMB-45 binds to gp100, an antigen expressed by melanocytes that can be useful in differentiating UM from nonmelanocytic tumours (Burnier et al, 1991).

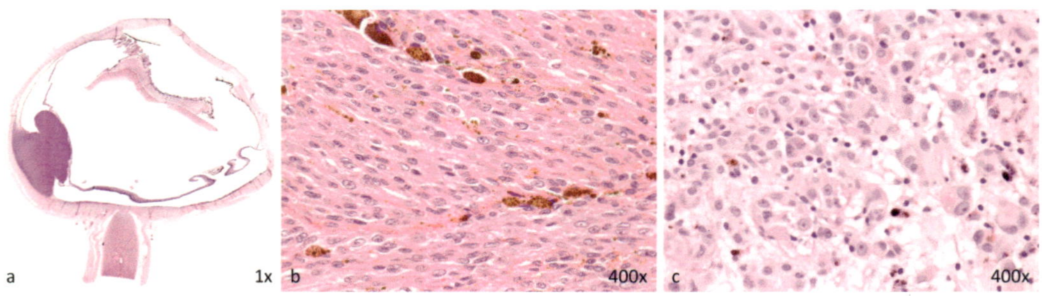

Figure 6. a: Haematoxylin and eosin staining of formalin fixed and paraffin embedded eye sample with a typical mushroom shaped melanoma.; 6b: Uveal melanoma tissue with spindle cell type characterised by elongated nuclei; 6c: Uveal melanoma tissue with epithelioid cells containing large pleomorphic nuclei and prominent eosinophilic nucleoli.

7. Genetic classification

Cytogenetic studies in solid tumours have been a greater challenge than in haematological malignancies since metaphase chromosome spreads of good quality are more difficult to obtain. Solid tumours frequently have highly complex chromosome alterations and are more heterogeneous. Despite this, UM has been well studied since the late eighties with different techniques, such as cytogenetic and fluorescent in situ hybridization (FISH) analysis. Over the years, we have learned that the majority of UMs contain non-random chromosomal anomalies on either the short arm (p) and or long arm (q) of chromosomes 1, 3, 6 and 8, which can serve as prognostic markers.

7.1. Cytogenetic and molecular techniques in UM research

To examine chromosomal changes in UM tissue several cytogenetic and molecular techniques are available. UMs are quite suitable for cytogenetic analysis because of their relatively simply karyotype. Large chromosomal gains, deletions and translocations can be visualized with conventional karyotyping and spectral karyotyping (SKY) (figure 7a). However, for the detection of smaller abnormalities other techniques are necessary, such as FISH (figure 7b), comparative genomic hybridization (CGH) or quantitative polymerase chain reaction (qPCR) based techniques. An approach is the multiplex ligation probe amplification (MLPA) which allows the relative quantification of multiple loci in one single reaction. MLPA can detect patients at risk for metastatic disease using the results for chromosome 3 and 8 with similar accuracy as FISH (Damato et al, 2009; Vaarwater et al, 2012). MLPA and other qPCR-based techniques as Multiplex Amplicon Quantification (MAQ) fill the gap between more expensive genome-wide screening assays and cheaper methods that only provide information on a single locus (Kumps et al, 2010). A different technique is microsatellite analysis (MSA). Microsatellites are tandem repeats of polymorphic sequences located in the non-coding regions of DNA. An extreme form of microsatellite instability was first described in hereditary nonpolyposis colorectal cancer syndrome (Thibodeau et al, 1993). This technique is used to study loss of heterozygosity (LOH) as an indicator of chromosomal loss. A drawback of MSA is that only a limited number of markers can be analyzed in one experiment.

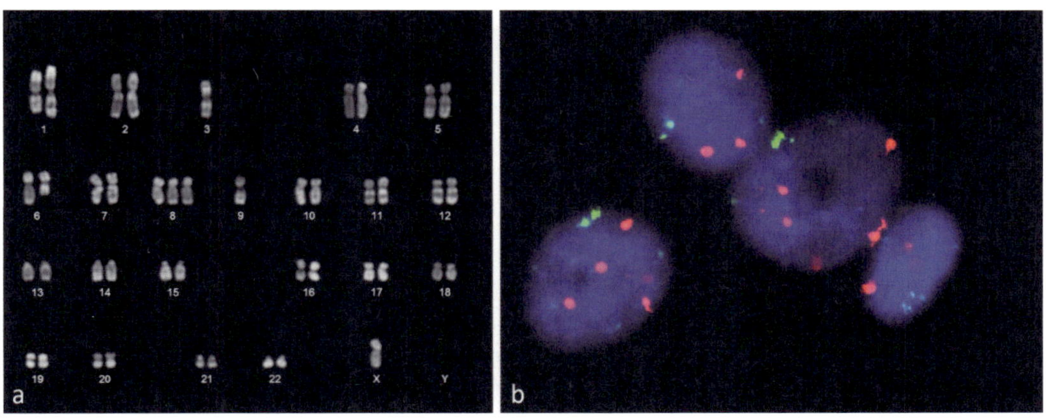

Figure 7. a: Example of a karyogram showing monosomy 3 and trisomy of chromosome 8; 7b: FISH analysis of a tumour demonstrates 1 signal for the probe on centromere 3 (green signals) and 3 to 4 signals of the probe on centromere 8 (red signals).

After completion of the human genome project, genome-wide DNA assays became available. Micro-assay based CGH, single nucleotide polymorphism (SNP) analysis and gene expression profiling (GEP) analysis are the frequently applied techniques. With the development of Next Generation Sequencing (NGS) technologies, the genome can be analyzed at base pair level. Genome-wide mutation analysis of tumour samples led to the discovery of a subset of genes in UM such as *GNAQ* and *BAP1*.

7.2. Chromosomal anomalies

7.2.1. Monosomy 3

Monosomy of chromosome 3 is observed in approximately 50% of the cases of UM and is strongly associated with clinical and histopathological prognostic factors and with metastatic death (Horsman et al, 1990; Prescher et al, 1990; Sisley et al, 1990). Prescher and associates were the first to find a strong correlation between loss of chromosome 3 and a poor prognosis of the patient (Prescher et al, 1996). Since then several groups have confirmed the prognostic value of monosomy 3 (Kilic et al, 2006; Sisley et al, 2000; Sisley et al, 1997; White et al, 1998). It is assumed that loss of chromosome 3 is a primary event, as it often occurs with other chromosomal aberrations in UM such as 1p loss, and gain of 6p and 8q (Prescher et al, 1995). Kiliç and colleagues established that tumours with concurrent loss of chromosome 1p and 3 are at higher risk of metastasizing than the tumours with other aberrations (Kilic et al, 2005). Mostly one entire copy of chromosome 3 is lost, although in some cases, isodisomy of chromosome 3 is acquired (Aalto et al, 2001; Scholes et al, 2001; White et al, 1998). Partial deletions or translocations have rarely been described on this chromosome making it difficult to map putative tumour suppressor genes. However, recently a mutation in the *BAP1* gene, located on chromosome 3, has been identified in UMs and this gene seems to play an important role in the tumour progression (Harbour et al, 2010). This gene will be discussed in more detail later in this chapter.

7.2.2. Chromosome 8

Abnormalities in chromosome 8, and in particular gain of 8q or an isochromosome 8q, are thought to be a secondary event in UM as variable copy numbers can be present in one melanoma (Horsman & White, 1993; Prescher et al, 1994). Gain of chromosome 8q is frequently found in tumours that also have loss of chromosome 3, and this is associated with a poor patient outcome (Aalto et al, 2001; Prescher et al, 1995; White et al, 1998). A SNP array analysis with this chromosome status is depicted in figure 8. The relationship between the percentages of aberrant copy numbers within UM cells and patient outcome has been investigated. A higher percentage of monosomy 3 and chromosome 8q gain in primary UM cells shows a strong relation with poor disease-free survival compared to low percentage aberrations (van den Bosch et al, 2012).

7.2.3. Chromosome 6

Rearrangements on chromosome 6 affect both arms of the chromosome, resulting in deletions of 6q and gains of 6p. The relative gain of chromosome 6p can occur either through an isochromosome of 6p or a deletion of 6q. Tumours with gain of 6p are thought to be a separate group within UM with an alternative genetic pathway in carcinogenesis, since gain of

6p is frequently found in tumours with disomy 3 (Ehlers et al, 2008; Hoglund et al, 2004; Sisley et al, 1997). However, this combination of gain of 6p with disomy 3 could not be confirmed by others (Mensink et al, 2009). Aberrations resulting in a relative increase of 6p have been found to be related with both a longer survival (White et al, 1998) or a decreased survival (Aalto et al, 2001). The effect of chromosome 6 aberrations on patient outcome is not conclusive.

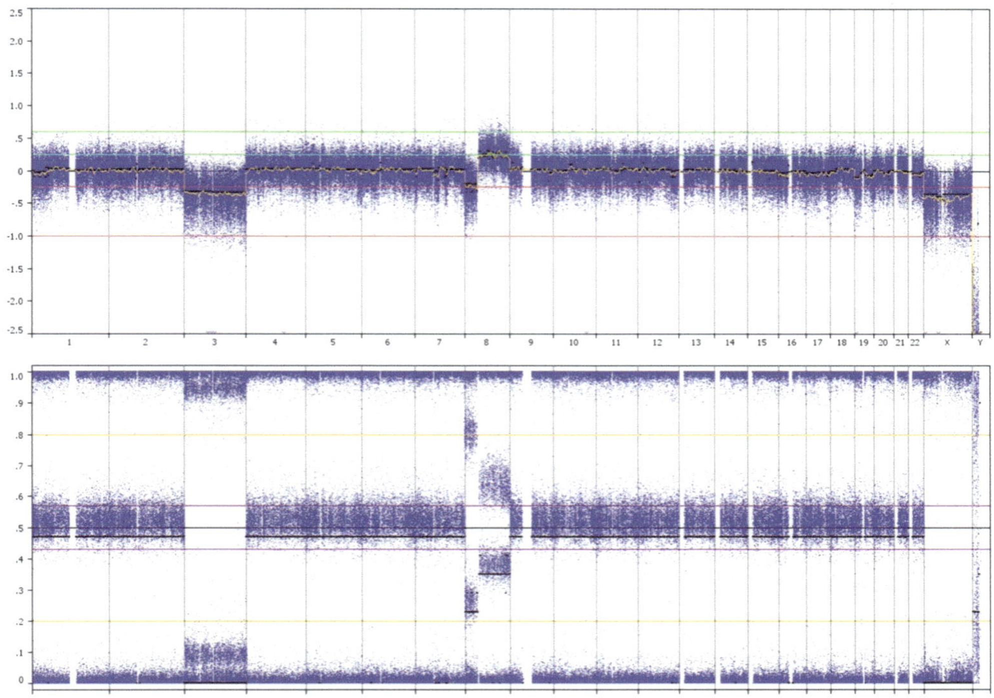

Figure 8. Single nucleotide polymorphism (SNP) array of an uveal melanoma. The upper panel (LogR ratio) shows loss of chromosome 3, partial loss of chromosome 8p and gain of chromosome 8q. The lower panel depicts the B-allele frequency representing allelic imbalance at these chromosomes.

7.2.4. Chromosome 1

In cutaneous melanoma rearrangements on the short arm of chromosome 1 are a common abnormality, occurring in about 80% of all cases (Fountain et al, 1990; Zhang et al, 1999). In UM this region on 1p is also frequently affected, giving rise to a deletion of 1p. However, these anomalies on chromosome 1 are less common than those in skin melanomas with a frequency of approximately 30% (Horsman & White, 1993; Parrella et al, 1999; Prescher et al, 1990; Prescher et al, 1995; Sisley et al, 2000).

Aberrations on other chromosomes have been explored, such as chromosome 9p21 (Scholes et al, 2001), chromosome 11q23 (Sisley et al, 2000), chromosome 18q22 (Mensink et al, 2008;

White et al, 2006), and chromosome 16q (Kilic et al, 2006; Vajdic et al, 2003). The impact on the prognosis, however, remains unclear due to contradictory findings.

7.2.5. Gene expression profiling

Using GEP UMs can be classified into two classes of tumours that correspond remarkably well with the ability of the tumour to metastasize. In a study of 25 UMs, class 1 tumours had a low risk of metastasizing and class 2 tumours had a high risk of developing metastasis (Onken et al, 2004). This molecular classification strongly predicts metastatic death and outperforms other clinical, histopathological and cytogenetic prognostic indicators (Petrausch et al, 2008; van Gils et al, 2008; Worley et al, 2007). Class 1 tumours predominantly show disomy of chromosome 3, whereas class 2 tumours consist mostly of monosomy 3 (Worley et al, 2007).

7.3. Candidate genes

After identifying the non-random chromosomal alterations in UM, the search for potential oncogenes and tumour suppressor genes followed. By narrowing down altered regions on chromosomes, researchers have tried to identify genes involved in tumourigenesis or progression towards metastasis. This way, studies have been conducted on chromosome 8q revealing potential oncogenes such as *MYC*, which is amplified in about 30% of the UMs (Parrella et al, 2001). Other oncogenes on chromosome 8q have been described, such as *DDEF1* and *NBS1* (now referred to as *ASAP1* and *NBN*, respectively) (Ehlers & Harbour, 2005; Ehlers et al, 2005). Yet, no specific oncogenic mutations on this region have been reported thus far. Other candidate genes were proposed, such as *HDM2*, *BCL-2* and *CCND1*. However, the pathogenic significance for any of these genes has not been established.

Mutations in certain genes have been well described for cutaneous melanoma. Examples of such genes are the oncogenes *NRAS*, *BRAF* and *AKT3*, and the tumour suppressors *CDKN2A*, *PTEN* and *TP53*. In contrast to skin melanomas, *PTEN* mutations were not observed in a study of nine cell lines (Naus et al, 2000). Nevertheless, in 15% of the UM cases mutations in *PTEN* were found resulting in activation of *AKT* and overexpression of the PI3K-PTEN-AKT pathway preventing apoptosis (Abdel-Rahman et al, 2006; Ehlers et al, 2008; Ibrahim & Haluska, 2009).

7.3.1. The RAS-RAF-MEK-ERK pathway

In a large proportion of the UMs the RAS-RAF-MEK-ERK pathway or mitogen-activated protein kinase (MAPK) pathway is constitutionally activated, leading to excessive cell proliferation and suggesting the presence of activating mutations upstream in the pathway (Weber et al, 2003; Zuidervaart et al, 2005). Mutation analysis on potential mutation sites in the *BRAF* gene were performed, since a single substitution (p.V600E) in *BRAF* occurs frequently in benign and premalignant cutaneous nevi (Davies et al, 2002; Pollock et al, 2003). However, *NRAS* and *BRAF* mutations have been reported in a few UMs but overall these mutations are rare (Cohen et al, 2003; Kilic et al, 2004; Mooy et al, 1991; Saldanha et al, 2004).

7.3.2. GNAQ and GNA11 gene

With the recent discovery of activating *GNAQ* and *GNA11* mutations new light has been shed on the MAPK pathway. Van Raamsdonk and co-workers demonstrated an alternative route to MAPK activation through G-protein signalling in melanocytic neoplasia including UMs. They reported a *GNAQ* mutation in 83% of blue naevi and in 46% of UM cases (Van Raamsdonk et al, 2009). Other studies confirmed these results, *GNAQ* mutations were found in half of the UM cases (Bauer et al, 2009; Onken et al, 2008). *GNAQ* and its paralog *GNA11* encode the heterotrimeric guanine nucleotide-binding protein G subunit alpha q and 11, respectively. Through mutations these subunits become activated and abrogate their intrinsic GTPase activity, which is required to return them to an inactive state. This oncogenic conversion is suggested to be the cause of constitutive MAPK pathway activation. A subsequent study reported that 83% of UM samples harboured Gα-protein mutations (*GNAQ* or *GNA11* mutations) affecting specific regions on either exon 4 or 5 (codon R183 or Q209, respectively) in a mutually exclusive pattern (Van Raamsdonk et al, 2010). There is no relation between *GNAQ* mutations and prognosis (Bauer et al, 2009). Hence, the presence of Gα-protein mutations in tumours at all stages of malignant progression and in melanocytic lesions of the choroid, suggests that they are early events in UM (Onken et al, 2008; Van Raamsdonk et al, 2009).

7.3.3. BAP1 gene

Exome genome sequencing led to the discovery of the BRCA1 associated protein 1 (*BAP1*) gene in UM (Harbour et al, 2010). *BAP1,* a nuclearly localized enzyme, was originally identified as an ubiquitin hydrolase that binds to the RING finger domain of BRCA1 (Farmer et al, 2005; Jensen et al, 1998). It has de-ubiquitinating activity and is involved in several biological processes, including regulation of cell cycle and cell growth, chromatin dynamics and DNA damage response (Farmer et al, 2005). *BAP1* is located on chromosome 3p21.1 and is thought to be a tumour suppressor gene (Ventii et al, 2008). Mutations in this gene first have been reported in a small number of breast and lung cancer cell lines (Jensen et al, 1998). Recently, inactivating somatic mutations were found in 84% of the metastasizing UMs. These mutations were only found in 1 out of 26 investigated class 1 tumours against 26 out of 31 class 2 tumours, implicating that *BAP1* mutations occur late in the UM progression (Harbour et al, 2010). In addition, co-segregating germline *BAP1* mutations have been described in several families with different range of diseases, such as cutaneous melanomas (Wiesner et al, 2011), malignant pleural mesotheliomas (Testa et al, 2011), and other cancers such as meningioma (Abdel-Rahman et al, 2011). Given the functional complexity of *BAP1,* different germline mutations in *BAP1* may predispose to divergent tumour types. To understand more about the impact of *BAP1* mutations on UM and other types of cancers, more extensive clinical, molecular genetic, and functional studies are ongoing.

8. Metastases

Irrespective of primary treatment of the UM nearly half of the patients develop metastases (Gilissen et al, 2011). UM spreads haematogenous, with a high tendency to metastasize to the liver in 90-95% of the patients. One explanation for the development of new distant metastasis years after the control of primary tumour is the presence of circulating tumour cells at time of the initial diagnosis (Manschot et al, 1995). In other words, the disease is often already disseminated at time of tumour diagnosis. Several pathways have been implicated in the preferential homing of tumour cells to the liver, such as hepatocyte growth factor (HGF) and it's corresponding receptor c-Met, insulin-like growth factor 1 (IGF-1), and chemokine CXCL12 (Bakalian et al, 2008). In case of liver metastasis prognosis is poor with a median survival of approximately 8 months (Eskelin et al, 2003).

Despite the fact that there a no therapeutic options for metastatic UM that improve survival or quality of life, the following methods can be used for screening of liver metastasis: liver function tests (gamma-glutamyl transpeptidase (γGT) and lactate dehydrogenase (LDH) from blood), liver imaging with US, CT and MRI. Although screening annually or semi-annually for liver metastasis by liver function tests are being widely used, there are reports of disseminated liver metastases and normal liver function tests (Donoso et al, 1985; Eskelin et al, 1999).

Patients have 97.5% chance or more of having no metastasis in the case of normal liver function tests, because of the high negative predictive value. However, isolated or combined liver function tests for aspartate aminotransferase (AST), alanine transaminase (ALT), yGT, LDH and phosphatidic acid (PA) are not indicated for detection of early liver metastasis (Mouriaux et al, 2012). Other upcoming screening options make use of serum markers, Among which S-100β (neural crest marker), melanoma inhibitory activity (MIA), tissue polypeptide specific antigen (TPS) and osteopontin (OPN). MIA and S-100β showed significant increase in levels before clinical diagnosis of metastasis (Barak et al, 2011). In a lead time of more than 6 months before clinical metastasis a significant increase in OPN and steeper trendlines in MIA and S-100β levels were demonstrated (Hendler et al, 2011).

9. Treatment of primary UM

Conservation of the eye in UM with useful vision has improved with advances in local irradiation (brachytherapy), heavy particle radiation techniques (proton and helium ion beam), stereotactic radiotherapy (SRT), endoresection, exoresection, transpupillary thermotherapy and photodynamic therapy (Spagnolo et al, 2012). If the tumours are larger, advanced and, in particular, if there is evidence of extraocular extension enucleation is advised (Spagnolo et al, 2012). In addition, enucleation is also performed after serious treatment induced complications (Hungerford, 1993; Shields et al, 1991). Choice of treatment depends on the location and size of the tumour and goals of therapy. Even though enucleation is sometimes required, eye-preserving approaches have shown to be equally successful regarding overall

http://dx.doi.org/10.5772/53631

survival and metastasis-free survival (Seddon et al, 1985; Seddon et al, 1990). Brachytherapy is the most common method for treating UM, and currently the ruthenium-106 (Ru-106) and iodine-125 (I-125) applicators are the most frequently used. Brachytherapy can be used in combination with other methods of treatment of UM, such as local resection or transpupillary thermotherapy (Pe'er, 2012). Local control with plaque radiotherapy has provided overall survival comparable to enucleation. Radiation-induced side effects have necessitated secondary enucleation in 10-22% of the patients (Bell & Wilson, 2004; Char et al, 1993; Finger, 1997; Garretson et al, 1987; Gunduz et al, 1999; Lommatzsch et al, 2000; Packer et al, 1992; Shields et al, 1991; Tjho-Heslinga et al, 1999; Vrabec et al, 1991). Local recurrences after brachytherapy are reported between 4 - 28%, depending on the size of the tumour and the follow up time (Damato & Foulds, 1996; Gragoudas, 1997; Karlsson et al, 1989; Seregard et al, 1997; Tjho-Heslinga et al, 1999; Wilson & Hungerford, 1999; Zografos et al, 1992). Radiation-induced complications include radiation retinopathy, radiation maculopathy, radiation opticopathy as well as recurrences (Gragoudas et al, 1999; Kinyoun et al, 1996; Summanen et al, 1996). Heavy particle radiation with positive charged particles (protons or helium-ions) enables treatment of small, medium- and large-choroidal melanomas. The local recurrence rate for proton beam irradiation is similar to brachytherapy and at 10 years is usually around 5% (Gragoudas, 1997; Zografos et al, 1992). Secondary enucleation is performed in 10 - 15% of patients either due to complications or local recurrence. Other complications, such as maculopathy, opticopathy, cataract, glaucoma, vitreous haemorrhage, retinal detachment and dryness have also been described (Desjardins et al, 2012). In concordance with proton beam irradiation radiogenic side effects are also reported after SRT. Side effects, such as radiation retinopathy, opticopathy and neovascular glaucoma are responsible for the majority of secondary visual loss and secondary enucleations after SRT (Mueller et al, 2000; Zehetmayer et al, 2000). The efficacy of SRT for UM has been proven in different studies with local tumour control rates reported over 90%, 5 and 10 years after treatment (Zehetmayer, 2012). Local resection (endoresection and exoresection) of UM aims to conserve the eye and remain a useful vision. The tumour can be removed in several manners, through the vitrous and retinal with a vitreous cutter, endoresection, or through a scleral opening exoresection. Variations of exoresection include iridectomy, iridocyclectomy, cyclochoroidectomy, and choroidectomy. Endoresection as well as exoresection can be used as a primary procedure, after another conservative therapy as a treatment option for recurrences or toxic tumour syndrome. An advantage of local resection is that eyes that would otherwise be inoperable can be preserved, while relative large tumour samples are available for prognostication and research (Damato & Foulds, 1996; Damato, 2012; Robertson, 2001).

10. Treatment of liver metastases

Although treatment options for small to medium sized melanoma improves visual outcome, there has not been any standardized therapy that improves survival in metastatic disease. Systemic treatment options, such as intravenous chemotherapy and immunotherapy do not seem to give promising results or survival benefit (Augsburger et al, 2009).

Several locoregional techniques are available, for example immunoembolization, chemoembolization, isolated liver perfusion and hepatic intra-arterial chemotherapy. In highly selected patients, surgical resection of liver metastases can be beneficial. Operating on patients with a time from diagnosis of the primary tumour to liver metastases of > 24 months, ≤ 4 liver metastatic lesions and absence of 'miliary' disease (multiple, diffuse, millimetre-sized, dark punctuate lesions on CT) is associated with prolonged survival. A median survival of 27 months has been described in patients with microscopically complete liver resection versus 14 months in patients with microscopically or macroscopically incomplete liver resection (Mariani et al, 2009).

11. Future prospects

With the discovery of *GNAQ* and *BAP1* mutations, new therapeutic strategies based on the specific mutated gene content seem promising. For tumours with Gα-protein mutations, the therapeutic goal is to inhibit downstream signalling molecules in the MAPK pathway that are activated. Preclinical studies show that inhibition of MAPK pathway in UM cell lines results in decreased cell proliferation (Van Raamsdonk et al, 2009). There are several key molecules in the MAPK pathway, which have been explored as potential therapeutic targets. One of such is MEK, and Gα-protein mutant UM cells showed to be mildly sensitive to the MEK inhibitor AZD6244 (Gill & Char, 2012). Another recent preclinical study proposed to target both the MAPK and PI3K/AKT pathway since both pathways are activated in UM. A combination of MEK and PI3K inhibition treatment resulted in induction of apoptosis in a Gα-mutant UM cells (Khalili et al, 2012). Other potential targets in the MAPK pathway are currently being investigated, including protein kinase C, which is a component of signalling from *GNAQ* to Erk1/2 (Wu et al, 2012).

Therapeutically targeting UMs with a *BAP1* mutation works in a different manner than the Gα-protein mutations, since *BAP1* acts as a tumour suppressor gene. Regaining lost functions of suppressor genes are in general more challenging than inhibiting an overactive oncogene. Nevertheless, ongoing studies show that histone deacetylase (HDAC) inhibitors may have therapeutic potential in UM. Landreville and colleagues established that HDAC inhibitors can reverse the histone H2A hyperubiquitination that occurs in cultured UM cells depleted of *BAP1*, and it induces morphologic differentiation, cell-cycle exit, and shifts to a differentiated, melanocytic GEP (Landreville et al, 2012). Examples of HDAC inhibitors are valproic acid, trichostatin A, LBH-589, and suberoylanilide hydroxamic acid. Clinical trials are needed to evaluate the effect of these compounds in UM patients, and hopefully UM specific treatment based on mutational content will lead to improved patient survival.

Abbreviations

UM: uveal melanoma

http://dx.doi.org/10.5772/53631

RPE: retina pigment epithelia

FAMM: familial atypical mole and melanoma syndrome

US: ultrasonography

OCT: optical coherence tomography

MRI: magnetic resonance imaging

CT: computed tomography

CHRPE: congenital hypertrophy of the retinal pigment epithelium

PEHC: peripheral exudative hemorrhagic chorioretinopathy

H&E: haematoxylin and eosin

PAS: Periodic-acid Schiff

FISH: fluorescent in situ hybridization

SKY: spectral karyotyping

CGH: comparative genomic hybridization

qPCR: quantitative polymerase chain reaction

MLPA: multiplex ligation probe amplification

MAQ: multiplex amplicon quantification

MSA: microsatellite analysis

LOH: loss of heterozygosity

SNP: single nucleotide polymorphism

GEP: gene expression profiling

NGS: next generation sequencing

MAPK: mitogen-activated protein kinase

HGF: hepatocyte growth factor

IGF-1: insulin-like growth factor 1

γGT: gamma-glutamyl transpeptidase

LDH: lactate dehydrogenase

AST: aspartate aminotransferase

ALT : alanine transaminase

PA: phosphatidic acid

MIA: melanoma inhibitory activity

TPS: tissue polypeptide specific antigen

OPN: osteopontin

SRT: stereotactic radiotherapy

Ru-106: ruthenium-106

I-125: iodine-125

HDAC: histone deacetylase

Author details

J.G.M. van Beek[1], A.E. Koopmans[1,2], R.M. Verdijk[3], N.C. Naus[1], A. de Klein[2] and E. Kilic[1]

1 Department of Ophthalmology, Erasmus MC, Rotterdam, The Netherlands

2 Department of Clinical Genetics, The Netherlands

3 Department of Pathology, The Netherlands

References

[1] Collaborative Ocular Melanoma Study Group (1997). Factors predictive of growth and treatment of small choroidal melanoma: COMS Report No. 5. *Arch Ophthalmol* 115: 1537-1544.

[2] Collaborative Ocular Melanoma Study Group (1998). Histopathologic characteristics of uveal melanomas in eyes enucleated from the Collaborative Ocular Melanoma Study. COMS report no. 6. *Am J Ophthalmol* 125: 745-766.

[3] Aalto Y, Eriksson L, Seregard S, Larsson O & Knuutila S (2001) Concomitant loss of chromosome 3 and whole arm losses and gains of chromosome 1, 6, or 8 in metastasizing primary uveal melanoma. *Invest Ophthalmol Vis Sci* 42: 313-317.

[4] Abdel-Rahman MH, Pilarski R, Cebulla CM, Massengill JB, Christopher BN, Boru G, Hovland P & Davidorf FH (2011) Germline BAP1 mutation predisposes to uveal melanoma, lung adenocarcinoma, meningioma, and other cancers. *J Med Genet* 48: 856-859.

[5] Abdel-Rahman MH, Yang Y, Zhou XP, Craig EL, Davidorf FH & Eng C (2006) High frequency of submicroscopic hemizygous deletion is a major mechanism of loss of expression of PTEN in uveal melanoma. *J Clin Oncol* 24: 288-295.

[6] Amer R, Pe'er J, Chowers I & Anteby I (2004) Treatment options in the management of choroidal metastases. *Ophthalmologica* 218: 372-377.

[7] Atmaca LS, Batioğlu F & Atmaca P. (1999). Fluorescein and indocyanine green videoangiography of choroidal melanomas. In *Jpn J Ophthalmol*, Vol. 43. pp. 25-30.

[8] Augsburger JJ, Corrêa ZM & Shaikh AH. (2009). Effectiveness of treatments for metastatic uveal melanoma. In *Am J Ophthalmol*, Vol. 148. pp. 119-127.

[9] Augsburger JJ, Schroeder RP, Territo C, Gamel JW & Shields JA. (1989). Clinical parameters predictive of enlargement of melanocytic choroidal lesions. In *Br J Ophthalmol*, Vol. 73. pp. 911-917.

[10] Bakalian S, Marshall JC, Logan P, Faingold D, Maloney S, Di Cesare S, Martins C, Fernandes BF & Burnier MN, Jr. (2008) Molecular pathways mediating liver metastasis in patients with uveal melanoma. *Clin Cancer Res* 14: 951-956.

[11] Barak V, Kaiserman I, Frenkel S, Hendler K, Kalickman I & Pe'er J (2011) The dynamics of serum tumor markers in predicting metastatic uveal melanoma (part 1). *Anticancer Res* 31: 345-349.

[12] Bauer J, Kilic E, Vaarwater J, Bastian BC, Garbe C & de Klein A (2009) Oncogenic GNAQ mutations are not correlated with disease-free survival in uveal melanoma. *Br J Cancer* 101: 813-815.

[13] Bell DJ & Wilson MW (2004) Choroidal melanoma: natural history and management options. *Cancer Control* 11: 296-303.

[14] Biswas J, Krishnakumar S & Shanmugam MP. (2002). Uveal melanoma in Asian Indians: a clinicopathological study. In *Arch Ophthalmol*, Vol. 120. pp. 522-523.

[15] Boldt HC, Byrne SF, Gilson MM, Finger PT, Green RL, Straatsma BR, Simpson ER & Hawkins BS (2008) Baseline echographic characteristics of tumors in eyes of patients enrolled in the Collaborative Ocular Melanoma Study: COMS report no. 29. *Ophthalmology* 115: 1390-1397, 1397 e1391-1392.

[16] Burnier MN, Jr., McLean IW & Gamel JW (1991) Immunohistochemical evaluation of uveal melanocytic tumors. Expression of HMB-45, S-100 protein, and neuron-specific enolase. *Cancer* 68: 809-814.

[17] Callender GR (1931) Malignant melanotic tumors of the eye: a study of histologic types in 111 cases. *Trans Am Acad Ophthalmol Otolaryngol* 36: 131-142.

[18] Campbell RJ, Sobin LH, Zimmerman LE & World Health Organization. (1998). *Histological typing of tumours of the eye and its adnexa*. International histological classification of tumours. Springer: Berlin ; London.

[19] Carreno E, Saornil MA, Garcia-Alvarez C, Lopez-Lara F, De Frutos-Baraja JM & Almaraz A (2012) Prevalence of ocular and oculodermal melanocytosis in Spanish population with uveal melanoma. *Eye (Lond)* 26: 159-162.

[20] Char DH, Kroll S, Stone RD, Harrie R & Kerman B. (1990). Ultrasonographic measurement of uveal melanoma thickness: interobserver variability. In *Br J Ophthalmol*, Vol. 74. pp. 183-185.

[21] Char DH & Miller T. (1995). Accuracy of presumed uveal melanoma diagnosis before alternative therapy. In *Br J Ophthalmol*, Vol. 79. pp. 692-696.

[22] Char DH, Quivey JM, Castro JR, Kroll S & Phillips T (1993) Helium ions versus iodine 125 brachytherapy in the management of uveal melanoma. A prospective, randomized, dynamically balanced trial. *Ophthalmology* 100: 1547-1554.

[23] Char DH, Stone RD, Irvine AR, Crawford JB, Hilton GF, Lonn LI & Schwartz A (1980) Diagnostic modalities in choroidal melanoma. *Am J Ophthalmol* 89: 223-230.

[24] Cohen Y, Goldenberg-Cohen N, Parrella P, Chowers I, Merbs SL, Pe'er J & Sidransky D (2003) Lack of BRAF mutation in primary uveal melanoma. *Invest Ophthalmol Vis Sci* 44: 2876-2878.

[25] Coleman DJ, Abramson DH, Jack RL & Franzen LA (1974) Ultrasonic diagnosis of tumors of the choroid. *Arch Ophthalmol* 91: 344-354.

[26] Collaborative Ocular Melanoma Study Group (2003) Comparison of clinical, echographic, and histopathological measurements from eyes with medium-sized choroidal melanoma in the collaborative ocular melanoma study: COMS report no. 21. *Arch Ophthalmol* 121: 1163-1171.

[27] Damato B (2010) Does ocular treatment of uveal melanoma influence survival? *Br J Cancer* 103: 285-290.

[28] Damato B, Dopierala J, Klaasen A, van Dijk M, Sibbring J & Coupland SE (2009) Multiplex ligation-dependent probe amplification of uveal melanoma: correlation with metastatic death. *Invest Ophthalmol Vis Sci* 50: 3048-3055.

[29] Damato B & Foulds WS (1996) Indications for trans-scleral local resection of uveal melanoma. *Br J Ophthalmol* 80: 1029-1030.

[30] Damato BE (2012) Local resection of uveal melanoma. *Dev Ophthalmol* 49: 66-80.

[31] Damato BE & Coupland SE (2012) Differences in uveal melanomas between men and women from the British Isles. *Eye (Lond)* 26: 292-299.

[32] Davies H, Bignell GR, Cox C, Stephens P, Edkins S, Clegg S, Teague J, Woffendin H, Garnett MJ, Bottomley W, Davis N, Dicks E, Ewing R, Floyd Y, Gray K, Hall S, Hawes R, Hughes J, Kosmidou V, Menzies A, Mould C, Parker A, Stevens C, Watt S, Hooper S, Wilson R, Jayatilake H, Gusterson BA, Cooper C, Shipley J, Hargrave D, Pritchard-Jones K, Maitland N, Chenevix-Trench G, Riggins GJ, Bigner DD, Palmieri G, Cossu A, Flanagan A, Nicholson A, Ho JW, Leung SY, Yuen ST, Weber BL, Seigler HF, Darrow TL, Paterson H, Marais R, Marshall CJ, Wooster R, Stratton MR & Futreal PA (2002) Mutations of the BRAF gene in human cancer. *Nature* 417: 949-954.

[33] Demirci H, Shields CL, Chao A-N & Shields JA. (2003). Uveal metastasis from breast cancer in 264 patients. In *Am J Ophthalmol*, Vol. 136. pp. 264-271.

[34] Desjardins L, Lumbroso-Le Rouic L, Levy-Gabriel C, Cassoux N, Dendale R, Mazal A, Delacroix S, Sastre X, Plancher C & Asselain B (2012) Treatment of uveal melanoma by accelerated proton beam. *Dev Ophthalmol* 49: 41-57.

[35] Diener-West M, Hawkins BS, Markowitz JA & Schachat AP. (1992). A review of mortality from choroidal melanoma. II. A meta-analysis of 5-year mortality rates following enucleation, 1966 through 1988. In *Arch Ophthalmol*, Vol. 110. pp. 245-250.

[36] Donoso LA, Shields JA, Augsburger JJ, Orth DH & Johnson P (1985) Metastatic uveal melanoma: diffuse hepatic metastasis in a patient with concurrent normal serum liver enzyme levels and liver scan. *Arch Ophthalmol* 103: 758.

[37] Edge SB & American Joint Committee on Cancer. (2010). *AJCC cancer staging manual.* Springer: New York ; London.

[38] Ehlers JP & Harbour JW (2005) NBS1 expression as a prognostic marker in uveal melanoma. *Clin Cancer Res* 11: 1849-1853.

[39] Ehlers JP, Worley L, Onken MD & Harbour JW (2005) DDEF1 is located in an amplified region of chromosome 8q and is overexpressed in uveal melanoma. *Clin Cancer Res* 11: 3609-3613.

[40] Ehlers JP, Worley L, Onken MD & Harbour JW (2008) Integrative genomic analysis of aneuploidy in uveal melanoma. *Clin Cancer Res* 14: 115-122.

[41] Eskelin S & Kivelä T. (2002). Mode of presentation and time to treatment of uveal melanoma in Finland. In *Br J Ophthalmol*, Vol. 86. pp. 333-338.

[42] Eskelin S, Pyrhonen S, Hahka-Kemppinen M, Tuomaala S & Kivela T (2003) A prognostic model and staging for metastatic uveal melanoma. *Cancer* 97: 465-475.

[43] Eskelin S, Pyrhönen S, Summanen P, Hahka-Kemppinen M & Kivelä T. (2000). Tumor doubling times in metastatic malignant melanoma of the uvea: tumor progression before and after treatment. In *Ophthalmology*, Vol. 107. pp. 1443-1449.

[44] Eskelin S, Pyrhonen S, Summanen P, Prause JU & Kivela T (1999) Screening for metastatic malignant melanoma of the uvea revisited. *Cancer* 85: 1151-1159.

[45] Farmer H, McCabe N, Lord CJ, Tutt AN, Johnson DA, Richardson TB, Santarosa M, Dillon KJ, Hickson I, Knights C, Martin NM, Jackson SP, Smith GC & Ashworth A (2005) Targeting the DNA repair defect in BRCA mutant cells as a therapeutic strategy. *Nature* 434: 917-921.

[46] Ferry AP (1964) Lesions Mistaken for Malignant Melanoma of the Posterior Uvea. A Clinicopathologic Analysis of 100 Cases with Ophthalmoscopically Visible Lesions. *Arch Ophthalmol* 72: 463-469.

[47] Finger PT (1997) Radiation therapy for choroidal melanoma. *Surv Ophthalmol* 42: 215-232.

[48] Folberg R, Rummelt V, Parys-Van Ginderdeuren R, Hwang T, Woolson RF, Pe'er J & Gruman LM (1993) The prognostic value of tumor blood vessel morphology in primary uveal melanoma. *Ophthalmology* 100: 1389-1398.

[49] Fountain JW, Bale SJ, Housman DE & Dracopoli NC (1990) Genetics of melanoma. *Cancer Surv* 9: 645-671.

[50] Frenkel S, Barzel I, Levy J, Lin AY, Bartsch DU, Majumdar D, Folberg R & Pe'er J (2008) Demonstrating circulation in vasculogenic mimicry patterns of uveal melanoma by confocal indocyanine green angiography. *Eye (Lond)* 22: 948-952.

[51] Garretson BR, Robertson DM & Earle JD (1987) Choroidal melanoma treatment with iodine 125 brachytherapy. *Arch Ophthalmol* 105: 1394-1397.

[52] Gass JD (1977) Problems in the differential diagnosis of choroidal nevi and malignant melanomas. The XXXIII Edward Jackson Memorial Lecture. *Am J Ophthalmol* 83: 299-323.

[53] Gilissen C, Hoischen A, Brunner HG & Veltman JA (2011) Unlocking Mendelian disease using exome sequencing. *Genome Biol* 12: 228.

[54] Gill HS & Char DH (2012) Uveal melanoma prognostication: from lesion size and cell type to molecular class. *Can J Ophthalmol* 47: 246-253.

[55] Gonder JR, Shields JA, Albert DM, Augsburger JJ & Lavin PT (1982) Uveal malignant melanoma associated with ocular and oculodermal melanocytosis. *Ophthalmology* 89: 953-960.

[56] Gragoudas ES (1997) 1996 Jules Gonin Lecture of the Retina Research Foundation. Long-term results after proton irradiation of uveal melanomas. *Graefes Arch Clin Exp Ophthalmol* 235: 265-267.

[57] Gragoudas ES, Li W, Lane AM, Munzenrider J & Egan KM (1999) Risk factors for radiation maculopathy and papillopathy after intraocular irradiation. *Ophthalmology* 106: 1571-1577; discussion 1577-1578.

[58] Collaborative Ocular Melanoma Study Group (1990). Accuracy of diagnosis of choroidal melanomas in the Collaborative Ocular Melanoma Study. COMS report no. 1. In *Arch Ophthalmol*, Vol. 108. pp. 1268-1273.

[59] Guenel P, Laforest L, Cyr D, Fevotte J, Sabroe S, Dufour C, Lutz JM & Lynge E (2001) Occupational risk factors, ultraviolet radiation, and ocular melanoma: a case-control study in France. *Cancer Causes Control* 12: 451-459.

[60] Gunduz K, Shields CL, Shields JA, Cater J, Freire JE & Brady LW (1999) Radiation complications and tumor control after plaque radiotherapy of choroidal melanoma with macular involvement. *Am J Ophthalmol* 127: 579-589.

[61] Guyer DR, Yannuzzi LA, Krupsky S, Slakter JS, Sorenson JA, Orlock D, Friedman E & Gragoudas ES (1993) Digital indocyanine-green videoangiography of intraocular tumors. *Semin Ophthalmol* 8: 224-229.

[62] Hammer H, Tóth-Molńar E, Oláh J & Dobozy A. (1995). Cutaneous dysplastic naevi: risk factor for uveal melanoma. In *Lancet*, Vol. 346. pp. 255-256.

[63] Harbour JW, Onken MD, Roberson ED, Duan S, Cao L, Worley LA, Council ML, Matatall KA, Helms C & Bowcock AM (2010) Frequent mutation of BAP1 in metastasizing uveal melanomas. *Science* 330: 1410-1413.

[64] Heindl LM, Mardin CY, Holbach LM, Naumann GO, Kruse FE & Knorr HL (2009) Vitreal seeding from uveal melanoma detected by high-resolution spectral-domain optical coherence tomography. *Arch Ophthalmol* 127: 1062-1064.

[65] Hendler K, Pe'er J, Kaiserman I, Baruch R, Kalickman I, Barak V & Frenkel S (2011) Trends in liver function tests: a comparison with serum tumor markers in metastatic uveal melanoma (part 2). *Anticancer Res* 31: 351-357.

[66] Hoglund M, Gisselsson D, Hansen GB, White VA, Sall T, Mitelman F & Horsman D (2004) Dissecting karyotypic patterns in malignant melanomas: temporal clustering of losses and gains in melanoma karyotypic evolution. *Int J Cancer* 108: 57-65.

[67] Holly EA, Aston DA, Char DH, Kristiansen JJ & Ahn DK. (1990). Uveal melanoma in relation to ultraviolet light exposure and host factors. In *Cancer Res.*, Vol. 50. pp. 5773-5777.

[68] Honavar SG, Singh AD, Shields CL, Shields JA & Eagle RC. (2000). Iris melanoma in a patient with neurofibromatosis. In *Surv Ophthalmol*, Vol. 45. pp. 231-236.

[69] Horsman DE, Sroka H, Rootman J & White VA (1990) Monosomy 3 and isochromosome 8q in a uveal melanoma. *Cancer Genet Cytogenet* 45: 249-253.

[70] Horsman DE & White VA (1993) Cytogenetic analysis of uveal melanoma. Consistent occurrence of monosomy 3 and trisomy 8q. *Cancer* 71: 811-819.

[71] Hosten N, Bornfeld N, Wassmuth R, Lemke AJ, Sander B, Bechrakis NE & Felix R (1997) Uveal melanoma: detection of extraocular growth with MR imaging and US. *Radiology* 202: 61-67.

[72] Hungerford JL (1993) Surgical treatment of ocular melanoma. *Melanoma Res* 3: 305-312.

[73] Ibrahim N & Haluska FG (2009) Molecular pathogenesis of cutaneous melanocytic neoplasms. *Annu Rev Pathol* 4: 551-579.

[74] Jensen DE, Proctor M, Marquis ST, Gardner HP, Ha SI, Chodosh LA, Ishov AM, Tommerup N, Vissing H, Sekido Y, Minna J, Borodovsky A, Schultz DC, Wilkinson KD, Maul GG, Barlev N, Berger SL, Prendergast GC & Rauscher FJ, 3rd (1998) BAP1: a novel ubiquitin hydrolase which binds to the BRCA1 RING finger and enhances BRCA1-mediated cell growth suppression. *Oncogene* 16: 1097-1112.

[75] Kanthan GL, Jayamohan J, Yip D & Conway RM. (2007). Management of metastatic carcinoma of the uveal tract: an evidence-based analysis. In *Clin Experiment Ophthalmol*, Vol. 35. pp. 553-565.

[76] Karlsson UL, Augsburger JJ, Shields JA, Markoe AM, Brady LW & Woodleigh R (1989) Recurrence of posterior uveal melanoma after 60Co episcleral plaque therapy. *Ophthalmology* 96: 382-388.

[77] Khalili JS, Yu X, Wang J, Hayes BC, Davies MA, Lizee G, Esmaeli B & Woodman SE (2012) Combination Small Molecule MEK and PI3K Inhibition Enhances Uveal Melanoma Cell Death in a Mutant GNAQ- and GNA11-Dependent Manner. *Clin Cancer Res* 18: 4345-4355.

[78] Khan J & Damato BE (2007) Accuracy of choroidal melanoma diagnosis by general ophthalmologists: a prospective study. *Eye (Lond)* 21: 595-597.

[79] Kilic E, Bruggenwirth HT, Verbiest MM, Zwarthoff EC, Mooy NM, Luyten GP & de Klein A (2004) The RAS-BRAF kinase pathway is not involved in uveal melanoma. *Melanoma Res* 14: 203-205.

[80] Kilic E, Naus NC, van Gils W, Klaver CC, van Til ME, Verbiest MM, Stijnen T, Mooy CM, Paridaens D, Beverloo HB, Luyten GP & de Klein A (2005) Concurrent loss of chromosome arm 1p and chromosome 3 predicts a decreased disease-free survival in uveal melanoma patients. *Invest Ophthalmol Vis Sci* 46: 2253-2257.

[81] Kilic E, van Gils W, Lodder E, Beverloo HB, van Til ME, Mooy CM, Paridaens D, de Klein A & Luyten GP (2006) Clinical and cytogenetic analyses in uveal melanoma. *Invest Ophthalmol Vis Sci* 47: 3703-3707.

[82] Kinyoun JL, Lawrence BS & Barlow WE (1996) Proliferative radiation retinopathy. *Arch Ophthalmol* 114: 1097-1100.

[83] Krohn J, Froystein T & Dahl O. (2008). Posterior uveal melanoma. Distribution of the sites of origin and patterns of tumour extent in the ocular fundus. In *Br J Ophthalmol*, Vol. 92. pp. 751-756.

[84] Kumps C, Van Roy N, Heyrman L, Goossens D, Del-Favero J, Noguera R, Vandesompele J, Speleman F & De Preter K (2010) Multiplex Amplicon Quantification (MAQ), a fast and efficient method for the simultaneous detection of copy number alterations in neuroblastoma. *BMC Genomics* 11: 298.

[85] Landreville S, Agapova OA, Matatall KA, Kneass ZT, Onken MD, Lee RS, Bowcock AM & Harbour JW (2012) Histone deacetylase inhibitors induce growth arrest and differentiation in uveal melanoma. *Clin Cancer Res* 18: 408-416.

[86] Lavinsky D, Belfort RN, Navajas E, Torres V, Martins MC & Belfort R, Jr. (2007) Fundus autofluorescence of choroidal nevus and melanoma. *Br J Ophthalmol* 91: 1299-1302.

[87] Lee CS, Bae JH, Jeon IH, Byeon SH, Koh HJ & Lee SC. (2010). Melanocytoma of the optic disk in the Korean population. In *Retina (Philadelphia, Pa)*, Vol. 30. pp. 1714-1720.

[88] Li W, Judge H, Gragoudas ES, Seddon JM & Egan KM. (2000). Patterns of tumor initiation in choroidal melanoma. In *Cancer Res.*, Vol. 60. pp. 3757-3760.

[89] Lommatzsch PK, Werschnik C & Schuster E (2000) Long-term follow-up of Ru-106/Rh-106 brachytherapy for posterior uveal melanoma. *Graefes Arch Clin Exp Ophthalmol* 238: 129-137.

[90] Mafee MF, Peyman GA, Grisolano JE, Fletcher ME, Spigos DG, Wehrli FW, Rasouli F & Capek V (1986) Malignant uveal melanoma and simulating lesions: MR imaging evaluation. *Radiology* 160: 773-780.

[91] Manschot WA, Lee WR & van Strik R (1995) Uveal melanoma: updated considerations on current management modalities. *Int Ophthalmol* 19: 203-209.

[92] Mantel I, Uffer S & Zografos L (2009) Peripheral exudative hemorrhagic chorioretinopathy: a clinical, angiographic, and histologic study. *Am J Ophthalmol* 148: 932-938 e931.

[93] Margo CE, Mulla Z & Billiris K. (1998). Incidence of surgically treated uveal melanoma by race and ethnicity. In *Ophthalmology*, Vol. 105. pp. 1087-1090.

[94] Mariani P, Piperno-Neumann S, Servois V, Berry MG, Dorval T, Plancher C, Couturier J, Levy-Gabriel C, Lumbroso-Le Rouic L, Desjardins L & Salmon RJ (2009) Surgical management of liver metastases from uveal melanoma: 16 years' experience at the Institut Curie. *Eur J Surg Oncol* 35: 1192-1197.

[95] Mashayekhi A, Siu S, Shields CL & Shields JA (2011) Slow enlargement of choroidal nevi: a long-term follow-up study. *Ophthalmology* 118: 382-388.

[96] McCluskey PJ, Watson PG, Lightman S, Haybittle J, Restori M & Branley M. (1999). Posterior scleritis: clinical features, systemic associations, and outcome in a large series of patients. In *Ophthalmology*, Vol. 106. pp. 2380-2386.

[97] Mensink HW, Kilic E, Vaarwater J, Douben H, Paridaens D & de Klein A (2008) Molecular cytogenetic analysis of archival uveal melanoma with known clinical outcome. *Cancer Genet Cytogenet* 181: 108-111.

[98] Mensink HW, Vaarwater J, Kilic E, Naus NC, Mooy N, Luyten G, Bruggenwirth HT, Paridaens D & de Klein A (2009) Chromosome 3 intratumor heterogeneity in uveal melanoma. *Invest Ophthalmol Vis Sci* 50: 500-504.

[99] Meyer D, Ge J, Blinder KJ, Sinard J & Xu S. (1999). Malignant transformation of an optic disk melanocytoma. In *Am J Ophthalmol*, Vol. 127. pp. 710-714.

[100] Mooy CM, Luyten GP, de Jong PT, Luider TM, Stijnen T, van de Ham F, van Vroonhoven CC & Bosman FT (1995) Immunohistochemical and prognostic analysis of apoptosis and proliferation in uveal melanoma. *Am J Pathol* 147: 1097-1104.

[101] Mooy CM, Van der Helm MJ, Van der Kwast TH, De Jong PT, Ruiter DJ & Zwarthoff EC (1991) No N-ras mutations in human uveal melanoma: the role of ultraviolet light revisited. *Br J Cancer* 64: 411-413.

[102] Mouriaux F, Diorio C, Bergeron D, Berchi C & Rousseau A (2012) Liver function testing is not helpful for early diagnosis of metastatic uveal melanoma. *Ophthalmology* 119: 1590-1595.

[103] Mueller AJ, Talies S, Schaller UC, Hoops JP, Schriever S, Kampik A, Wowra B, Horstmann G & Mack A (2000) [Stereotaxic precision irradiation of large uveal melanomas with the gamma knife]

[104] Die stereotaktische Prazisionsbestrahlung grosser uvealer Melanome mit dem Gamma-Knife. *Ophthalmologe* 97: 537-545.

[105] Muscat S, Parks S, Kemp E & Keating D (2004) Secondary retinal changes associated with choroidal naevi and melanomas documented by optical coherence tomography. *Br J Ophthalmol* 88: 120-124.

[106] Muscat S, Srinivasan S, Sampat V, Kemp E, Parks S & Keating D (2001) Optical coherence tomography in the diagnosis of subclinical serous detachment of the macula secondary to a choroidal nevus. *Ophthalmic Surg Lasers* 32: 474-476.

[107] Nakamura S, Hikita, Yamakawa, Moriya, Yano, Furusato, Cameron & Rushing. (2012). A clinically challenging diagnosis of adenoma of the retinal pigment epithelium presenting with clinical features of choroidal hemangioma. In *OPTH* pp. 497.

[108] Naus NC, Zuidervaart W, Rayman N, Slater R, van Drunen E, Ksander B, Luyten GP & Klein A (2000) Mutation analysis of the PTEN gene in uveal melanoma cell lines. *Int J Cancer* 87: 151-153.

[109] Onken MD, Worley LA, Ehlers JP & Harbour JW (2004) Gene expression profiling in uveal melanoma reveals two molecular classes and predicts metastatic death. *Cancer Res* 64: 7205-7209.

[110] Onken MD, Worley LA, Long MD, Duan S, Council ML, Bowcock AM & Harbour JW (2008) Oncogenic mutations in GNAQ occur early in uveal melanoma. *Invest Ophthalmol Vis Sci* 49: 5230-5234.

[111] Packer S, Stoller S, Lesser ML, Mandel FS & Finger PT (1992) Long-term results of iodine 125 irradiation of uveal melanoma. *Ophthalmology* 99: 767-773; discussion 774.

[112] Pane AR & Hirst LW (2000) Ultraviolet light exposure as a risk factor for ocular melanoma in Queensland, Australia. *Ophthalmic Epidemiol* 7: 159-167.

[113] Parrella P, Caballero OL, Sidransky D & Merbs SL (2001) Detection of c-myc amplification in uveal melanoma by fluorescent in situ hybridization. *Invest Ophthalmol Vis Sci* 42: 1679-1684.

[114] Parrella P, Sidransky D & Merbs SL (1999) Allelotype of posterior uveal melanoma: implications for a bifurcated tumor progression pathway. *Cancer Res* 59: 3032-3037.

[115] Pe'er J (2012) Ruthenium-106 brachytherapy. *Dev Ophthalmol* 49: 27-40.

[116] Petrausch U, Martus P, Tonnies H, Bechrakis NE, Lenze D, Wansel S, Hummel M, Bornfeld N, Thiel E, Foerster MH & Keilholz U (2008) Significance of gene expression

analysis in uveal melanoma in comparison to standard risk factors for risk assessment of subsequent metastases. *Eye (Lond)* 22: 997-1007.

[117] Peyster RG, Augsburger JJ, Shields JA, Satchell TV, Markoe AM, Clarke K & Haskin ME (1985) Choroidal melanoma: comparison of CT, fundoscopy, and US. *Radiology* 156: 675-680.

[118] Pollock PM, Harper UL, Hansen KS, Yudt LM, Stark M, Robbins CM, Moses TY, Hostetter G, Wagner U, Kakareka J, Salem G, Pohida T, Heenan P, Duray P, Kallioniemi O, Hayward NK, Trent JM & Meltzer PS (2003) High frequency of BRAF mutations in nevi. *Nat Genet* 33: 19-20.

[119] Prescher G, Bornfeld N & Becher R (1990) Nonrandom chromosomal abnormalities in primary uveal melanoma. *J Natl Cancer Inst* 82: 1765-1769.

[120] Prescher G, Bornfeld N & Becher R (1994) Two subclones in a case of uveal melanoma. Relevance of monosomy 3 and multiplication of chromosome 8q. *Cancer Genet Cytogenet* 77: 144-146.

[121] Prescher G, Bornfeld N, Friedrichs W, Seeber S & Becher R (1995) Cytogenetics of twelve cases of uveal melanoma and patterns of nonrandom anomalies and isochromosome formation. *Cancer Genet Cytogenet* 80: 40-46.

[122] Prescher G, Bornfeld N, Hirche H, Horsthemke B, Jockel KH & Becher R (1996) Prognostic implications of monosomy 3 in uveal melanoma. *Lancet* 347: 1222-1225.

[123] Ratanatharathorn V, Powers WE, Grimm J, Steverson N, Han I, Ahmad K & Lattin PB (1991) Eye metastasis from carcinoma of the breast: diagnosis, radiation treatment and results. *Cancer Treat Rev* 18: 261-276.

[124] Richter MN, Bechrakis NE, Stoltenburg-Didinger G & Foerster MH. (2003). Transscleral resection of a ciliary body leiomyoma in a child: case report and review of the literature. In *Graefes Arch Clin Exp Ophthalmol*, Vol. 241. pp. 953-957.

[125] Richtig E, Langmann G, M uuml llner K & Smolle J. (2004). Ocular Melanoma: Epidemiology, Clinical Presentation and Relationship with Dysplastic Nevi. In *Neuropsychobiology*, Vol. 218. pp. 111-114.

[126] Robertson DM (2001) Melanoma endoresection: a perspective. *Retina* 21: 403-407.

[127] Ross JJ & Kemp EG (2009) Large choroidal osteoma with macular decalcification. *Retina* 29: 413-414.

[128] Rosset A, Zografos L, Coucke P, Monney M & Mirimanoff RO (1998) Radiotherapy of choroidal metastases. *Radiother Oncol* 46: 263-268.

[129] Rottinger EM, Heckemann R, Scherer E, Vogel M & Meyer-Schwickerath G (1976) Radiation therapy of choroidal metastases from breast cancer. *Albrecht Von Graefes Arch Klin Exp Ophthalmol* 200: 243-250.

[130] Saldanha G, Purnell D, Fletcher A, Potter L, Gillies A & Pringle JH (2004) High BRAF mutation frequency does not characterize all melanocytic tumor types. *Int J Cancer* 111: 705-710.

[131] Schaudig U, Hassenstein A, Bernd A, Walter A & Richard G (1998) Limitations of imaging choroidal tumors in vivo by optical coherence tomography. *Graefes Arch Clin Exp Ophthalmol* 236: 588-592.

[132] Schmidt-Pokrzywniak A, Jöckel K-H, Bornfeld N, Sauerwein W & Stang A. (2009). Positive interaction between light iris color and ultraviolet radiation in relation to the risk of uveal melanoma: a case-control study. In *Ophthalmology*, Vol. 116. pp. 340-348.

[133] Scholes AG, Liloglou T, Maloney P, Hagan S, Nunn J, Hiscott P, Damato BE, Grierson I & Field JK (2001) Loss of heterozygosity on chromosomes 3, 9, 13, and 17, including the retinoblastoma locus, in uveal melanoma. *Invest Ophthalmol Vis Sci* 42: 2472-2477.

[134] Scott IU, Murray TG & Hughes JR (1998) Evaluation of imaging techniques for detection of extraocular extension of choroidal melanoma. *Arch Ophthalmol* 116: 897-899.

[135] Seddon JM, Gragoudas ES, Albert DM, Hsieh CC, Polivogianis L & Friedenberg GR (1985) Comparison of survival rates for patients with uveal melanoma after treatment with proton beam irradiation or enucleation. *Am J Ophthalmol* 99: 282-290.

[136] Seddon JM, Gragoudas ES, Egan KM, Glynn RJ, Howard S, Fante RG & Albert DM (1990) Relative survival rates after alternative therapies for uveal melanoma. *Ophthalmology* 97: 769-777.

[137] Seregard S, aft Trampe E, Lax I, Kock E & Lundell G (1997) Results following episcleral ruthenium plaque radiotherapy for posterior uveal melanoma. The Swedish experience. *Acta Ophthalmol Scand* 75: 11-16.

[138] Shah CP, Weis E, Lajous M, Shields JA & Shields CL. (2005). Intermittent and Chronic Ultraviolet Light Exposure and Uveal Melanoma. In *Ophthalmology*, Vol. 112. pp. 1599-1607.

[139] Shields CL, Bianciotto C, Pirondini C, Materin MA, Harmon SA & Shields JA. (2008). Autofluorescence of choroidal melanoma in 51 cases. In *Br J Ophthalmol*, Vol. 92. pp. 617-622.

[140] Shields CL, Cater J, Shields JA, Singh AD, Santos MC & Carvalho C (2000) Combination of clinical factors predictive of growth of small choroidal melanocytic tumors. *Arch Ophthalmol* 118: 360-364.

[141] Shields CL, Furuta M, Berman EL, Zahler JD, Hoberman DM, Dinh DH, Mashayekhi A & Shields JA (2009a) Choroidal nevus transformation into melanoma: analysis of 2514 consecutive cases. *Arch Ophthalmol* 127: 981-987.

[142] Shields CL, Furuta M, Thangappan A, Nagori S, Mashayekhi A, Lally DR, Kelly CC, Rudich DS, Nagori AV, Wakade OA, Mehta S, Forte L, Long A, Dellacava EF, Kaplan

B & Shields JA. (2009b). Metastasis of uveal melanoma millimeter-by-millimeter in 8033 consecutive eyes. In *Arch Ophthalmol*, Vol. 127. pp. 989-998.

[143] Shields CL, Kaliki S, Furuta M, Mashayekhi A & Shields JA (2012) Clinical spectrum and prognosis of uveal melanoma based on age at presentation in 8,033 cases. *Retina* 32: 1363-1372.

[144] Shields CL, Salazar PF, Mashayekhi A & Shields JA. (2009c). Peripheral Exudative Hemorrhagic Chorioretinopathy Simulating Choroidal Melanoma in 173 Eyes. In *Ophthalmology*, Vol. 116. pp. 529-535. American Academy of Ophthalmology.

[145] Shields CL, Salazar PF, Mashayekhi A & Shields JA (2009d) Peripheral exudative hemorrhagic chorioretinopathy simulating choroidal melanoma in 173 eyes. *Ophthalmology* 116: 529-535.

[146] Shields CL, Shields JA, Gross NE, Schwartz GP & Lally SE (1997) Survey of 520 eyes with uveal metastases. *Ophthalmology* 104: 1265-1276.

[147] Shields CL, Shields JA, Kiratli H, De Potter P & Cater JR. (1995). Risk factors for growth and metastasis of small choroidal melanocytic lesions. In *Trans Am Ophthalmol Soc*, Vol. 93. pp. 259-275- discussion 275-259.

[148] Shields CL, Sun H, Demirci H & Shields JA. (2005a). Factors predictive of tumor growth, tumor decalcification, choroidal neovascularization, and visual outcome in 74 eyes with choroidal osteoma. In *Arch Ophthalmol*, Vol. 123. pp. 1658-1666.

[149] Shields JA. (1973). Lesions simulating malignant melanoma of the posterior uvea. In *Arch Ophthalmol*, Vol. 89. pp. 466-471.

[150] Shields JA, Demirci H, Mashayekhi A, Eagle Jr. RC & Shields CL. (2006). Melanocytoma of the optic disk: a review. In *Surv Ophthalmol*, Vol. 51. pp. 93-104.

[151] Shields JA, Demirci H, Mashayekhi A & Shields CL. (2004). Melanocytoma of optic disc in 115 cases. In *Ophthalmology*, Vol. 111. pp. 1739-1746.

[152] Shields JA, Eagle RC, Shields CL, Brown GC & Lally SE. (2009e). Malignant Transformation of Congenital Hypertrophy of the Retinal Pigment Epithelium. In *OPHTHA*, Vol. 116. pp. 2213-2216. Elsevier Inc.

[153] Shields JA, Mashayekhi A, Ra S & Shields CL (2005b) Pseudomelanomas of the posterior uveal tract: the 2006 Taylor R. Smith Lecture. *Retina* 25: 767-771.

[154] Shields JA, Shields CL & Donoso LA (1991) Management of posterior uveal melanoma. *Surv Ophthalmol* 36: 161-195.

[155] Shields JA, Shields CL, Eagle RC & De Potter P. (1994). Observations on seven cases of intraocular leiomyoma. The 1993 Byron Demorest Lecture. In *Arch Ophthalmol*, Vol. 112. pp. 521-528.

[156] Singh AD, Bergman L & Seregard S. (2005a). Uveal melanoma: epidemiologic aspects. In *Ophthalmol Clin North Am*, Vol. 18. pp. 75-84- viii.

[157] Singh AD, Damato BE, Pe'er J, Murphee AL & Perry JD. (2009). Essentials of Ophthalmic Oncology pp. 288. Slack Incorporated.

[158] Singh AD, De Potter P, Fijal BA, Shields CL, Shields JA & Elston RC (1998) Lifetime prevalence of uveal melanoma in white patients with oculo(dermal) melanocytosis. *Ophthalmology* 105: 195-198.

[159] Singh AD, Kalyani P & Topham A (2005b) Estimating the risk of malignant transformation of a choroidal nevus. *Ophthalmology* 112: 1784-1789.

[160] Singh AD, Rennie IG, Seregard S, Giblin M & McKenzie J. (2004). Sunlight exposure and pathogenesis of uveal melanoma. In *Surv Ophthalmol*, Vol. 49. pp. 419-428.

[161] Singh AD, Shields CL, De Potter P, Shields JA, Trock B, Cater J & Pastore D. (1996). Familial uveal melanoma. Clinical observations on 56 patients. In *Arch Ophthalmol*, Vol. 114. pp. 392-399.

[162] Singh AD, Shields CL, Shields JA, Eagle RC & De Potter P. (1995). Uveal melanoma and familial atypical mole and melanoma (FAM-M) syndrome. In *Ophthalmic Genet.*, Vol. 16. pp. 53-61.

[163] Singh AD & Topham A (2003) Incidence of uveal melanoma in the United States: 1973-1997. *Ophthalmology* 110: 956-961.

[164] Singh AD, Turell ME & Topham AK. (2011). Uveal Melanoma: Trends in Incidence, Treatment, and Survival. In *Ophthalmology*, Vol. 118. pp. 1881-1885. Elsevier Inc.

[165] Singh N, Kulkarni P, Aggarwal AN, Mittal BR, Gupta N, Behera D & Gupta A. (2012). Choroidal Metastasis as a Presenting Manifestation of Lung Cancer. In *Medicine*, Vol. 91. pp. 179-194.

[166] Sisley K, Parsons MA, Garnham J, Potter AM, Curtis D, Rees RC & Rennie IG (2000) Association of specific chromosome alterations with tumour phenotype in posterior uveal melanoma. *Br J Cancer* 82: 330-338.

[167] Sisley K, Rennie IG, Cottam DW, Potter AM, Potter CW & Rees RC (1990) Cytogenetic findings in six posterior uveal melanomas: involvement of chromosomes 3, 6, and 8. *Genes Chromosomes Cancer* 2: 205-209.

[168] Sisley K, Rennie IG, Parsons MA, Jacques R, Hammond DW, Bell SM, Potter AM & Rees RC (1997) Abnormalities of chromosomes 3 and 8 in posterior uveal melanoma correlate with prognosis. *Genes Chromosomes Cancer* 19: 22-28.

[169] Sobottka B, Schlote T, Krumpaszky HG & Kreissig I. (1998). Choroidal metastases and choroidal melanomas: comparison of ultrasonographic findings. In *Br J Ophthalmol*, Vol. 82. pp. 159-161.

[170] Spagnolo F, Caltabiano G & Queirolo P. (2012). Uveal melanoma. In *Cancer Treatment Reviews*, Vol. 38. pp. 549-553. Elsevier Ltd.

[171] Stanga PE, Lim JI & Hamilton P (2003) Indocyanine green angiography in chorioretinal diseases: indications and interpretation: an evidence-based update. *Ophthalmology* 110: 15-21; quiz 22-13.

[172] Sumich P, Mitchell P & Wang JJ. (1998). Choroidal nevi in a white population: the Blue Mountains Eye Study. In *Arch Ophthalmol*, Vol. 116. pp. 645-650.

[173] Summanen P, Immonen I, Kivela T, Tommila P, Heikkonen J & Tarkkanen A (1996) Radiation related complications after ruthenium plaque radiotherapy of uveal melanoma. *Br J Ophthalmol* 80: 732-739.

[174] Testa JR, Cheung M, Pei J, Below JE, Tan Y, Sementino E, Cox NJ, Dogan AU, Pass HI, Trusa S, Hesdorffer M, Nasu M, Powers A, Rivera Z, Comertpay S, Tanji M, Gaudino G, Yang H & Carbone M (2011) Germline BAP1 mutations predispose to malignant mesothelioma. *Nat Genet* 43: 1022-1025.

[175] Thibodeau SN, Bren G & Schaid D (1993) Microsatellite instability in cancer of the proximal colon. *Science* 260: 816-819.

[176] Tjho-Heslinga RE, Davelaar J, Kemme HM, de Vroome H, Oosterhuis JA, Bleeker JC & Leer JW (1999) Results of ruthenium irradiation of uveal melanomas: the Dutch experience. *Radiother Oncol* 53: 133-137.

[177] Toth-Molnar E, Hammer H & Olah J (2000) Cutaneous dysplastic naevi in uveal melanoma patients: markers for prognosis? *Melanoma Res* 10: 36-39.

[178] Tsina EK, Lane AM, Zacks DN, Munzenrider JE, Collier JM & Gragoudas ES (2005) Treatment of metastatic tumors of the choroid with proton beam irradiation. *Ophthalmology* 112: 337-343.

[179] Vaarwater J, van den Bosch T, Mensink HW, van Kempen C, Verdijk RM, Naus NC, Paridaens D, Bruggenwirth HT, Kilic E & de Klein A (2012) Multiplex ligation-dependent probe amplification equals fluorescence in-situ hybridization for the identification of patients at risk for metastatic disease in uveal melanoma. *Melanoma Res* 22: 30-37.

[180] Vajdic CM, Hutchins AM, Kricker A, Aitken JF, Armstrong BK, Hayward NK & Armes JE (2003) Chromosomal gains and losses in ocular melanoma detected by comparative genomic hybridization in an Australian population-based study. *Cancer Genet Cytogenet* 144: 12-17.

[181] Vajdic CM, Kricker A, Giblin M, McKenzie J, Aitken J, Giles GG & Armstrong BK (2002) Sun exposure predicts risk of ocular melanoma in Australia. *Int J Cancer* 101: 175-182.

[182] van den Bosch T, van Beek JG, Vaarwater J, Verdijk RM, Naus NC, Paridaens D, de Klein A & Kilic E (2012) Higher percentage of FISH-determined monosomy 3 and 8q amplification in uveal melanoma cells relate to poor patient prognosis. *Invest Ophthalmol Vis Sci* 53: 2668-2674.

[183] van Gils W, Lodder EM, Mensink HW, Kilic E, Naus NC, Bruggenwirth HT, van Ijcken W, Paridaens D, Luyten GP & de Klein A (2008) Gene expression profiling in uveal melanoma: two regions on 3p related to prognosis. *Invest Ophthalmol Vis Sci* 49: 4254-4262.

[184] van Hees CL, de Boer A, Jager MJ, Bleeker JC, Kakebeeke HM, Crijns MB, Vandenbroucke JP & Bergman W (1994) Are atypical nevi a risk factor for uveal melanoma? A case-control study. *J Invest Dermatol* 103: 202-205.

[185] Van Raamsdonk CD, Bezrookove V, Green G, Bauer J, Gaugler L, O'Brien JM, Simpson EM, Barsh GS & Bastian BC (2009) Frequent somatic mutations of GNAQ in uveal melanoma and blue naevi. *Nature* 457: 599-602.

[186] Van Raamsdonk CD, Griewank KG, Crosby MB, Garrido MC, Vemula S, Wiesner T, Obenauf AC, Wackernagel W, Green G, Bouvier N, Sozen MM, Baimukanova G, Roy R, Heguy A, Dolgalev I, Khanin R, Busam K, Speicher MR, O'Brien J & Bastian BC (2010) Mutations in GNA11 in uveal melanoma. *N Engl J Med* 363: 2191-2199.

[187] Ventii KH, Devi NS, Friedrich KL, Chernova TA, Tighiouart M, Van Meir EG & Wilkinson KD (2008) BRCA1-associated protein-1 is a tumor suppressor that requires deubiquitinating activity and nuclear localization. *Cancer Res* 68: 6953-6962.

[188] Verbeek AM (1985) Differential diagnosis of intraocular neoplasms with ultrasonography. *Ultrasound Med Biol* 11: 163-170.

[189] Virgili G, Gatta G, Ciccolallo L, Capocaccia R, Biggeri A, Crocetti E, Lutz J-M & Paci E. (2007). Incidence of Uveal Melanoma in Europe. In *Ophthalmology*, Vol. 114. pp. 2309-2315.e2302.

[190] Vrabec TR, Augsburger JJ, Gamel JW, Brady LW, Hernandez C & Woodleigh R (1991) Impact of local tumor relapse on patient survival after cobalt 60 plaque radiotherapy. *Ophthalmology* 98: 984-988.

[191] Weber A, Hengge UR, Urbanik D, Markwart A, Mirmohammadsaegh A, Reichel MB, Wittekind C, Wiedemann P & Tannapfel A (2003) Absence of mutations of the BRAF gene and constitutive activation of extracellular-regulated kinase in malignant melanomas of the uvea. *Lab Invest* 83: 1771-1776.

[192] Wei W, Mo J, Jie Y & Li B (2010) Adenoma of the retinal pigment epithelium: a report of 3 cases. *Can J Ophthalmol* 45: 166-170.

[193] White JS, McLean IW, Becker RL, Director-Myska AE & Nath J (2006) Correlation of comparative genomic hybridization results of 100 archival uveal melanomas with patient survival. *Cancer Genet Cytogenet* 170: 29-39.

[194] White VA, Chambers JD, Courtright PD, Chang WY & Horsman DE (1998) Correlation of cytogenetic abnormalities with the outcome of patients with uveal melanoma. *Cancer* 83: 354-359.

[195] Wiesner T, Obenauf AC, Murali R, Fried I, Griewank KG, Ulz P, Windpassinger C, Wackernagel W, Loy S, Wolf I, Viale A, Lash AE, Pirun M, Socci ND, Rutten A, Pal-

medo G, Abramson D, Offit K, Ott A, Becker JC, Cerroni L, Kutzner H, Bastian BC & Speicher MR (2011) Germline mutations in BAP1 predispose to melanocytic tumors. *Nat Genet* 43: 1018-1021.

[196] Wilder HC (1946) Intra-ocular tumors in soldiers, World War II. *Mil Surg* 99: 459-490.

[197] Wilson MW & Hungerford JL (1999) Comparison of episcleral plaque and proton beam radiation therapy for the treatment of choroidal melanoma. *Ophthalmology* 106: 1579-1587.

[198] Worley LA, Onken MD, Person E, Robirds D, Branson J, Char DH, Perry A & Harbour JW (2007) Transcriptomic versus chromosomal prognostic markers and clinical outcome in uveal melanoma. *Clin Cancer Res* 13: 1466-1471.

[199] Wu X, Zhu M, Fletcher JA, Giobbie-Hurder A & Hodi FS (2012) The protein kinase C inhibitor enzastaurin exhibits antitumor activity against uveal melanoma. *PLoS One* 7: e29622.

[200] Yang SS, Fu AD, McDonald HR, Johnson RN, Ai E & Jumper JM (2003) Massive spontaneous choroidal hemorrhage. *Retina* 23: 139-144.

[201] Zehetmayer M (2012) Stereotactic photon beam irradiation of uveal melanoma. *Dev Ophthalmol* 49: 58-65.

[202] Zehetmayer M, Kitz K, Menapace R, Ertl A, Heinzl H, Ruhswurm I, Georgopoulos M, Dieckmann K & Potter R (2000) Local tumor control and morbidity after one to three fractions of stereotactic external beam irradiation for uveal melanoma. *Radiother Oncol* 55: 135-144.

[203] Zhang J, Glatfelter AA, Taetle R & Trent JM (1999) Frequent alterations of evolutionarily conserved regions of chromosome 1 in human malignant melanoma. *Cancer Genet Cytogenet* 111: 119-123.

[204] Zografos L, Bercher L, Egger E, Chamot L, Gailloud C, Uffer S, Perret C & Markovits C (1992) [Treatment of eye tumors by accelerated proton beams. 7 years experience]

[205] Le traitement des tumeurs oculaires par faisceau de protons acceleres. 7 ans d'experience. *Klin Monbl Augenheilkd* 200: 431-435.

[206] Zuidervaart W, van Nieuwpoort F, Stark M, Dijkman R, Packer L, Borgstein AM, Pavey S, van der Velden P, Out C, Jager MJ, Hayward NK & Gruis NA (2005) Activation of the MAPK pathway is a common event in uveal melanomas although it rarely occurs through mutation of BRAF or RAS. *Br J Cancer* 92: 2032-2038.

Chapter 6

Recombinant DNA Technology in Emerging Modalities for Melanoma Immunotherapy

Vitali Alexeev, Alyson Pidich,
Daria Marley Kemp and Olga Igoucheva

Additional information is available at the end of the chapter

http://dx.doi.org/10.5772/55357

1. Introduction

The history of immunotherapy of cancer dates back to 1890s when New York surgeon William Coley used Streptococcus and Serratia bacterial extracts to treat cancer. Up to the mid-1930s 'Coley's mixed toxins,'' were used to treat various tumors. Better understanding of the human immune system led to the identification of a number of tumor-associated antigens (TAAs) in the 1980s [1] and development of various immunotherapeutic approaches. Of particular relevance to melanoma immunotherapy was the identification of various antigens expressed specifically in melanocytes and, respectively, in the majority of melanomas. These melanoma-associated antigens include tyrosinase (Tyr), a key enzyme in melanin biosynthesis, tyrosinase-related proteins 1 and 2 (TRP1, TRP2), gp100 (aka pmel17), Melan-a, and MART1. These and several other melanoma-associated antigens formed the basis for the immunologic targeting of the tumor. Up to date, multiple peptide, dendritic cell, adjuvant, lymphocyte, antibody, DNA and virus-based strategies were tested in pre-clinical and clinical studies with varying degrees of success. In recent years, identification of the specific antigenic MHC class I epitopes, advancements in genetic engineering, gene delivery, and cell-based therapeutic approaches allowed development of the novel melanoma-targeting immuno-therapeutics.

2. Genetic engineering of antigen-specific T cells

2.1. Recombinant T cell receptors

Identification of the tumor-reactive T cells among a population of the tumor-infiltrating lymphocytes led to the development of the T cell-based therapies, particularly to the strategy known as adoptive T cells transfer. This strategy is based on the isolation of the tumor-infiltrating lymphocytes following analysis of their ability to target tumor cells and clonal expansion of tumor-reactive T cells via stimulation of cell proliferation with anti-CD3 and antiCD28 antibodies in the presence of IL-2. Upon obtaining a large quantity (> 10^8 cells), these cells are infused back to a tumor-bearing patient along with the lymphodepleting chemotherapy to temporary knock down circulating immunocytes and repetitive administration of the IL-2 (Fig. 1).

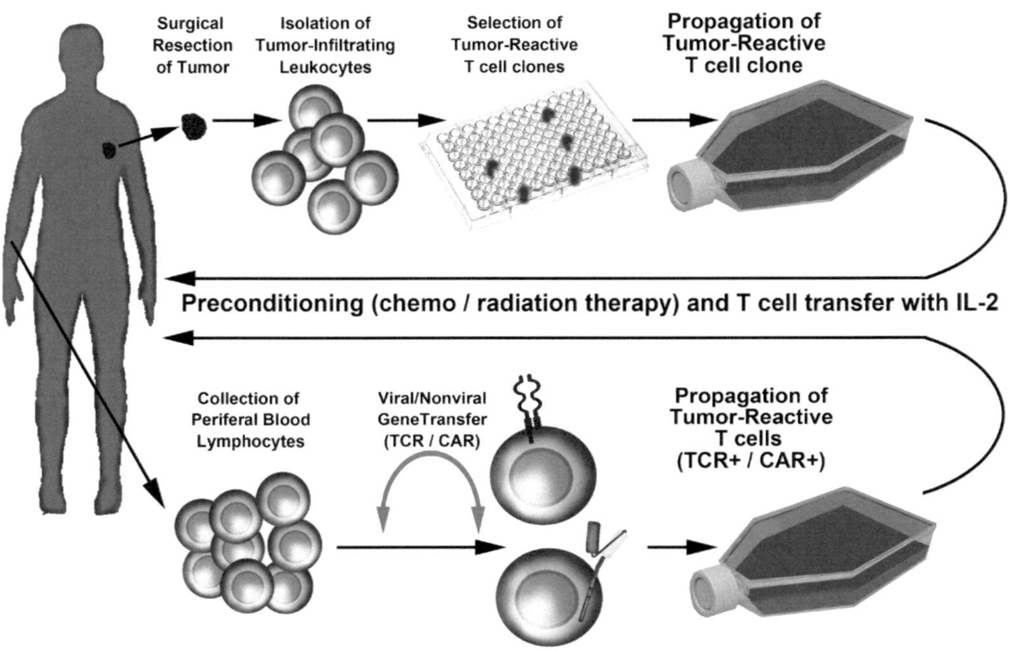

Figure 1. Clinical application of the T cell-mediated tumor immunotherapy. Diagram on the top depicts application of the Tumor-Infiltrating Lymphocytes (TILs). Diagram on the bottom illustrates application of the genetically engineered (TCR and CAR-modified) T cells.

Presently, 87 clinical trials using TIL are completed or on-going. These clinical trials are aimed at treatment of multiple cancers including: Malignant Melanoma, Nasopharyngeal Carcinoma, Hepatocellular Carcinoma, Breast Carcinoma, Leukemia, Lymphoma, Multiple Myeloma, Plasma Cell Neoplasm, Kidney Cancer, Metastatic Colorectal Cancer, Metastatic Gastric Cancer, Metastatic Pancreatic Cancer, Metastatic Hepatocellular Carcinoma, Cervical Cancer, Oropharyngeal Cancer, Vaginal Cancer, Anal Cancer, Penile Cancer, Non-Small Cell Lung Cancer, Brain and Central Nervous System Tumors. Several completed clinical trials on malignant melanoma clearly demonstrated that infusing TILs along with IL-2 and preconditioning with reduced-intensity circulating lymphocyte-depleting chemotherapy mediates tumor-targeting immune response in up to 50% of patients [2]. The highest response rate up to 70 % with up to 30% complete remission lasting for up to 3 years was reported when radiation sensitization was used in conjunction with the transfer of the tumor-reactive TILs.

Despite the success of the pioneering studies at the Surgery Branch of the US National Cancer Institute and the consequent clinical trials, this approach, although holding much promise in treating melanoma, is facing several challenges that limit broad application of the TIL-based immunotherapy. As TILs are isolated from resected tumors, the first and foremost requirement is the eligibility for surgery, which should be conducted, preferably, in the facility equipped for the isolation of TILs, identification and expansion of the tumor-reactive T cells. *Ex vivo* stimulation and propagation of TILs to large quantities required for the effective immunotherapy is time-consuming, labor-retaining, and expensive. Although recent clinical studies showed that infusion of the minimally cultured TILs without pre-selection for tumor reactivity provide a rather high response rate [3], the search for a better melanoma-targeting strategy is on-going.

Nevertheless, isolation of the individual melanoma-reactive T cell clones allowed the development of another immunotherapeutic approach – generation of the T cells expressing recombinant antigen specific T cell receptors (TCRs). TCRs are members of the immunoglobulin family proteins. Each TCR consists of 2 different membrane-anchored chains that are joined by the disulfide bridges to form heterodimer. About 95% of the T cells are characterized by the expression of the α and β chains, whereas the remaining 5% express γ and δ chains. Respectively, T cells expressing these receptors are often referred to as α/β and γ/δ T cells. Each chain is comprised of the variable and constant regions. The variable domain of both α- and β-chains have three hypervariable regions also known as complementarity determining regions (CDR), however, the β-chain has an additional area of hypervariability that is not involved in antigen binding. TCR α and γ chains are generated within T cells by VJ recombination, whereas β and δ chains by the V(D)J recombination. Currently, the majority of the TILs selected for the ability to target tumors are α/β T cells expressing respective TCR chains that determine T cell specificity to an antigenic peptides presented by the major histocompatability complex (MHC) proteins. Therefore, it was proposed that sequences encoding tumor antigen recognizing TCR chains can be obtained from tumor-reactive T cells and then used for the gene transfer into patient-derived lymphocytes, thereby creating large quantities of tumor-reactive T cells. The first TCRs specific to melanocytic antigens MART-1 and gp-100 were cloned in 1990s. Pioneering clinical studies using human peripheral blood lymphocytes transduced with these TCRs demonstrated melanoma regression in lymphodepleted patients [4] (Fig. 1). Although these and other initial clinical studies demonstrated a feasibility of the recombinant T cells-based approach, they also revealed multiple challenges. For example, the ability of recombinant TCR chains to interact and pair with the endogenous chains could lead to the generation of 4 different TCRs in a single cell (Fig. 2). Chain misparing decreases the expression of the function, tumor-reactive TCRs and therefore reduces T cell-mediated tumor targeting. To overcome misparing, several strategies were proposed. Recent pre-clinical and clinical studies demonstrated that replacement of the human TCR constant region with murine counterpart reduced misparing and allowed enhanced expression of the functional TCRs and improved T cell functional activity [5]. It was also reported that targeted mutagenesis and generation of the additional cystein residues in recombinant α and β chains permitted stronger pairing of these chains, higher expression of functional TCRs and improved T cell function [6, 7]. Recent studies also showed that targeting of the endogenous chains by siRNA allows higher expression of the functional recombinant TCR. Of particular interest is the proposed approach to encode siRNA along with the TCR chains to concurrently express recombinant and inhibit translation of the endogenous chains [8]. Protein engineering was also employed to improve pairing of the recombinant chains. Thus, substitution of specific amino acids within constant regions of the antigen-specific TCRs supported paring and enhanced functional activity of these receptors [9]. It remains to be determined which of these recombinant DNA-based methods will provide better targeting of melanoma (Fig. 2). Nevertheless, recent studies using chimeric murine-human hybrid highly avid tyrosinase-specific TCR demonstrated a favorable clinical outcome [10].

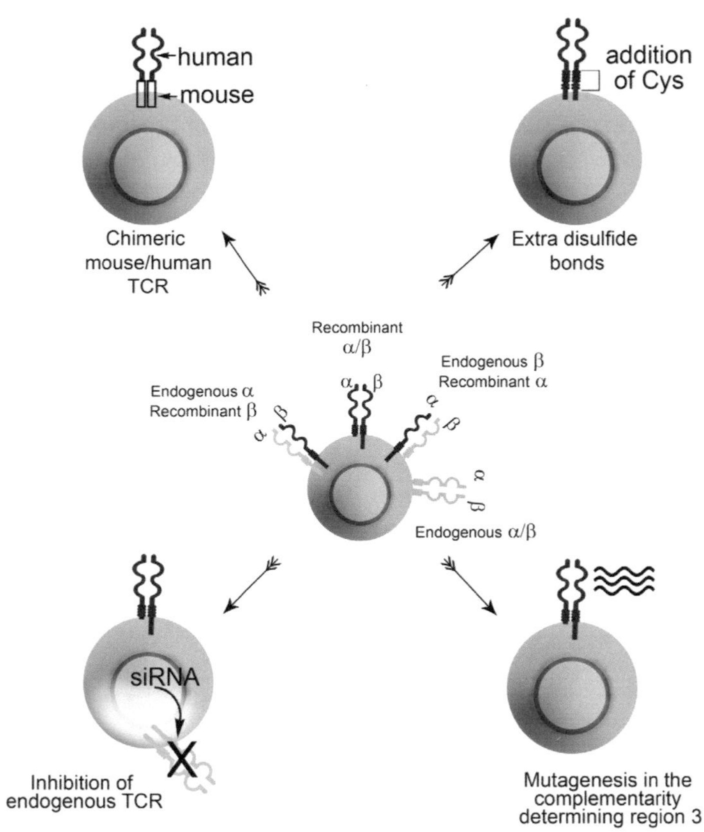

Figure 2. Strategies aimed at the improvement of the recombinant TCR pairing. Expression of the recombinant TCR may lead to the generation of 4 different TCRs within a cell (center). Different strategies designed to improve tumor-specific recombinant TCR pairing and activity include: generation of hybrid molecules containing the constant region from murine TCR, addition of disulfide bonds, alteration of the amino acid sequence within the TCR chains, and siRNA-mediated inhibition of the endogenous TCR gene expression (see text for details).

It is apparent that both α and β chains of the antigen-specific TCR should be expressed in each individual T cell. To date, internal ribosomal entry site (IRES) elements [11], double promoters [12], or co-infection with several viral vectors [13] were used to express several heterologous proteins in cells. However, these methods have their imperfections. For instance, in IRES-mediated co-expression, the upstream protein is usually more strongly transcribed than the downstream protein. Expression of the proteins from two different or biscistronic promoters or the use of multiples viruses also do not provide equal concurrent expression of multiple transgenes. A more promising approach involves the use of the self-processing viral peptide bridges such as 2A or 2A-like peptides described in Picornaviridae [14]. In picornavirus, these sequences share a highly conservative 18 amino acids motif mediating cleavage between C-terminal glycine and N-terminal proline of the 2B peptide. At present 2a and 2A-like sequences are commonly refer to as *cis*-acting hydrolase elements that allows ribosome skipping and cellular expression of multiple, discrete proteins in essentially equimolar quantities derived from a single ORF. To ensure concurrent expression of both α and β chains of the transgenic TCR an A2 sequence is most commonly used for quantitative co-expression of these heterologous proteins.

Transfer of the recombinant TCR genes into the T cells is another somewhat limiting factor for the broad application of the genetically engineered T cells for melanoma immuno-targeting. Currently, for human applications, a gene transfer platform that can mediate stable transfer of the TCR genes is retroviral system [15]. Lentiviral vectors and transposons were also tested [16, 17]. Use of retroviruses provided several advantages including a rather high infectivity and rapid integration of the transgene into host genome. With multiple vector backbones, virus packaging cell lines, and well-established GMP protocols, a retroviral system offers relative simplicity of viral vector construction and production of viruses. Since retroviruses can infect only dividing cells, stimulation of the T cell proliferation must be done prior to the gene transfer. Also, these viruses have limited capacity for the packaging. For instance, high virus titers cannot be obtained with larger retroviral vectors. Although an average size of a viral vector encoding typical α/β TCR is around 7 kb, this limits possible alternative approaches such as inclusion of various regulatory elements or another transgenes that may enhance T cell activation. Use of the viral system also presents certain safety concerns relevant to the random integration of the transgenes into the host genome that may result in the activation of oncogenes or inactivation of tumor suppressors. This may lead to the various adverse invents including development of a lymphoproliferative disease resembling leukemia due, in part, to the integration of the retroviral gene transfer vehicle near an oncogene [18, 19]. Thus far, the development of lymphoma-like symptoms has not been reported in patients treated with recombinant T cells. It is also essential to note that production of the TCR-encoding cGMP virus substantially increases the cost of the treatment with recombinant T cells. On the contrary to the retrovirus-based gene transfer, lentiviruses can infect non-dividing cells and therefore can be used for the gene transfer into quiescent T cells. Although "safe" lentiviral systems are developed to minimize the chance of producing replication-competent virus (eg. ViaraSafe from Cell Biolabs), transduction of patient-derived T cells for the adoptive transfer will always present some degree of risk.

Besides viral approaches, non-viral gene transfer may also be used for the expression of the TCRs in T cells. Recently, a Sleeping Beauty Transposon System was tested for the transduction of the T cells [17]. Sleeping Beauty Transposon System consists of two components - the transposon, composed of inverted terminal repeat sequences (IRs) with desired genetic material in between, and a SB transposase enzyme. Most recently, a number of IRs and hyperactive transposases with increasing enzymatic activities were developed to mediate transposition of transposon-encoding proteins into the genomic DNA [20]. Although transposition of SB transposons appears to be unregulated, it has certain advantages over viral based approaches. For instance, expression of transgenes, TCRs in particular, could be regulated by specific promoters that provide either T cell specific expression (eg. CD3 promoter; [21, 22]), or high level of expression (eg. elongation factor 1 promoter; [23,24]. Promoters may also be selected for further specific applications (discussed below). On the contrary to the viral gene transfer, non-viral systems also permit significantly simpler production of the cGMP-grade material (plasmid DNA) and lesser safety testing. Up to date, the Sleeping Beauty transposon-mediated approach was shown to mediate a long-term stable integration of the T-cell receptor genes targeting melanoma-derived antigen, MART-1, in laboratory settings (Fig. 3b). This system provided 50% efficiency of the TCR integration into the genome of the T cells and sustained functional reactivity of lymphocytes to the antigen-positive melanoma [25].

Other non-viral strategies could be useful in genetic engineering of the T cells. For example, integrase-mediated insertion of the genetic material may provide stable, site-directed integration of the transgenes (TCRs) into T cell genome. This strategy involves integrase from the *Streptomyces* phage ΦC31 that catalyzes unidirectional recombination between attP motifs in phage and attB sites in bacterial genomes. Usually attP and attB sites are cleaved and joined to each other, generating two hybrid sequences (attL and attR) that flank the integrated phage genome. However, ΦC31 integrase can also recognize several endogenous sequences in eukaryotic chromosomes as attP sites and integrate attB-bearing transgenes into them (Fig. 3c). Such pseudo attP sites were found in every mammalian genome with more than 100 ΦC31 integration sites identified in human cells. Thus far, only three preferred sites located in human Xq22.1, 8p22, 19q13.31 loci are commonly used by this enzyme [26, 27]. Therefore, ΦC31-integrase-based system is somewhat similar to the SB transposone system (Fig. 3b, c). Yet, it provides better specificity of the transgene integration. We recently tested whether ΦC31 can efficiently integrate transgenes into the T cells. Our initial data using GFP-encoding reporter plasmid with short (34bp) attB site demonstrated that nucleofection reaction provides rather efficient transduction of the transgene and ΦC31 integrase-encoding plasmids into T cells (Fig. 4a) and stable, integrase-dependent insertion of the reporter into both CD4+ and CD8+ T cells (Fig. 4b). Transduction of the T cells with tyrosinase-specific TCR (described in 10) ligated into the attB-harboring mammalian expression vector also resulted in the sustained expression of this melanoma-specific TCR and the ability of the T cells to target antigen-positive melanoma cells *in vitro* (Fig. 4c)

Collectively, viral and non-viral strategies for the genetic engineering of the T cells expressing melanoma-specific TCRs are suitable for the *ex vivo* production of large quantities (more than 10^8 cells) of the tumor-specific T cells that can be used for the adoptive T cell transfer. However, clinical utility of the non-viral approaches remains to be elucidated. In spite of T cell trans-

http://dx.doi.org/10.5772/55357

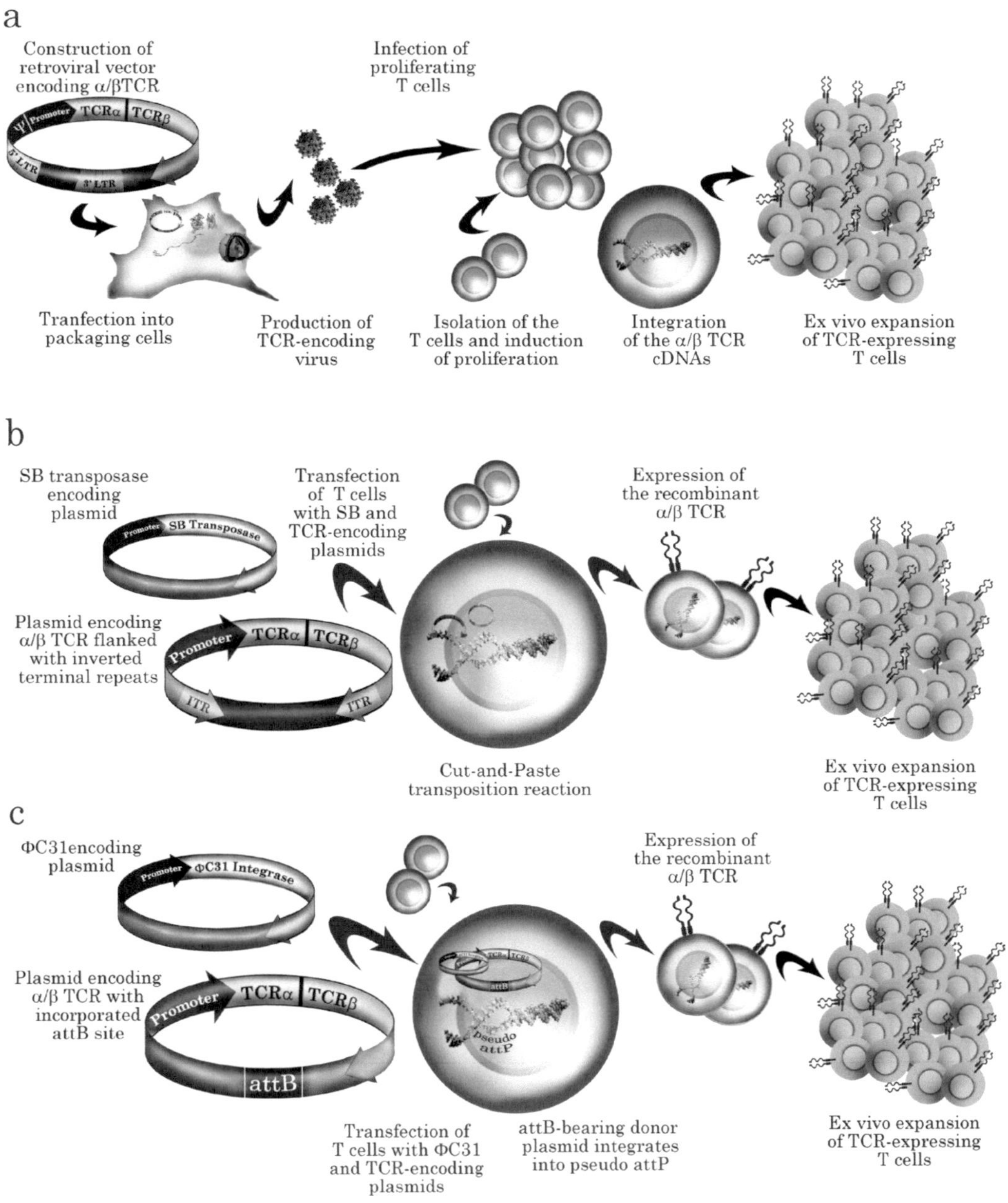

Figure 3. Schematic diagram depicting genetic engineering of the tumor-targeting T cells expressing recombinant TCR. Diagrams depict generation of the recombinant T cells via (a) retrovirus-mediated gene transfer, (b) Sleeping Beauty transposon-mediated gene transposition, and (c) ΦC31 integrase-mediated gene insertion (see text for details).

duction strategy, it is clear that the ability to generate melanoma-specific recombinant T cell receptors allowed significant advancement in the development of the clinically-applicable TCR-based approach for melanoma immunotherapy. Its primary advantages are in the use of

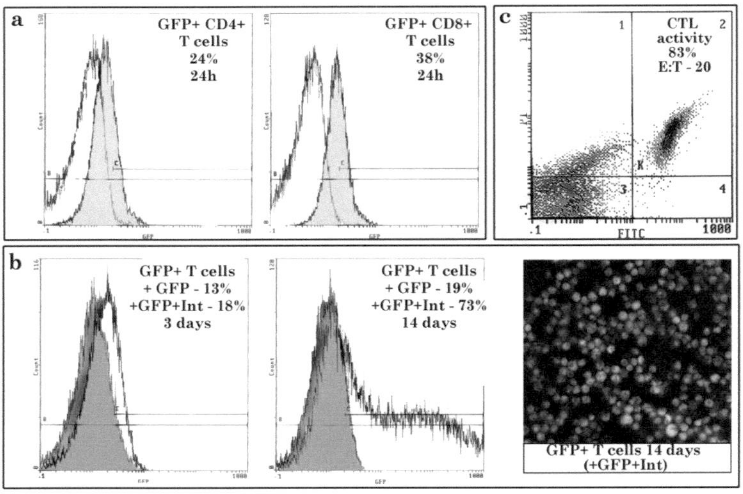

Figure 4. ΦC31 integrase-mediated genetic modification of the T cells. (a) Example showing typical nucleofection reaction of the reporter gene (GFP) into freshly isolated T cells 24 hours post Nucleofection (representative FACS profiles). (b) Analysis of the GFP expression after Nucleofection of the T cells in the presence of absence of the ΦC31 integrase-encoding plasmid (representative profiles and the direct fluorescent microscopy) 3 and 14 days after Nucleofection. (c) FACS-based analysis of the CTL activity of the recombinant T cells generated to express tyrosinase-specific TCR against human melanoma in vitro (representative profile). Times and percentages are indicated in the panels; Shaded Profiles – GFP-positive cells (see text for details).

a natural and a rather well-understood mechanism of the T cell function and the ability to select/generate multiple melanoma-reactive TCRs that can be used alone or in combination. Currently, several melanoma-targeting TCRs specific to tyrosinase, MART-1, and gp100 were cloned. One can envision generation of TCR-encoding cDNA banks that could be utilized for the generation of different melanoma-reacting T cells from the pool of patient-derived T cells to target several TAAs. However, this strategy has several disadvantages including restriction of specific TCRs to one HLA type, dependence from the expression and presentation of an antigen, limited intracellular signaling from the recombinant α/β TCRs, misparing of TCR chains, and the inability to target non-protein tumor antigens.

At present time, about 20 clinical studies involving melanoma-specific T cells expressing recombinant TCR were conducted in US alone (some of them reviewed in [28]). The result of some of the completed trials opened new perspectives for the improvement of the TCR-based strategies. For instance, adoptive transfer of the T cells genetically engineered to express highly avid MART-1-specific TCR has achieved objective clinical responses in a 13% of treated patients [29]. Analysis of CTL-resistant tumor cell revealed that these resistant clones exhibited hyperactivation of the NF-κB survival pathway and overexpression of the antiapoptotic Bcl-2, Bcl-x, Bcl-$_{xL}$, and Mcl-1 genes [30]. These studies suggest that sensitivity of melanoma to the recombinant T cells could be increased by the pharmacological inhibition of the NF-κB pathway and/or Bcl-2 family members. Multiple investigative studies are on-going to further improve recombinant TCR-based approach.

2.2. Chimeric antigen receptors

Independently, an alternative approach involving recombinant DNA technology was developed to generate tumor-targeting T cells. It utilizes fusion of the variable chain of the tumor-antigen-specific antibody, TCR constant region, and intracellular signaling domains. Initially, these structures were called T-bodies [31]. They are comprise of the single-chain antibody (sFv), TCR transmembrane domain and the intracellular signaling domain of the TCR-ζ. One of the first tumor associated antigens targeted by T cells expressing T-bodies was erbB2 (HER2/neu) receptor that is over-expressed in multiple cancers [32]. Later, a more general term – chimeric antigen receptors or CARs emerged. As compared to the TCRs, CARs allow overcoming dependency on HLA type, antigen presentation, and restricted intracellular signaling of the recombinant α/β TCRs. Initial studies with T-bodies (and recombinant TCRs) demonstrated a rather short lifespan of the engineered T cells and the inability of the recombinant receptors to fully support persistence of the T cell. To address this issue, several studies were conducted to identify the most potent CAR structures by testing several signaling molecules involved in T cell activation (Fig. 5). It was demonstrated that fusion of TCR-ζ with the intracellular domain of CD28 can augment cytokine production by CAR-expressing T cells upon encountering antigen and enhance antitumor efficacy [33]. Inclusion of CD134 (OX-40) into CAR structure also led to the elevated tumoricidal activity of the recombinant T cells [34]. Comparative analysis of the different CARs comprised of TCR-ζ signal transduction domain, CD28 and/or CD137 (4-1BB) intracellular domains demonstrated that addition of the CD137 supports T cell function to a greater extent as compared to other constructs [35]. Collectively, addition of these signaling domains to the CAR structure allowed overcoming (to certain extent) inefficient effector function and anergic status of the T cells.

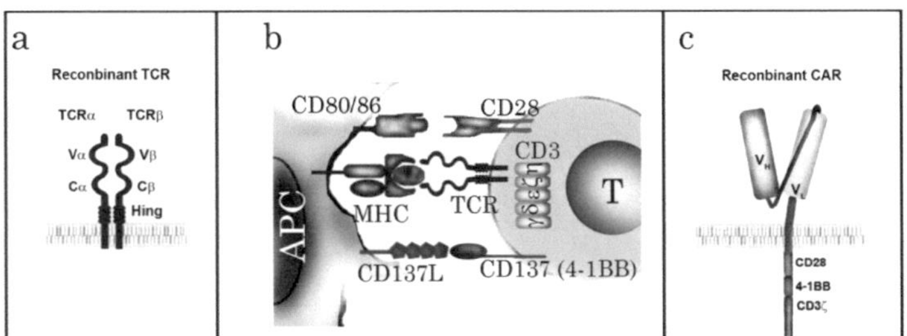

Figure 5. Recombinant TCR and CAR structures. (a) Diagram depicting recombinant TCR structure. (b) Diagram illustrating molecular interactions involved in TCR-mediated pro-proliferation and pro-survival intracellular signaling including engagement of the CD28, CD3, and CD137 (4-1BB). (c) Diagram depicting recombinant CAR structure with CD3ξ, CD137 (4-1BB), and CD28 signaling domains (see text for details).

As recognition of target cells by CAR depends on the antibody, CARs can recognize not only polypeptides but also non-protein molecules such as tumor-associated glycolipids and carbohydrates. However, antibody-mediated binding require surface expression of an antigen and strict selection of TAAs to avoid autoimmune side effects. Also, use of the mouse monoclonal antibody sequences in CAR design may lead to the unwanted immune recognition of the CAR-expressing T cells and limit long-term clinical use [36, 37]. Nevertheless, existence of a large number of the tumor antigen-specific antibodies and robust anti-tumor response by CAR-expressing T cells suggest great clinical utility of these recombinant molecules. Currently, in US alone there are 18 clinical trials aimed at treatment of various malignancies with CAR-engineered leukocytes, with 16 trials in the recruitment phase. Eight of them are aimed at targeting different B cell malignancies with anti-CD19-CAR. Three trials are intended to test HER2-specific CAR-modified T cells for the treatment of sarcoma, glioblastoma, and advanced Her2-positive lung malignancy.

With regard to melanoma, several CAR designs were tested for the ability to target this malignancy. Thus, recent studies demonstrated that treatment of melanoma xenografts in nude mice using engineered T cells expressing tandem CAR (CD28/TCRζ) specific to ganglioside GD3 with IL2 supplementation led to complete remissions of the established tumors in 50 % of treated animals [38]. As GD3 is often over-expressed in melanoma, this approach could be potent in eliminating melanoma in human patients.

Another attractive target for the CAR-mediated T cell therapy for melanoma is a high molecular weight melanoma-associated antigen (HMW-MAA) encoded by CSPG4 gene. This is a cell-surface proteoglycan expressed on more than 90% of the tumors. Recent studies on targeting of this antigen using CAR that is comprised of the anti- HMW-MAA antibody chain and intracellular signaling domains of the CD28, CD137, and CD3ζ demonstrated that T cell genetically modified to express this CAR were cytolytic to the HMW-MAA–positive melanoma cells, produced cytokine and proliferate *in vitro* [39]. The potential clinical utility of the CAR-mediated HMW-MAA targeting was emphasized by another recent animal study [40]. Analysis of a few human melanoma biopsies revealed the presence of less than 2% of specific tumor cells co-expressing CD20 and HMW-MAA. Implantation of tumors containing these CD20+ HMW-MAA+ cells into immuno-deficient mice resulted in a rapid growth of tumors. Targeting of these pre-established lesions with T cells expressing either CD20 or HMW-MAA-directed CAR showed elimination of lesions in nearly 90% of treated animals. CD20-specific engineered T cells were unable to eradicated melanoma lesions artificially expressing CD20 suggesting that native expression of the antigen is required for effective targeting. These studies provided additional evidence that direction of the T cells toward HMW-MAA via genetic engineering can permit effective elimination of tumor lesions.

As progression of most tumors including melanoma depends on the microenvironment, T-cell mediated targeting of the microenvironmental components could also be a viable strategy for melanoma immunotherapy. Particularly, tumor survival was shown to be dependent on the *de novo* formation of the intratumoral blood vessels characterised by high levels of the vascular endothelial growth factor receptor 2 (VEGFR2/KDR). Also, a number of studies associated high levels of VEGFR2 expression with various tumor stroma cells including subsets of macrophages, immature monocytes, immature dendritic cells and immuno-suppressive CD4+CD25+ regulatory T cells (Treg) [41-46]. Therefore, it was suggested that targeting of VEGFR2 – positive cells in tumor stroma may provide clinical benefits and tumor regression. In support of this notion, recent studies demonstrated that the direction of the T cells toward VEGFR-2 via CAR provide an effective means to eliminate pre-established experimental melanoma.

Thus, using an animal model, it was shown that after systemic transplantation, anti–VEGFR-2 CAR and IL-12–co-transduced T cells infiltrated the tumors, expanded and persisted within tumor mass leading to tumor regression [47]. The anti-tumor effect was dependent on targeting of IL-12–responsive host cells via activation of anti–VEGFR-2 CAR-T cells and release of IL-12. Based on this data, one clinical trial aimed at the assessment of safety and effectiveness of cell therapy was initiated to treat recurrent and relapsed cancer by using anti-VEGFR2 CAR-modified T cells.

Presently, there is an accumulating body of evidence suggesting clinical utility of the T cell genetically engineered to express melanoma antigen-specific CARs. It is likely that in the near future CAR-mediated targeting of different melanoma antigens will evolve into general practice of cancer immunotherapy.

3. DNA vaccination

Another immunotherapeutic approach directly relevant to recombinant DNA is genetic or DNA vaccination. The original idea of DNA vaccination emanated from the observations that intramuscular injection of DNA encoding influenza A virus protein resulted in the robust activation of the immune responses that protected the host from viral challenge [48]. Generally, DNA-mediated activation of immune response involves multiple processes. First, plasmid DNA should be delivered intracellularly and expressed in the host cells. Next, in most of cases the antigen has to be secreted from the cells and picked up by the dendritic cells (DC), processed and presented in the context of the MHC class II to the CD4+ T helper (Th) cells. Alternatively, if the antigen is expressed directly in the DCs, it could be processed intracellularly and presented via MHC class I molecules, leading to the activation of the CD8+ T cells and induction of the cytotoxic immune responses. Initial studies on DNA vaccination were carried out using an intramuscular route of vaccine administration (Fig. 6). This allowed high levels of antigen expression and secretion from the elongated muscle cells into perimysium, the resident site of the intramuscular DCs. Later, DNA vaccination through the skin was suggested to be superior over the intramuscular route. Skin has evolved as a barrier to prevent the entry of pathogens, with efficient immune surveillance complex including Langerhans cells, dendritic cells, lymphocytes, and other leukocytes. Skin is also rich in lymphatic vasculature network that provides an efficient route for DC and T cell trafficking. Depending on the physical methods of into-skin DNA delivery, DNA-based vaccines can be targeted to specific locations in the skin [49].

The DNA vaccination approach has several advantages over other types of vaccinations: (i) multiple expression vectors coding for different antigen and co-stimulatory molecules can be concurrently delivered into the skin (or the muscle); (ii) the use of cell-type-specific promoters can provide specificity of protein expression; (iii) protein expression from designed plasmids can be controlled by inducible promoters, the use of ubiquitous chromatin opening elements (UCOE), or chemically (e.g. sodium butyrate). Also of note is the relative simplicity and inexpensiveness of the cGMP grade DNA vaccine production and pre-clinical testing. These

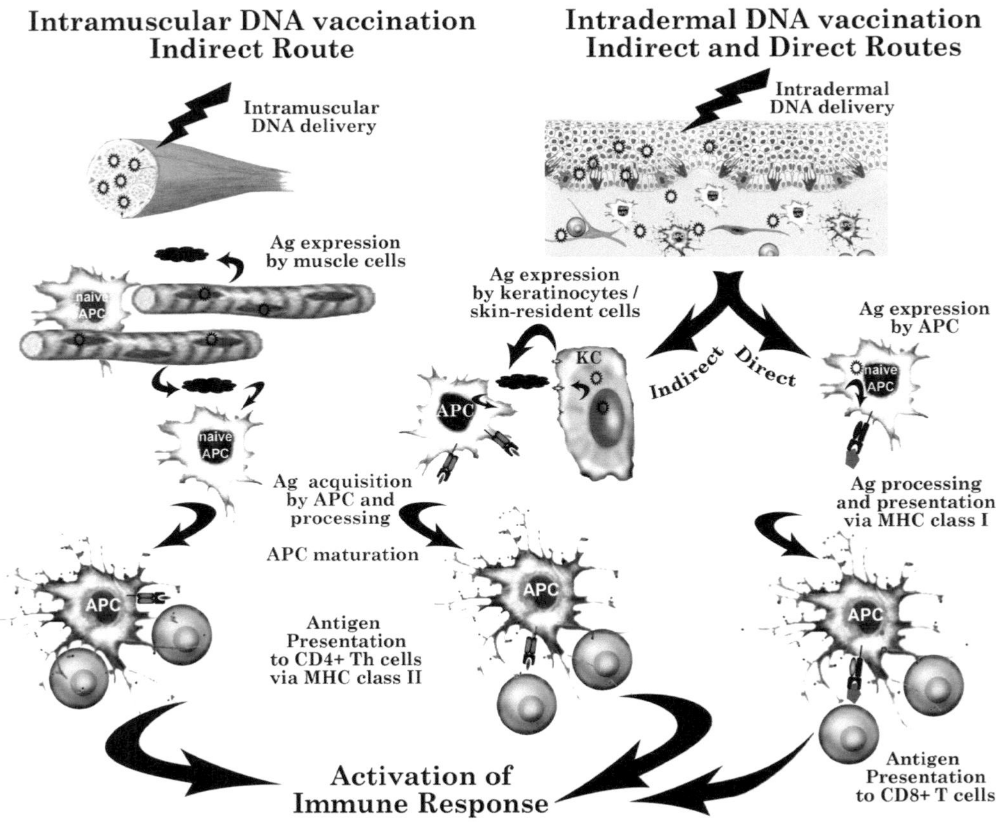

Figure 6. Intramuscular and Intradermal DNA vaccination. Intramuscular and intradermal sites are used for DNA vaccination. The former allows high level of antigen (Ag) expression in muscle cells and MHC class II Ag processing and presentation whereas the latter permits expression of the Ag in the Antigen-Presenting Cells (APC) and direct presentation of the antigenic peptides to the CD8+ cytotoxic T cells (see text for details).

attractive characteristics of DNA vaccines have prompted extensive research within the past 10 years.

Multiple studies on pre-clinical animal models of melanoma and other cancers have been conducted. Studies on the canine model of aggressive and metastatic melanoma (stages II-IV) demonstrated that xenogeneic vaccination of dogs with DNA vaccine coding for human tyrosinase led to an excellent clinical response in the majority of vaccinated dogs. A long-term survival of dogs with advanced stage IV disease with bulky lung metastases (on average 400 days) was observed [50]. Vaccinated dogs with stage II/III disease also had long-term survivals (on average 500 days) with no evidence of melanoma on necropsy. Overall, median survival time for all treated dogs was 389 days. Another canine model study [51] showed that xenogeneic DNA vaccination induces melanoma-specific antibody response, which coincides with observed clinical responses. As a result, in 2010 Merial, an animal health company has gained full-licensure from the U.S. Department of Agriculture (USDA) for ONCEPT™ Canine

Melanoma DNA Vaccine. Up to date, ONCEPT is the first and only USDA-approved therapeutic vaccine for the treatment of cancer in either animals or humans. (The first DNA vaccine was licensed by the USDA in 2005 for prevention of West Nile virus infection in horses).

However, presently only a few human clinical trials on DNA vaccination were conducted. One of such study, aimed at the evaluation of the immune response in patients with hormone-refractory prostate cancer showed that DNA vaccination with a prostate-specific antigen (PSA) encoding plasmid given with GM-CSF and IL-2 is safe in doses of up to 900 μg, and that the vaccination can induce cellular and humoral immune responses [52].

Similar to the reference above canine studies, DNA vaccines were shown to be effective in mouse melanoma models when mice were vaccinated with heterologous DNA encoding human melanoma-associated antigen gp-100 [53]. This vaccination regimen was augmented by the GM-CSF and was most effective in the prophylactic setting. It was also effective in suppressing pre-established melanoma. However, vaccinations with autologous mouse melanoma antigens were less successful. Nevertheless, the relative simplicity of modifying recombinant DNA allowed testing of various genetic alterations aimed at breaking the immunologic tolerance and enhancing immune responses to DNA vaccines. For example, concurrent vaccination with DNA encoding several melanoma-specific epitopes can be used. This approach was tested in several studies with different degree of success. As a result, vaccination of mice with $gp100_{25-33}$ and $TRP\text{-}2_{181-188}$ encoding minigene was effective in preventing melanoma development [54]. As many of the melanoma MHC class I epitopes were characterized for melanoma including those derived from tyrosinase, TRP1, TRP2, gp-100, MART-1, and MC-1R (some of them shared between mouse and human MHC molecules [55], one can envision generation of an ultimate genetic immunogen capable of targeting several melanoma-associated antigens.

Recombinant DNA technology has also allowed introduction of immuno-augmentation sequences into the DNA vaccine composition. Identified universal pan HLA DR helper binding epitope (PADRE; KXVAAWYLKA) was shown to enhance immunogenicity of both peptide and DNA vaccines [56, 57]. Other studies demonstrated augmentation of melanoma-specific immune responses via direct fusion of the DNA vaccine with the VP22 protein of the herpes simplex virus-1 [58].

Besides introducing immuno-enhancing alteration to the DNA vaccine, other strategies could be employed to enhance DNA vaccination efficacy including addition of the immuno-enhancing molecules to vaccine composition, alteration of the microenvironment at vaccine administration site, and use of the prime-boost immunization regimens. Recent studies demonstrated that antibody-mediated inhibition of the cytotoxic T lymphocyte antigen 4 (CTLA-4) enhances melanoma-specific immune response. This strategy was recently tested in treatment of stage III-IV melanoma and the drug (Ipilimumam) was approved by the FDA as first anti-melanoma immunotherapeutic [59, 60]. CTLA-4 presents its immuno-inhibitory function during activation of the T cells by the antigen-presenting cells. It also inhibits TCR-mediated intracellular signaling in activated T cells and down-modulating T cell mediated immunity. Therefore, it is possible that inhibition of CTLA-4 in conjunction with DNA vaccination may provide significant enhancement of the vaccine-mediated immune response induction. Although providing CTLA-4 inhibiting antibodies like Ipilimumab along with DNA vaccination is not feasible, other options could be explored. For example, recently characterized genetically engineered lipocalin (LCN2) exhibits a strong cross-species antagonistic activity to CTLA-4 [61]. It is likely that this molecule could be included into DNA vaccine composition to enhance DC-mediated activation of the T cells. Other immuno-modulatory strategies may include addition of CD40 ligand, which was shown to stimulate expression of maturation markers CD80, CD86 and IL-12 in APC [62, 63] and its ability to activate $CD8^+$ T cells and increase cell-mediated immunity [64, 65]. Addition of different cytokines and growth factors including GM-CSF, IL-2, IL12 for stimulation/support of the T cells was also tested in several studies (as exemplified in preceding paragraphs) and could be further explored. Alteration of microenvironment via application chemokines to recruit specific sets of the leukocytes to the vaccine administration site may also provide a favorable milieu for the launch of the effective DNA-vaccine induced immune response [66, 67]. These and many other strategies can be proposed; however, the clinical utility of the DNA vaccination combination with other approaches remains to be determined. Nevertheless, presently in the US alone, 10 clinical studies utilizing xenogenic (mouse) or human DNA vaccines coding for melanoma associated antigens have been completed. In these trials, tyrosinase, gp75, gp100, and TRP2 were used as antigens. Although most of these studies are already completed, currently no study results are posted nor are follow-up reports available on patient survival and characterization of immune response. Nevertheless, DNA vaccination remains to be a promising modality that could provide cost-effective and generic immunotherapy for patients with melanoma and other cancers.

4. Other strategies involving recombinant DNA technology

At the present time, almost every immuno-therapeutic approach utilizes recombinant DNA in one way or another. Understanding of the immuno-regulatory functions of DCs and the molecular mechanisms involved in the capture, processing and presentation of antigens by DCs allowed the development of the DC-based vaccines. Initially, in the mid 1990's, several pre-clinical and clinical studies were conducted using autologous DCs pulsed with melanoma-associated antigens. These studies demonstrated that antigen-loaded DC can trigger active melanoma specific immune responses [68, 69]. However, it became apparent that enforced expression of the antigens in DC rather than loading of these cells with peptides allows for presentation of the tumor-derived antigens via MHC class I complex and priming of the CD8+ T cells to elicit cytotoxic immune response. Moreover, to provide DC specific expression of the antigens, long and short CD11c promoters were characterized and used in several studies [70, 71]. These promoters allow effective and cell type specific expression of the antigens in DCs, as well as more efficient priming and activation of the T cells *in vitro* and *in vivo*. Considering a necessity of the direct interaction of the DC with T lymphocytes, application of T cell recruiting chemokines was also explored recently. These pioneering studies demonstrate that forced expression of the secondary lymphoid chemokine, CCL21, in antigen loaded DCs enhances their ability to recruit and activate T cells [72, 73]. One clinical phase I clinical trial

http://dx.doi.org/10.5772/55357

using CCL21 transduced DCs pulsed with MART-1 and gp100 was completed in 2012. Altogether, a total of 64 clinical trials aimed at targeting of melanoma using dendritic cells are listed. Thirty nine of them are completed with no reports yet available. The majority of these trials in some way utilize recombinant DNA technology.

5. Conclusion

During last decade, various melanoma-specific immunotherapeutics that utilize recombinant DNA have been developed and tested in pre-clinical and clinical studies with varying degrees of clinical success. Many of these approaches, including recombinant TCRs and CARs, have already demonstrated promising clinical results, thus providing us with the hope that in the near future melanoma immunotherapy will become curable for melanoma patients.

Acknowledgements

Presented here data regarding clinical trials was obtained through registry and results database of publicly and privately supported clinical studies (clinicaltrials.gov). Experimental data presented on Fig. 4 was obtained in Dr. Alexeev's laboratory. Plasmid DNA encoding tyrosinase-specific TCR was kindly provided by Dr. S.A. Rosenberg (NCI, NIH). ΦC31 integrase-encoding plasmid was obtained from Dr. M.P. Calos (Stanford University, CA).

Author details

Vitali Alexeev[1*], Alyson Pidich[2], Daria Marley Kemp[1] and Olga Igoucheva[1]

*Address all correspondence to: vitali.alexeev@jefferson.edu

1 Department of Dermatology and Cutaneous Biology, Jefferson Medical College, Thomas Jefferson University, Philadelphia, Pennsylvania, USA

2 Temple University School of Medicine, Philadelphia, Pennsylvania, USA

References

[1] Knuth, A., Wolfel, T., Klehmann, E., Boon, T. and Meyer zum Buschenfelde, K.H. (1989) Cytolytic T-cell clones against an autologous human melanoma: specificity study and definition of three antigens by immunoselection. *Proceedings of the National Academy of Sciences of the United States of America*, 86, 2804-2808.

[2] Dudley, M.E., Yang, J.C., Sherry, R., Hughes, M.S., Royal, R., Kammula, U., Robbins, P.F., Huang, J., Citrin, D.E., Leitman, S.F. *et al.* (2008) Adoptive cell therapy for patients with metastatic melanoma: evaluation of intensive myeloablative chemoradiation preparative regimens. *J Clin Oncol*, 26, 5233-5239.

[3] Dudley, M.E., Gross, C.A., Langhan, M.M., Garcia, M.R., Sherry, R.M., Yang, J.C., Phan, G.Q., Kammula, U.S., Hughes, M.S., Citrin, D.E. *et al.* CD8+ enriched "young" tumor infiltrating lymphocytes can mediate regression of metastatic melanoma. *Clinical cancer research : an official journal of the American Association for Cancer Research*, 16, 6122-6131.

[4] Goff, S.L., Johnson, L.A., Black, M.A., Xu, H., Zheng, Z., Cohen, C.J., Morgan, R.A., Rosenberg, S.A. and Feldman, S.A. Enhanced receptor expression and in vitro effector function of a murine-human hybrid MART-1-reactive T cell receptor following a rapid expansion. *Cancer immunology, immunotherapy : CII*, 59, 1551-1560.

[5] Cohen, C.J., Zhao, Y., Zheng, Z., Rosenberg, S.A. and Morgan, R.A. (2006) Enhanced antitumor activity of murine-human hybrid T-cell receptor (TCR) in human lymphocytes is associated with improved pairing and TCR/CD3 stability. *Cancer research*, 66, 8878-8886.

[6] Cohen, C.J., Li, Y.F., El-Gamil, M., Robbins, P.F., Rosenberg, S.A. and Morgan, R.A. (2007) Enhanced antitumor activity of T cells engineered to express T-cell receptors with a second disulfide bond. *Cancer research*, 67, 3898-3903.

[7] Kuball, J., Dossett, M.L., Wolfl, M., Ho, W.Y., Voss, R.H., Fowler, C. and Greenberg, P.D. (2007) Facilitating matched pairing and expression of TCR chains introduced into human T cells. *Blood*, 109, 2331-2338.

[8] Okamoto, S., Mineno, J., Ikeda, H., Fujiwara, H., Yasukawa, M., Shiku, H. and Kato, I. (2009) Improved expression and reactivity of transduced tumor-specific TCRs in human lymphocytes by specific silencing of endogenous TCR. *Cancer research*, 69, 9003-9011.

[9] Govers, C., Sebestyen, Z., Coccoris, M., Willemsen, R.A. and Debets, R. T cell receptor gene therapy: strategies for optimizing transgenic TCR pairing. *Trends Mol Med*, 16, 77-87.

[10] Frankel, T.L., Burns, W.R., Peng, P.D., Yu, Z., Chinnasamy, D., Wargo, J.A., Zheng, Z., Restifo, N.P., Rosenberg, S.A. and Morgan, R.A. Both CD4 and CD8 T cells mediate equally effective in vivo tumor treatment when engineered with a highly avid TCR targeting tyrosinase. *J Immunol*, 184, 5988-5998.

[11] Douin, V., Bornes, S., Creancier, L., Rochaix, P., Favre, G., Prats, A.C. and Couderc, B. (2004) Use and comparison of different internal ribosomal entry sites (IRES) in tricistronic retroviral vectors. *BMC biotechnology*, 4, 16.

[12] Baron, U., Freundlieb, S., Gossen, M. and Bujard, H. (1995) Co-regulation of two gene activities by tetracycline via a bidirectional promoter. *Nucleic acids research*, 23, 3605-3606.

[13] Mastakov, M.Y., Baer, K., Kotin, R.M. and During, M.J. (2002) Recombinant adeno-associated virus serotypes 2- and 5-mediated gene transfer in the mammalian brain: quantitative analysis of heparin co-infusion. *Molecular therapy : the journal of the American Society of Gene Therapy*, 5, 371-380.

[14] Ryan, M.D., King, A.M. and Thomas, G.P. (1991) Cleavage of foot-and-mouth disease virus polyprotein is mediated by residues located within a 19 amino acid sequence. *J Gen Virol*, 72 (Pt 11), 2727-2732.

[15] Baum, C., Schambach, A., Bohne, J. and Galla, M. (2006) Retrovirus vectors: toward the plentivirus? *Molecular therapy : the journal of the American Society of Gene Therapy*, 13, 1050-1063.

[16] Frecha, C., Levy, C., Cosset, F.L. and Verhoeyen, E. (2010) Advances in the field of lentivector-based transduction of T and B lymphocytes for gene therapy. *Molecular therapy : the journal of the American Society of Gene Therapy*, 18, 1748-1757.

[17] Hackett, P.B., Largaespada, D.A. and Cooper, L.J. (2010) A transposon and transposase system for human application. *Molecular therapy : the journal of the American Society of Gene Therapy*, 18, 674-683.

[18] Hacein-Bey-Abina, S., von Kalle, C., Schmidt, M., Le Deist, F., Wulffraat, N., McIntyre, E., Radford, I., Villeval, J.L., Fraser, C.C., Cavazzana-Calvo, M. *et al.* (2003) A serious adverse event after successful gene therapy for X-linked severe combined immunodeficiency. *The New England journal of medicine*, 348, 255-256.

[19] Nam, C.H. and Rabbitts, T.H. (2006) The role of LMO2 in development and in T cell leukemia after chromosomal translocation or retroviral insertion. *Molecular therapy : the journal of the American Society of Gene Therapy*, 13, 15-25.

[20] Mates, L. (2011) Rodent transgenesis mediated by a novel hyperactive Sleeping Beauty transposon system. *Methods Mol Biol*, 738, 87-99.

[21] Chatterjee, M., Hedrich, C.M., Rauen, T., Ioannidis, C., Terhorst, C. and Tsokos, G.C. (2012) CD3-T Cell Receptor Co-stimulation through SLAMF3 and SLAMF6 Receptors Enhances RORgammat Recruitment to the IL17A Promoter in Human T Lymphocytes. *The Journal of biological chemistry*, 287, 38168-38177.

[22] Clevers, H., Lonberg, N., Dunlap, S., Lacy, E. and Terhorst, C. (1989) An enhancer located in a CpG-island 3' to the TCR/CD3-epsilon gene confers T lymphocyte-specificity to its promoter. *The EMBO journal*, 8, 2527-2535.

[23] Hahm, S.H., Yi, Y., Lee, D.K., Noh, M.J., Yun, L., Hwang, S. and Lee, K.H. (2004) Construction of retroviral vectors with enhanced efficiency of transgene expression. *Journal of virological methods*, 121, 127-136.

[24] Morita, S., Kojima, T. and Kitamura, T. (2000) Plat-E: an efficient and stable system for transient packaging of retroviruses. *Gene therapy*, 7, 1063-1066.

[25] Peng, P.D., Cohen, C.J., Yang, S., Hsu, C., Jones, S., Zhao, Y., Zheng, Z., Rosenberg, S.A. and Morgan, R.A. (2009) Efficient nonviral Sleeping Beauty transposon-based TCR gene transfer to peripheral blood lymphocytes confers antigen-specific antitumor reactivity. *Gene therapy*, 16, 1042-1049.

[26] Sclimenti, C.R., Thyagarajan, B. and Calos, M.P. (2001) Directed evolution of a recombinase for improved genomic integration at a native human sequence. *Nucleic acids research*, 29, 5044-5051.

[27] Groth, A.C., Olivares, E.C., Thyagarajan, B. and Calos, M.P. (2000) A phage integrase directs efficient site-specific integration in human cells. *Proceedings of the National Academy of Sciences of the United States of America*, 97, 5995-6000.

[28] Park, T.S., Rosenberg, S.A. and Morgan, R.A. (2011) Treating cancer with genetically engineered T cells. *Trends in biotechnology*, 29, 550-557.

[29] Morgan, R.A., Dudley, M.E., Wunderlich, J.R., Hughes, M.S., Yang, J.C., Sherry, R.M., Royal, R.E., Topalian, S.L., Kammula, U.S., Restifo, N.P. *et al.* (2006) Cancer regression in patients after transfer of genetically engineered lymphocytes. *Science*, 314, 126-129.

[30] Jazirehi, A.R., Baritaki, S., Koya, R.C., Bonavida, B. and Economou, J.S. (2011) Molecular mechanism of MART-1+/A*0201+ human melanoma resistance to specific CTL-killing despite functional tumor-CTL interaction. *Cancer research*, 71, 1406-1417.

[31] Eshhar, Z. (1997) Tumor-specific T-bodies: towards clinical application. *Cancer immunology, immunotherapy : CII*, 45, 131-136.

[32] Moritz, D., Wels, W., Mattern, J. and Groner, B. (1994) Cytotoxic T lymphocytes with a grafted recognition specificity for ERBB2-expressing tumor cells. *Proceedings of the National Academy of Sciences of the United States of America*, 91, 4318-4322.

[33] Koehler, H., Kofler, D., Hombach, A. and Abken, H. (2007) CD28 costimulation overcomes transforming growth factor-beta-mediated repression of proliferation of redirected human CD4+ and CD8+ T cells in an antitumor cell attack. *Cancer research*, 67, 2265-2273.

[34] Finney, H.M., Akbar, A.N. and Lawson, A.D. (2004) Activation of resting human primary T cells with chimeric receptors: costimulation from CD28, inducible costimulator, CD134, and CD137 in series with signals from the TCR zeta chain. *J Immunol*, 172, 104-113.

[35] Milone, M.C., Fish, J.D., Carpenito, C., Carroll, R.G., Binder, G.K., Teachey, D., Samanta, M., Lakhal, M., Gloss, B., Danet-Desnoyers, G. *et al.* (2009) Chimeric receptors containing CD137 signal transduction domains mediate enhanced survival of T cells

and increased antileukemic efficacy in vivo. *Molecular therapy : the journal of the American Society of Gene Therapy*, 17, 1453-1464.

[36] Kershaw, M.H., Westwood, J.A., Parker, L.L., Wang, G., Eshhar, Z., Mavroukakis, S.A., White, D.E., Wunderlich, J.R., Canevari, S., Rogers-Freezer, L. *et al.* (2006) A phase I study on adoptive immunotherapy using gene-modified T cells for ovarian cancer. *Clinical cancer research : an official journal of the American Association for Cancer Research*, 12, 6106-6115.

[37] Lamers, C.H., Willemsen, R., van Elzakker, P., van Steenbergen-Langeveld, S., Broertjes, M., Oosterwijk-Wakka, J., Oosterwijk, E., Sleijfer, S., Debets, R. and Gratama, J.W. (2011) Immune responses to transgene and retroviral vector in patients treated with ex vivo-engineered T cells. *Blood*, 117, 72-82.

[38] Lo, A.S., Ma, Q., Liu, D.L. and Junghans, R.P. (2010) Anti-GD3 chimeric sFv-CD28/T-cell receptor zeta designer T cells for treatment of metastatic melanoma and other neuroectodermal tumors. *Clinical cancer research : an official journal of the American Association for Cancer Research*, 16, 2769-2780.

[39] Burns, W.R., Zhao, Y., Frankel, T.L., Hinrichs, C.S., Zheng, Z., Xu, H., Feldman, S.A., Ferrone, S., Rosenberg, S.A. and Morgan, R.A. (2010) A high molecular weight melanoma-associated antigen-specific chimeric antigen receptor redirects lymphocytes to target human melanomas. *Cancer research*, 70, 3027-3033.

[40] Schmidt, P., Kopecky, C., Hombach, A., Zigrino, P., Mauch, C. and Abken, H. (2011) Eradication of melanomas by targeted elimination of a minor subset of tumor cells. *Proceedings of the National Academy of Sciences of the United States of America*, 108, 2474-2479.

[41] Duignan, I.J., Corcoran, E., Pennello, A., Plym, M.J., Amatulli, M., Claros, N., Iacolina, M., Youssoufian, H., Witte, L., Samakoglu, S. *et al.* Pleiotropic stromal effects of vascular endothelial growth factor receptor 2 antibody therapy in renal cell carcinoma models. *Neoplasia (New York, N.Y*, 13, 49-59.

[42] Larrivee, B., Pollet, I. and Karsan, A. (2005) Activation of vascular endothelial growth factor receptor-2 in bone marrow leads to accumulation of myeloid cells: role of granulocyte-macrophage colony-stimulating factor. *J Immunol*, 175, 3015-3024.

[43] Murdoch, C., Muthana, M., Coffelt, S.B. and Lewis, C.E. (2008) The role of myeloid cells in the promotion of tumour angiogenesis. *Nature reviews*, 8, 618-631.

[44] Suzuki, H., Onishi, H., Wada, J., Yamasaki, A., Tanaka, H., Nakano, K., Morisaki, T. and Katano, M. VEGFR2 is selectively expressed by FOXP3high CD4+ Treg. *European journal of immunology*, 40, 197-203.

[45] Udagawa, T., Puder, M., Wood, M., Schaefer, B.C. and D'Amato, R.J. (2006) Analysis of tumor-associated stromal cells using SCID GFP transgenic mice: contribution of local and bone marrow-derived host cells. *Faseb J*, 20, 95-102.

[46] Zhang, N., Fang, Z., Contag, P.R., Purchio, A.F. and West, D.B. (2004) Tracking angiogenesis induced by skin wounding and contact hypersensitivity using a Vegfr2-luciferase transgenic mouse. *Blood*, 103, 617-626.

[47] Chinnasamy, D., Yu, Z., Kerkar, S.P., Zhang, L., Morgan, R.A., Restifo, N.P. and Rosenberg, S.A. Local delivery of interleukin-12 using T cells targeting VEGF receptor-2 eradicates multiple vascularized tumors in mice. *Clinical cancer research : an official journal of the American Association for Cancer Research*, 18, 1672-1683.

[48] Ulmer, J.B., Donnelly, J.J., Parker, S.E., Rhodes, G.H., Felgner, P.L., Dwarki, V.J., Gromkowski, S.H., Deck, R.R., DeWitt, C.M., Friedman, A. *et al.* (1993) Heterologous protection against influenza by injection of DNA encoding a viral protein. *Science*, 259, 1745-1749.

[49] Alexeev, V. and Uitto, J. (2005) *DNA pharmaceuticals for skin diseases*. Wiley-VCH, Weinheim.

[50] Bergman, P.J., McKnight, J., Novosad, A., Charney, S., Farrelly, J., Craft, D., Wulderk, M., Jeffers, Y., Sadelain, M., Hohenhaus, A.E. *et al.* (2003) Long-term survival of dogs with advanced malignant melanoma after DNA vaccination with xenogeneic human tyrosinase: a phase I trial. *Clinical cancer research : an official journal of the American Association for Cancer Research*, 9, 1284-1290.

[51] Liao, J.C., Gregor, P., Wolchok, J.D., Orlandi, F., Craft, D., Leung, C., Houghton, A.N. and Bergman, P.J. (2006) Vaccination with human tyrosinase DNA induces antibody responses in dogs with advanced melanoma. *Cancer Immun*, 6, 8.

[52] Pavlenko, M., Roos, A.K., Lundqvist, A., Palmborg, A., Miller, A.M., Ozenci, V., Bergman, B., Egevad, L., Hellstrom, M., Kiessling, R. *et al.* (2004) A phase I trial of DNA vaccination with a plasmid expressing prostate-specific antigen in patients with hormone-refractory prostate cancer. *British journal of cancer*, 91, 688-694.

[53] Rakhmilevich, A.L., Imboden, M., Hao, Z., Macklin, M.D., Roberts, T., Wright, K.M., Albertini, M.R., Yang, N.S. and Sondel, P.M. (2001) Effective particle-mediated vaccination against mouse melanoma by coadministration of plasmid DNA encoding Gp100 and granulocyte-macrophage colony-stimulating factor. *Clin Cancer Res*, 7, 952-961.

[54] Xiang, R., Lode, H.N., Chao, T.H., Ruehlmann, J.M., Dolman, C.S., Rodriguez, F., Whitton, J.L., Overwijk, W.W., Restifo, N.P. and Reisfeld, R.A. (2000) An autologous oral DNA vaccine protects against murine melanoma. *Proceedings of the National Academy of Sciences of the United States of America*, 97, 5492-5497.

[55] Parkhurst, M.R., Fitzgerald, E.B., Southwood, S., Sette, A., Rosenberg, S.A. and Kawakami, Y. (1998) Identification of a shared HLA-A*0201-restricted T-cell epitope from the melanoma antigen tyrosinase-related protein 2 (TRP2). *Cancer research*, 58, 4895-4901.

[56] Bettahi, I., Dasgupta, G., Renaudet, O., Chentoufi, A.A., Zhang, X., Carpenter, D., Yoon, S., Dumy, P. and BenMohamed, L. (2009) Antitumor activity of a self-adjuvanting glyco-lipopeptide vaccine bearing B cell, CD4+ and CD8+ T cell epitopes. *Cancer immunology, immunotherapy : CII*, 58, 187-200.

[57] del Guercio, M.F., Alexander, J., Kubo, R.T., Arrhenius, T., Maewal, A., Appella, E., Hoffman, S.L., Jones, T., Valmori, D., Sakaguchi, K. *et al.* (1997) Potent immunogenic short linear peptide constructs composed of B cell epitopes and Pan DR T helper epitopes (PADRE) for antibody responses in vivo. *Vaccine*, 15, 441-448.

[58] Engelhorn, M.E., Guevara-Patino, J.A., Merghoub, T., Liu, C., Ferrone, C.R., Rizzuto, G.A., Cymerman, D.H., Posnett, D.N., Houghton, A.N. and Wolchok, J.D. (2008) Mechanisms of immunization against cancer using chimeric antigens. *Molecular therapy : the journal of the American Society of Gene Therapy*, 16, 773-781.

[59] Hodi, F.S., O'Day, S.J., McDermott, D.F., Weber, R.W., Sosman, J.A., Haanen, J.B., Gonzalez, R., Robert, C., Schadendorf, D., Hassel, J.C. *et al.* Improved survival with ipilimumab in patients with metastatic melanoma. *The New England journal of medicine*, 363, 711-723.

[60] Schartz, N.E., Farges, C., Madelaine, I., Bruzzoni, H., Calvo, F., Hoos, A. and Lebbe, C. Complete regression of a previously untreated melanoma brain metastasis with ipilimumab. *Melanoma research*, 20, 247-250.

[61] Schonfeld, D., Matschiner, G., Chatwell, L., Trentmann, S., Gille, H., Hulsmeyer, M., Brown, N., Kaye, P.M., Schlehuber, S., Hohlbaum, A.M. *et al.* (2009) An engineered lipocalin specific for CTLA-4 reveals a combining site with structural and conformational features similar to antibodies. *Proceedings of the National Academy of Sciences of the United States of America*, 106, 8198-8203.

[62] Feder-Mengus, C., Schultz-Thater, E., Oertli, D., Marti, W.R., Heberer, M., Spagnoli, G.C. and Zajac, P. (2005) Nonreplicating recombinant vaccinia virus expressing CD40 ligand enhances APC capacity to stimulate specific CD4+ and CD8+ T cell responses. *Human gene therapy*, 16, 348-360.

[63] Sato, T., Terai, M., Yasuda, R., Watanabe, R., Berd, D., Mastrangelo, M.J. and Hasumi, K. (2004) Combination of monocyte-derived dendritic cells and activated T cells which express CD40 ligand: a new approach to cancer immunotherapy. *Cancer immunology, immunotherapy : CII*, 53, 53-61.

[64] Peter, I., Nawrath, M., Kamarashev, J., Odermatt, B., Mezzacasa, A. and Hemmi, S. (2002) Immunotherapy for murine K1735 melanoma: combinatorial use of recombinant adenovirus expressing CD40L and other immunomodulators. *Cancer gene therapy*, 9, 597-605.

[65] Rousseau, R.F., Biagi, E., Dutour, A., Yvon, E.S., Brown, M.P., Lin, T., Mei, Z., Grilley, B., Popek, E., Heslop, H.E. *et al.* (2006) Immunotherapy of high-risk acute leukemia

with a recipient (autologous) vaccine expressing transgenic human CD40L and IL-2 after chemotherapy and allogeneic stem cell transplantation. *Blood*, 107, 1332-1341.

[66] Guo, J.H., Fan, M.W., Sun, J.H. and Jia, R. (2009) Fusion of antigen to chemokine CCL20 or CXCL13 strategy to enhance DNA vaccine potency. *International immunopharmacology*, 9, 925-930.

[67] Novak, L., Igoucheva, O., Cho, S. and Alexeev, V. (2007) Characterization of the CCL21-mediated melanoma-specific immune responses and in situ melanoma eradication. *Molecular cancer therapeutics*, 6, 1755-1764.

[68] Nestle, F.O., Alijagic, S., Gilliet, M., Sun, Y., Grabbe, S., Dummer, R., Burg, G. and Schadendorf, D. (1998) Vaccination of melanoma patients with peptide- or tumor lysate-pulsed dendritic cells. *Nature medicine*, 4, 328-332.

[69] 69.Thurner, B., Haendle, I., Roder, C., Dieckmann, D., Keikavoussi, P., Jonuleit, H., Bender, A., Maczek, C., Schreiner, D., von den Driesch, P. *et al.* (1999) Vaccination with mage-3A1 peptide-pulsed mature, monocyte-derived dendritic cells expands specific cytotoxic T cells and induces regression of some metastases in advanced stage IV melanoma. *The Journal of experimental medicine*, 190, 1669-1678.

[70] Brocker, T., Riedinger, M. and Karjalainen, K. (1997) Targeted expression of major histocompatibility complex (MHC) class II molecules demonstrates that dendritic cells can induce negative but not positive selection of thymocytes in vivo. *The Journal of experimental medicine*, 185, 541-550.

[71] Ni, J., Nolte, B., Arnold, A., Fournier, P. and Schirrmacher, V. (2009) Targeting antitumor DNA vaccines to dendritic cells via a short CD11c promoter sequence. *Vaccine*, 27, 5480-5487.

[72] Mule, J.J. (2009) Dendritic cell-based vaccines for pancreatic cancer and melanoma. *Annals of the New York Academy of Sciences*, 1174, 33-40.

[73] Terando, A., Roessler, B. and Mule, J.J. (2004) Chemokine gene modification of human dendritic cell-based tumor vaccines using a recombinant adenoviral vector. *Cancer gene therapy*, 11, 165-173.

Chapter 7

Acquired Resistance to Targeted MAPK Inhibition in Melanoma

Kavitha Gowrishankar, Matteo S. Carlino and Helen Rizos

Additional information is available at the end of the chapter

http://dx.doi.org/10.5772/53629

1. Introduction

The worldwide incidence of cutaneous melanoma has steadily increased in fair-skinned individuals over recent decades with estimates suggesting a doubling of melanoma incidence every 10-20 years [1]. Melanoma remains the major cause of skin cancer related deaths [2], with survival rates averaging less than six months for patients with metastases in visceral organs [3]. Conventional systemic therapies, including single agent dacarbazine and temozolamide, produce response rates of less than 10%, and are not proven to improve survival (reviewed in [4]). Recently, however, the treatment of melanoma has been revolutionized by therapies targeting the RAF-MEK-ERK mitogen activated protein kinase (MAPK) pathway. This pathway is constitutively activated in the majority of melanomas via oncogenic mutations in the BRAF kinase or its upstream regulator, N-RAS [5, 6].

Most BRAF mutations produce a single amino acid substitution of valine by glutamic acid at amino acid 600 (V600E), and this leads to a 500-fold increase in kinase activity [5, 7]. Targeting this mutant BRAF with the highly specific inhibitors, vemurafenib (PLX4032) and dabrafenib (GSK2118436) has produced response rates above 50% and improved progression-free survival in patients with BRAF-mutant metastatic melanoma [8-12]. Both BRAF inhibitors are active against melanoma brain metastases [13, 14] and vemurafenib treatment prolongs overall survival compared with dacarbazine [11]. Despite the marked initial responses to BRAF inhibitors, tumor re-growth occurs in most patients with a median progression-free survival of 5 to 6 months [8, 11, 15].

The U.S Food and Drug Administration (FDA) approved the use of vemurafenib for the treatment of BRAF-mutant melanoma in 2011, and submissions for the use of dabrafenib in the treatment of BRAF-mutant melanoma were made in late 2012. We are now beginning to understand the complex pathways regulating the response and side-effect profiles of these targeted inhibitors. The challenge is to define the molecular drivers and pathways of resistance and response and to translate these molecular findings into rational strategies for clinical testing and improved therapies. In the following chapter we describe the molecular mechanisms that contribute to BRAF inhibitor resistance *in vitro* and *in vivo*. We also highlight the current strategies employed to dissect resistance drivers and explore the future of targeted therapies in the long-term treatment of melanoma.

2. The BRAF kinase and the MAPK pathway

Aberrant activation of the MAPK pathway is present in over 80% of primary cutaneous melanomas [16]. MAPK signalling is driven by mutated N-RAS and activating mutations in the downstream RAS effector, BRAF, in 20% and 60% of melanomas, respectively (Figure 1) [16]. Of cutaneous melanomas with no mutations in BRAF or N-RAS, many activate MAPK signalling via oncogenic mutations in the receptor tyrosine kinase, c-Kit [17], activating mutations in the Rac1 GTPase or inactivating mutations in the N-RAS inhibitor NF1 [18].

Among the BRAF mutations identified in melanoma, over 80% involve a single nucleotide mutation resulting in the substitution of valine for glutamic acid at amino acid 600. This mutation is also present in up to 80% of benign, growth-arrested nevi [19], implicating BRAF as an initiating event that co-operates with additional genetic lesions to promote melanoma. Over 60 other mutations in BRAF have been described in melanoma; most affect codon 600 (V600E, V600K, V600R and V600D), lie within the kinase domain and show elevated kinase activity. In particular, alterations affecting codon 600 show 150- ($BRAF^{V600K}$) to 700- ($BRAF^{V600D}$) fold more kinase activity than the wild type BRAF protein [7].

A wealth of preclinical data has demonstrated the critical role of $BRAF^{V600E}$ as an oncogene in melanoma. The specific silencing of BRAF with short interfering (si)RNA resulted in decreased ERK signalling, diminished proliferation and regression of BRAF mutant melanomas [20-23]. More importantly, class I RAF inhibitors, which target the activated form of RAF kinases, show remarkable antitumor activity; both vemurafenib and dabrafenib have shown response rates of 50% in patients with BRAF-mutant melanoma [8-12]. In addition, the selective inhibition of the BRAF target proteins, MEK1/2, with trametinib (GSK11202212) improved rates of progression-free and overall survival amongst patients with BRAF mutant melanoma when compared to dacarbazine [9, 15, 24, 25].

3. Mechanisms of acquired BRAF inhibitor resistance in melanoma

Despite the marked initial responses to single-agent BRAF inhibitors, tumor re-growth occurs in most patients and 5-20% of individuals fail to respond early during treatment [8, 10, 11, 26]. The acquisition of resistance to targeted therapy is common and resistance has been observed with trastuzumab in HER2-amplified breast cancer, imatinib in gastrointestinal stromal tumors (GISTs) and chronic myelogenous leukemia (CML), epidermal growth factor receptor (EGFR) inhibitors in lung cancer and hedgehog inhibitors in medulloblastoma [27]. Resistance mechanisms to these drugs are complex but include the acquisition of secondary mutations in the target oncogene that prevent drug binding, up-regulation of signalling pathways downstream of the target and the induction of alternate, secondary survival pathways. Defining the mechanisms of melanoma resistance to targeted inhibitors is a high priority, as it can guide the selection of appropriate drug combinations and advance the development of new and improved drugs. This is best demonstrated for imatinib-resistant leukemias. The identification of secondary Bcr-Abl mutations in these resistant cancers promoted the development of the potent, next-generation receptor tyrosine kinase inhibitors dasatanib and nilotinib [28].

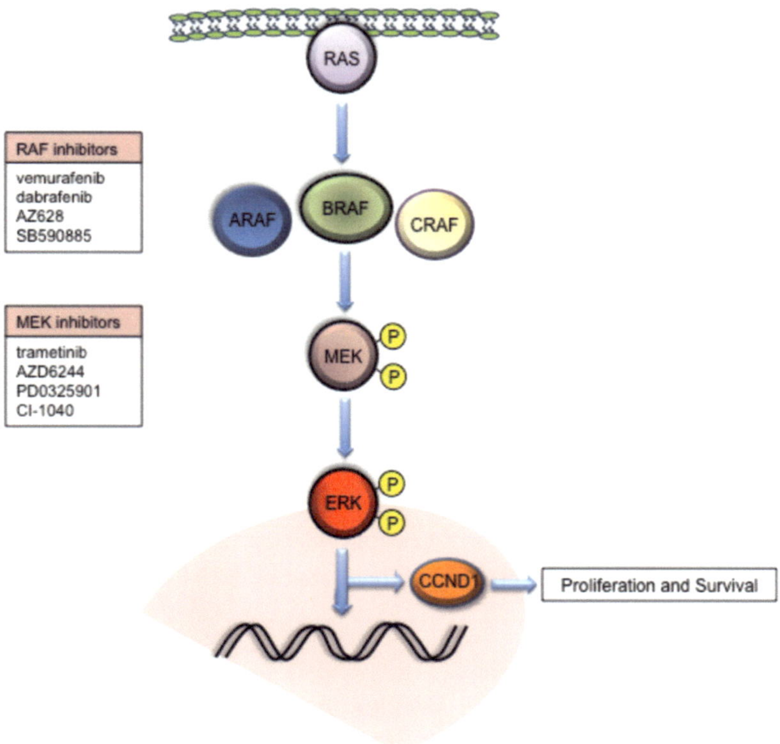

Figure 1. MAPK signalling cascade. Activation of the RAS GTPase promotes the kinase activity of the RAF serine/threonine protein kinases, ARAF, BRAF and CRAF. Activated RAF kinases promote the sequential phosphorylation and activation of the MEK1/2 and ERK1/2 kinases. The ERK proteins translocate into the nucleus and stimulate the translation of proteins and the activities of many transcription factors. This leads to a series of gene expression changes, including elevated CCND1 that promotes cell proliferation and survival. Specific inhibitors to RAF and MEK kinases are indicated. ARAF, v-raf murine sarcoma 3611 viral oncogene homolog; BRAF, v-raf murine sarcoma viral oncogene B1; CCND1, cyclin D1; CRAF, v-raf-1 murine leukemia viral oncogene homolog 1; ERK, extracellular signal-regulated kinase; MEK mitogen-activated protein kinase kinase.

4. Alterations affecting BRAF

Drug resistance is often associated with the acquisition of so-called gatekeeper mutations in the target oncogene that prevent drug binding. In a series of detailed reports, deep sequencing of melanoma biopsies derived from patients progressing on vemurafenib treatment did not find any secondary BRAF mutations. Moreover, immunoprecipitated BRAF from vemurafenib-resistant melanomas retained drug sensitivity in an *in vitro* kinase assay, confirming drug-target binding was maintained [29].

4.1. BRAF copy number gain

The amplification and overexpression of $BRAF^{V600E}$ is associated with BRAF inhibitor resistance in melanoma [30] (Figure 2). In a sequencing screen of 20 pairs of patient-matched baseline (before BRAF inhibitor therapy) and progressing (acquired resistance to BRAF inhibition) melanoma tissue, 20% showed $BRAF^{V600E}$ copy-number gains, ranging from 2- to 14- fold. These copy-number gains, which are likely underestimates due to non-tumor cell contamination, correlated with increased BRAF protein expression in tumor specimens. Moreover, preclinical melanoma cell models with ectopically expressed $BRAF^{V600E}$ confirmed that cells overexpressing mutant BRAF developed resistance to vemurafenib and that this resistance could be overcome by increasing the dose of vemurafenib, applying MEK inhibitors (AZD6244) or concurrently inhibiting both MEK and BRAF (Figure 1) [30].

Unlike melanoma cell models [30], BRAF-mutant colorectal cancer cells with amplification of the BRAF gene (2- to 7- fold) were resistance to the MEK inhibitor AZD6244 [31]. In these colon cancer cells, the increased expression of mutant BRAF resulted in excess activation of MEK and ERK, rendering cells unresponsive to MEK inhibition. In the presence of the BRAF inhibitor, AZ628, however, the abundance of activated MEK was reduced and the allosteric MEK inhibitor AZD6244 prevented ERK phosphorylation [31]. Thus, the concurrent inhibition of MEK and BRAF overcomes resistance mediated by BRAF amplification in both melanoma and colorectal cancers.

Intriguingly, BRAF copy-number gains (3- to 4-fold) were also identified in baseline (drug-naive) melanoma and colorectal tumor samples. In one such colorectal tumor only 28% of cells showed BRAF amplification and 10% of these tumor cells had more than 10 copies of BRAF [30, 31]. These data indicate that cell sensitivity to MEK and BRAF inhibition is likely to reflect the level of BRAF amplification and resistance may arise from the expansion of a limited number of cells with pre-existing BRAF gains. This notion is consistent with a recent study showing that K-RAS mutations conferring resistance to EGFR inhibitors were likely to be present in a clonal subpopulation of the colorectal tumor cells prior to the initiation of targeted therapy. These results may explain resistance to RAF inhibitors and other targeted therapies occurs in a highly reproducible fashion within 5 to 6 months [32].

http://dx.doi.org/10.5772/53629

4.2. BRAF splicing variants

In other melanomas, resistance to vemurafenib was acquired via the expression of splice variant isoforms of BRAF^{V600E}. Three of five vemurafenib-resistant clones of the SKMEL-238 melanoma cells expressed a novel 61kDa variant of BRAF^{V600E}. This p61BRAF^{V600E} splice variant, lacked exons 4-8, a region encoding the RAS binding domain, and was sufficient to render MEK activation resistant to vemurafenib (Figure 3). The variant appears to arise from a splicing defect as no intragenic somatic deletions within the BRAF gene were detected [33].

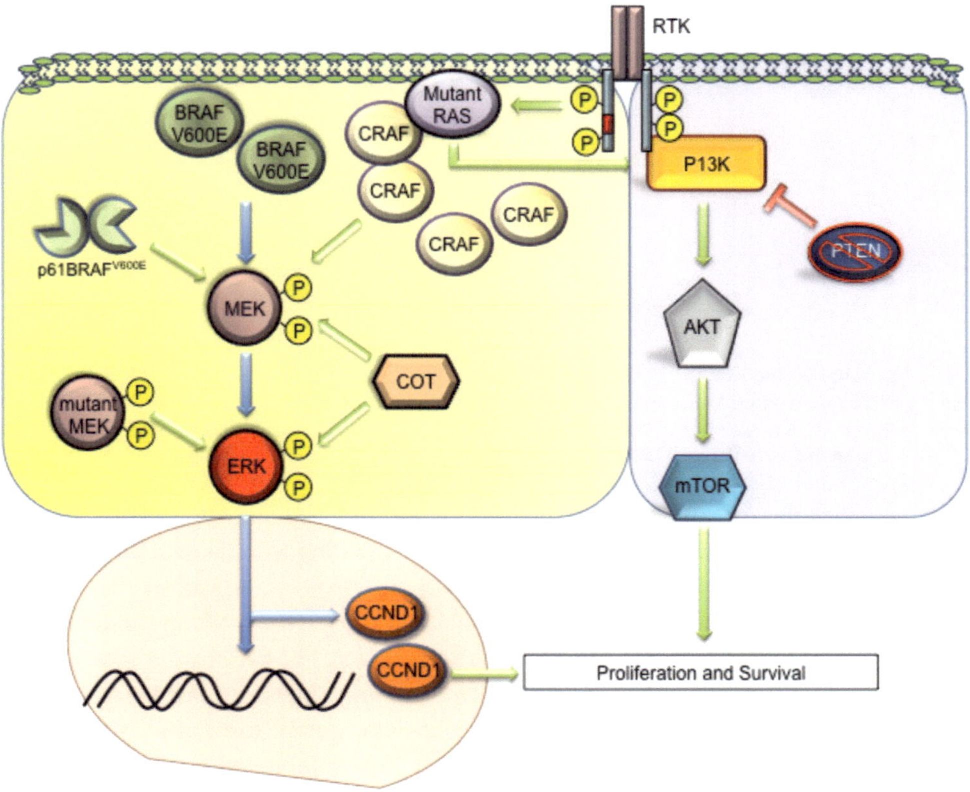

Figure 2. Mechanisms of resistance to BRAF inhibition. MAPK re-activation, in the presence of RAF inhibitors, can occur via A. the mutational activation and amplification of RAS, B. the upregulation of RTKs such as PDGFRß and IGF-1R, C. elevated expression of CRAF, COT or CCND1, D. MEK mutations, or E. the expression and dimerization of BRAF^{V600E} splice variants, such as p61BRAFV600E. Mutant RAS and upregulated RTKs also activate the PI3K/mTOR survival pathway, which is further activated by the loss of PTEN (adapted from [87]). AKT, v-akt murine thymoma viral oncogene; BRAF, v-raf murine sarcoma viral oncogene B1; CCND1, cyclin D1; CRAF, v-raf-1 murine leukemia viral oncogene homolog 1; ERK, extracellular signal-regulated kinase; COT, mitogen-activated protein kinase kinase kinase 8; MEK mitogen-activated protein kinase kinase; mTOR, mechanistic target of rapamycin; PI3K, phosphoinositide-3-kinase PTEN, phosphatase and tensin homolog; RTK, receptor tyrosine kinase.

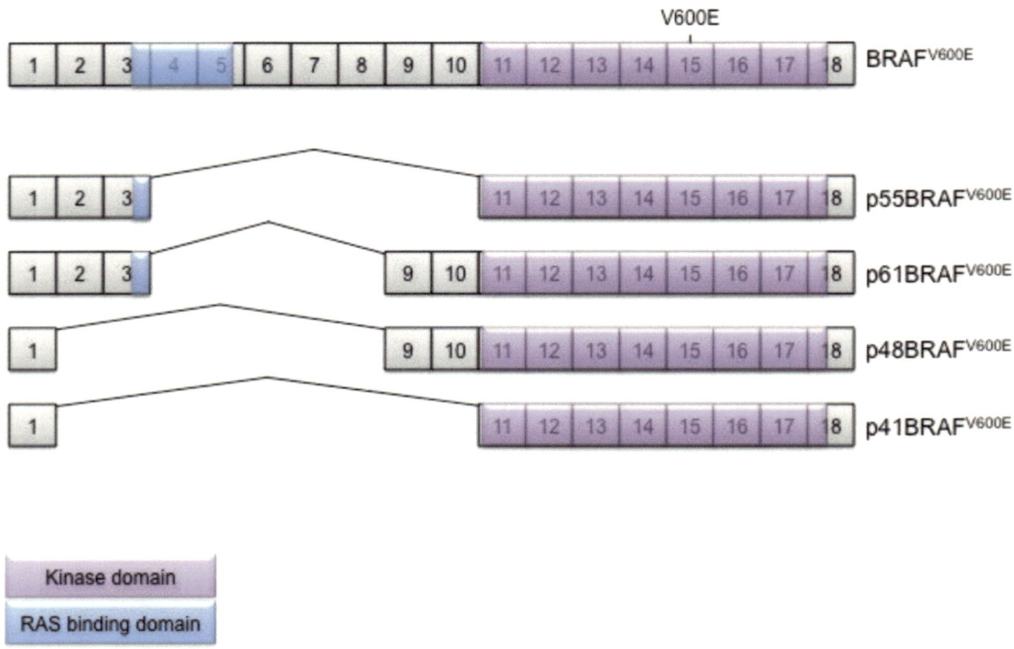

Figure 3. Aberrant splicing of BRAF^{V600E} confers RAF inhibitor resistance. Several in frame BRAF^{V600E} splice variants lacking the RAS binding domain have been detected in vemurafenib-resistant melanoma tumor specimens. The exon structure of full-length and spice variant forms of BRAF are shown. The location of the activating V600E mutation, the RAS binding and kinase domains are highlighted (adapted from [33]).

It is known that the amino terminus of BRAF negatively regulates its kinase activity by masking the carboxy-terminal catalytic domain. Upon binding to activated RAS, the amino-terminal regulatory domain of RAF proteins unfolds to expose the carboxy terminal sites that are required for dimerization and full kinase activity. The in-frame deletion in the p61BRAF^{V600E} variant leads to the constitutive dimerization of BRAF in the absence of activated RAS [34]. Dimerization of p61BRAF^{V600E} was shown to be critical for mediating BRAF-inhibitor resistance, as the R509H dimerization-deficient mutant form of p61BRAF^{V600E} was sensitive to vemurafenib and monomeric p61BRAF^{V600E} was inhibited by vemurafenib *in vitro*. Thus, it has been proposed that binding of vemurafenib to one p61BRAF^{V600E} protomer elicits an allosteric change in the other, drug-free protomer, thereby decreasing its affinity for the drug (Figure 4). Four independent BRAF splicing variants were also detected in tumors derived from six of nineteen patients with acquired resistance to vemurafenib (Figure 3). In each case, the alternative splice variants were in frame, lacked the RAS binding domain and were confined to the mutant allele [33]. This indicates that BRAF missplicing is likely due to a mutation or epigenetic change that specifically impacts the BRAF^{V600E} allele. Importantly, no splice BRAF variants were detected in 27 melanomas resected from vemurafenib-naive patients [33].

http://dx.doi.org/10.5772/53629

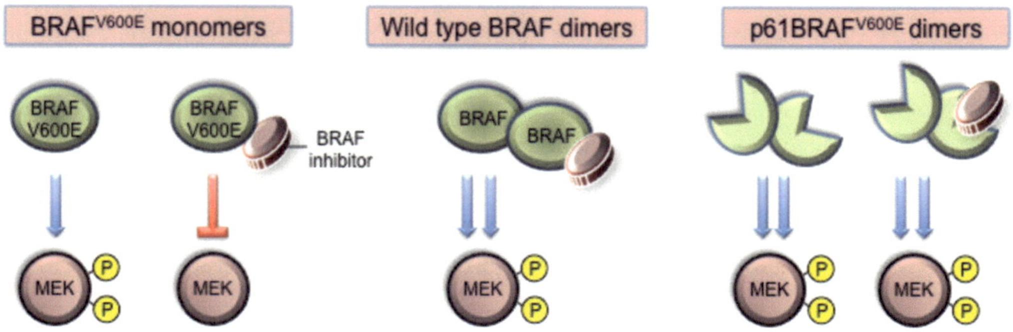

Figure 4. BRAF dimerization, RAF inhibitor binding and MAPK signalling. Mutant BRAF functions as a monomer and is effectively inhibited at low RAF inhibitor concentrations. In cells with activated RAS, the binding of RAS to RAF kinases promotes the homo- and heterodimerization (not shown) of wild type RAF proteins. In the presence of low BRAF inhibitor concentrations, one protomer of the RAF dimer binds inhibitor and this promotes the transactivation of the second, inhibitor-free RAF protomer. Thus in RAS-activated cells, BRAF inhibitor can induce the activation of RAF dimers and promote elevated MAPK signalling. Similarly, dimers of p61BRAF^{V600E} splicing variant are resistant to BRAF inhibition because binding of the drug to one protomer, allosterically alters the second protomer and diminishes its affinity for the RAF inhibitor. Much higher concentrations of RAF inhibitor are required to bind both protomers in a RAF dimer and inhibit ERK signalling.

5. N-RAS mutations

In the normal physiological setting, activated RAS signalling promotes the dimerization and activation of RAF proteins. In the presence of BRAF inhibitors and RAS signalling, the binding of drug to one molecule in a non-mutated RAF dimer can promote activation of the second RAF molecule (Figure 4). Thus, in the presence of RAS activation, the activity of homo- and heterodimeric RAF complexes can be paradoxically activated by RAF inhibitors [35-37].

In melanomas with BRAF^{V600E}, any alterations promoting RAF dimerization are predicted to confer resistance to RAF inhibitors. As expected, activating N-RAS mutations mediate resistance to vemurafenib [29] and dabrafenib [38]. Oncogenic N-RAS^{Q61K} was detected in a single vemurafenib-resistant clone derived from the M249 melanoma cells. This resistant subclone maintained ERK activation in the presence of vemurafenib, presumably via a kinase switch from BRAF to CRAF (Figure 1) [39, 40]. These cells were also sensitive to inhibition with the MEK inhibitor, AZD6244 in the presence or absence of vemurafenib, suggesting that in this cell clone oncogenic N-RAS confers resistance by principally engaging the MAPK cascade. Oncogenic N-RAS mutations were also detected in a patient with acquired resistance to vemurafenib; separate N-RAS mutations (Q61K and Q61R) were detected in two melanoma biopsies taken on initial progression and six months after initial progression. Both mutations were associated with copy-number amplification and N-RAS overexpression [29].

In a second study, oncogenic N-RAS^{Q61H} was detected in two of six dabrafenib resistant subclones, generated from the MelRMu cell line. In contrast to the initial report [29], these two N-RAS mutant, MelRMu sublines showed diminished sensitivity to MEK inhibitor, trametinib and to the combined inhibition of BRAF and MEK, when compared to the parental cells. Moreover, ectopic expression of N-RAS^{Q61K} in the MelRMu cells diminished the efficacy of combined MEK and BRAF inhibition [38]. A third report also identified N-RAS mutations (N-RAS^{Q61K} and N-RAS^{A146T}) in two melanoma sublines with acquired resistance to dabrafenib. These mutations were shown to confer dabrafenib resistance, and induced the heterodimerization of BRAF^{V600E} with C-RAF in the presence of drug [41]. These N-RAS mutant clones showed partial sensitivity to trametinib and to the concurrent inhibition of BRAF and MEK proteins [41]. It is known that mutant N-RAS can signal via multiple pathways including the PI3K/AKT/mTOR survival cascade [42] and consequently, N-RAS mutant dabrafenib-resistant melanoma cells were responsive to the simultaneous inhibition of MEK and the PI3K/mTOR pathway [41].

There are some discrepancies in the literature regarding the role of activated RAS in selectively sensitizing cancer cells to MEK inhibition. Certainly, N-RAS mutation status did not predict MEK inhibitor sensitivity in melanoma cell lines [43], and MEK inhibitors show only modest clinical activity in patients with RAS-mutant tumors [9, 44]. It seems likely that the impact of mutant N-RAS on MEK inhibitor responses reflects its expression and activity and ultimately the network of activated N-RAS-dependent effectors. This is in agreement with a recent report demonstrating that K-RAS^{13D}-mutant HCT116 colorectal cancer cells became resistant to MEK inhibition upon amplification of the driving K-RAS^{13D} oncogene [45].

6. CRAF overexpression

Increased expression of the CRAF kinase has also been associated with BRAF inhibitor resistance (Figure 2). Villanueva et al. (2010) observed increased CRAF protein levels in melanoma cells chronically treated with the BRAF inhibitor SB-590885. In this cell model MAPK signalling driven by persistent insulin growth factor receptor (IGF-1R) activity, was rewired to utilise both CRAF and ARAF (Figure 1), and the inhibition of all three RAF isoforms was required to inhibit the proliferation of these 885-resistant cells [46]. This is in contrast to melanoma sublines rendered resistant to the pan-RAF inhibitor AZ628. These AZ628-resistant cells showed elevated basal levels of CRAF protein, but the knockdown of CRAF alone strongly inhibited cell proliferation, in the absence of AZ628 treatment [47]. These cells switched from BRAF to CRAF dependence, and the precise mechanism of CRAF-mediated AZ628 resistance remains unclear, as this inhibitor strongly suppresses both BRAF^{V600E} and CRAF [48]. The role of CRAF in conferring RAF-inhibitor resistance may reflect the distinct genetic profiles of the melanoma cells used, the pathway rewiring involved in resistance, the mechanism of drug action and its impact on the RAF protein dimerization.

http://dx.doi.org/10.5772/53629

7. MEK mutations

Mutations in mitogen activated protein kinase, MEK1 have also been shown to confer resistance to MAPK inhibitors. A random mutagenesis screen of MEK1 revealed that mutations interfering with target-drug binding (e.g. I99T, G128D, L215P) and mutations that upregulate MEK1 intrinsic activity (e.g. Q56P, P124S) conferred resistance to the allosteric MEK inhibitor AZD6244 [49]. The G128D MEK1 mutation also conferred resistance to the BRAF inhibitor PLX4720 [50] (Figure 5).

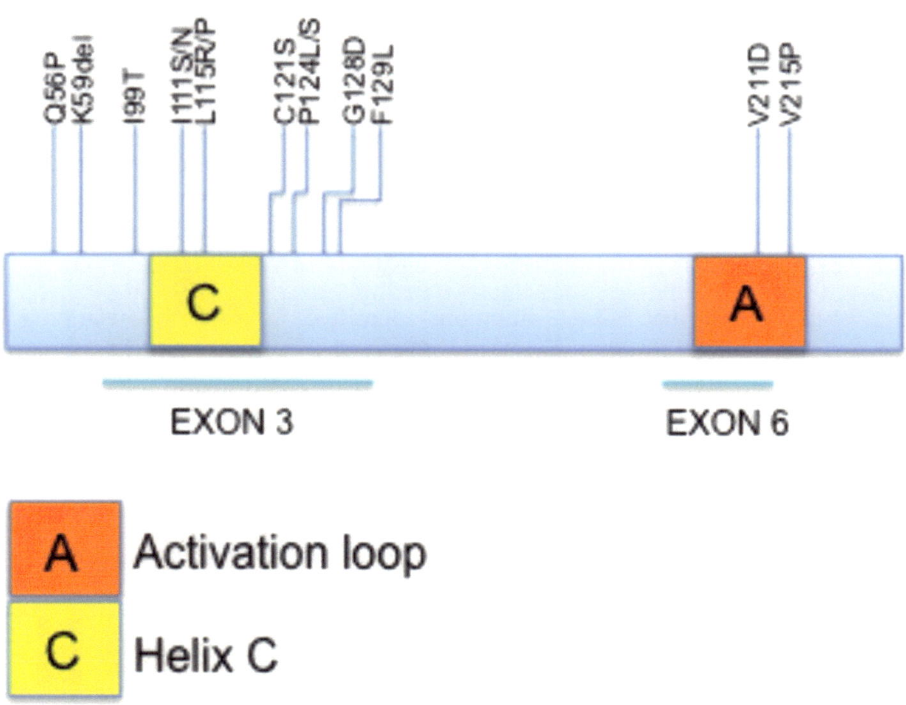

Figure 5. MEK1 mutations associated with MAPK inhibitor resistance. Allosteric MEK inhibitors binds to the MEK1 hydrophobic pocket that includes residues from helix C and the activation loop. Primary MEK1 mutations affect this drug-binding pocket (e.g. I99T, I111N/S, L115P/R, G128D, F129L, V211D and L215P) and can directly perturb the allosteric binding of the MEK inhibitor. Secondary MEK1 mutations reside outside the drug-binding region and include mutations near the amino terminus (e.g. Q56P) and proximal to the helix C (C121S, P124S/L). These secondary MEK1 mutations increase MEK1 kinase activity. The C121S and P124L MEK1 mutation have been detected in MEK inhibitor resistant patient tumors [50], whereas P124S and I111S MEK1 mutations were identified in pre-treatment melanomas [54]. Shi et al. found that of the P124S, I111S and C121S, only C121S conferred vemurafenib resistance in melanoma cells.

Deep sequencing of tumors from five patients progressing on AZD6244 treatment, identified the MEK1^{P124L} mutation in the progressing, but not pre-treatment tumor sample from one patient. The existence of this MEK1 mutation was independently verified in *ex vivo* cell lines established from tumor material, and its activity in conferring MEK- and BRAF-inhibitor resistance validated in transfected melanoma cells. As with BRAF truncation and amplification, alterations in MEK1 protein did not alter the sensitivity of melanoma cells to the combined inhibition of BRAF and MEK inhibitors. A $MEK1^{C121S}$ mutation was detected via mutational profiling in a melanoma sample from a patient with acquired resistance to vemurafenib. This mutation was not detected in the pre-treatment biopsy, showed increased intrinsic kinase activity and conferred resistance to BRAF and MEK inhibition *in vitro* [50]. BRAFi-resistant YUSIT1 melanoma cells also acquired a MEK1 mutation with increased kinase activity (K59del). These cells were dependent on MEK1 for proliferation and displayed higher ERK phosphorylation following treatment with dabrafenib [41].

Resistance to the allosteric MEK inhibitor PD0325901 in breast and colorectal cancer cell lines was also consistently associated with MEK mutations in the allosteric binding domain. MEK-inhibitor resistant sublines derived from the MDA-MB-231 breast and HCT-116 colon cancer cells gained the $MEK1^{L115P}$ and $MEK1^{F129L}$ mutations, respectively and the MEK-inhibitor resistant LoVo colorectal cells acquired a $MEK2^{V215E}$ mutation (homologous to V211D mutations in MEK1) (Figure 5). The L115P and V211D mutations abrogated MEK inhibitor binding, while F129L increased the intrinsic activity of MEK and showed enhanced interaction with CRAF [51, 52]. Cell lines expressing mutant $MEK1^{K57N}$, which was identified in two lung adenocarcinomas, also showed decreased sensitivity to MEK inhibition [53].

A recent study found that MEK1 mutations identified in resistant melanoma lesions might not predict BRAF-inhibitor sensitivity. Shi *et al* found that five of 31 melanomas excised pre-BRAF inhibitor treatment carried concurrent somatic BRAF and MEK1 ($MEK1^{P124S}$ and MEK^{I111S}) activating mutations and that three of these five patients showed objective tumor responses. When the P124S, I111S and C121S MEK1 mutants were stably introduced into a series of melanoma cell lines, only the $MEK1^{C121S}$ mutant restored p-ERK levels in the presence of vemurafenib, even though all mutants showed intrinsically enhanced kinase activity [54] (Figure 5). Thus, the relative impact of MEK1 mutations may vary depending on the type of mutation, tumor genetic background and the dependence on BRAF. For instance, YUSIT1 cells were dependent on the $MEK1^{K59del}$ for proliferation, and the $MEK1^{F129L}$ mutant may induce a BRAF to CRAF kinase switch [41, 51]. Finally, a more detailed tumor profile, correlating tumor response with the relative proportion of double-BRAF/MEK1 mutant cells within metastases, will help clarify the precise role of MEK1 in mediating BRAF-inhibitor resistance.

8. COT overexpression

A recent gain of function screen tested the activity of 597 kinases (75% of the annotated human kinases) in conferring vemurafenib resistance in the A375 melanoma cell line. Nine candidates, including receptor tyrosine kinases (Axl, ERBB2), conferred significant resistance with the mitogen activated protein kinase kinase kinase 8 (the gene encoding COT/Tpl2) emerging as the top candidate. Overexpression of COT resulted in constitutive ERK activation in the presence of vemurafenib (Figure 2). COT activated ERK via MEK-dependent and

-independent mechanisms and ectopic COT expression conferred decreased sensitivity to the MEK inhibitors CI-1040 and AZD6244. COT expression was also elevated in two of three patient samples obtained early in the course of treatment and further increased in a relapsing specimen relative to its pre-treatment and on-treatment controls. Considering that inhibition of $BRAF^{V600E}$ increases COT expression, it is possible that COT accumulation may reflect secondary responses to BRAF inhibition and resistance. Nevertheless, the silencing and inhibition of COT in the RPMI-7951 melanoma cells, which express increased COT, decreased ERK phosphorylation and suppressed cell viability [55].

9. Activation of receptor tyrosine kinases

An emerging theme in BRAF inhibitor resistance is the upregulation and activation of receptor tyrosine kinases. Garraway and co-workers demonstrated that ectopically expressed receptor tyrosine kinases Axl and ERBB2, circumvented vemurafenib activity [55], and two independent reports detected increased expression and activity of the platelet derived growth factor (PDGFRß) and IGF-1R in vemurafenib-resistant melanoma sublines [29, 46] (Figure 2). Vemurafenib-resistant tumor biopsies derived from patients also showed overexpression of PDGFRß (4 of 11 patients) and IGF-1R (2 of 5 patients) compared to the corresponding pre-treatment tumor specimens [29, 46]. The knockdown or inhibition of PDGFRß and IGF-1R overcame vemurafenib resistance in cell lines, but resistance was not due to activation of ERK alone [29, 46]. Instead, receptor tyrosine kinase-upregulated, vemurafenib resistant melanoma cell lines, showed phosphorylation of both ERK and PI3K/AKT (Figure 2), and the concurrent and sustained inhibition of the MAPK and PI3K/AKT/mTOR pathways was required to overcome PDGFRß- and IGF-1R-mediated vemurafenib resistance [46, 56]. The upregulation and activation of these receptors was not due to gene amplification or genetic alterations within the coding sequence [29, 46].

These studies predict that RTK activation via increased autocrine tumor cell ligand secretion, or paracrine ligand production from stromal cells may confer resistance to MAPK inhibition. A recent report found increased activation of the fibroblast growth factor (FGF) receptor 3 was associated with elevated levels of autocrine secreted FGF2 ligand in vemurafenib resistant melanoma sublines [57]. Moreover the secretion of growth factors from co-cultured fibroblast cells conferred vemurafenib resistance to BRAF-mutant melanoma cell lines. Stromal cell secretion of the hepatocyte growth factor (HGF) correlated best with vemurafenib resistance in this cell screen, and HGF was detected in tumor-associated stromal cells in 23 of 34 melanoma tumors resected from patients prior to MAPK inhibitor treatment. Critically, these 23 patients also showed activation of the HGF receptor MET in their tumor biopsies, and had a poorer response to MAPK-inhibitor treatment compared to patients whose stromal cells lacked HGF expression [58]. Increased plasma HGF levels in 126 metastatic melanoma patients, prior to treatment with vemurafenib, was also associated with a reduction in the progression-free and overall survival rates [59]. The stromal cell secretion of HGF resulted in reactivation of the MAPK and PI3K/mTOR signalling pathways and immediate (innate) resistance to RAF inhibition. Whether activation of MET also has a role in acquired resistance to RAF inhibitors remains to be determined, but activating somatic MET mutations and amplifications have been detected in human cancers [60-62]. Regardless, of the mechanism of MET activation, the sensitivity of MET-activated melanoma cells can be restored by the simultaneous inhibition of RAF and either HGF or MET [58]. Finally, it is worth noting that although activation of PDGFRß and IGF-1R are associated with vemurafenib resistance [29, 46], the ligand activation of these two receptors appears insufficient to drive sustained pathway activation or vemurafenib resistance [58, 59].

10. Other regulators of response to MAPK inhibitors

Typically, the suppression of MAPK signalling promotes cell cycle arrest that is associated with increased expression of the CDK inhibitor $p27^{Kip1}$ and inhibition of cyclin D1 expression (Figure 1). Cyclin D1 is a regulator of the cyclin dependent kinases (CDKs) 4 and 6 and the formation of binary cyclin D-CDK4/6 complexes promote the phosphorylation of the retinoblastoma protein (pRb) and cell cycle progression [63-65]. Cyclin D1 is commonly amplified in melanoma and often in conjunction with mutated BRAF [66, 67]. The clinical significance of this genotype was demonstrated in BRAF-mutant melanoma cell lines with increased cyclin D1 protein expression. These cells showed intrinsic resistance to the growth-arresting effects of the RAF inhibitor, SB590885 and the ectopic expression of cyclin D1 conferred RAF-inhibitor resistance, which was enhanced by the dual overexpression of CDK4 and cyclin D1 [67]. These data confirm that the MAPK-independent expression of critical MAPK downstream targets will regulate RAF-inhibitor response and may diminish the dependence of cells to oncogenic BRAF.

Several independent studies have shown that loss of the phosphatase and tensin homolog (PTEN) tumor suppressor, which occurs in over 10% of melanoma tumors, is predictive of attenuated RAF-inhibitor mediated cytotoxicity [68, 69]. Cells lacking PTEN remain dependent on MAPK for proliferation but utilise increased AKT signalling for survival (Figure 2). Elevated AKT promotes the nuclear exclusion of the FOXO3a transcription factor, which leads to the downstream suppression of the FOXO3a pro-apoptotic target BIM [69, 70]. Predictably, ectopic expression of activated AKT3 also prevented BRAF inhibitor induced BIM and apoptosis [71] and MEK inhibitor-sensitive cancer cell lines show significantly higher FOXO3a and BIM protein levels compared to resistant cell lines [70]. Similar to RTK-induced resistance, the simultaneous inhibition of the MAPK and AKT pathways is required to restore PTEN-null cell sensitivity to MAPK inhibitors [68]. Finally, homozygous PTEN loss and increased pAKT levels were associated with vemurafenib resistance in a progressing biopsy derived from a single patient [46].

Considering the independent roles of cyclin D and PTEN in diminishing dependence on MAPK signalling and engaging the AKT survival cascade, it is anticipated that the concurrent alteration of these cell cycle regulators would confer increased levels of resistance to MAPK inhibitors. In a recent study, vemurafenib was shown to have purely cytostatic effects in melanoma cells with either PTEN or pRb loss; pRb deleted cells should behave as cells with elevated cyclinD1/CDK4 overexpression. $BRAF^{V600E}$ cells with concurrent loss of both pRb and PTEN were completely resistant to RAF inhibition, and these cells continued proliferating in the presence of this RAF inhibitor [68]. The clinical significance of pRb loss in conferring MAPK inhibitor resistance is uncertain, however, as pRb loss is uncommon in melanoma [72].

Finally, activation of the STAT3 pathway was found to be associated with AZD6244 resistance in a panel of lung cancer cell lines. STAT3 activity was shown to decrease BIM accumulation through the upregulation of miR-17, and the inhibition of STAT3 or miR-17 upregulated BIM and sensitized resistant cells to MEK inhibition [73].

11. Therapies to overcome MAPK inhibitor resistance

Irrespective of the precise mechanisms of resistance to class I RAF inhibitors, tumors that acquire resistance or are inherently insensitive to these inhibitors often maintain some dependency on the MAPK pathway [29, 33, 38, 55, 57, 74]. These data suggest that further inhibition of the MAPK cascade at the downstream MEK or ERK nodes may be effective in treating resistance to single agent BRAF inhibitors. Despite the preclinical evidence of MEK-inhibitor sensitivity in cells with acquired resistance to BRAF inhibitors [38], clinical trials applying this strategy have been disappointing. The MEK inhibitor trametinib showed minimal activity (response rates of 3%) in patients previously treated with a BRAF inhibitor [75]. Clinical benefit was observed, however, when patients who progressed on prior BRAF inhibitor were treated with a combination of BRAF and MEK inhibitors. Partial responses were observed in 17% of patients, suggesting that dual MAPK blockade can abrogate some BRAF inhibitor resistance mechanisms [76]. The triaging of patients, based on BRAF inhibitor resistance drivers, may also improve the clinical benefit of second line MAPK inhibitor therapies. For instance, melanoma cells expressing BRAF splice variants are sensitive to MEK inhibition [33], whereas cells with BRAF copy number gains respond to the concurrent inhibition of BRAF and MEK [30, 31]. Finally, specific inhibitors of ERK have recently become available, and these show anti-proliferative activity in MEK-inhibitor resistant cells and synergise with MEK inhibitors to prevent or delay the emergence of acquired resistance [52].

Sustained and significant responses have also been observed when RAF-inhibitor resistant cell lines are treated with combination MAPK and PI3K/mTOR inhibitors. For instance, in RTK-expressing vemurafenib-resistant cells, inhibition of PI3K/mTOR activity in combination with vemurafenib showed potent synergy. Compensatory signalling via MEK permitted survival in the presence of PI3K/mTOR/MAPK inhibition, but cytotoxicity was restored using a combination of MEK inhibitor with the dual PI3K/mTOR inhibitor BEZ235 [56]. A number of combinations of MEK and PI3K/mTOR pathway inhibitors combinations have entered early phase clinical trials, however their benefit in the setting of BRAF/MEK inhibitor resistance remains untested.

Many of the proteins involved in melanoma development and RAF-inhibitor resistance are targets of the heat shock protein (Hsp)-90 family of chaperones. Hsp90 proteins regulate the conformation, stability and function of many RTKs and kinases, including IGF-1R, BRAF, CRAF, CDK4, AKT and cyclin D1 [77, 78]. The pharmacological inhibition of Hsp90 using the selective inhibitor, XL888 abrogated acquired and intrinsic vemurafenib resistance. XL888 induced apoptosis in melanoma cells with mutant N-RAS, elevated PDGFRß, COT, IGF-1R, CRAF and cyclin D1. Apoptosis was associated with diminished accumulation of the resistance driver, nuclear accumulation of FOXO3a and an increase in BIM expression. Moreover, Hsp90 inhibition was a more effective apoptotic inducer when combined with MEK and PI3K inhibition [79]. Hsp90 inhibitors have shown promising results in ERBB2-amplified breast cancers [80], but lacked clinical activity in vemurafenib-naive melanoma patients [81]. Evaluation of pre- and post treatment melanoma biopsies confirmed incomplete degradation of $BRAF^{V600E}$, when the inhibitor was given on a weekly schedule. Whether Hsp90 inhibition will prove effective when administered more frequently, in RAF-inhibitor resistant melanoma patients, or in combination with MAPK inhibitors remains to be tested.

12. Conclusions

BRAF-targeted therapy has recently emerged as the standard treatment for patients with BRAF-mutant melanoma. Responses are not durable, however and studies of acquired resistance to BRAF inhibition reveal a diversity of resistance mechanism but a common resistance theme. Melanoma cells adapt by re-engaging MAPK signalling and activating parallel survival networks. The management and prevention of BRAF inhibitor resistance is likely to be achieved through combination therapies. The combination of BRAF and MEK inhibitors has shown better response than single agent therapy [25] and is currently being evaluated in phase III clinical trials compared to vemurafenib (NCT01597908) or dabrafenib (NCT01584648) in treatment naive patients with $BRAF^{V600E}$ mutant melanoma. Trials combining MEK with AKT inhibitors (NCT01021748), the pan-RAF inhibitor sorafenib and MEK inhibition (NCT0034999206), testing HDAC inhibition with vorinostat (NCT006670820) are also under way. Further, Phase I trials for inhibition of PDGFRβ, FGFR and other tyrosine kinases using Dovitinib in patients with advanced melanoma has shown promising results [82]. Finally, rechallenging patients with selective BRAF inhibitors after a treatment-free interval provided clinical benefit to two patients who had previously progressed on MAPK inhibitors [83]. Additional studies are required to determine the significance of rechallenging patients after treatment interruption.

It has been suggested that a detailed catalogue of resistance mechanism in an individual's tumor should inform effective second line therapy [84]. This strategy may not prove sufficient, as it does not account for stromal-mediated resistance drivers, the heterogeneous nature of melanoma and the fact that melanoma tumors from a single patient may develop multiple mechanisms of resistance. For instance, two independent vemurafenib-resistant nodal metastases derived from a single patient, harboured distinct N-RAS activating mutations

[29] and intra-tumoral heterogeneity has been observed in a progressing BRAF-mutant melanoma metastases from patients treated with BRAF inhibitors [85, 86].

Nevertheless, defining the mechanisms of RAF-inhibitor resistance is a critical step in understanding the signalling pathways required to circumvent therapy. At present, up to 40% of RAF-inhibitor resistant melanomas have undefined resistance drivers, and the role of MAPK and PI3K signalling needs to be assessed in this subgroup. The fact that half of all melanoma patients have wild type BRAF melanoma, further highlights the need for an integrated preclinical and clinical approach to guide rational design of effective initial and second-line treatment options.

Acknowledgements

This work is supported by Program Grant 633004 and project grants of the National Health and Medical Research Council of Australia (NHMRC) and an infrastructure grant to Westmead Millennium Institute by the Health Department of NSW through Sydney West Area Health Service. HR is a recipient of a Cancer Institute New South Wales, Research Fellowship and a NHMRC Senior Research Fellowship. MSC is supported by a Rotary Health Australia scholarship

Author details

Kavitha Gowrishankar, Matteo S. Carlino and Helen Rizos

*Address all correspondence to: helen.rizos@sydney.edu.au

Westmead Institute for Cancer Research, University of Sydney at Westmead Millennium Institute and Melanoma Institute Australia, Westmead Hospital, Westmead, Australia

References

[1] Jemal A, Siegel R, Xu J, Ward E. Cancer statistics, 2010. CA Cancer J Clin. 2010;60(5): 277-300.

[2] Cummins DL, Cummins JM, Pantle H, Silverman MA, Leonard AL, Chanmugam A. Cutaneous malignant melanoma. Mayo Clin Proc. 2006;81(4):500-7.

[3] Balch CM, Gershenwald JE, Soong SJ, Thompson JF, Atkins MB, Byrd DR, et al. Final version of 2009 AJCC melanoma staging and classification. J Clin Oncol. 2009;27(36): 6199-206..

[4] Thompson JF, Scolyer RA, Kefford RF. Cutaneous melanoma. Lancet. 2005;365:687-701.

[5] Davies H, Bignell GR, Cox C, Stephens P, Edkins S, Clegg S, et al. Mutations of the BRAF gene in human cancer. Nature. 2002;417(6892):949-54.

[6] Lee JH, Choi JW, Kim YS. Frequencies of BRAF and NRAS mutations are different in histological types and sites of origin of cutaneous melanoma: a meta-analysis. Br J Dermatol. 2011;164(4):776-84.

[7] Wan PT, Garnett MJ, Roe SM, Lee S, Niculescu-Duvaz D, Good VM, et al. Mechanism of activation of the RAF-ERK signaling pathway by oncogenic mutations of B-RAF. Cell. 2004;116(6):855-67.

[8] Flaherty KT, Puzanov I, Kim KB, Ribas A, McArthur GA, Sosman JA, et al. Inhibition of mutated, activated BRAF in metastatic melanoma. N Engl J Med. 2010;363(9): 809-19.

[9] Falchook GS, Lewis KD, Infante JR, Gordon MS, Vogelzang NJ, Demarini DJ, et al. Activity of the oral MEK inhibitor trametinib in patients with advanced melanoma: a phase 1 dose-escalation trial. Lancet Oncol. 2012;13(8):782-9.

[10] Hauschild A, Grob JJ, Demidov LV, Jouary T, Gutzmer R, Millward M, et al. Dabrafenib in BRAF-mutated metastatic melanoma: a multicentre, open-label, phase 3 randomised controlled trial. Lancet. 2012;380(9839):358-65.

[11] Chapman PB, Hauschild A, Robert C, Haanen JB, Ascierto P, Larkin J, et al. Improved Survival with Vemurafenib in Melanoma with BRAF V600E Mutation. N Engl J Med. 2011;364:2507-16.

[12] Sosman JA, Kim KB, Schuchter L, Gonzalez R, Pavlick AC, Weber JS, et al. Survival in BRAF V600-mutant advanced melanoma treated with vemurafenib. N Engl J Med. 2012;366(8):707-14.

[13] Long GV, Trefzer U, Davies MA, Kefford RF, Ascierto PA, Chapman PB, et al. Dabrafenib in patients with Val600Glu or Val600Lys BRAF-mutant melanoma metastatic to the brain (BREAK-MB): a multicentre, open-label, phase 2 trial. Lancet Oncol. 2012 (in press).

[14] Dummer R, Rinderknecht J, Goldinger S, Wagner I, Mitchell L, Veronese M, et al. An open-label pilot study of vemurafenib in previously treated metastatic melanoma patients with brain metastases. J Clin Oncol. 2011;29:(suppl; abstr 8548).

[15] Falchook GS, Long GV, Kurzrock R, Kim KB, Arkenau TH, Brown MP, et al. Dabrafenib in patients with melanoma, untreated brain metastases, and other solid tumours: a phase 1 dose-escalation trial. Lancet. 2012;379:1893-901.

[16] Platz A, Egyhazi S, Ringborg U, Hansson J. Human cutaneous melanoma; a review of NRAS and BRAF mutation frequencies in relation to histogenetic subclass and body site. Mol Oncol. 2008;1(4):395-405.

[17] Curtin JA, Busam K, Pinkel D, Bastian BC. Somatic activation of KIT in distinct subtypes of melanoma. Journal of clinical oncology : official journal of the American Society of Clinical Oncology. 2006;24(26):4340-6.

[18] Krauthammer M, Kong Y, Ha BH, Evans P, Bacchiocchi A, McCusker JP, et al. Exome sequencing identifies recurrent somatic RAC1 mutations in melanoma. Nat Genet. 2012;29(10).

[19] Pollock PM, Harper UL, Hansen KS, Yudt LM, Stark M, Robbins CM, et al. High frequency of BRAF mutations in nevi. Nat Genet. 2003;33(1):19-20.

[20] Hingorani SR, Jacobetz MA, Robertson GP, Herlyn M, Tuveson DA. Suppression of BRAF(V599E) in human melanoma abrogates transformation. Cancer Res. 2003;63:5198-202.

[21] Karasarides M, Chiloeches A, Hayward R, Niculescu-Duvaz D, Scanlon I, Friedlos F, et al. B-RAF is a therapeutic target in melanoma. Oncogene. 2004;23(37):6292-8.

[22] Hoeflich KP, Gray DC, Eby MT, Tien JY, Wong L, Bower J, et al. Oncogenic BRAF is required for tumor growth and maintenance in melanoma models. Cancer Res. 2006;66(2):999-1006.

[23] Sumimoto H, Miyagishi M, Miyoshi H, Yamagata S, Shimizu A, Taira K, et al. Inhibition of growth and invasive ability of melanoma by inactivation of mutated BRAF with lentivirus-mediated RNA interference. Oncogene. 2004;23(36):6031-9.

[24] Flaherty KT, Robert C, Hersey P, Nathan P, Garbe C, Milhem M, et al. Improved survival with MEK inhibition in BRAF-mutated melanoma. N Engl J Med. 2012;367(2): 107-14.

[25] Flaherty KT, Infante JR, Daud A, Gonzalez R, Kefford RF, Sosman J, et al. Combined BRAF and MEK Inhibition in Melanoma with BRAF V600 Mutations. N Engl J Med. 2012 (in press)

[26] Kefford R, Arkenau H-T, Brown MP, Millward M, Infante J, Long G, et al., editors. Selective inhibition of oncogenic BRAF V600E/K/D by GSK2118436: Evidence of clinical activity in subjects with metastatic melanoma. 7th International Melanoma Research Congress; 2010; Sydney, Australia.

[27] Ellis LM, Hicklin DJ. Resistance to Targeted Therapies: Refining Anticancer Therapy in the Era of Molecular Oncology. Clin Cancer Res. 2009;15(24):7471-8.

[28] Bixby D, Talpaz M. Seeking the causes and solutions to imatinib-resistance in chronic myeloid leukemia. Leukemia. 2011;25(1):7-22.

[29] Nazarian R, Shi H, Wang Q, Kong X, Koya RC, Lee H, et al. Melanomas acquire resistance to B-RAF(V600E) inhibition by RTK or N-RAS upregulation. Nature. 2010;468(7326):973-7.

[30] Shi H, Moriceau G, Kong X, Lee MK, Lee H, Koya RC, et al. Melanoma whole-exome sequencing identifies (V600E)B-RAF amplification-mediated acquired B-RAF inhibitor resistance. Nat Commun. 2012;3(724):724.

[31] Corcoran RB, Dias-Santagata D, Bergethon K, Iafrate AJ, Settleman J, Engelman JA. BRAF Gene Amplification Can Promote Acquired Resistance to MEK Inhibitors in Cancer Cells Harboring the BRAF V600E Mutation. Sci Signal. 2010;3(149):ra84.

[32] Diaz LA, Jr., Williams RT, Wu J, Kinde I, Hecht JR, Berlin J, et al. The molecular evolution of acquired resistance to targeted EGFR blockade in colorectal cancers. Nature. 2012;486(7404):537-40.

[33] Poulikakos PI, Persaud Y, Janakiraman M, Kong X, Ng C, Moriceau G, et al. RAF inhibitor resistance is mediated by dimerization of aberrantly spliced BRAF(V600E). Nature. 2011;480:387-90.

[34] Weber CK, Slupsky JR, Kalmes HA, Rapp UR. Active Ras induces heterodimerization of cRaf and BRaf. Cancer Res. 2001;61(9):3595-8.

[35] Heidorn SJ, Milagre C, Whittaker S, Nourry A, Niculescu-Duvas I, Dhomen N, et al. Kinase-dead BRAF and oncogenic RAS cooperate to drive tumor progression through CRAF. Cell. 2010;140(2):209-21.

[36] Poulikakos PI, Zhang C, Bollag G, Shokat KM, Rosen N. RAF inhibitors transactivate RAF dimers and ERK signalling in cells with wild-type BRAF. Nature. 2010;464(7287):427-30.

[37] Hatzivassiliou G, Song K, Yen I, Brandhuber BJ, Anderson DJ, Alvarado R, et al. RAF inhibitors prime wild-type RAF to activate the MAPK pathway and enhance growth. Nature. 2010;464(7287):431-5.

[38] Gowrishankar K, Snoyman S, Pupo GM, Becker TM, Kefford RF, Rizos H. Acquired Resistance to BRAF Inhibition Can Confer Cross-Resistance to Combined BRAF/MEK Inhibition. J Invest Dermatol. 2012;132(7):1850-9.

[39] Dumaz N, Hayward R, Martin J, Ogilvie L, Hedley D, Curtin JA, et al. In melanoma, RAS mutations are accompanied by switching signaling from BRAF to CRAF and disrupted cyclic AMP signaling. Cancer Res. 2006;66(19):9483-91.

[40] Jaiswal BS, Janakiraman V, Kljavin NM, Eastham-Anderson J, Cupp JE, Liang Y, et al. Combined targeting of BRAF and CRAF or BRAF and PI3K effector pathways is required for efficacy in NRAS mutant tumors. PLoS ONE. 2009;4(5):e5717.

[41] Greger J, Eastman S, Zhang V, Bleam MR, Hughes A, Smitheman KN, et al. Combinations of BRAF, MEK, and PI3K/mTOR inhibitors overcome acquired resistance to the BRAF inhibitor GSK2118436 dabrafenib, mediated by NRAS or MEK mutations. Mol Cancer Ther. 2012;11(4):909-20.

[42] Smalley KS. Understanding melanoma signaling networks as the basis for molecular targeted therapy. J Invest Dermatol. 2010;130(1):28-37.

[43] Solit DB, Garraway LA, Pratilas CA, Sawai A, Getz G, Basso A, et al. BRAF mutation predicts sensitivity to MEK inhibition. Nature. 2006;439(7074):358-62.

[44] Nissan MH, Solit DB. The "SWOT" of BRAF Inhibition in Melanoma: RAF Inhibitors, MEK Inhibitors or Both? Curr Oncol Rep. 2011;13(6):479-87.

[45] Little AS, Balmanno K, Sale MJ, Newman S, Dry JR, Hampson M, et al. Amplification of the Driving Oncogene, KRAS or BRAF, Underpins Acquired Resistance to MEK1/2 Inhibitors in Colorectal Cancer Cells. Sci Signal. 2011;4(166):ra17.

[46] Villanueva J, Vultur A, Lee JT, Somasundaram R, Fukunaga-Kalabis M, Cipolla AK, et al. Acquired resistance to BRAF inhibitors mediated by a RAF kinase switch in melanoma can be overcome by cotargeting MEK and IGF-1R/PI3K. Cancer Cell. 2010;18(6):683-95.

[47] Montagut C, Sharma SV, Shioda T, McDermott U, Ulman M, Ulkus LE, et al. Elevated CRAF as a potential mechanism of acquired resistance to BRAF inhibition in melanoma. Cancer Res. 2008;68(12):4853-61.

[48] Shen M, Wu A, Aquila B, Lyne P, Drew L, editors. Linking molecular characteristics to the pharmacological response of a panel of cancer cell lines to the BRAF inhibitor, AZ628. AACR 98th Meeting; 2007 June 9, 2011; Los Angeles.

[49] Emery CM, Vijayendran KG, Zipser MC, Sawyer AM, Niu L, Kim JJ, et al. MEK1 mutations confer resistance to MEK and B-RAF inhibition. Proc Natl Acad Sci U S A. 2009;106(48):20411-6.

[50] Wagle N, Emery C, Berger MF, Davis MJ, Sawyer A, Pochanard P, et al. Dissecting Therapeutic Resistance to RAF Inhibition in Melanoma by Tumor Genomic Profiling. J Clin Oncol. 2011;29(22):3085-96.

[51] Wang H, Daouti S, Li WH, Wen Y, Rizzo C, Higgins B, et al. Identification of the MEK1(F129L) activating mutation as a potential mechanism of acquired resistance to MEK inhibition in human cancers carrying the B-RafV600E mutation. Cancer Res. 2011;71(16):5535-45.

[52] Hatzivassiliou G, Liu B, O'Brien C, Spoerke JM, Hoeflich KP, Haverty PM, et al. ERK inhibition overcomes acquired resistance to MEK inhibitors. Mol Cancer Ther. 2012;11(5):1143-54.

[53] Marks JL, Gong Y, Chitale D, Golas B, McLellan MD, Kasai Y, et al. Novel MEK1 mutation identified by mutational analysis of epidermal growth factor receptor signaling pathway genes in lung adenocarcinoma. Cancer Res. 2008;68(14):5524-8.

[54] Shi H, Moriceau G, Kong X, Koya RC, Nazarian R, Pupo GM, et al. Preexisting MEK1 Exon 3 Mutations in V600E/KBRAF Melanomas Do Not Confer Resistance to BRAF Inhibitors. Cancer Discov. 2012;2(5):414-24.

[55] Johannessen CM, Boehm JS, Kim SY, Thomas SR, Wardwell L, Johnson LA, et al. COT drives resistance to RAF inhibition through MAP kinase pathway reactivation. Nature. 2010;468:968-72.

[56] Shi H, Kong X, Ribas A, Lo RS. Combinatorial treatments that overcome PDGFRbeta-driven resistance of melanoma cells to V600EB-RAF inhibition. Cancer Res. 2011;71(15):5067-74.

[57] Yadav V, Zhang X, Liu J, Estrem S, Li S, Gong XQ, et al. Reactivation of Mitogen-Activated Protein Kinase (MAPK) Pathway by FGF Receptor 3 (FGFR3)/Ras Mediates Resistance to Vemurafenib in Human B-RAF V600E Mutant Melanoma. J Biol Chem. 2012;287(33):28087-98.

[58] Straussman R, Morikawa T, Shee K, Barzily-Rokni M, Qian ZR, Du J, et al. Tumour micro-environment elicits innate resistance to RAF inhibitors through HGF secretion. Nature. 2012;487(7408):500-4.

[59] Wilson TR, Fridlyand J, Yan Y, Penuel E, Burton L, Chan E, et al. Widespread potential for growth-factor-driven resistance to anticancer kinase inhibitors. Nature. 2012 Jul 4;487(7408):505-9.

[60] Puri N, Ahmed S, Janamanchi V, Tretiakova M, Zumba O, Krausz T, et al. c-Met is a potentially new therapeutic target for treatment of human melanoma. Clin Cancer Res. 2007;13(7):2246-53.

[61] Lorenzato A, Olivero M, Patane S, Rosso E, Oliaro A, Comoglio PM, et al. Novel somatic mutations of the MET oncogene in human carcinoma metastases activating cell motility and invasion. Cancer Res. 2002;62(23):7025-30.

[62] Engelman JA, Zejnullahu K, Mitsudomi T, Song Y, Hyland C, Park JO, et al. MET amplification leads to gefitinib resistance in lung cancer by activating ERBB3 signaling. Science. 2007;316(5827):1039-43.

[63] Sherr CJ, Roberts JM. CDK inhibitors: positive and negative regulators of G1-phase progression. Genes Dev. 1999;13(12):1501-12.

[64] Lavoie JN, L'Allemain G, Brunet A, Muller R, Pouyssegur J. Cyclin D1 expression is regulated positively by the p42/p44MAPK and negatively by the p38/HOGMAPK pathway. J Biol Chem. 1996;271(34):20608-16.

[65] Donovan JC, Milic A, Slingerland JM. Constitutive MEK/MAPK activation leads to p27(Kip1) deregulation and antiestrogen resistance in human breast cancer cells. J Biol Chem. 2001;276(44):40888-95.

[66] Lazar V, Ecsedi S, Szollosi AG, Toth R, Vizkeleti L, Rakosy Z, et al. Characterization of candidate gene copy number alterations in the 11q13 region along with BRAF and NRAS mutations in human melanoma. Mod Pathol. 2009;22(10):1367-78.

[67] Smalley KS, Lioni M, Dalla Palma M, Xiao M, Desai B, Egyhazi S, et al. Increased cyclin D1 expression can mediate BRAF inhibitor resistance in BRAF V600E-mutated melanomas. Mol Cancer Ther. 2008;7(9):2876-83.

[68] Xing F, Persaud Y, Pratilas CA, Taylor BS, Janakiraman M, She QB, et al. Concurrent loss of the PTEN and RB1 tumor suppressors attenuates RAF dependence in melanomas harboring (V600E)BRAF. Oncogene. 2012;31(4):446-57.

[69] Paraiso KH, Xiang Y, Rebecca VW, Abel EV, Chen A, Munko AC, et al. PTEN loss confers BRAF inhibitor resistance to melanoma cells through the suppression of BIM expression. Cancer Res. 2011;71:2750-60.

[70] Yang JY, Chang CJ, Xia W, Wang Y, Wong KK, Engelman JA, et al. Activation of FOXO3a is sufficient to reverse mitogen-activated protein/extracellular signal-regulated kinase kinase inhibitor chemoresistance in human cancer. Cancer Res. 2010;70(11):4709-18.

[71] Shao Y, Aplin AE. Akt3-mediated resistance to apoptosis in B-RAF-targeted melanoma cells. Cancer Res. 2010;70(16):6670-81.

[72] Saenz-Santamaria MC, McNutt NS, Shea CR. Immunohistochemical expression of retinoblastoma protein in cutaneous melanomas. Br J Dermatol. 1995;133(6):890-5.

[73] Dai B, Meng J, Peyton M, Girard L, Bornmann WG, Ji L, et al. STAT3 mediates resistance to MEK inhibitor through microRNA miR-17. Cancer Res. 2011;71(10):3658-68.

[74] Paraiso KH, Fedorenko IV, Cantini LP, Munko AC, Hall M, Sondak VK, et al. Recovery of phospho-ERK activity allows melanoma cells to escape from BRAF inhibitor therapy. Br J Cancer. 2010;102(12):1724-30.

[75] Kim KB, Lewis K, Pavlick AC, Infante JR, Ribas A, Sosman JA, et al., editors. A phase II study of the MEK1/MEK2 inhibitor GSK1120212 in metastatic BRAF-V600E or K mutant cutaneous melanoma patients previously treated with or without a BRAF inhibitor. International Melanoma Congress; 2011; Tampa, Florida, USA: Pigment Cell Res.

[76] Flaherty K, Infante JR, Falchook G, Weber JD, Daud A, Hamid O, et al., editors. Phase I/II expansion cohort of BRAF inhibitor GSK2118436 + MEK inhibitor GSK1120212 in patients with BRAF mutant metastatic melanoma who progressed on a prior BRAF inhibitor. International Melanoma Congress; 2011; Tampa, Florida, USA: Pigment Cell Res.

[77] Den RB, Lu B. Heat shock protein 90 inhibition: rationale and clinical potential. Ther Adv Med Oncol. 2012;4(4):211-8.

[78] Whitesell L, Santagata S, Lin NU. Inhibiting HSP90 to treat cancer: a strategy in evolution. Curr Mol Med. 2012;17:17.

[79] Paraiso KH, Haarberg E, Wood E, Rebecca VW, Chen YA, Xiang Y, et al. The heat shock protein-90 inhibitor XL888 overcomes BRAF inhibitor resistance mediated through diverse mechanisms. Clin Cancer Res. 2012;18(9):2502-14.

[80] Modi S, Stopeck A, Linden H, Solit D, Chandarlapaty S, Rosen N, et al. HSP90 inhibition is effective in breast cancer: a phase II trial of tanespimycin (17-AAG) plus trastuzumab in patients with HER2-positive metastatic breast cancer progressing on trastuzumab. Clin Cancer Res. 2011;17(15):5132-9.

[81] Solit DB, Osman I, Polsky D, Panageas KS, Daud A, Goydos JS, et al. Phase II trial of 17-allylamino-17-demethoxygeldanamycin in patients with metastatic melanoma. Clin Cancer Res. 2008 Dec 15;14(24):8302-7.

[82] Nikolaou VA, Stratigos AJ, Flaherty KT, Tsao H. Melanoma: new insights and new therapies. J Invest Dermatol. 2012;132(3 Pt 2):854-63.

[83] Neyns B, Seghers AC, Wilgenhof S, Lebbe C. Successful rechallenge in two patients with BRAF-V600-mutant melanoma who experienced previous progression during treatment with a selective BRAF inhibitor. Melanoma Res. 2012 (in press).

[84] Alcala AM, Flaherty KT. BRAF Inhibitors for the Treatment of Metastatic Melanoma: Clinical Trials and Mechanisms of Resistance. Clin Cancer Res. 2012;18(1):33-9.

[85] Wilmott JS, Tembe V, Howle JR, Sharma R, Thompson JF, Rizos H, et al. Intratumoral molecular heterogeneity in a BRAF-mutant, BRAF inhibitor-resistant melanoma: a case illustrating the challenges for personalized medicine. Molecular cancer therapeutics. 2012 (in press)

[86] Richtig E, Schrama D, Ugurel S, Fried I, Niederkorn A, Massone C, et al. BRAF mutation analysis of only one single metastatic lesion can restrict the treatment of melanoma - a case report. Br J Dermatol. 2012;7(10):1365-2133.

[87] Catalanotti F, Solit DB. Will Hsp90 inhibitors prove effective in BRAF-mutant melanomas? Clin Cancer Res. 2012;18(9):2420-2.

Chapter 8

Pars Plana Vitrectomy Associated with or Following Plaque Brachytherapy for Choroidal Melanoma

John O. Mason and Sara Mullins

Additional information is available at the end of the chapter

http://dx.doi.org/10.5772/53630

1. Introduction

There are underlying concerns regarding the safety of vitrectomy surgery in eyes with intraocular malignancy. These concerns are associated with vitrectomy, both with or without plaque brachytherapy for choroidal melanoma. These include the possibility of local tumor dissemination, extension of malignant cells to the ocular surface and orbit, and remote metastasis. The purpose of this chapter is to discuss the safety and efficacy of employing pars plana vitrectomy in the setting of choroidal melanoma, whether concurrent with treatment or post radiation treatment.

Uveal melanomas are the most common primary intraocular malignancy and, besides the skin, the uvea is the area most commonly affected by melanoma. The incidence of ocular melanoma in the United States is approximately six cases per one million population each year with a median age of onset of 55 years. [1,2] Distant metastasis peaks two to three years after enucleation with uveal melanomas, and patients with remote metastasis seldom survive longer than one year. [3]

Currently, treatments for remote metastasis include immunotherapy, hepatic chemoembolization, as well as experimental treatment modalities. Unfortunately, survival has not dramatically increased with any of the current treatment modalities for metastatic choroidal melanoma. Many factors have been suggested as being of prognostic value including larger tumor size, anterior tumor margin, cellular pleomorphism, extrascleral extension, and genetics including monosomy 3 and genetic expression profiling. These will be discussed in later paragraphs.

The indications for pars plana vitrectomy (PPV) have increased exponentially since its inception in the 1970s. Traditionally, 20-gauge PPV has caused delayed wound healing, requirement of sclerotomy sutures, postoperative astigmatism, and patient discomfort. Recently, small gauge PPV has been introduced. The 25-gauge transconjunctival sutureless PPV system enables sutureless three-port PPV without the need for conjunctival peritomies, decreases mean operative times, reduces post surgical patient discomfort, and decreases surgically-induced trauma at sclerotomy sites. [4] Decreased traumatic conjunctival and scleral manipulation with less postop inflammation, as well as less induced astigmatism, allows for more rapid postoperative visual recovery. The self-sealing nature of the incisions in sutureless PPV, however, does pose potential concerns for the possibility of vitreous incarceration, postoperative endophthalmitis, and hypotony. [5-7]

Posterior uveal melanomas can cause visual disturbances secondary to vitreous hemorrhage, exudative retinal detachments, and radiation-related complications. Treatment consisted of enucleation prior to the Collaborative Ocular Melanoma Study (COMS), which found that at twelve years, there were no significant differences in survival between enucleation and plaque brachytherapy with regards to medium size choroidal melanomas. [8] Radiation has resulted in a new set of complications, some of which are amenable to the use of vitrectomy surgery in the setting of a treated choroidal melanoma. This chapter will discuss the safety and efficacy of vitrectomy regarding diagnosis and biopsy, endoresection, and radiation-induced complications.

2. Pars plana vitrectomy for diagnostic biopsy as well as molecular genetic testing

The diagnosis of posterior choroidal melanoma is often made clinically, as well as aided by ancillary testing, such as ultrasonography, optical coherence tomography, transillumination, and angiography. Choroidal melanoma rarely requires a biopsy to make the diagnosis. With the advent of cytogenetic and molecular genetic studies, there has been a recent effort to obtain fresh tumor tissue. Early cytogenetic studies suggested that certain chromosomes (chromosome 3, 6, and 8) abnormalities were associated with a higher likelihood for metastatic disease. In the early 1990s, it was recognized that a chromosomal 3 alteration was closely associated with metastatic disease. The most important was monosomy 3 (loss of one copy of chromosome 3), which is closely associated with metastatic disease. [9,10]

Other chromosomal changes have been associated with metastatic disease including loss of 1p and 8p as well as gain of 8q, loss of 6q, and gain of 6p. These have been linked statistically to metastatic death in choroidal melanoma. [11]

This cytogenetic information has become increasingly accessible to physicians, and the risk of misinterpreting this information has also increased. Cytogenetic analysis for choroidal melanoma was first performed with standard karyotyping, in which direct visualization was used and chromosomal abnormalities identified by morphologic changes and chromosome banding pattern and size. However, this technique required the need for a highly trained cytogeneticist, led to sampling error due to analysis of only a few tumor cells, and had an inability to detect small changes. There are other techniques that rely on direct analy-

http://dx.doi.org/10.5772/53630

sis of chromosomes including spectral karyotyping (SKY), fluorescence in situ hybridization (FISH), and comparative genomic hybridization (CGH).

The above techniques were superior to clinical and histopathologic variables alone in predicting which patients will develop metastatic disease. However, these techniques had limitations including false positives and negatives, a high rate of failure due to the amount of tissue required, the variability of technique from center to center, and intratumoral heterogeneity. Perhaps the most limiting factor in the accuracy of monosomy 3 analysis is due to heterogeneity. A single choroidal melanoma can be comprised of a mixture of cells, some of which contain one copy of chromosome 3 and others that contain the normal two copies. Sampling one portion of the tumor can often produce the wrong test result.

Recently, thousands of genes could be monitored simultaneously for micro-RNA (mRNA) expression. [12] With the advent of newer software, massive amounts of data could be analyzed and multidimensional analysis could provide new heights of biologic information that were previously unobtainable. This was seen in cancer, where gene expression profiling (GEP) revealed many types of cancer that were thought to be uniform based on their common tissue source, but were instead composed of multiple subtypes of molecularly distinct cancers. This was the case with choroidal melanoma. GEP has helped to simplify our molecular understanding of choroidal melanoma. Rather than many different molecular subtypes, there are only two major choroidal melanoma subtypes, class 1 and class 2. GEP is extremely accurate for predicting patient metastatic rates. Class 1 tumors have a very low risk and class 2 have a very high risk of metastatic disease. [12]

The superiority of GEP over monosomy 3 has been verified by multiple groups. [12] In the past, the major disadvantage of GEP was the expense and limited availability. [13] However, once the value of GEP became clear, considerable effort was devoted to optimizing it for application and use. With regards to choroidal melanoma, GEP evaluates 15 different genetic abnormalities resulting in a class 1 or class 2 classification. This small number of genes has allowed a commercially available, relatively inexpensive assay. This is a polymerase chain reaction based assay, which requires a much smaller biopsy sample and has a very low failure rate. With this technology, we can now identify uveal melanoma patients who are likely to develop metastatic disease. But the question remains, what is the role of vitrectomy with regards to biopsying choroidal melanoma?

Obtaining cells for analysis requires a fine-needle aspiration biopsy (FNAB). Techniques for performing biopsy may be transvitreal or transscleral. Newer techniques even involve the use of small gauge vitrectomy. Transscleral biopsy involves the use of a 27- or 30-gauge needle that is inserted tangentially through the sclera at the base of the tumor. Traditionally following transscleral biopsy, a radioactive plaque is then placed. Transvitreal biopsy may also be performed with a 25- or 27-gauge needle via a pars plana approach. The needle is inserted into the tumor and tumor cells are aspirated. [14] Paul Finger, M.D. was a pioneer in introducing the 25-gauge vitrector to biopsy ocular melanomas. He first used the technique to aspirate cells from an iris melanoma. [13] More recently with the advent of sutureless vitrectomy, newer techniques include performing a 25-gauge vitrectomy followed by inserting a

25- or 27-gauge needle through the 25-gauge cannula and into the center of the tumor, followed by aspiration of tumor cells. [15]

Potential complications of biopsy include vitreous hemorrhage, retinal detachment, and the potential for intraocular or extraocular tumor dissemination. In a series of 500 fine needle biopsy procedures, there were no cases of local recurrence or intraocular dissemination. [16] However, follow up was only three years. There were no cases of extrascleral extension due to FNAB. In another publication by Shields et al, they focused on the outcome of each patient after FNAB. [17] Each patient was treated with plaque brachytherapy at the time of FNAB, and there were no enucleations as all biopsy specimens were obtained by needle sampling. There were no complications in this study as well. Twenty-five-gauge PPV using the vitrector to obtain cells has also resulted in no intraocular dissemination or increased metastasis to date. [13,15]

Most recently, investigators at the Jules Stein Eye Institute performed an Institutional Review Board approved retrospective study to evaluate local and systemic outcomes in patients undergoing FNAB at the time of plaque surgery for choroidal melanoma. Included were all patients with choroidal melanoma treated with Iodine-125 brachytherapy and intraoperative transscleral FNAB from 2005 to 2010. [18] The study included 170 consecutive patients. The technique used for FNAB involved transscleral approach using a 30-gauge needle. They found no cases of treatment failure and there were no cases of orbital dissemination. Metastatic disease developed in 14 of the 170 patients. The metastatic rate in their study was similar to the metastatic rate in the COMS. The COMS did not include FNAB of tumors. In this study, when compared with the largest multicenter prospective study ever performed in ocular oncology, performing FNAB did not increase the risk of developing metastatic disease from choroidal melanoma.

3. Pars plana vitrectomy for treatment of choroidal melanoma using endoresection

Removal of a tumor using an internal approach (endoresection) was first investigated for posterior choroidal melanomas in the 1980s, primarily for small juxtapapillary melanomas that were not amenable to other forms of treatment including brachytherapy at that time. Endoresection has never gained widespread popularity. However, studies have investigated the use of endoresection as an alternative to plaque brachytherapy to avoid radiation related complications such as radiation retinopathy, optic neuropathy, and retinal ischemia. Surgical techniques vary dependent upon surgeon, however the basic principles remain. A three-port PPV is performed with posterior hyaloid dissection. Diathermy or endolaser is used around the periphery of the tumor, followed by creation of a retinotomy. The vitreous cutter is used to excise the tumor to bare sclera. Photocoagulation is then used followed by gas or silicone oil tamponade to flatten the retina. This surgical technique has many complications including retinal detachment, proliferative vitreoretinopathy, severe bleeding, and cataract. The results for local tumor control and metastasis have been favorable, with complications ranging from 2% to 9.4%. [19-22] A very large risk and potential drawback has been the question of whether this procedure results in liberating active tumor causing a potential increase in orbital recurrence and metastatic disease. This question will be answered by the studies cited below.

Kertes et al, in the *British Journal of Ophthalmology,* followed 32 consecutive patients that were treated with endoresection. The patient's choroidal melanoma was pathologically confirmed and all patients were followed for a mean of 40.1 months. At the time, this was the longest follow up and largest series reporting on endoresection for posterior uveal melanoma. [19] The authors found that only three patients developed distant metastasis and died of malignant melanoma. In one case, distant metastasis developed in association with an intraocular recurrence. The most common complications the authors encountered were vitreous hemorrhage in 37.5% of patients, cataract in eight of 32 eyes, and three cases of retinal detachment. With an average of almost three and one-half years follow up, the authors concluded that their results, with regards to metastatic disease, were no worse than patients treated with plaque brachytherapy. They stated that their experience did not support the contention that surgical manipulation of malignant choroidal melanoma promotes metastasis. Furthermore, endoresection is a reasonable and safe alternative to the management of posterior uveal melanoma. Approximately 50% of uveal melanomas occur less than 3mm from the optic nerve or fovea, and the authors felt that their technique was particularly well suited to the treatment of choroidal melanomas that are in close proximity to the optic nerve and fovea.

Damato and associates, in a 1998 *British Journal of Ophthalmology* article, reported on 52 patients undergoing endoresection for choridal melanoma. Their technique involved vitrectomy, retinal incision, hemostasis by raising intraocular pressure and by moderate hypotensive anesthesia, endoresection using the vitrector, endodiathermy, endolaser, and fluid-air exchange to reattach the retina. [20] They used adjunctive ruthenium plaque radiotherapy in selected cases. Their patients had a mean tumor thickness of 3.9 mm. Most of the choroidal melanomas extended to within two disc diameters of the optic nerve. Follow up was a median of 20 months. The main complications included retinal detachment in 16 of 52 patients and cataract in 25 of 52 patients. Twenty-three of the 52 patients had 20/200 or better vision postoperatively. No patients developed local tumor recurrence. Only one of the 52 patients undergoing endoresection developed metastatic disease, 41 months postoperatively. The authors concluded that endoresection did not increase the rate of metastatic disease.

Garcia-Arumi and associates reported on 25 consecutive patients undergoing vitreoretinal surgery with endoresection for high posterior choroidal melanomas. [21] The tumor thickness ranged from 9.1 mm to 12.8 mm. The authors employed standard endoresection technique, but did use a 120-degree anterior retinotomy prior to endoresecting the melanoma and reattaching the retina. The postoperative complications included cataract in 40%, retinal detachment in 16%, epiretinal macular proliferation in 8%, and submacular hemorrhage in 4%. The final visual acuity postoperatively ranged from hand motion to 20/30, with a mean of 20/100. Remarkably, no tumors recurred, and there was no evidence of metastatic disease in follow up, which ranged from 12 to 72 months. The authors state that the reason for having such a low rate of retinal detachment was due to modifying their technique, including trimming the vitreous base, examining the peripheral retina carefully for breaks, and avoiding high infusion pressure. These authors also concluded that endoresection was efficacious and did not increase the rate of metastatic disease.

Most recently, Karkhaneh and associates reported on 20 patients undergoing endoresection for medium size posterior choroidal melanoma. [22] Tumor thickness ranged from 5.5 mm to 11 mm. Preoperative visual acuity ranged from hand motion to 20/40, while postoperative visual acuity ranged from no light perception to 20/30. The authors stated that for tumors with thickness less than 9 mm in their study, they could have been treated with radiotherapy, but endoresection of the tumor may be an alternative approach in some parts of the world where radiotherapy is not readily available. Of the authors' patients, 6.7% had 20/40 or better vision at three years, while 73% had 20/200 or less. Only one in 20 patients died of metastatic disease in a mean follow up of 89.5 months. This is the longest follow up of all case series of patients undergoing endoresection for choroidal melanoma. This rate of metastatic disease is certainly lower than the metastatic rate seen in the COMS.

In contrast to enucleation, endoresection of posterior choroidal melanoma is designed to preserve vision and maintain a cosmetically acceptable eye. In contrast to brachytherapy, endoresection has fewer long-term complications such as radiation optic neuropathy or radiation retinopathy. Immediate complications of endoresection can be severe, including vitreous hemorrhage, retinal detachment, cataract, and proliferative vitreoretinopathy. [19-22] The primary goal of endoresection is to eradicate the tumor while preserving vision. However, the question of cutting into a malignant tumor and liberating cells, some of which may lead to local tumor recurrence or orbital tumor recurrence and/or distant metastasis, needed to be answered. There is no current evidence that endoresection of posterior choroidal melanoma is different from enucleation or brachytherapy with regard to patient survival and metastatic disease, seen in the above detailed literature. [19-22]

4. Pars plana vitrectomy for exudative retinal detachment secondary to choroidal melanoma

Exudative retinal detachment is the most common etiology of vision loss from untreated, recently diagnosed choroidal melanoma. Historically, management has been conservative, as the exudative retinal detachment will often resolve following brachytherapy for choroidal melanoma. However, large exudative retinal detachments secondary to choroidal melanoma often will not resolve and can lead to irreversible vision loss from photoreceptor damage during the several months needed for post brachytherapy resolution. The consistency of subretinal fluid associated with exudative retinal detachment from choroidal melanoma is found to be more viscous compared to subretinal fluid in rhegmatogenous retinal detachments, which can explain the longer duration of reabsorption leading to limited visual recovery. [23]

http://dx.doi.org/10.5772/53630

Gibran and Kapoor reported on six consecutive patients with choroidal melanoma and secondary exudative retinal detachment that underwent radiation therapy, transretinal biopsy with the 25-gauge vitrector, and surgical treatment of the exudative retinal detachment, including vitrectomy and drainage of subretinal fluid with retinal tamponade. [23] All patients had a successful reattachment of the retina with significant restoration of vision. There were no recurrences of exudative retinal detachment. Five of the six patients had 20/40 or better vision postoperatively. More importantly, there were no cases of extrascleral extension or metastatic disease.

5. Pars plana vitrectomy for complications after brachytherapy for choroidal melanoma

Posterior choroidal melanoma treated by brachytherapy can often result in decreased visual acuity due to retinal detachment, vitreous hemorrhage, radiation retinopathy, radiation optic neuropathy, radiation macular ischemia, epimacular proliferation, vitreous debris, and cataract. Potential indications for vitrectomy following melanoma brachytherapy include exudative retinal detachment, tractional and rhegmatogenous retinal detachment, vitreous hemorrhage, vitreous debris, and epimacular proliferation.

There is controversy regarding surgical treatment of eyes harboring a melanoma, whether treated or untreated, and whether there are viable tumor cells that may increase intraocular recurrence, extraocular recurrence, and metastatic disease. This question will be answered by the articles discussed below, as well as our data at Retina Consultants of Alabama/The University of Alabama at Birmingham School of Medicine, Department of Ophthalmology.

Foster and associates reported on nine patients undergoing 20-gauge PPV in eyes containing a treated posterior uveal melanoma. [24] In their series, vitrectomy was performed for vitreous hemorrhage in five patients, macular pucker in two patients, macular hole in one patient, and rhegmatogenous retinal detachment in one patient. Vitrectomy was performed at a mean 24.7 months after melanoma radiation treatment. Dispersion of tumor cells during vitrectomy was not observed in any patient. One patient had melanoma cells detected in the vitreous aspirate. This patient had intratumoral and vitreous hemorrhage before plaque brachytherapy, underwent combined cataract extraction and vitrectomy, and developed intraocular tumor dissemination 56 months after vitrectomy. No other patients developed intraocular tumor dissemination. None of the nine patients developed systemic metastatic disease.

More recently, Bansal et al reported on the author's experience with vitrectomy for vitreous hemorrhage in eyes with posterior choroidal melanoma. [25] They reviewed the medical records of 47 patients who underwent vitrectomy for vitreous hemorrhage following Iodine-125 brachytherapy for posterior choroidal melanoma. The primary outcome of their analysis included rates of intraocular tumor dissemination, extrascleral extension, local tumor recurrence, and systemic metastasis. The average time to develop vitreous hemorrhage was 22 months following brachytherapy. With a mean follow up of five years, only four of the 47 patients (8%) developed metastatic disease, and no cases had intraocular tumor dissemination or extraocular extension.

In 2012, Sisk and Murray reported on combined phacoemulsification and sutureless vitrectomy for complex vitreoretinal diseases. [26] In their retrospective review of 114 eyes that had vitrectomy and cataract extraction, 72 of these eyes had a diagnosis of melanoma post radiation treatment. The authors' primary outcome measures were visual acuity and perioperative complications. They did not report on tumor recurrence or metastatic disease.

We at Retina Consultants of Alabama/The University of Alabama at Birmingham School of Medicine, Department of Ophthalmology reviewed the medical records of 155 consecutive patients with choroidal melanoma treated with Iodine-125 brachytherapy. [15] We identified 20 patients that subsequently underwent 25-gauge PPV following brachytherapy. The average age was 64. The etiology for 25-gauge PPV was epimacular proliferation in one patient, vitreous debris in two patients, rhegmatogenous retinal detachment in three patients, exudative retinal detachment in one patient, and vitreous hemorrhage in 13 patients. The average interval from plaque brachytherapy to 25-gauge vitrectomy was 59 months (range 16 to 98 months). Patients were followed after their 25-gauge PPV an average of 36 months (range nine to 100 months). We found one of 20 patients to have local intraocular recurrence. One patient subsequently was enucleated for a blind painful eye secondary to neovascular glaucoma. Sixteen of the 20 patients had improvement in vision following PPV. Most importantly, no systemic metastatic disease was reported in any of the 20 patients at their last visit, which was a mean of 36 months following their 25-gauge PPV.

In summary, the reports by Foster et al, [24] Bansal et al, [25] and Mason and Mullins [15] reveal the safety of performing vitrectomy in patients who have been treated with brachytherapy for choroidal melanoma. The combined reports by Foster and Mason found zero of 29 patients developed metastatic disease following vitrectomy, while Bansal found only four of 47 patients to have developed metastatic disease following vitrectomy in patients with treated choroidal melanoma. This meta-analysis certainly reveals a much lower incidence of metastatic disease than previous reports, including the COMS (which did not include PPV following brachytherapy). [8] Our current findings based on the above literature, are the following: sutureless vitrectomy may be performed safely in patients having post brachytherapy complications, sutureless vitrectomy does not increase the rate of metastatic disease, and, patients may take comfort that vitrectomy following brachytherapy for choroidal melanoma may result in an increase in vision with no threat of increasing metastatic disease.

6. Conclusion

With the advent of globe salvaging techniques regarding management of choroidal melanoma, ocular oncologists face challenges in the care of these patients. Tumor biopsy is gaining widespread acceptance to obtain tissue for genetic analyses, allowing for more precise determination of metastatic disease prognosis. The use of vitrectomy with regards to tumor biopsy, endoresection, and post radiation complications has expanded rapidly.

http://dx.doi.org/10.5772/53630

Fortunately, all literature to date has shown PPV to be very efficacious and safe in the setting of a patient with choroidal melanoma. Furthermore, there has been no increased rate of metastasis of choroidal melanoma when vitrectomy has been employed prior to or following treatment of the tumor.

Author details

John O. Mason[1*] and Sara Mullins[2]

*Address all correspondence to: masonallmason@yahoo.com

1 Retina Consultants of Alabama, P.C. and the University of Alabama at Birmingham School of Medicine, Department of Ophthalmology, Birmingham, Alabama, USA

2 University of Alabama at Birmingham School of Medicine, Department of Ophthalmology, Birmingham, Alabama, USA

References

[1] Scotto J, Fraumeni JF Jr, Lee JAH. Melanomas of the Eye and Other Noncutaneous Sites: Epidemiologic Aspects. Journal of National Cancer Institute 1976;56 489-491.

[2] Seddon JM, Egan KM, Gragoudas ES. Epidemiology of Uveal Melanoma. In: Ryan SJ. (ed.) Retina. Volume 1. Second Edition. St. Louis: CV Mosby; 1994. p717-724.

[3] Zimmerman LE, McLean IW. An Evaluation of Enucleation in the Management of Uveal Melanomas. American Journal of Ophthalmology 1979;87 741-760.

[4] Fujii GY, de Juan E Jr, Humayun MS, et al. Initial Experience Using the Transconjuctival Sutureless Vitrectomy System for Vitreoretinal Surgery. Ophthalmology 2002;109 1814-1820.

[5] Taylor SR, Aylward GW. Endophthalmitis Following 25-Gauge Vitrectomy. Eye 2005;19 1228-1229.

[6] Taban M, Ufret-Vincenty RL, Sears JE. Endophthalmitis After 25-Gauge Transconjunctival Sutureless Vitrectomy. Retina 2006;26 830-831.

[7] Magasso L, Maia A, Maia Mauricio, et al. Endophthalmitis After 25-Gauge Pars Plana Vitrectomy. Retinal Cases and Brief Reports 2007;1 185-187.

[8] The Collaborative Ocular Melanoma Study Randomized Trial of Iodine 125 Brachytherapy for Choroidal Melanoma: V. Twelve-Year Mortality Rates and Prognostic Factors: COMS Report No. 28. Archives of Ophthalmology 2006;124 1684-1693.

[9] Kilic E, Naus NC, van Gils W, et al. Concurrent Loss of Chromosome Arm 1p and Chromosome 3 Predicts a Decreased Disease-Free Survival in Uveal Melanoma Patients. Investigative Ophthalmology and Visual Science 2005;46(7) 2253-2257.

[10] Maat W, Jordanova ES, van Zelderen-Bhola SL, et al. The Heterogeneous Distribution of Monosomy 3 in Uveal Melanomas: Implications for Prognostication Based on Fine-Needle Aspiration Biopsies. Archives of Pathology and Laboratory Medicine 2007;131(1) 91-96.

[11] Sisley K, Rennie IG, Cottam DW, Potter AM, Potter CW, Rees RC. Cytogenetic Findings in Six Posterior Uveal Melanomas: Involvement of Chromosomes 3, 6, and 8. Genes Chromosomes and Cancer 1990;2(3) 205-209.

[12] Harbour JW, Onken MD, Roberson ED, et al. Frequent Mutation of BAP1 in Metastasizing Uveal Melanomas. Science 2010;330 1410-1413.

[13] Finger PT. A New Technique for 25-Gauge Iridotomy, Iridectomy, and Tumor Biopsy: The Finger Iridectomy Technique May be a Flexible and Safe Way to Biopsy Tumors. Retinal Physician 2006;May/Jun 73-76, 95.

[14] Faulkner-Jones BE, Foster WJ, Harbour JW, Smith ME, Davila RM. Fine Needle Aspiration Biopsy with Adjunct Immunohistochemistry in Intraocular Tumor Management. Acta Cytologica 2005;49 297-308.

[15] Mason JO III, Mullins S. Risk and Benefit of Pars Plana Vitrectomy in Eyes Treated with Plaque Therapy for Choroidal Melanoma: Proceedings of the University of Alabama at Birmingham School of Medicine, Department of Ophthalmology Annual Clinical and Research Symposium 2012, 27-28 April 2012, Birmingham, Alabama, United States of America.

[16] Shields CL, Ganguly A, Bianciotto CG, Turaka K, Tavallali A, Shields JA. Prognosis of Uveal Melanoma in 500 Cases Using Genetic Testing of Fine-Needle Aspiration Biopsy Specimens. Ophthalmology 2011;118 396-401.

[17] Shields CL, Ganguly A, Materin MA, Teixeira L, Mashayekhi A, Swanson LA, Marr BP, Shields JA. Chromosome 3 Analysis of Uveal Melanoma Using Fine-Needle Aspiration Biopsy at the Time of Plaque Radiotherapy in 140 Consecutive Cases. Transamerican Ophthalmological Society 2007;105 43-52.

[18] Johansson CC, Mougiakakos D, Trocme E, et al. Expression and Prognostic Significance of iNO8 in Uveal Melanoma. International Journal of Cancer 2010;126 2682-2689.

[19] Kertes PJ, Johnson JC, Peyman GA. Internal Resection of Posterior Uveal Melanomas. British Journal of Ophthalmology 1998;82 1147-1153.

[20] Damato B, Groenewald C, McGalliard J, Wong D. Endoresection of Choroidal Melanoma. British Journal of Ophthalmology 1998;82 213-218.

[21] Garcia-Arumi J, Sararols L, Martinez V, Corcostegui B. Vitreoretinal Surgery and Endoresection in High Posterior Choroidal Melanomas. Retina 2001;21(5) 445-452.

[22] Karkhaneh R, Chams H, Amoli FA, Riazi-Esfahani M, et al. Long-Term Surgical Outcome of Posterior Choroidal Melanoma Treated by Endoresection. Retina 2007;27(7) 908-914.

[23] Gibran SK, Kapoor KG. Management of Exudative Retinal Detachment in Choroidal Melanoma. Clinical and Experimental Ophthalmology 2009;37 654-659.

[24] Foster WJ, Harbour W, Holekamp NM, Shah GK, Thomas MA. Pars Plana Vitrectomy in Eyes Containing a Treated Posterior Uveal Melanoma. American Journal of Ophthalmology 2003;136 471-476.

[25] Bansal AS, Bianciotto C, Maguire JI, Regillo CD, Shields JA, Shields CA. Pars Plana Vitrectomy in Eyes with Treated Posterior Uveal Melanoma. Retina Today 2011;Nov/Dec 54-56.

[26] Sisk RA, Murray TG. Combined Phacoemulsification and Sutureless 23-Gauge Pars Plana Vitrectomy for Complex Vitreoretinal Diseases. British Journal of Ophthalmology 2010;94 1028-1032.

Chapter 9

Combination Therapies to Improve Delivery of Protective T Cells into the Melanoma Microenvironment

Devin B. Lowe, Jennifer L. Taylor and
Walter J. Storkus

Additional information is available at the end of the chapter

http://dx.doi.org/10.5772/53634

1. Introduction

Incidence rates for melanoma continue to rise between 2-3% each year in the United States [1]. Although melanoma accounts for 5% of new cancer cases, the disease is responsible for most deaths resulting from skin cancer. Five-year survival rates for localized disease have historically been greater than 95% after successfully excising tumors that are less than 1 mm thick [2]. Yet, despite intense efforts in the field, the ability to improve patient survival with invasive forms of the disease has changed little over the past two decades. Current five-year prognostic rates for regional and metastatic melanoma are approximately 66% and 15%, respectfully [1].

FDA-approved agents dacarbazine (DTIC), interferon-α, and high-dose IL-2 have long been employed as palliative therapies in advanced-stage melanoma patients (albeit with significant adverse side effects) [3]. Recent exciting data from large multicenter clinical trials has helped usher in the FDA approval of two new therapies that significantly improve upon the efficacy of existing first-line treatments such as DTIC. Ipilimumab is a humanized monoclonal antibody that functionally blocks the CTLA-4 molecule involved in suppressing T cell activation. In a randomized, double-blind phase III study, metastatic melanoma patients with unresectable stage III or IV disease were administered ipilimumab, ipilimumab plus a peptide vaccine specific to the melanosomal antigen gp100, or gp100 vaccine alone [4]. Ipilimumab therapy resulted in at least a 10 month median overall survival compared to 6.4 months for the gp100 vaccine treatment arm, but no statistical differences were observed between the ipilimumab treatment groups. In a follow-up phase III trial, patients with treatment-naive stage III or IV melanoma received DTIC alone or combined ipilimumab and DTIC therapy [5]. Although there was an improvement to median overall survival (9.1 versus 11.2 months, respectively), treatment with ipilimumab/DTIC significantly improved survival rates in patients at 3 years of follow-up. Vemurafenib is a small molecule drug that inhibits the activity of mutant BRAF (BRAF V600E) molecules in melanoma cells that constitutively signal via the MAPK pathway, promoting tumor cell proliferation and preventing cancer cell apoptosis [6]. Patients with previously untreated metastatic melanoma were first screened for the BRAF V600E mutation and then randomized to receive vemurafenib or DTIC in a phase III clinical trial [7]. At 6 months post therapy, vemurafenib resulted in an improved overall survival rate of 84% relative to 64% for DTIC treatment. Objective responses were also observed in 48% of vemurafenib-treated patients compared to 5% confirmed responses in the DTIC treatment arm. Although these preliminary findings are promising, the follow-up time of the study was inadequate to address the final objective and evaluation of progression-free survival rates for these patients is currently ongoing [8]. In a similarly structured phase II trial, vemurafenib administration in previously-treated BRAF V600E-selected melanoma patients led to a median overall survival of 15.9 months, which exceeds that previously observed for standard first-line treatments in patients with metastatic melanoma [9]. Unfortunately, the current level of care for metastatic melanoma remains far below the general expectations of wide-spread durable responses since most patients relapse from the above mentioned therapeutic interventions and eventually succumb to disease.

2. Supposed barriers to effective treatment

Improving tumor stage classification, candidate drug/therapy selection, and prediction of a patient's outcome to treatment could result from defining molecular events involved in the transformation of normal melanocytes into melanomas [2]. The delineation of these molecular patterns has proven difficult, however, since melanoma contains high frequencies of dissimilar gene mutations, deletions, duplications, and translocations across the range of patients evaluated [10]. A number of inherited events have been illuminated (transmissible through genetic or epigenetic means) that appear directly involved in initiating a melanocyte's pathway to malignancy by first inducing the clonal selection and outgrowth of cells [11]. Examples include alterations in the kinases BRAF and KIT and the tumor suppressor protein PTEN. The activating BRAF (BRAF-V600E) point mutation occurs in approximately 50% of melanomas (more commonly in cutaneous melanomas) and constitutively drives the MAPK pathway - without upstream RAS activation - leading to cell proliferation and survival [12]. The frequency of BRAF mutations is also preserved among primary and metastatic melanoma lesions, supporting the hypothesis that genetic disruption of BRAF is an early event that does not drive metastasis alone [12, 13]. KIT alterations account for up to 25% of acral and mucosal melanoma subtypes [6, 14]. The most common genetic change in KIT is an activating point mutation that stimulates the MAPK and PI3K-AKT signaling pathways, promoting cell growth and migration and preventing apoptosis [15]. Additional common melanoma defects are cells disrupted/deficient in the gene encoding PTEN. Under normal physiologic conditions, growth factors bind their respective cell surface receptor tyrosine kinase (RTK) and induce PI3K activity. PTEN serves to block PI3K function by preventing phosphorylation of PIP2 to PIP3, which ultimately drives signaling events through the PI3K-AKT pathway. In the absence of the phosphatase activity of PTEN, the AKT signaling cascade is unrestrained, driving the cell into a pro-survival mode. Simultaneous PTEN and BRAF alterations are two of the more widely documented correlative markers in late-stage melanoma patients and highlight the importance of the overlapping and non-overlapping functions of the AKT and MAPK pathways, respectively, in maintaining a malignant state. The common melanoma genetic aberrations (e.g., BRAF, KIT, PTEN) are not currently utilized for clinical diagnosis or prognosis, though, considering the seemingly paradoxical instances where gene markers do not correlate with independent classifiers of tumorigenesis [2]. For example, PTEN expression profiles have been reported to predict more aggressive forms of melanoma in cases of PTEN gene disruption [16] or activation [17] alongside clinico-pathological results. Drug-candidate discovery and testing has instead flourished with the improved knowledge of recurring primary genetic aberrations that appear to induce melanoma, as highlighted above for the FDA-approved BRAF inhibitor vemurafenib. Many other potential therapies have entered into clinical trials and have been well-described in a recent review [6]. One such promising drug is the RTK inhibitor dasatinib. With regard to melanoma, dasatinib targets KIT (and a limited range of alternate RTKs), leading to the disruption of the MAPK and PI3K signaling pathways. In a recently completed phase I trial, unselected patients with stage III or IV metastatic melanoma were administered dasatinib along with DTIC [18]. Combined treatment resulted in an objective response rate of 13.8% and median progression free survival of 13.4 weeks and appeared to be more active than either agent applied alone based on historical controls. Although these results are promising and support follow-up studies with this TKI, clinical evidence suggests that dasatinib preferably inhibits mutated KIT (occurring at exon 11 or 13) versus overexpressed wild-type KIT in melanoma patients [19-21]. It will, therefore, be of interest to closely monitor the differential anti-tumor efficacy of dasatinib treatment in melanoma patients harboring KIT mutations in future trials in order to select the most suitable patient population for clinical trial accrual.

Monotherapeutic use of drugs specific to the more commonly disrupted signaling pathways in melanoma has several drawbacks. At best, known drug/molecular target combinations are available for no more than 50% of melanoma patients (as in the case with vemurafenib and mutated BRAF), which severely limits treatment options for excluded patients. Drug resistance also presents a major concern in melanoma patients treated under these regimes. Tumor cells are capable of thwarting the benefits of targeted molecular approaches based on a number of innate and acquired mechanisms that include utilizing compensatory cell signaling pathways [22] and survival signals provided by the supportive TME [23]. In the instance of vemurafenib treatment, most BRAF-V600E-selected patients respond to therapy in the short-term (~80%) but fail to maintain durable responses [24]. Such clinical observations are not specific to melanoma but describe a wider phenomenon of eventually developing resistance to molecularly-targeted approaches in solid tumors [25, 26]. It has been hypothesized that therapy administration actually promotes the natural selection of a resistant tumor mass in the host [27]. These problematic corollaries will have to be overcome through the prudent use of combinational strategies that coordinately attack tumor cells and/or the tumor stroma at multiple, non-redundant levels. As one example, tyrosine kinase inhibitor (TKI) drugs (e.g., sunitinib, axitinib, dasatinib) remain attractive front-line agents to improve the efficacy of other co-applied strategies such as immunotherapy since these small molecule inhibitors may enable heightened responses to immune intervention based on the removal of suppression pathways inherent in the TME (as discussed in subsequent sections).

The initial driver mutations occurring in a melanocyte (e.g., BRAF, KIT, PTEN) are directly implicated in arresting cell cycle control points and promoting the clonal selection and expansion of cells that may disseminate systemically [11]. These primary genetic aberrations also induce an array of secondary events – all of which may contribute to molecular intra- and inter-patient heterogeneity. The pattern of tumor growth typically follows a course, whereby, melanomas transition from a benign radial phase in the epidermis (i.e., nevus) to vertical growth into the dermis and eventual systemic spread [28]. Upon reaching a size of 1-2 mm, a primary tumor nodule is growth-limited based on the need to develop a blood supply capable of providing sufficient nutrients to cells and effectively discharging metabolic waste [29]. To progress beyond this 1-2 mm limit, molecular signals in the tumor must be initiated to promote neovascularization. Hypoxia serves as one stimulus to initiate the expression of vascular endothelial growth factor (VEGF) by melanoma cells [30]. VEGF secretion by tumor cells can also result from inflammatory cytokines derived from infiltrating immunosuppressive cell populations such as tumor-associated macrophages (TAMs) and myeloid-derived suppressor cells (MDSCs). In general terms, locoregional VEGF production recruits endothelial precursor cells by binding its cognate high affinity receptor VEGFR2 [29, 30]. Endothelial cells in turn promote pericyte trafficking and coverage via elaboration of platelet-derived growth factor (PDGF). The effects of angiogenic pathways induced under conditions of tumor growth, however, do not resemble normal physiologic conditions. There is no hierarchical structure of arterioles to venules to capillaries. Instead, the tumor blood supply consists of a chaotic distribution of immature and mature endothelial cells, which are partly due to continued VEGF signaling by melanoma and endothelial cells and pericytes. Chronic VEGF expression serves to antagonize the interaction of endothelial cells and pericytes (by inhibiting PDGF/PDGFR binding) as well as to promote an ongoing cycle of endothelial cell recruitment and proliferation. The end-results are blood vessels comprised of loosely connected endothelial cells with little-to-no pericyte coverage. Consequently, blood flow is severely restricted in areas of the tumor while fluid build-up (e.g., plasma protein extravasation) occurs in the tumor interstitium, all of which contributes to heightened hypoxia, acidosis, and interstitial pressure. These TME dynamics in late-stage disease may help account for melanoma's intrinsic resistance to chemo/radiotherapies [31]. First, the delivery of anti-tumor strategies is impaired due to deficiencies in the tumor-derived blood supply and increased interstitial pressure. The hypoxic environment also directly contributes to a reduced efficacy of drug function such as in the case of radiotherapies. Lastly, conventional strategies that incorporate cytotoxic drugs have a diminished effect on tumor cells selected for growth under hypoxic and acidic conditions.

3. Improving treatment strategies

3.1. Vascular reconditioning hypothesis

Correcting deficiencies in the tumor vasculature could potentially circumvent many of the problems that serve to limit the effective treatment of late-stage metastatic melanoma patients as outlined above. Historically, vasculature disruption was hypothesized to starve tumors, leading to apoptosis/necrosis and lesional regression. In reality, anti-vasculature measures appear to primarily modulate the overall tumor blood vessel architecture through actions on immature endothelial cells [32]. These effects lead to transient improvements in blood flow (thereby, diminishing hypoxia and acidosis) and reduced interstitial pressure in the tumor mass [31]. In phase II clinical trials, patients with either metastatic melanoma or colorectal cancer have experienced improved response rates when bevacizumab (an anti-VEGF monoclonal antibody therapy) was combined with a standard of care treatment such as chemotherapy [33-37]. Although bevacizumab monotherapy exhibits minimal clinical impact [38], the antibody appears to exert a helper action by improving the bioavailability/activity of co-delivered cytotoxic drugs via its disruption of the melanoma-associated vasculature. This overarching paradigm has been formally tested in a number of preclinical models showing the improved distribution and efficacy of anti-tumor agents subsequent to tumor blood vessel "normalization" [29]. One caveat to this strategy is the need to consider the optimal schedule for application of each modality to yield superior anti-tumor efficacy. Our laboratory has recently reported that delayed TKI administration in a therapeutic melanoma mouse model negated protection from a dendritic cell (DC) vaccine based on subcutaneous tumor growth kinetics [39]. These studies and others indicate a window of therapeutic opportunity where anti-vasculature measures are highly effective in enhancing co-administered anti-tumor therapies. Melanomas, however, would be expected to become refractory to the action of anti-vascular drugs based on the selection of mature blood vessels that are effectively stabilized by pericytes [32]. As noted with molecular targeting strategies, tumor cells are also likely selected based on their ability to induce angiogenesis via alternate signaling pathways that do not overlap those sensitive to the originally-administered agents. In the absence of an effective second line strategy, increased tumor growth following anti-vasculature monotherapy may instead occur [40].

3.2. Immunotherapy and melanoma

The immune system provides a promising platform for consideration of inclusion in combined anti-melanoma therapies as it holds many theoretical advantages over standard treatment options such as chemotherapy or bulk cytokine (biologic modifier) administration. Namely, immunotherapies can be tailored to specifically target and kill tumor cells while leaving the surrounding normal tissue intact. Immune memory (recall) can also aid in sustained therapeutic action as a result of active vaccination, allowing for the maintenance of sub-clinical residual disease (in the adjuvant setting) or the prevention of recurrent tumor variants (i.e., through mechanisms of immune cross-priming and epitope spreading in the protective T cell repertoire). Several clinical studies have highlighted the proof-of-principle for immunotherapy in mediating objective clinical responses in melanoma patients. Therapies incorporating ipilimumab and bevacizumab have been discussed in preceding sections. Impressive clinical results have also been obtained using *ex vivo* expanded tumor infiltrating lymphocytes (TIL; T cells) in combination with rhIL-2 and non-lethal irradiation therapy, although this is a highly specialized process limited to a few locations worldwide [41, 42]. Durable complete responses (CR) (RECIST) have been observed in 22% of patients undergoing this form of treatment and most responses have been durable for > 3 years irrespective of prior treatments. Not all patients are suited to this approach, however, due to the technical constraints of resecting and culturing TIL (approximately 45% of patients are eligible at this stage) and severe toxicities associated with IL-2 administration and lymphodepletion.

The general failure of immunotherapeutic strategies to date likely involves a number of issues. As noted, melanoma is a vascularized cancer that maintains an aberrant blood vessel system. Immunologic strategies that rely on the anti-tumor properties of effector cells such as CD8+ T cells or antibodies may be unable to penetrate areas of the tumor based on the abnormal dynamics of blood flow and high interstitial pressure. Other melanoma characteristics such as reduced oxygen content and low pH serve to further reduce the function of cytotoxic CD8+ T cells if they should even be recruited into the TME. First-line strategies that recondition the melanoma-associated vasculature would be expected to overcome such obstacles and allow for the improved delivery and cytotoxic action of immunotherapeutic moieties.

Melanoma is an inherently immunogenic tumor, given the anti-tumor properties of resected TIL *in vitro* [43] and clinical observations that patients with higher frequencies of TIL have improved overall survival [43, 44]. However, the late-stage TME is also quite immunosuppressive. Due in part to the hypoxic nature of the TME, immunosuppressive cells such as regulatory T cells (Tregs), TAMs, and MDSCs become enriched within the tumor and reinforce their own survival/function while coordinately opposing the survival/function of protective T effector cells and Type-1 polarized DCs via soluble mediators and direct cell-to-cell contact [45, 46]. Elaboration of cytokines such as IL-10 and TGF-β sustain Tregs and inhibit T cell Type-1 polarization and DC maturation [47-49]. T cells are further suppressed by MDSC secretion of reactive oxygen and nitrogen species, TGF-β, VEGF, and arginase (i.e., through L-arginine depletion) [50]. Additionally, melanoma cells can express inhibitory molecules such as PD-L1 on their cell surface that interacts with T cell-expressed PD1, leading to T cell dysfunction and death [51]. Melanoma cells might also prevent DC processing/presentation or T cell targeting through defects in the antigen presenting machinery and/or antigen loss. Therefore, combined immunotherapies must counteract the suppressive TME at some level (e.g., ipilimumab's anti-CTLA-4 mode of action). By reversing the balance of immunosuppression toward inflammatory Type-1 immunity, one can envision improved clinical benefits for coordinately-applied cancer vaccines. Yet, the optimization of the vaccine sub-component of such regimens remains an area of intense study [52].

3.3. Focus on dendritic cell vaccination

DCs provide a theoretical advantage over other vaccine types since they potently stimulate antigen-specific *de novo* and memory recall T cell responses [47]. Under steady-state conditions, a mature DC first migrates out of the periphery and into the TME where antigen is sampled and processed/presented in the form of MHC class I/II-peptide complexes [53]. After upregulating CCR7 expression, antigen-loaded DC become competent to migrate to tissue-draining lymph nodes, where it may provide an antigenic target, costimulation (e.g., DC CD80/86 binding the T cell receptor CD28), and cytokines to allow for the activation of antigen-specific CD4+ and/or CD8+ T cells. These educated effector T cells then return to the blood circulation where a portion of these cells may enter the tumor and perform anti-tumor activities.

Effective vaccination against melanoma antigens (many of which are non-mutated and expressed by normal melanocytes) presents a formidable challenge. Indeed, most tumor-associated antigens are on the whole less immunogenic than tumor specific antigens that arise as a result of viral infection (e.g., HPV induced cervical cancer). Assuming that host central and peripheral tolerance mechanisms have not deleted the appropriate T cell repertoire, the maturation status of the DC may be key to whether specific anti-melanoma T cell responses can be invoked at all. For example, improperly matured DCs may engage responder T cells and induce either anergy or death rather than T cell activation, expansion, and differentiation into effector cells. In addition, the immunosuppressive TME can adversely condition both endogenous DC and T cell survival/function. Immuno-oncologists have attempted to tackle these confounding issues by adoptive transfer of *ex vivo* manipulated DCs (and T cells) that exhibit preferred (normal) bioactivity. In the case of DCs, these cells may be harvested as blood precursors from cancer patients and subsequently polarized to a Type-1 phenotype through genetic manipulation or exposure to a cocktail of inflammatory-prone soluble mediators in culture. After further loading with target antigens associated with tumor cell growth and progression, this cellular vaccine may be reinfused back into the patient. Fully-mature DCs generated in this fashion are able to efficiently home to draining lymph nodes and activate/instruct resident effector-prone T cells while remaining functionally-resistant to TME inhibitory factors such as IL-10, TGF-β, VEGF, IL-6, and PGE_2 [54]. The framework for the autologous DC delivery strategy in cancer patients has been validated to some degree with the FDA-approved cellular immunotherapy designated sipuleucel-T. In this protocol, peripheral blood mononuclear cells (PBMCs) are harvested from men with castration-resistant prostate cancer and incubated with a fusion protein containing prostatic acid phosphatase and GM-CSF, a cytokine important for DC maturation [55, 56]. The stimulated PBMCs are then delivered back into patients every two weeks for a total of three injections. In a phase III double-blind multicenter trial, sipuleucel-T resulted in a median survival advantage of 4.1 months in 22% of individuals versus the placebo group [55]. Sipuleucel-T promoted heightened Type-I T cell and antibody responses against the vaccine fusion protein in a majority of patients presumably due to the enhanced maturation state of infused activated DCs [56]. Overall survival correlated with improved specific immunity in responding patients suggesting that sipuleucel-T's mechanism of action includes immune targeting of prostate carcinoma cells by vaccine-induced T cells.

Many clinical studies have highlighted the ability of DC-based adoptive therapy to boost resident anti-tumor T cell responses and to mediate corollary clinical activity in patients with melanoma [57-65]. In one of the first reported DC-based therapy trials in the melanoma setting, DCs were harvested from patients (regardless of their HLA type), cultured in the presence of rhGM-CSF and rhIL-4 for one week, and pulsed with melanoma-associated peptides (e.g., HLA-A2 restricted gp100, tyrosinase, and Melan-A/MART1 peptides) or autologous tumor lysates [59]. The cellular vaccines were delivered into tumor uninvolved inguinal lymph nodes at least 4 times at weekly intervals. Eleven out of 16 (69%) enrolled patients developed DTH reactions to intradermal injections of DCs loaded with either vaccine-derived peptides or tumor lysates following DC vaccine therapy. Subsequent analysis of infiltrating T cells in representative biopsied DTH sites revealed peptide-specific reactivity to antigenic components of the vaccine. Overall, 2 CR and 3 PR were observed with these same patients also exhibiting vaccine-specific reactivity as evidenced in DTH testing. In a separate phase I clinical trial reported by Ribas and colleagues, GM-CSF/IL-4 *ex vivo* cultured DCs were loaded with a Melan-A/MART1 peptide and delivered intradermally into metastatic melanoma patients a total of 3 times every 2 weeks alongside tremelimumab (anti-CTLA-4) treatment [66]. Tetramer and ELISPOT analysis revealed increases in the frequency of peripheral Melan-A/MART1-reactive CD8+ T cells as a consequence of specific vaccination in 9 of 15 (60%) individuals, although tremelimumab therapy did not appear to enhance Melan-A/MART1 T cell frequency and function. Four vaccinated patients experienced objective clinical responses (2 CR, 2 PR) with 3 individuals also displaying an improved MART-1 T cell response post-DC vaccination. Although such studies provide proof-of principle, major improvements are still needed in order to achieve durable clinical responses and prolonged survival rates in a majority of patients undergoing autologous DC therapy. A potential improvement to DC activity *in vivo* may reside with how DCs are manipulated *ex vivo* following leukopheresis. In cases where DCs are stimulated to an underwhelmed (use of GM-CSF/IL-4) or exhausted (use of PGE_2) Type-1 state, effector T cells suffer from an inability to effectively mediate anti-tumor responses [49]. One promising DC polarizing method incorporates IL-1β, TNF-α, IFN-α, IFN-γ, and poly-I:C in the *ex vivo* culturing phase to effectively mature DCs (designated α-DC1). Twenty-two patients with recurrent malignant glioma were administered up to 4 vaccinations intranodally of α-DC1 loaded with glioma associated antigens at 2 week intervals [67]. At the conclusion of the immunization cycle, 58% of evaluable patients demonstrated a response to at least one antigenic component of the vaccine based on PBMC specific activity through IFN-γ ELISPOT or tetramer analysis. Upregulated gene expression profiles of Type-1 cytokines (e.g., IFN-α, IFN-γ) and chemokines (e.g., CXCL10) were also observed in PBMCs from α-DC1 treated patients, suggesting that the vaccine therapy enhanced the cytolytic activity and trafficking ability of immune cells. Progression free survival was extended to 12 months in 9 of 22 patients receiving the α-DC1 vaccine. The ability of α-DC1 to produce IL-12 (and, hence, stimulate CD4+ and CD8+ T cell function) correlated to prolonged progression free survival. Based on the safety profile and relative success of this trial, the α-DC1 generation protocol is currently being evaluated in a phase I trial in patients with metastatic melanoma (NCT00390338).

Another way to improve the immunogenicity of autologous DC-based therapy involves the choice of antigenic target for presentation to T cells (i.e., therapeutic selection of the responding anti-tumor T cell repertoire for expansion). Most DC-based vaccine trials have incorporated melanoma-associated antigens such as gp100, tyrosinase, Melan-A/MART1 and MAGE in the vaccine formulation. Despite the surprisingly high immunogenic nature of these "self" antigens in vaccinated patients, tumor cells can continue to grow progressively by evading the effector T cell system via various well-described mechanisms [46, 48, 53]. For instance, the tumor mass is composed of a heterogeneous mixture of cancer cells that exhibit a range of defects/deficiencies in the antigen presentation machinery that limits effective presentation of tumor antigen-derived peptides in MHC complexes and leads to poor recognition by the immune system. As such, a fraction of tumor cells may become "invisible" to the adaptive immune system, resulting in the negative selection of treatment-resistant tumor cells in progressor lesions [68]. This scenario can be avoided in part by the use of vaccines incorporating antigens that represent proteins required for maintenance of the transformed state, progressive growth, or metastasis. Alternatively, one may consider the inclusion of antigens expressed not by tumor cells themselves but by the supportive stromal cells (whose phenotype is uniquely modified by the TME) that enable the formation of large bulk tumors. We hypothesize that peptides associated with tumor angiogenesis (summarized in Table 1) may provide an ideal source of targets for DC/peptide vaccine design. In effect, targeting the underlying tumor stroma (e.g., vascular cells, pericytes) would disrupt melanoma growth and promote tumor-specific immunity and protection. Our laboratory has previously demonstrated the ability to successfully treat HLA-A2+ transgenic mice bearing established colon carcinoma or melanomas using DC-based vaccines containing antigens differentially associated with the tumor vasculature [69]. Animals administered peptide-loaded DC vaccines displayed enhanced protection from established tumor growth and ability, in instances of complete regression, to provide durable protection from dormant disease. Interestingly, active vaccination against tumor stromal antigens led to the corollary cross-priming of T cell responses directed against alternate vascular-associated antigens that were not originally comprised in the vaccine therapy as well as *bona fide* tumor cell-associated antigens. Normal donors and melanoma patients also exhibited immune reactivity to many of the stromal antigens upon *in vitro* sensitization, indicating that operational tolerance to such "self" antigens may be broken using a DC/peptide-based vaccination approach [70]. Importantly, this vaccine strategy appears safe in treated mice since we have not observed deleterious immunologic responses against the normal tissue vasculature, disruptions to the normal cutaneous wound healing process, or aberrations in the fertility/litter size of pre-vaccinated female animals [69, 70].

Stromal antigen	Cell expression	AA positions	Peptide sequence	CD8+ T cell response		
				HLA-A2+ transgenic mice	HLA-A2+ normal donors	HLA-A2+ melanoma patients
DLK1	P	269-277	RLTPGVHEL	++	+	++
		310-318	ILGVLTSLV	++	+	++
		328-336	FLNKCETWV	+++	+	++
EphA2	VEC	883-891	TLADFDPRV	+++	+	++
HBB	P	31-39	RLLVVYPWT	+	+	++
		105-114	RLLGNVLVCV	+	+	+
NG2	P	770-778	TLSNLSFPV	-	-	++
		2238-2246	LILPLLFYL	+	-	++
NP1	P	331-339	GLLRFVTAV	+	+	+++
		433-441	GMLGMVSGL	++	+	+++
		869-877	VLLGAVCGV	+++	+	+
NP2	P	214-222	DIWDGIPHV	-	-	++
		328-336	YLQVDLRFL	-	-	++
PDGFRβ	P	890-898	ILLWEIFTL	+++	+	+
PSMA	VEC	441-450	LLQERGVAYI	+	-	+
RGS5	P	5-13	LAALPHSCL	+	-	++
TEM1	VEC/P	691-700	LLVPTCVFLV	+	++	++
VEGFR1	VEC/P	770-778	TLFWLLLTL	++	+	+

Table 1. Candidate melanoma-associated vascular peptides for DC vaccine design. CD8+ T cell response summaries are provided from previous work by our laboratory [69, 70]. Naïve HLA-A2+ transgenic mice were vaccinated bi-weekly with DCs pre-pulsed with the appropriate antigen-derived peptide. One week following the second DC vaccine, splenic CD8+ T cells were harvested and co-cultured 48 hours with the HLA-A2+ T2 cell line pulsed with the relevant peptide. CD8+ T cell elaboration of IFN-γ (as a read-out for Type-1 activity) was then determined through ELISA. Human CD8+ T cell responses to stromal peptides were determined by first isolating PBMCs and stimulating cells in the presence of antigen-loaded autologous DCs for 1 week. Normal donor samples underwent 2 rounds of IVS while PBMCs obtained from melanoma patients were subjected to 1 round of IVS. CD8+ T cell IFN-γ expression was assessed as similarly described for HLA-A2+ transgenic mice. Abbreviations used: AA, amino acid; P, pericyte; VEC, vascular endothelial cell; -, No observed activity; +, low activity; ++, medium activity; +++, high activity; IVS, *in vitro* sensitization

3.4. Combining small molecule drugs with DC vaccination

In addition to empirically improving DC vaccine design (e.g., via the *ex vivo* conditioning of the APC and a rationale selection of the included antigenic targets), the effectiveness of such treatments would be expected to improve by mitigating the functional constraints on vaccine-induced T effector cells imposed by the generally suppressive TME. As previously mentioned, the aberrant dynamics of the tumor vascular architecture and enrichment of regulatory cell populations (e.g., MDSC, Treg) in the TME consort to diminish the recruitment, vitality, and tumoricidal activity of immune cells *in situ*. Therefore, the conditional abrogation of the negative attributes of the TME would be predicted to improve infiltration and function of vaccine-expanded T cell populations, leading to more durable objective clinical responses in melanoma patients as diagramed in Figure 1. What follows are examples of three FDA-approved TKI drugs that could be utilized in DC-based vaccine combination immunotherapies to achieve this goal.

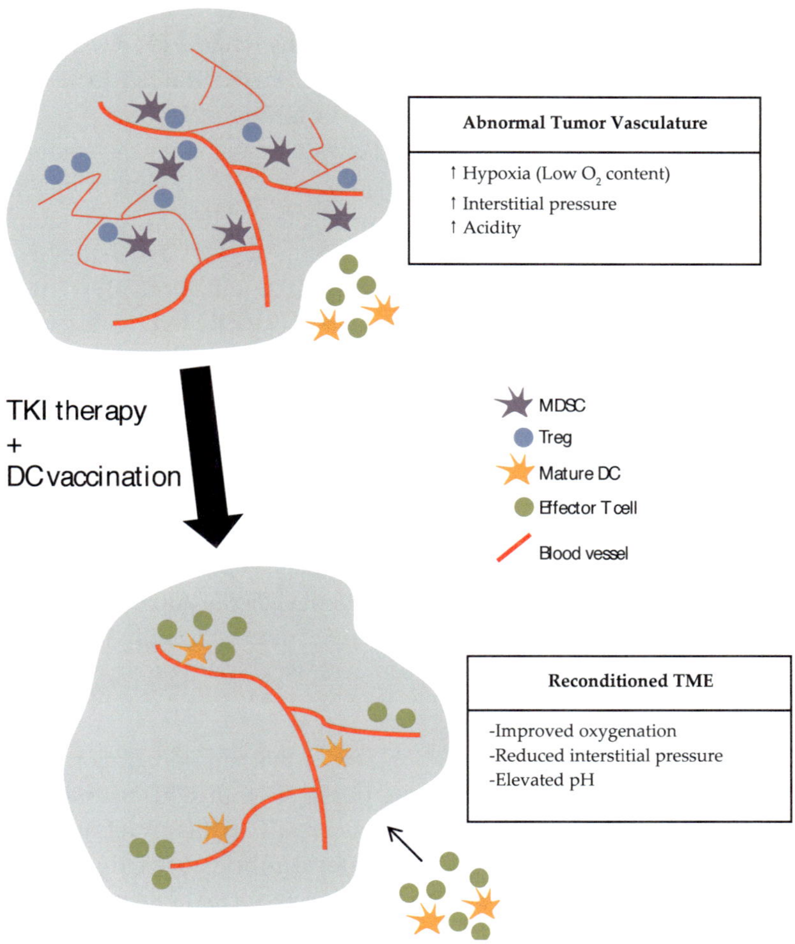

Figure 1. Paradigm for effective combination treatment of melanoma. Established vascularized cancers such as melanoma are entrenched with a chaotic blood vessel network and immunosuppressive cell populations. These TME properties serve to prevent the intratumoral delivery and function of single-agent cytotoxic therapies, including specific active vaccination. In cases of combined therapeutic strategies where the melanoma-associated vasculature is first modulated through TKI drug sensitization, for example, immature blood vessels (i.e., endothelial cells loosely decorated by or absent in pericyte coverage) may be disrupted, resulting in a normoxic TME with reduced interstitial pressure and acidity. Frequencies of MDSC and Treg cells are also minimized through mechanisms that are not entirely clear.

Consequently, vaccine-initiated effector T cells can better traffick into tumors and exert their anti-tumor functions. Mature DCs are also able to infiltrate the tumor lesion and sample material from dying cells or necrotic tissue for cross-presentation purposes to unknown/untargeted tumor associated antigens, leading to activation of a broad T cell repertoire that is competent to promote durable anti-tumor immunity. Abbreviations used: TKI, tyrosine kinase inhibitor; MDSC, myeloid-derived suppressor cell; Treg, regulatory T cell; DC, dendritic cell; TME, tumor microenvironment

Sunitinib binds to and inhibits a range of tyrosine kinases including the vascular associated molecules VEGFR and PDGFR. The drug is approved for use in patients with metastatic renal cell carcinoma (mRCC) or gastrointestinal stromal tumors, where most patients respond favorably to treatment in the short-term [71, 72]. In one recently reported phase I trial, metastatic melanoma patients harboring KIT mutations were administered sunitinib using the FDA-approved regimen of 50 mg/day for 4 weeks followed by 2 weeks off drug [73]. Out of 10 evaluable patients, 1 individual had a CR that lasted 15 months while 2 PR endured between 1-7 months. A separate clinical study, reported on the ability of sunitinib to work in concert with docetaxel therapy in patients with solid tumors including melanoma [74]. Two PR were confirmed in a total of 12 metastatic melanoma patients treated with the combination regimen, supporting a potential tumor vascular "reconditioning" role of sunitinib in improving the delivery and function of cytotoxic therapies within the TME. Our own animal studies support a similar paradigm for combination immunotherapies [39]. Protection from established melanoma progression (based on tumor growth kinetics and survival) were enhanced in mice receiving both sunitinib and DC/peptide-based vaccination versus either agent administered as a monotherapy. Sunitinib co-treatment facilitated the recruitment of DC-"primed" Type-1 CD8+ T cells into melanoma lesions based in part on the upregulated expression of VCAM-1 (on vascular endothelial cells) and CXCR3 ligand chemokines (e.g., CXCL9, CXCL10, CXCL11) within the TME. This TKI also reduced frequencies of immunosuppressive cell populations such as MDSC and Tregs in the tumor and tumor draining lymph node (TDLN), which was associated with increased cytotoxic potential mediated by vaccine-induced CD8+ T cells. Sunitinib therapy has similarly been reported to prevent the peripheral accumulations of MDSCs and Tregs in mRCC patients [75-77]. Although the molecular mechanism underlying these alterations remains an open question, sunitinib inhibits STAT3 activation (via inhibition of upstream tyrosine kinases) which may prove core to its perceived anti-tumor actions [39, 75].

Axitinib is a potent TKI targeting VEGFRs (VEGFR1, 2, and 3) that support tumor angiogenesis [30, 78]. Following the completion of a recent phase III trial [79], axitinib was granted approval by the FDA as a second-line therapy for mRCC patients refractory to first-line treatment options including sunitinib. Axitinib has also been used to treat patients with melanoma. Pre-clinical studies have supported a role for axitinib monotherapy to disrupt angiogenesis and tumor formation in xenograft melanoma models [80]. A multicenter phase II trial also justified the continued use of axitinib-based treatment in metastatic melanoma patients [81]. Individuals receiving this TKI experienced reductions of VEGFR2 and VEGFR3 and increased levels of soluble VEGF in their plasma. Treatment with axitinib was associated with an overall objective response rate of 18.8%, which is comparable to historical response rates for chemotherapy and IL-2-based therapies. Given the relative clinical success for axitinib monotherapy, we assessed the impact of axitinib on DC/peptide-based vaccination on established melanoma growth in murine models [82]. Melanoma-bearing mice administered axitinib and specific vaccines were protected from tumor growth and displayed enhanced survival for up to 80 days following melanoma implantation. Axitinib-sensitization improved the trafficking and retention of vaccine-induced CD8+ T cells in the TME, with the Type-1 functionality (as assessed by IFNγ expression) of CD8+ T cells elevated in both the tumor site and the TDLN. Similar to our observations with sunitinib [39], axitinib reduced systemic frequencies of MDSCs and Tregs and promoted a Type-1 TME, as evidenced by the upregulated expression of Tbet, IFN-γ, CXCR3, and CXCL10 gene transcripts.

Dasatinib has already been reported to selectively abrogate mutated KIT activity in human melanomas [19, 83]. This TKI also inhibits other tyrosine kinases such as the Src family of kinases (impacting PI3K-AKT signaling) involved in melanoma adhesion, motility, and invasion [84, 85]. As a monotherapy, dasatinib was well-tolerated in melanoma patients, yielding an objective response rate comparable to alternate current first-line treatment options [18]. Dasatinib diminishes tumor angiogenesis by inhibiting the tyrosine kinases EphA2 and PDGFR that play significant roles in endothelial and pericyte biology, respectively [84]. In unpublished results from our laboratory, dasatinib mediates anti-TME effects that are similar to sunitinib and axitinib in melanoma-bearing mice [39, 82]. Animals treated with dasatinib undergo a restructuring of the tumor vasculature in association with reduced hypoxia and MDSC/Treg frequencies and increased accumulation of T effector cells in the TME, particularly when combined with a DC/peptide-based vaccine. The combined therapy also yielded greatest objective clinical benefit when compared with either monotherapeutic approach. Overall, these studies have supported the design of a pilot phase II trial (dasatinib + DC/tumor stromal antigen-based vaccine) at the University of Pittsburgh planned to begin enrolling patients in Q4 2012. In this trial, HLA-A2+ patients with advanced-stage melanoma will be administered dasatinib and an autologous αDC1/peptide vaccine, with frequencies of antigen-specific T cells monitored in patient blood and tumor biopsies over time along with objective clinical responses.

4. Conclusions

The emergence of ipilimumab and vemurafenib as treatment alternatives to the long-standing DTIC-, IL-2-, and IFN-α-based therapies attests to progress made in treating patients with metastatic melanoma. Although the genetic heterogeneity of melanoma cells has confounded high-throughput sequencing technologies, patterns of molecular aberrations are becoming clearer and help support the clinical application of FDA-approved small molecule drugs (such as TKIs) as therapeutic options in eligible patients. Select TKIs (e.g., sunitinib, axitinib, dasatinib) not only directly inhibit melanoma growth and progression by specifically disrupting cell intrinsic signaling pathways, but these drugs indirectly perturb tumorigenesis based on their "normalizing" effects on the TME. Central to this therapeutic paradigm is the ability of the drugs to recondition the chaotic architecture and fluid dynamics of the blood vasculature in the TME. The short-term consequences of TKI sensitization are impressive and include a reversal of hypoxia, acidosis, and interstitial pressure in the TME, which allows for a corollary improvement in the accumulation and action of co-applied cytotoxic therapies (including immunotherapies).

Combinational immunotherapies hold great promise in minimizing/preventing the emergence and progression of (same) therapy-resistant melanoma populations, as has typically been observed in cases of single-agent treatment strategies. These approaches also have potential to result in a state of perpetual disease dormancy which may extend patient overall survival [69]. The current challenge to the field is to determine the best combination (dosing and scheduling) of agents to best affect a state of durable clinical benefit in the advance-stage disease setting. From our work, and that of many others, immunotherapy represents one promising component of such combined treatment strategies, particularly when integrated with agents that act as immune adjuvants, inhibitors of immune regulatory cells, and "normalizers" of the TME. Preclinical studies have clearly justified the combined strategy of TKI drug therapy alongside specific DC/peptide-based vaccination. In particular, TKI administration essentially serves as an "immune adjuvant" by reversing the inherent immunosuppression of the TME upon diminishing frequencies of suppressive cell populations and physically manipulating the tumor vasculature architecture. Vaccine-initiated effector T cells are then able to more effectively infiltrate a tumor lesion in order to perform their clinically-beneficial cytolytic functions. Prospective clinical trials will test the validity of this operational biologic paradigm on patient outcome and define a series of safe and effective combination treatment options for melanoma patients.

Acknowledgments

This work was supported by NIH grants P01 CA100327, R01 CA114071, R01 CA140375 and P50 CA121973 (to W.J.S.) and the University of Pittsburgh Cancer Center Support Grant (CCSG; P30 CA047904). D.B.L. was supported by a Postdoctoral Fellowship (PF-11-151-01-LIB) from the American Cancer Society.

Author details

Devin B. Lowe[1], Jennifer L. Taylor[1] and Walter J. Storkus[1,2*]

*Address all correspondence to: storkuswj@upmc.edu

1 Dermatology and Immunology, University of Pittsburgh School of Medicine, Pittsburgh, PA, USA

2 University of Pittsburgh Cancer Institute, Pittsburgh, PA, USA

References

[1] American Cancer Society. http://www.cancer.org/Research/CancerFactsFigures/CancerFactsFigures/cancer-facts-figures-2012 (accessed 14 August 2012).

[2] Tremante E, Ginebri A, Lo Monaco E, Frascione P, Di Filippo F, Terrenato I, et al. Melanoma molecular classes and prognosis in the postgenomic era. Lancet Oncol. 2012;13(5) e205-11.

[3] Lacy KE, Karagiannis SN, Nestle FO. Advances in the treatment of melanoma. Clin Med. 2012;12(2) 168-71.

[4] Hodi FS, O'Day SJ, McDermott DF, Weber RW, Sosman JA, Haanen JB, et al. Improved survival with ipilimumab in patients with metastatic melanoma. N Engl J Med. 2010;363(8) 711-23.

[5] Robert C, Thomas L, Bondarenko I, O'Day S, M DJ, Garbe C, et al. Ipilimumab plus dacarbazine for previously untreated metastatic melanoma. N Engl J Med. 2011;364(26) 2517-26.

[6] Flaherty KT, Hodi FS, Fisher DE. From genes to drugs: targeted strategies for melanoma. Nat Rev Cancer. 2012;12(5) 349-61.

[7] Chapman PB, Hauschild A, Robert C, Haanen JB, Ascierto P, Larkin J, et al. Improved survival with vemurafenib in melanoma with BRAF V600E mutation. N Engl J Med. 2011;364(26) 2507-16.

[8] Ernstoff MS. Been there, not done that--melanoma in the age of molecular therapy. N Engl J Med. 2011;364(26) 2547-8.

[9] Sosman JA, Kim KB, Schuchter L, Gonzalez R, Pavlick AC, Weber JS, et al. Survival in BRAF V600-mutant advanced melanoma treated with vemurafenib. N Engl J Med. 2012;366(8) 707-14.

[10] Hoek KS. Exploring melanoma's massively parallel universe. Pigment Cell Melanoma Res. 2010;23(3) 306-7.

[11] Bennett DC. How to make a melanoma: what do we know of the primary clonal events? Pigment Cell Melanoma Res. 2008;21(1) 27-38.

[12] Mehnert JM, Kluger HM. Driver Mutations in Melanoma: Lessons Learned From Bench-to-Bedside Studies. Curr Oncol Rep. 2012;14(5) 449-57.

[13] Colombino M, Capone M, Lissia A, Cossu A, Rubino C, De Giorgi V, et al. BRAF/NRAS Mutation Frequencies Among Primary Tumors and Metastases in Patients With Melanoma. J Clin Oncol. 2012;30(20) 2522-9.

[14] Furney SJ, Turajlic S, Fenwick K, Lambros MB, MacKay A, Ricken G, et al. Genomic characterisation of acral melanoma cell lines. Pigment Cell Melanoma Res. 2012;25(4) 488-92.

[15] Jazirehi AR, Wenn PB, Damavand M. Therapeutic implications of targeting the PI3Kinase/AKT/mTOR signaling module in melanoma therapy. Am J Cancer Res. 2012;2(2) 178-91.

[16] Mikhail M, Velazquez E, Shapiro R, Berman R, Pavlick A, Sorhaindo L, et al. PTEN expression in melanoma: relationship with patient survival, Bcl-2 expression, and proliferation. Clin Cancer Res. 2005;11(14) 5153-7.

[17] Meyer S, Fuchs TJ, Bosserhoff AK, Hofstadter F, Pauer A, Roth V, et al. A seven-marker signature and clinical outcome in malignant melanoma: a large-scale tissue-microarray study with two independent patient cohorts. PLoS One. 2012;7(6) e38222.

[18] Algazi AP, Weber JS, Andrews SC, Urbas P, Munster PN, DeConti RC, et al. Phase I clinical trial of the Src inhibitor dasatinib with dacarbazine in metastatic melanoma. Br J Cancer. 2012;106(1) 85-91.

[19] Woodman SE, Trent JC, Stemke-Hale K, Lazar AJ, Pricl S, Pavan GM, et al. Activity of dasatinib against L576P KIT mutant melanoma: molecular, cellular, and clinical correlates. Mol Cancer Ther. 2009;8(8) 2079-85.

[20] Kluger HM, Dudek AZ, McCann C, Ritacco J, Southard N, Jilaveanu LB, et al. A phase 2 trial of dasatinib in advanced melanoma. Cancer. 2011;117(10) 2202-8.

[21] Woodman SE, Lazar AJ, Aldape KD, Davies MA. New strategies in melanoma: molecular testing in advanced disease. Clin Cancer Res. 2012;18(5) 1195-200.

[22] Wilson TR, Fridlyand J, Yan Y, Penuel E, Burton L, Chan E, et al. Widespread potential for growth-factor-driven resistance to anticancer kinase inhibitors. Nature. 2012;487(7408) 505-9.

[23] Straussman R, Morikawa T, Shee K, Barzily-Rokni M, Qian ZR, Du J, et al. Tumour micro-environment elicits innate resistance to RAF inhibitors through HGF secretion. Nature. 2012;487(7408) 500-4.

[24] Flaherty KT, Puzanov I, Kim KB, Ribas A, McArthur GA, Sosman JA, et al. Inhibition of mutated, activated BRAF in metastatic melanoma. 2010;N Engl J Med. 363(9) 809-19.

[25] Rini BI, Atkins MB. Resistance to targeted therapy in renal-cell carcinoma. Lancet Oncol. 2009;10(10) 992-1000.

[26] Montemurro M, Bauer S. Treatment of gastrointestinal stromal tumor after imatinib and sunitinib. Curr Opin Oncol. 2011;23(4) 367-72.

[27] Puzanov I, Burnett P, Flaherty KT. Biological challenges of BRAF inhibitor therapy. Mol Oncol. 2011;5(2) 116-23.

[28] Leong SP, Mihm MC, Jr., Murphy GF, Hoon DS, Kashani-Sabet M, Agarwala SS, et al. Progression of cutaneous melanoma: implications for treatment. Clin Exp Metastasis. In press, 2012.

[29] Goel S, Duda DG, Xu L, Munn LL, Boucher Y, Fukumura D, et al. Normalization of the vasculature for treatment of cancer and other diseases. Physiol Rev. 2011;91(3) 1071-121.

[30] Carmeliet P, Jain RK. Molecular mechanisms and clinical applications of angiogenesis. Nature. 2011;473(7347) 298-307.

[31] Jain RK. Normalization of tumor vasculature: an emerging concept in antiangiogenic therapy. Science. 2005;307(5706) 58-62.

[32] Helfrich I, Scheffrahn I, Bartling S, Weis J, von Felbert V, Middleton M, et al. Resistance to antiangiogenic therapy is directed by vascular phenotype, vessel stabilization, and maturation in malignant melanoma. J Exp Med. 2010;207(3) 491-503.

[33] Hurwitz H, Fehrenbacher L, Novotny W, Cartwright T, Hainsworth J, Heim W, et al. Bevacizumab plus irinotecan, fluorouracil, and leucovorin for metastatic colorectal cancer. N Engl J Med. 2004;350(23) 2335-42.

[34] Del Vecchio M, Mortarini R, Canova S, Di Guardo L, Pimpinelli N, Sertoli MR, et al. Bevacizumab plus fotemustine as first-line treatment in metastatic melanoma patients: clinical activity and modulation of angiogenesis and lymphangiogenesis factors. Clin Cancer Res. 2010;16(23) 5862-72.

[35] Hainsworth JD, Infante JR, Spigel DR, Peyton JD, Thompson DS, Lane CM, et al. Bevacizumab and everolimus in the treatment of patients with metastatic melanoma: a phase 2 trial of the Sarah Cannon Oncology Research Consortium. Cancer. 2010;116(17) 4122-9.

[36] Perez DG, Suman VJ, Fitch TR, Amatruda T, 3rd, Morton RF, Jilani SZ, et al. Phase 2 trial of carboplatin, weekly paclitaxel, and biweekly bevacizumab in patients with unresectable stage IV melanoma: a North Central Cancer Treatment Group study, N047A. Cancer. 2009;115(1) 119-27.

[37] Vihinen PP, Hernberg M, Vuoristo MS, Tyynela K, Laukka M, Lundin J, et al. A phase II trial of bevacizumab with dacarbazine and daily low-dose interferon-alpha2a as first line treatment in metastatic melanoma. Melanoma Res. 2010;20(4) 318-25.

[38] Giantonio BJ, Catalano PJ, Meropol NJ, O'Dwyer PJ, Mitchell EP, Alberts SR, et al. Bevacizumab in combination with oxaliplatin, fluorouracil, and leucovorin (FOLFOX4) for previously treated metastatic colorectal cancer: results from the Eastern Cooperative Oncology Group Study E3200. J Clin Oncol. 2007;25(12) 1539-44.

[39] Bose A, Taylor JL, Alber S, Watkins SC, Garcia JA, Rini BI, et al. Sunitinib facilitates the activation and recruitment of therapeutic anti-tumor immunity in concert with specific vaccination. Int J Cancer. 2011;129(9) 2158-70.

[40] Ebos JM, Lee CR, Cruz-Munoz W, Bjarnason GA, Christensen JG, Kerbel RS. Accelerated metastasis after short-term treatment with a potent inhibitor of tumor angiogenesis. Cancer Cell. 2009;15(3) 232-9.

[41] Rosenberg SA, Yang JC, Sherry RM, Kammula US, Hughes MS, Phan GQ, et al. Durable complete responses in heavily pretreated patients with metastatic melanoma using T-cell transfer immunotherapy. Clin Cancer Res. 2011;17(13) 4550-7.

[42] Restifo NP, Dudley ME, Rosenberg SA. Adoptive immunotherapy for cancer: harnessing the T cell response. Nat Rev Immunol. 2012;12(4) 269-81.

[43] Yannelli JR, Wroblewski JM. On the road to a tumor cell vaccine: 20 years of cellular immunotherapy. Vaccine. 2004;23(1) 97-113.

[44] Clemente CG, Mihm MC, Jr., Bufalino R, Zurrida S, Collini P, Cascinelli N. Prognostic value of tumor infiltrating lymphocytes in the vertical growth phase of primary cutaneous melanoma. Cancer. 1996;77(7) 1303-10.

[45] Ostrand-Rosenberg S, Sinha P, Beury DW, Clements VK. Cross-talk between myeloid-derived suppressor cells (MDSC), macrophages, and dendritic cells enhances tumor-induced immune suppression. Semin Cancer Biol. 2012;22(4) 275-81.

[46] Lowe DB, Storkus WJ. Chronic inflammation and immunologic-based constraints in malignant disease. Immunotherapy. 2011;3(10) 1265-74.

[47] Karthaus N, Torensma R, Tel J. Deciphering the message broadcast by tumor-infiltrating dendritic cells. Am J Pathol. 2012;181(3) 733-42.

[48] Mayer CT, Berod L, Sparwasser T. Layers of dendritic cell-mediated T cell tolerance, their regulation and the prevention of autoimmunity. Front Immunol. 2012;3 183.

[49] Kalinski P, Edington H, Zeh HJ, Okada H, Butterfield LH, Kirkwood JM, et al. Dendritic cells in cancer immunotherapy: vaccines or autologous transplants? Immunol Res. 2011;50(2-3) 235-47.

[50] Lechner MG, Liebertz DJ, Epstein AL. Characterization of cytokine-induced myeloid-derived suppressor cells from normal human peripheral blood mononuclear cells. J Immunol. 2010;185(4) 2273-84.

[51] Topalian SL, Drake CG, Pardoll DM. Targeting the PD-1/B7-H1(PD-L1) pathway to activate anti-tumor immunity. Curr Opin Immunol. 2012;24(2) 207-12.

[52] Klebanoff CA, Acquavella N, Yu Z, Restifo NP. Therapeutic cancer vaccines: are we there yet? Immunol Rev. 2011;239(1) 27-44.

[53] Palucka K, Banchereau J. Cancer immunotherapy via dendritic cells. Nat Rev Cancer. 2012;12(4) 265-77.

[54] Kalinski P. Regulation of immune responses by prostaglandin E2. J Immunol. 2012;188(1) 21-8.

[55] Kantoff PW, Higano CS, Shore ND, Berger ER, Small EJ, Penson DF, et al. Sipuleucel-T immunotherapy for castration-resistant prostate cancer. N Engl J Med. 2010;363(5) 411-22.

[56] Sheikh NA, Petrylak D, Kantoff PW, Dela Rosa C, Stewart FP, Kuan LY, et al. Sipuleucel-T immune parameters correlate with survival: an analysis of the randomized phase 3 clinical trials in men with castration-resistant prostate cancer. Cancer Immunol Immunother. In press, 2012.

[57] Palucka AK, Ueno H, Connolly J, Kerneis-Norvell F, Blanck JP, Johnston DA, et al. Dendritic cells loaded with killed allogeneic melanoma cells can induce objective clinical responses and MART-1 specific CD8+ T-cell immunity. J Immunother. 2006;29(5) 545-57.

[58] O'Rourke MG, Johnson M, Lanagan C, See J, Yang J, Bell JR, et al. Durable complete clinical responses in a phase I/II trial using an autologous melanoma cell/dendritic cell vaccine. Cancer Immunol Immunother. 2003;52(6) 387-95.

[59] Nestle FO, Alijagic S, Gilliet M, Sun Y, Grabbe S, Dummer R, et al. Vaccination of melanoma patients with peptide- or tumor lysate-pulsed dendritic cells. Nat Med. 1998;4(3) 328-32.

[60] Thurner B, Haendle I, Roder C, Dieckmann D, Keikavoussi P, Jonuleit H, et al. Vaccination with mage-3A1 peptide-pulsed mature, monocyte-derived dendritic cells expands specific cytotoxic T cells and induces regression of some metastases in advanced stage IV melanoma. J Exp Med. 1999;190(11) 1669-78.

[61] Salcedo M, Bercovici N, Taylor R, Vereecken P, Massicard S, Duriau D, et al. Vaccination of melanoma patients using dendritic cells loaded with an allogeneic tumor cell lysate. Cancer Immunol Immunother. 2006;55(7) 819-29.

[62] Schuler-Thurner B, Schultz ES, Berger TG, Weinlich G, Ebner S, Woerl P, et al. Rapid induction of tumor-specific type 1 T helper cells in metastatic melanoma patients by vaccination with mature, cryopreserved, peptide-loaded monocyte-derived dendritic cells. J Exp Med. 2002;195(10) 1279-88.

[63] Ridolfi L, Petrini M, Fiammenghi L, Granato AM, Ancarani V, Pancisi E, et al. Dendritic cell-based vaccine in advanced melanoma: update of clinical outcome. Melanoma Res. 2011;21(6) 524-9.

[64] Steele JC, Rao A, Marsden JR, Armstrong CJ, Berhane S, Billingham LJ, et al. Phase I/II trial of a dendritic cell vaccine transfected with DNA encoding melan A and gp100 for patients with metastatic melanoma. Gene Ther. 2011;18(6) 584-93.

[65] Ribas A, Camacho LH, Lee SM, Hersh EM, Brown CK, Richards JM, et al. Multicenter phase II study of matured dendritic cells pulsed with melanoma cell line lysates in patients with advanced melanoma. J Transl Med. 2010;8 89.

[66] Ribas A, Comin-Anduix B, Chmielowski B, Jalil J, de la Rocha P, McCannel TA, et al. Dendritic cell vaccination combined with CTLA4 blockade in patients with metastatic melanoma. Clin Cancer Res. 2009;15(19) 6267-76.

[67] Okada H, Kalinski P, Ueda R, Hoji A, Kohanbash G, Donegan TE, et al. Induction of CD8+ T-cell responses against novel glioma-associated antigen peptides and clinical

activity by vaccinations with {alpha}-type 1 polarized dendritic cells and polyinosinic-polycytidylic acid stabilized by lysine and carboxymethylcellulose in patients with recurrent malignant glioma. J Clin Oncol. 2011;29(3) 330-6.

[68] Schreiber RD, Old LJ, Smyth MJ. Cancer immunoediting: integrating immunity's roles in cancer suppression and promotion. Science. 2011;331(6024) 1565-70.

[69] Zhao X, Bose A, Komita H, Taylor JL, Chi N, Lowe DB, et al. Vaccines targeting tumor blood vessel antigens promote CD8(+) T cell-dependent tumor eradication or dormancy in HLA-A2 transgenic mice. J Immunol. 2012;188(4) 1782-8.

[70] Zhao X, Bose A, Komita H, Taylor JL, Kawabe M, Chi N, et al. Intratumoral IL-12 gene therapy results in the crosspriming of Tc1 cells reactive against tumor-associated stromal antigens. Mol Ther. 2011;19(4) 805-14.

[71] Najjar YG, Rini BI. Novel agents in renal carcinoma: a reality check. Ther Adv Med Oncol. 2012;4(4) 183-94.

[72] Koshenkov VP, Rodgers SE. Adjuvant therapy of gastrointestinal stromal tumors. Curr Opin Oncol. 2012;24(4) 414-8.

[73] Minor DR, Kashani-Sabet M, Garrido M, O'Day SJ, Hamid O, Bastian BC. Sunitinib therapy for melanoma patients with KIT mutations. Clin Cancer Res. 2012;18(5) 1457-63.

[74] de Jonge MJ, Dumez H, Kitzen JJ, Beuselinck B, Verweij J, Courtney R, et al. Phase I safety and pharmacokinetic study of SU-014813 in combination with docetaxel in patients with advanced solid tumours. Eur J Cancer. 2011;47(9) 1328-35.

[75] Ko JS, Rayman P, Ireland J, Swaidani S, Li G, Bunting KD, et al. Direct and differential suppression of myeloid-derived suppressor cell subsets by sunitinib is compartmentally constrained. Cancer Res. 2010;70(9) 3526-36.

[76] Ko JS, Zea AH, Rini BI, Ireland JL, Elson P, Cohen P, et al. Sunitinib mediates reversal of myeloid-derived suppressor cell accumulation in renal cell carcinoma patients. Clin Cancer Res. 2009;15(6) 2148-57.

[77] Finke JH, Rini B, Ireland J, Rayman P, Richmond A, Golshayan A, et al. Sunitinib reverses type-1 immune suppression and decreases T-regulatory cells in renal cell carcinoma patients. Clin Cancer Res. 2008;14(20) 6674-82.

[78] Olsson AK, Dimberg A, Kreuger J, Claesson-Welsh L. VEGF receptor signalling - in control of vascular function. Nat Rev Mol Cell Biol. 2006;7(5) 359-71.

[79] Rini BI, Escudier B, Tomczak P, Kaprin A, Szczylik C, Hutson TE, et al. Comparative effectiveness of axitinib versus sorafenib in advanced renal cell carcinoma (AXIS): a randomised phase 3 trial. Lancet. 2011;378(9807) 1931-9.

[80] Hu-Lowe DD, Zou HY, Grazzini ML, Hallin ME, Wickman GR, Amundson K, et al. Nonclinical antiangiogenesis and antitumor activities of axitinib (AG-013736), an or-

al, potent, and selective inhibitor of vascular endothelial growth factor receptor tyrosine kinases 1, 2, 3. Clin Cancer Res. 2008;14(22) 7272-83.

[81] Fruehauf J, Lutzky J, McDermott D, Brown CK, Meric JB, Rosbrook B, et al. Multicenter, phase II study of axitinib, a selective second-generation inhibitor of vascular endothelial growth factor receptors 1, 2, and 3, in patients with metastatic melanoma. Clin Cancer Res. 2011;17(23) 7462-9.

[82] Bose A, Lowe DB, Rao A, Storkus WJ. Combined vaccine+axitinib therapy yields superior antitumor efficacy in a murine melanoma model. Melanoma Res. 2012;22(3) 236-43.

[83] Antonescu CR, Busam KJ, Francone TD, Wong GC, Guo T, Agaram NP, et al. L576P KIT mutation in anal melanomas correlates with KIT protein expression and is sensitive to specific kinase inhibition. Int J Cancer. 2007;121(2) 257-64.

[84] Buettner R, Mesa T, Vultur A, Lee F, Jove R. Inhibition of Src family kinases with dasatinib blocks migration and invasion of human melanoma cells. Mol Cancer Res. 2008;6(11) 1766-74.

[85] Jilaveanu LB, Zito CR, Aziz SA, Chakraborty A, Davies MA, Camp RL, et al. In vitro studies of dasatinib, its targets and predictors of sensitivity. Pigment Cell Melanoma Res. 2011;24(2) 386-9.

Section 2

Melanoma Treatment Approaches

Chapter 10

Management of In-Transit Malignant Melanoma

Paul J. Speicher, Douglas S. Tyler and Paul J. Mosca

Additional information is available at the end of the chapter

http://dx.doi.org/10.5772/53618

1. Introduction

In-transit melanoma is a unique pattern of recurrence that occurs in up to ten percent of patients with melanoma. In-transit disease denotes multifocal tumor deposits occurring between the site of the primary lesion and its regional draining lymph node basin [1, 2]. It is an independent adverse prognostic factor and is frequently associated with distant metastasis. This pattern of recurrence represents a challenging management problem, but provides unique treatment modalities as well. In addition, studying in-transit melanoma has the potential to shed additional light on melanoma biology. The goal of this chapter is to discuss the presentation, underlying disease biology, and various current treatment strategies for this unique pattern of recurrence in melanoma.

2. Background

2.1. Nomenclature and staging

The nomenclature used for in-transit melanoma can be confusing, in part because a number of different terms have traditionally been used in the literature to describe what is most likely the same oncologic process. Historically, terms such as locoregional recurrence, satellitosis, and in-transit disease have all been used with varying definitions and intentions. Historically, satellitosis has been defined as locoregional recurrence, not lying within the regional nodal basin, that is located within either 5cm of the initial lesion or 2cm of the excision scar, whereas the term in-transit disease has been defined as such a recurrence occurring at greater distances from the initial lesion or scar, respectively. In either case, such lesions likely represent tumor deposits growing along routes of lymphatic drainage. More recently, it has become apparent that for locoregional recurrence, distance from the primary lesion to the site of recurrence does not carry significant prognostic value [3-6]. Accordingly, the most recent AJCC staging system for melanoma does not differentiate between in-transit lesions and satellitosis in the assignment of stage, both being designated as N2 or N3 disease, depending on regional node status [7]. Thus, in an effort to address the ambiguity arising from nomenclature, many authors have advocated for eliminating the term satellitosis, instead referring to all regional non-nodal metastatic disease as in-transit disease.

Stage	T	N	M
IIIA	Any depth, *Without* ulceration	1-3 nodes (not clinically detectable)	No distant disease
IIIB	Any depth, *With* ulceration	1-3 nodes (not clinically detectable)	No distant disease
	Any depth, *Without* ulceration	1-3 nodes (clinically detectable), *OR* in-transit lesions	No distant disease
IIIC	Any depth, *With* ulceration	1-3 nodes (clinically detectable), *OR* in-transit lesions, *OR* any combination of positive nodes and in-transit disease, *OR* greater than 4 positive nodes	No distant disease

Table 1. Breakdown of AJCC staging for stage III melanoma [7].

An additional and equally important point of clarification is the distinction between actual local recurrence and in-transit disease. True local recurrence is defined as a primary tumor that recurs as a result of incomplete primary excision, and is confined to or contiguous with an excision scar and bearing an in situ component [8]. As this carries a much better prognosis, it must be distinguished from potentially similar appearing in-transit disease found in close proximity to a prior excisional scar.

2.2. Presentation

By definition, in-transit melanoma represents advanced stage disease, and such recurrences are typically discovered months after the initial management of a primary lesion. In most series, this disease-free interval to recurrence as in-transit disease ranges from 12-16 months [9, 10]. The clinical presentation can be quite variable, but usually involves anywhere from one to upwards of one-hundred small cutaneous or subcutaneous nodules. The lesions themselves can differ significantly in size, ranging from sub-millimeter diameter to well over one centimeter. They may take the form of superficial cutaneous (also called epidermotropic) or deeper subcutaneous tumors. For extremity-based disease, the lesions may be clustered near the primary lesion, or may involve the entire extremity extending between the primary tumor and its lymphatic drainage basin. For non-extremity disease, the distribution can be even more variable, with widespread tumor burden on the head, neck or trunk, depending on the location of the primary melanoma.

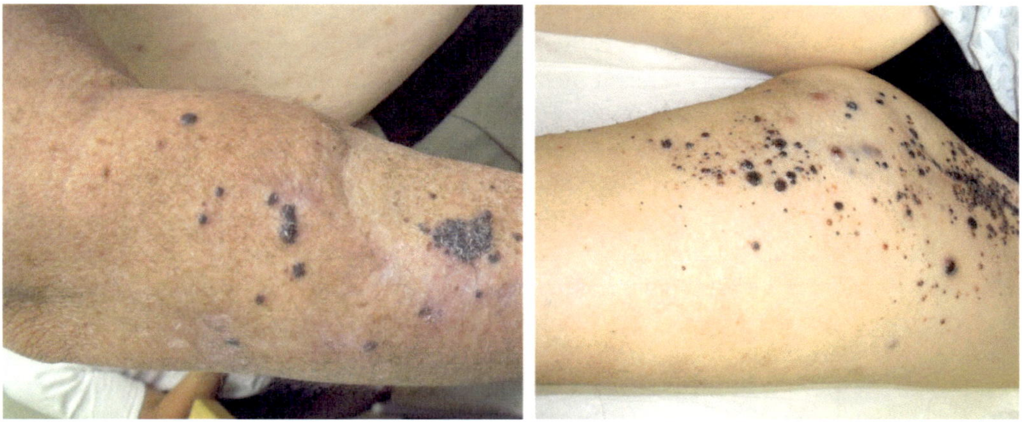

Figure 1. Examples of in-transit melanoma of the arm (left) and leg (right). Note the distribution and extent of disease, making these presentations very poor candidates for surgical excision. On the left, there is evidence of in-transit metastases both within the area of previous skin flap, as well as extending more proximally along its course of lymphatic drainage. On the right, there is extensive disease extending up to the inguinal crease.

2.3. Incidence

In-transit melanoma is a relatively uncommon phenomenon, with fewer than 10% of melanomas recurring as in-transit disease [1, 11]. This accounts for approximately 12-22% of all recurrences, although this number is difficult to determine with accuracy due to ambiguity regarding terminology used to describe local recurrence versus regional in-transit disease [12-14]. Stage of disease appears to be the most important factor that predicts the development of in-transit metastasis. The presence of associated nodal disease significantly increases risk of in-transit recurrence, with one study reporting incidence as high as 31% when three or more positive nodes were present [12]. Location itself also appears to be a factor, with a higher incidence of in-transit disease in the lower extremities compared to the upper extremities [15]. Of note, some earlier authors observed that surgical lymph node dissection may lead to increased risk of recurrence as in-transit disease, an area of some debate. This is postulated to be a result of lymphatic trapping, whereby dissection of the draining lymph node basin removes the potential outflow of lymphatic tumor deposits, possibly leading to increased likelihood of in-transit disease. In larger, more recent studies, however, neither sentinel lymph node biopsy nor lymphadenectomy were found to have any effect on the incidence of in-transit metastases [16-19].

2.4. Outcomes

The presence of in-transit metastases indicates either N2 or N3 status under the current AJCC TNM system, and is classified as stage IIIB or C disease, respectively. In-transit melanoma carries a poor prognosis, with 5-year survival rates ranging from 25% to 30% in most reports [12, 20, 21]. Additionally, the presence or absence of regional lymph node disease is of significant prognostic value; the combination of nodal metastasis and in-transit melanoma comprise stage IIIC disease, which is associated with a poorer outcome than stage IIIB (40% vs. 59% five-year survival, respectively) [7]. There is a high incidence of occult distant metastasis in the presence of in-transit melanoma, but this is not universally the case. Studies examining the outcomes of major amputation for the treatment of this pattern of recurrence have identified a number of patients who experience a complete and durable response and have demonstrated five-year survival rates ranging from 21-32% [22-26]. This indicates that a significant minority of patients with in-transit metastases have disease that is truly limited to the extremity at the time of detection. Nonetheless, it is essential that distant metastases be ruled out when staging patients with in-transit melanoma, since treatment options and prognosis may differ substantially when measurable distant disease is present.

3. Biology of in-transit disease

The underlying biology of in-transit melanoma is believed to be related to lymphatic dissemination of small tumor emboli along the lymphatic drainage from the primary tumor. It is generally accepted that these migrating tumor cells become trapped in the dermal and subdermal lymphatics, typically, though not always, somewhere between the primary lesion and the draining regional lymph nodes. These cells are thought to remain static along this route, eventually progressing to a clinically detectable lesion. Consistent with this theory, in-transit melanoma is often described as an ongoing process, with increasing disease burden over time. Although the lymphatic route is the most likely biological explanation, some authors have suggested other mechanisms. One alternate explanation describes in-transit disease as a manifestation of systemic disease resulting from hematogenous spread, similar to distant metastases [27, 28]. Proponents of this argue that in the lymphatic theory, wider margins of primary excision would be expected to include more static occult cells, with subsequent improved clinical outcomes, yet this has not been shown to be the case. It is difficult to reconcile this theory, however, with the significant differences in survival observed in stage III versus stage IV melanoma.

4. Therapy for in-transit disease

Treatment of locoregionally recurrent melanoma depends on a number of important factors, including tumor size, multiplicity, and anatomic location. Although in-transit melanoma is often followed by metastatic disease, it is important that the surgeon choose an appropriate therapy based on clinical presentation, history, technical experience, and patient preference.

4.1. Local management

Distinguishing in-transit disease from true local recurrence is of great importance, as the management and prognosis differ substantially. Local recurrence, or tumor confined to or contiguous with an excision scar and bearing an in situ component, should be managed similarly to the primary lesion with wide local excision. For in-transit disease, however, it is generally accepted that the wide local excision margin guidelines applicable to primary melanomas need not be applied. In-transit metastases are generally very clearly demarcated histologically from surrounding tissue, and complete macroscopic excision with negative surgical margins is usually all that is required.

In addition to wide local excision, there has been significant interest in other forms of local therapy for melanoma lesions, including laser ablation, external beam radiation, and intralesional injections. Irrespective of modality, these should all be thought of as equivalents to local surgical excision regarding indications and prognosis.

Laser therapy was first described in 1973, and has gained favor in the local treatment of in-transit disease that is not amenable to surgical excision, such as when the disease is too extensive [29]. It is most useful in patients with a large number of small in-transit lesions, but its advantages and utility decrease as lesions increase in size [30]. For tumors smaller than approximately 3mm, the entire lesion can be ablated using a carbon dioxide laser, though larger lesions must be circumscribed using the laser and subsequently excised with forceps.

Intralesional injections have also been used in the treatment of in-transit melanoma with some success. The most commonly used therapies include bacillus Calmette-Guérin (BCG), dinitrochlorobenzene (DNCB), and interferon-alpha (INF-α), and IL-2. Small studies have demonstrated complete response rates of 31-63% (overall response 45-91%), although long-term survival, when reported, remained unfortunately low [31-33]. This suggests that if surgical excision is not a viable option, intralesional injection is a reasonable alternative. More recently, electrochemotherapy (ECT) has gained popularity as local alternative to radiotherapy and laser ablation. This technique relies on using high intensity electric pulses to allow intracellular delivery of cytotoxic drugs, such as cisplatin and bleomycin, via intralesional injection [34]. Complete response rates have been reported as 53-89% (overall response 84-99%), with minimal systemic toxicity [35-37]. Unfortunately, regardless of which method is employed, local management of in-transit melanoma remains suboptimal in many situations.

4.2. Radiation therapy

Early in-vitro and clinical studies suggested that melanoma tumors exhibited significant intrinsic resistance to ionizing radiation, and as such, radiotherapy has not traditionally been considered to have a major role in the treatment of in-transit melanoma [38, 39]. More recent studies, however, have suggested radiotherapy may be of value in certain subsets of individuals, particularly those with one or few metastatic lesions that are not amenable to surgical excision [40]. As a primary treatment, radiotherapy is largely reserved for palliation of patients with incurable symptomatic lesions, particularly in cases that are not amenable to surgical excision. Generally speaking, when unresectable in-transit melanoma is amenable to regional chemotherapy, this should be considered prior to employing radiotherapy.

While some studies have demonstrated potential benefit of adjuvant radiation therapy in patients with nodal melanoma metastases, there are very little data regarding the use of adjuvant radiation therapy in the setting of in-transit disease [41, 42]. Treatment depends on area and location of involvement. While not routine practice, adjuvant radiotherapy should be considered in patients with head and neck disease, and in those with positive margins that are not amenable to re-excision [43-45].

4.3. Regional therapy

Given the high rate of local treatment failure and frequently increased burden of in-transit disease, regionally focused modalities offer potential strategies to obtain more durable treatment responses. Regional chemotherapy is a promising therapeutic option for suitable patients with extremity in-transit melanoma and is currently the focus of exciting research. This modality involves vascular isolation of the affected area, after which chemotherapy is then delivered at doses 10-20 times higher than doses that can be achieved and tolerated systemically, with dosing based on affected limb volume. As regional therapy requires complete vascular isolation of the affected body area, obvious anatomic limitations are involved. The inflow and outflow vessels to the area of interest must be selectively cannulated, and the treatment region must then be isolated from the systemic circulation, usually by means of a tourniquet.

There remains significant debate as to whether regional chemotherapy produces an overall survival benefit over other therapeutic modalities, but studies have demonstrated a survival benefit in patients who exhibited a clinical response [46-48]. Originally described in the 1950s, two primary forms of regional chemotherapy have evolved: hyperthermic isolated limb perfusion (HILP) and isolated limb infusion (ILI).

	HILP	ILI
Drug delivery	Cardiopulmonary bypass	Manual pump with three-way stopcock
Circuit pressure	High; with significant risk for systemic leak	Low; significantly reduced risk of systemic leak
Vessel access	Open surgical exposure; large diameter cannulas	Percutaneous access under fluoroscopic guidance, smaller diameter cannulas
Limb pH	Physiologic	Acidotic
Limb oxygenation	Active membrane oxygenation	No external oxygenation; profound hypoxia
Temperature	39-40°C	37.8-38.5°C
Duration of treatment	60 minutes	30 minutes
Technical demand	Technically complex, difficult re-operation	Technically simpler, re-do operation without difficulty

Table 2. Comparison of technique and parameters between hyperthermic isolated limb perfusion (HILP) and isolated limb infusion (ILI).

4.4. Regional chemotherapy agents

Melphalan is typically the drug of choice for regional chemotherapy. It is an alkylating agent derived from phenylalanine, an amino acid preferentially taken up by melanocytes due to its key role in melanin synthesis. Theoretically, melphalan should produce selective toxicity in melanocytes and melanin-containing melanoma cells. As a systemic agent, however, melphalan is ineffective despite its theoretical benefits, as its allowable dose is significantly less than its effective dose. For regional therapy, in contrast, this much higher effective dose is achieved without systemic toxicity.

Other agents have been employed either alone or in combination with melphalan in the treatment of in-transit melanoma. An essential quality of any agent considered for regional therapy is the constraint that it must not require metabolic transformation to take on a biologically active form. Cisplatin is another alkylating agent that held significant promise in preclinical studies of regional chemotherapy. Early clinical reports were favorable regarding response rates, but were plagued by concerns over toxicity [49-51]. Subsequent studies confirmed significant limb-threatening toxicity with the use of cisplatin, and as such most authors recommend against its routine use in regional therapy [52, 53]. Similarly, TNFα has exhibited some potential, particularly when combined with interferon-gamma, but widespread use of TNFα-based regimens have been tempered by significant concerns regarding toxicity [54]. The 2006 ACOSOG Z0020 trial comparing melphalan with melphalan plus TNFα was terminated early after interim analysis demonstrated a significant increase in toxicity with the addition of TNFα and yet a similar clinical response rate compared to melphalan alone [55]. Temozolomide is a newer alkylating agent that could have potential application in regional chemotherapy, as it also does not require hepatic conversion to become active. Early results in animal models reported superior tumor growth delay compared to regional melphalan, and a phase 1 clinical trial is currently underway, enrolling patients at Duke University Medical Center [56].

4.5. Isolated limb perfusion

Isolated limb perfusion (ILP) was first described in Creech and colleagues in 1958, basing their technique on advances in cardiopulmonary bypass developed for cardiac surgery in the 1950s [57]. They utilized an extracorporeal oxygenator as part of the isolated limb circuit to deliver high dose chemotherapy while maintaining normal oxygen tension and pH of the treated limb. Ten years later, Stehlin and coworkers added the effects of hyperthermia to the treatment protocol, now called hyperthermic isolated limb perfusion (HILP), enhancing the cytotoxicity of the chemotherapy and increasing efficacy [58]. The technical aspects of HILP vary somewhat among surgeons and institutions, but the basic technique is similar.

The procedure is performed under general anesthesia, and the vasculature supplying the affected limb is exposed and cannulated. During this exposure, one typically performs a regional lymphadenectomy, which aids vascular exposure (particularly in the case of the iliac vessels) and is often indicated from an oncologic standpoint. The target limb is isolated from the systemic circulation using a proximal tourniquet. Perfusion is then initiated via the cannulated vessels, utilizing a membrane oxygenator and cardiopulmonary bypass apparatus to maintain limb oxygen tension and pH at physiologic levels. The perfusion treatment is generally continued for 60 to 90 minutes, depending on the protocol. External warming blankets and heated melphalan perfusate are used to achieve hyperthermia. During HILP, it is important to monitor for leakage of the perfusate into the systemic circulation, particularly when high dose TNF-alpha is employed, as systemic leakage can lead to significant morbidity or mortality. Traditionally this monitoring was performed using intravenous fluorescein and watching for staining proximal to the tourniquet. A more precise method involves the administration of radiolabeled tracer into the HILP circuit, followed by continuously monitored systemic radiation exposure using a gamma probe placed over the chest. After completion of chemotherapy perfusion, a 30-minute washout period with crystalloids follows to remove the active agents.

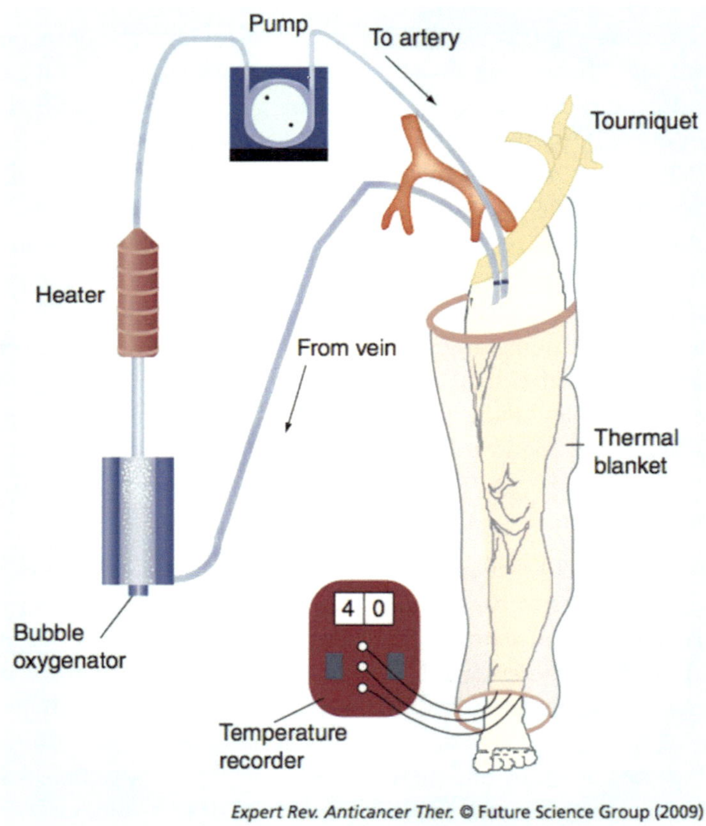

Figure 2. Hyperthermic isolated limb perfusion. Surgical exposure of the proximal vasculature is followed by cannulation and circulation of chemotherapy perfusate. Acid-base status and oxygenation is maintained throughout the procedure. Reproduced with permission.

Results of HILP vary widely, perhaps depending on the patient population and adjunctive agents employed. In single-center studies, overall response rates of 81-100% and complete response rates of 39-82% [46, 48, 59-62] have been reported. However, the previously mentioned multi-center ACOSOG Z0020 study demonstrated complete response rates of only 25%, significantly lower than what had been previously reported [55]. Overall, recurrence rates are 50-60% within one year, and overall 5-year survival rates remain in the 30-40% range [63]. As such, while HILP may be the best treatment option for suitable patients with in-transit extremity melanoma, there remains significant room for therapeutic improvement.

Study (year) [ref]	Patients (n)	CR (%)	PR (%)	OR (%)
Minor (1985) [60]	18	82	18	100
Storm (1985) [62]	26	50	31	81
Di Filippo (1989) [59]	69	39	43	82
Cornett (2006) [55]	58	25	39	64
Sanki (2007) [48]	120	69	15	84
Raymond (2011) [61]	62	55	26	81

Table 3. Response rates following HILP in patients with in-transit melanoma. Adapted with permission from Coleman et al., Expert Rev. Anticancer Ther. 2009;9(11):1599-1602. CR: Complete response; PR: Partial response; OR: Overall response.

4.6. Isolated limb infusion

Isolated limb infusion (ILI) was developed by Thompson and coworkers at the Sydney Melanoma Unit as a less invasive alternative to HILP. This technique employs percutaneous catheters inserted under fluoroscopic guidance as a means to cannulate the target limb vessels. An external tourniquet is used to isolate the limb, which is then wrapped in heating blankets. The key difference with ILI as compared to HILP is the lack of a perfusion pump and membrane oxygenator. The melphalan solution is instead manually circulated via the arterial catheter using a syringe and three-way stopcock. Consequently, during ILI the limb is not maintained at normal pH and oxygen tension, and becomes markedly hypoxic and acidotic during the course of the procedure. Some authors propose that the acidosis and hypoxia may serve to augment melphalan action [64]. In addition, while external and internal warming are performed in ILI, limb temperatures achieved with ILI are lower than those in HILP and generally do not exceed 38.5 degrees centigrade [65, 66].

From a technical standpoint, ILI is appreciably simpler and easier to perform and learn. The infusion treatment is continued for about 30 minutes, followed by a similar washout period with crystalloid. Lower doses of melphalan are typically used, often in combination with dactinomycin, and regional morbidity is reduced, particularly with respect to incidence of severe toxicity. In light of these factors, ILI is generally well tolerated, and is often offered to frail patients with multiple comorbidities who would not tolerate the longer and more invasive groin exposure required for HILP. Along similar lines, due to its simplicity and lower morbidity, ILI can be safely offered as a repeat procedure. Although theoretically attractive as a means of obtaining fractionated regional chemotherapy, elective repeat ILI has not been shown to improve survival compared to single ILI [67]. However, repeat ILI can be very valuable in the management of recurrent or progressive in-transit disease after primary regional therapy.

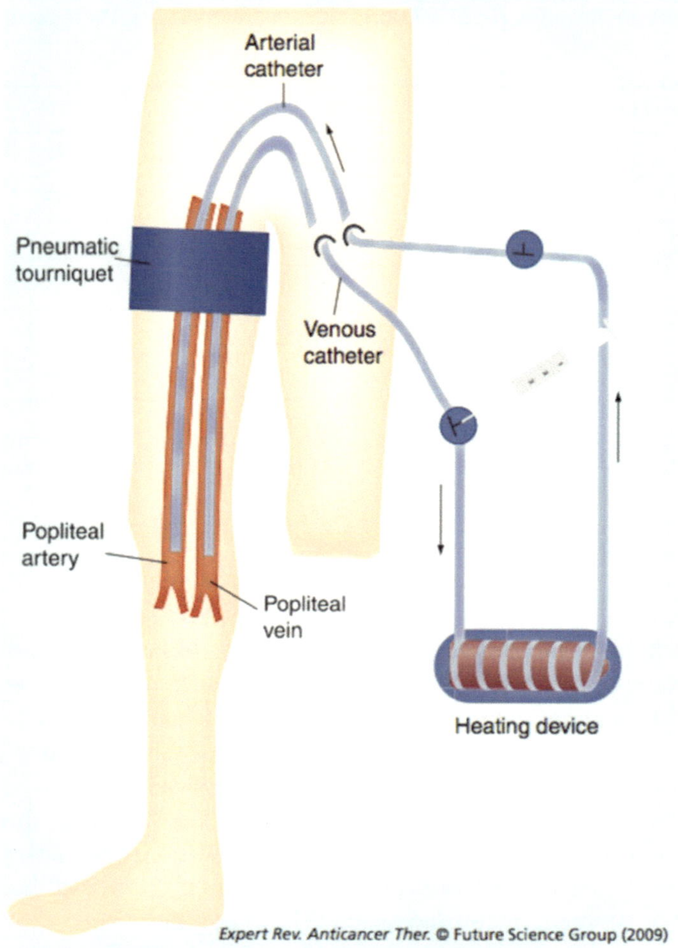

Figure 3. Isolated limb infusion. Catheters are placed percutaneously, and chemotherapy is circulated by hand without active oxygenation, leading to profound hypoxia and acidosis.

Outcomes after ILI are generally inferior to HILP, with complete response ranging from 23-44% and overall response ranging from 43-100% [47, 61, 65, 66, 68-70]. In one of the largest studies explicitly comparing patterns of recurrence, ILI was found to have both significantly higher probability of recurrence (85% vs. 65%) and shorter time to first recurrence (8 months vs. 23 months) as compared to HILP [71]. Notably, there was no statistically significant difference in overall survival between the two groups, although there was a trend in favor of HILP.

Study (year) [ref]	Patients (n)	CR (%)	PR (%)	OR (%)
Mian (2001) [70]	9	44	56	100
Lindner (2002) [66]	128	41	44	85
Brady (2006) [69]	22	23	27	50
Kroon (2008) [47]	185	38	46	84
Beasley (2009) [68]	128	31	33	64
Raymond (2011) [61]	126	30	13	43

Table 4. Response rates following ILI in patients with in-transit melanoma. Adapted with permission from Coleman et al., Expert Rev. Anticancer Ther. 2009;9(11):1599-1602. CR: Complete response; PR: Partial response; OR: Overall response.

4.7. Post-treatment complications

As a result of the high concentration of chemotherapies administered in regional therapy, some degree of tissue toxicity is often seen. Multiple grading systems have been developed to score regional toxicity after treatment, with one of the most prominent being that developed by Wieberdink and colleagues. In this system scores range from Grade I, or no evidence of significant reaction, to Grade V, representing reaction severe enough to warrant possible amputation [72]. Up to 85% of patients will exhibit Grade I or II level of toxicity, but as a result of careful drug dosing based on limb volume rather than total body weight, fortunately overall less than 1% of patients develop Grade V toxicity [73]. While the spectrum of toxicity is similar between patients undergoing ILI and HILP, the risk of significant toxicity is greater among those undergoing HILP. Furthermore, HILP carries a higher risk of limb loss from amputation as compared to ILI. Regardless of modality, most adverse reactions are transient, with almost all patients demonstrating some skin erythema and edema that peaks in the first month post-operatively. Rare but more serious complications include severe muscle toxicity and the development of compartment syndrome, necessitating fasciotomy.

4.8. Amputation

Amputation is almost never indicated in the standard treatment of in-transit melanoma. As mentioned previously, historical treatment of in-transit disease by means of limb amputation has led to long-term survival rates of 20-30 percent, which would suggest that a significant minority of patients with locoregional disease have recurrence that is in fact confined entirely to the affected extremity. Recent advancements in aggressive local management, regional therapy and systemic treatment have rendered extremity amputation obsolete except for the most intractable disease, particularly in light of comparable five-year survival rates among patients undergoing these therapies. Thus, amputation should generally only be offered with palliative intent or in patients who refuse or are not candidates for regional chemotherapy or other less morbid therapies [22, 26].

4.9. Systemic treatment

While a comprehensive discussion regarding systemic therapy for the treatment of melanoma is beyond the scope of this chapter, when appropriate this modality should be considered in the management of in-transit disease. Systemic therapy is typically applied in cases of in-transit disease in the presence of distant metastases – that is, stage IV disease [74]. Similarly, patients with non-extremity in-transit metastases – such as in-transit disease involving the head and neck, truncal or genitalia – present a difficult management problem and are often palliated best with systemic treatment options. Systemic therapy should also be considered for in-transit metastases in patients with recurrent or progressive disease who are not candidates for repeat local or regional therapy. Unfortunately, systemic therapy for the treatment of patients with advanced melanoma has historically been quite poor. A large meta-analysis of 42 trials of systemic treatments demonstrating a median progression free survival of 1.7 months with only 14.5% of patients being progression-free at 6 months [75]. Despite this poor track record, newer approaches to systemic treatment of regional disease may hold promise, including vascular regulating agents, signal targeting therapies and immune modulation therapy.

Current strategies have focused on attempting to increase tumor sensitivity to chemotherapeutics, improve local drug delivery, or target apoptotic pathways in an attempt to augment response to regional therapy. The BRAF enzyme inhibitor vemurafenib, as well as the immune modulating anti-CTLA-4 antibody ipilimumab, have recently shown promise in phase III trials, although neither is likely to provide durable disease-free survival [76, 77]. Another newer agent is bevacizumab, a monoclonal antibody to vascular endothelial growth factor (VEGF), which is believed to normalize immature and shunt-dominated tumor vasculature, leading to improved delivery of chemotherapeutics to tumor cells. A recent preclinical animal study demonstrated that systemic treatment with bevacizumab prior to regional therapy increased delivery of melphalan to the tumors of interest [78]. Another vascular targeting agent of recent interest is ADH-1, a pentapeptide that targets and disrupts N-cadherin adhesion complexes, which are predominantly expressed by melanocytes after malignant transition into melanoma [79, 80]. ADH-1 is believed to increase blood vessel permeability, increasing chemotherapy drug delivery [81]. A recent phase II clinical trial studying pre-treatment systemic ADH-1 administration prior to ILI with melphalan demonstrated a reassuring complete response rate of 38% and an overall response rate of 60%, although no significant progression free survival was appreciated [82]. The role of all of these agents as systemic adjuncts to regional chemotherapy remains to be seen, and is being defined in ongoing trials.

5. Conclusions

In-transit melanoma is a distinctive form of tumor recurrence, and is an indicator of late-stage disease. It is very distressing to patients, often requiring multiple treatments, procedures and hospitalizations. As such, management of this disease can be challenging and frustrating to clinicians as well. Similar to systemic melanoma, in-transit disease is notoriously resistant to chemotherapy, and treatment outcomes remain unsatisfactorily poor. Local therapies often tout impressive initial response rates, but are plagued by recurrence. Over the past half-century, advances have been made in regional approaches to chemotherapy, including isolated limb perfusion and isolated limb infusion. While some of these methods have demonstrated limited success, significant improvements in patient outcomes will require further advances in both regional and systemic treatment of melanoma.

Author details

Paul J. Speicher, Douglas S. Tyler and Paul J. Mosca

Division of Surgical Oncology, Department of Surgery, Duke University Medical Center, Durham, USA

References

[1] Pawlik TM, Ross MI, Johnson MM, Schacherer CW, McClain DM, Mansfield PF, et al. Predictors and natural history of in-transit melanoma after sentinel lymphadenectomy. Annals of surgical oncology. 2005;12(8):587-96. Epub 2005/07/16.

[2] Meier F, Will S, Ellwanger U, Schlagenhauff B, Schittek B, Rassner G, et al. Metastatic pathways and time courses in the orderly progression of cutaneous melanoma. The British journal of dermatology. 2002;147(1):62-70. Epub 2002/07/09.

[3] Singletary SE, Tucker SL, Boddie AW, Jr. Multivariate analysis of prognostic factors in regional cutaneous metastases of extremity melanoma. Cancer. 1988;61(7):1437-40. Epub 1988/04/01.

[4] Karakousis CP, Temple DF, Moore R, Ambrus JL. Prognostic parameters in recurrent malignant melanoma. Cancer. 1983;52(3):575-9. Epub 1983/08/01.

[5] Roses DF, Karp NS, Oratz R, Dubin N, Harris MN, Speyer J, et al. Survival with regional and distant metastases from cutaneous malignant melanoma. Surgery, gynecology & obstetrics. 1991;172(4):262-8. Epub 1991/04/01.

[6] Haffner AC, Garbe C, Burg G, Buttner P, Orfanos CE, Rassner G. The prognosis of primary and metastasising melanoma. An evaluation of the TNM classification in 2,495 patients. British journal of cancer. 1992;66(5):856-61. Epub 1992/11/01.

[7] Balch CM, Gershenwald JE, Soong SJ, Thompson JF, Atkins MB, Byrd DR, et al. Final version of 2009 AJCC melanoma staging and classification. Journal of clinical oncolo-

gy : official journal of the American Society of Clinical Oncology. 2009;27(36): 6199-206. Epub 2009/11/18.

[8] Brown CD, Zitelli JA. The prognosis and treatment of true local cutaneous recurrent malignant melanoma. Dermatologic surgery : official publication for American Society for Dermatologic Surgery [et al]. 1995;21(4):285-90. Epub 1995/04/01.

[9] Lee YT. Loco-regional recurrent melanoma: I natural history. Cancer treatment reviews. 1980;7(2):59-72. Epub 1980/06/01.

[10] Wong JH, Cagle LA, Kopald KH, Swisher SG, Morton DL. Natural history and selective management of in transit melanoma. Journal of surgical oncology. 1990;44(3): 146-50. Epub 1990/07/01.

[11] Roses DF, Harris MN, Rigel D, Carrey Z, Friedman R, Kopf AW. Local and in-transit metastases following definitive excision for primary cutaneous malignant melanoma. Annals of surgery. 1983;198(1):65-9. Epub 1983/07/01.

[12] Cascinelli N, Bufalino R, Marolda R, Belli F, Nava M, Galluzzo D, et al. Regional nonnodal metastases of cutaneous melanoma. European journal of surgical oncology : the journal of the European Society of Surgical Oncology and the British Association of Surgical Oncology. 1986;12(2):175-80. Epub 1986/06/01.

[13] McCarthy WH, Shaw HM, Thompson JF, Milton GW. Time and frequency of recurrence of cutaneous stage I malignant melanoma with guidelines for follow-up study. Surgery, gynecology & obstetrics. 1988;166(6):497-502. Epub 1988/06/01.

[14] Soong SJ, Harrison RA, McCarthy WH, Urist MM, Balch CM. Factors affecting survival following local, regional, or distant recurrence from localized melanoma. Journal of surgical oncology. 1998;67(4):228-33. Epub 1998/05/14.

[15] Karakousis CP, Balch CM, Urist MM, Ross MM, Smith TJ, Bartolucci AA. Local recurrence in malignant melanoma: long-term results of the multiinstitutional randomized surgical trial. Annals of surgical oncology. 1996;3(5):446-52. Epub 1996/09/01.

[16] Kang JC, Wanek LA, Essner R, Faries MB, Foshag LJ, Morton DL. Sentinel lymphadenectomy does not increase the incidence of in-transit metastases in primary melanoma. Journal of clinical oncology : official journal of the American Society of Clinical Oncology. 2005;23(21):4764-70. Epub 2005/07/22.

[17] Morton DL, Thompson JF, Cochran AJ, Mozzillo N, Elashoff R, Essner R, et al. Sentinel-node biopsy or nodal observation in melanoma. The New England journal of medicine. 2006;355(13):1307-17. Epub 2006/09/29.

[18] Pawlik TM, Ross MI, Thompson JF, Eggermont AM, Gershenwald JE. The risk of in-transit melanoma metastasis depends on tumor biology and not the surgical approach to regional lymph nodes. Journal of clinical oncology : official journal of the American Society of Clinical Oncology. 2005;23(21):4588-90. Epub 2005/07/22.

[19] van Poll D, Thompson JF, Colman MH, McKinnon JG, Saw RP, Stretch JR, et al. A sentinel node biopsy does not increase the incidence of in-transit metastasis in pa-

tients with primary cutaneous melanoma. Annals of surgical oncology. 2005;12(8): 597-608. Epub 2005/07/16.

[20] Calabro A, Singletary SE, Balch CM. Patterns of relapse in 1001 consecutive patients with melanoma nodal metastases. Archives of surgery (Chicago, Ill : 1960). 1989;124(9):1051-5. Epub 1989/09/01.

[21] Zogakis TG, Bartlett DL, Libutti SK, Liewehr DJ, Steinberg SM, Fraker DL, et al. Factors affecting survival after complete response to isolated limb perfusion in patients with in-transit melanoma. Annals of surgical oncology. 2001;8(10):771-8. Epub 2002/01/05.

[22] Jaques DP, Coit DG, Brennan MF. Major amputation for advanced malignant melanoma. Surgery, gynecology & obstetrics. 1989;169(1):1-6. Epub 1989/07/01.

[23] Karakousis CP, Choe KJ, Holyoke ED. Biologic behavior and treatment of intransit metastasis of melanoma. Surgery, gynecology & obstetrics. 1980;150(1):29-32. Epub 1980/01/01.

[24] McPeak CJ, McNeer GP, Whiteley HW, Booher RJ. Amputation for Melanoma of the Extremity. Surgery. 1963;54:426-31. Epub 1963/09/01.

[25] Pack GT, Gerber DM, Scharnagel IM. End results in the treatment of malignant melanoma; a report of 1190 cases. Annals of surgery. 1952;136(6):905-11. Epub 1952/12/01.

[26] Turnbull A, Shah J, Fortner J. Recurrent melanoma of an extremity treated by major amputation. Archives of surgery (Chicago, Ill : 1960). 1973;106(4):496-8. Epub 1973/04/01.

[27] Griffiths RW, Briggs JC. Incidence of locally metastatic ('recurrent') cutaneous malignant melanoma following conventional wide margin excisional surgery for invasive clinical stage I tumours: importance of maximal primary tumour thickness. The British journal of surgery. 1986;73(5):349-53. Epub 1986/05/01.

[28] Heenan PJ, Ghaznawie M. The pathogenesis of local recurrence of melanoma at the primary excision site. British journal of plastic surgery. 1999;52(3):209-13. Epub 1999/09/04.

[29] Kaplan I, Ger R, Sharon U. The carbon dioxide laser in plastic surgery. British journal of plastic surgery. 1973;26(4):359-62. Epub 1973/10/01.

[30] Strobbe LJ, Nieweg OE, Kroon BB. Carbon dioxide laser for cutaneous melanoma metastases: indications and limitations. European journal of surgical oncology : the journal of the European Society of Surgical Oncology and the British Association of Surgical Oncology. 1997;23(5):435-8. Epub 1997/12/11.

[31] Green DS, Bodman-Smith MD, Dalgleish AG, Fischer MD. Phase I/II study of topical imiquimod and intralesional interleukin-2 in the treatment of accessible metastases in malignant melanoma. The British journal of dermatology. 2007;156(2):337-45. Epub 2007/01/17.

[32] Radny P, Caroli UM, Bauer J, Paul T, Schlegel C, Eigentler TK, et al. Phase II trial of intralesional therapy with interleukin-2 in soft-tissue melanoma metastases. British journal of cancer. 2003;89(9):1620-6. Epub 2003/10/30.

[33] von Wussow P, Block B, Hartmann F, Deicher H. Intralesional interferon-alpha therapy in advanced malignant melanoma. Cancer. 1988;61(6):1071-4. Epub 1988/03/15.

[34] Testori A, Faries MB, Thompson JF, Pennacchioli E, Deroose JP, van Geel AN, et al. Local and intralesional therapy of in-transit melanoma metastases. Journal of surgical oncology. 2011;104(4):391-6. Epub 2011/08/23.

[35] Glass LF, Pepine ML, Fenske NA, Jaroszeski M, Reintgen DS, Heller R. Bleomycin-mediated electrochemotherapy of metastatic melanoma. Archives of dermatology. 1996;132(11):1353-7. Epub 1996/11/01.

[36] Heller R, Jaroszeski MJ, Reintgen DS, Puleo CA, DeConti RC, Gilbert RA, et al. Treatment of cutaneous and subcutaneous tumors with electrochemotherapy using intralesional bleomycin. Cancer. 1998;83(1):148-57. Epub 1998/07/09.

[37] Mir LM, Glass LF, Sersa G, Teissie J, Domenge C, Miklavcic D, et al. Effective treatment of cutaneous and subcutaneous malignant tumours by electrochemotherapy. British journal of cancer. 1998;77(12):2336-42. Epub 1998/07/02.

[38] Adair FE. Treatment of melanoma: report of four hundred cases. Surgery, gynecology & obstetrics. 1936;62:406-8.

[39] Barranco SC, Romsdahl MM, Humphrey RM. The radiation response of human malignant melanoma cells grown in vitro. Cancer research. 1971;31(6):830-3. Epub 1971/06/01.

[40] Overgaard J, Gonzalez Gonzalez D, Hulshof MC, Arcangeli G, Dahl O, Mella O, et al. Hyperthermia as an adjuvant to radiation therapy of recurrent or metastatic malignant melanoma. A multicentre randomized trial by the European Society for Hyperthermic Oncology. International journal of hyperthermia : the official journal of European Society for Hyperthermic Oncology, North American Hyperthermia Group. 1996;12(1):3-20. Epub 1996/01/01.

[41] Burmeister BH, Henderson MA, Ainslie J, Fisher R, Di Iulio J, Smithers BM, et al. Adjuvant radiotherapy versus observation alone for patients at risk of lymph-node field relapse after therapeutic lymphadenectomy for melanoma: a randomised trial. The lancet oncology. 2012;13(6):589-97. Epub 2012/05/12.

[42] Corry J, Smith JG, Bishop M, Ainslie J. Nodal radiation therapy for metastatic melanoma. International journal of radiation oncology, biology, physics. 1999;44(5): 1065-9. Epub 1999/07/27.

[43] Ballo MT, Bonnen MD, Garden AS, Myers JN, Gershenwald JE, Zagars GK, et al. Adjuvant irradiation for cervical lymph node metastases from melanoma. Cancer. 2003;97(7):1789-96. Epub 2003/03/26.

[44] O'Brien CJ, Petersen-Schaefer K, Stevens GN, Bass PC, Tew P, Gebski VJ, et al. Adjuvant radiotherapy following neck dissection and parotidectomy for metastatic malignant melanoma. Head & neck. 1997;19(7):589-94. Epub 1997/10/10.

[45] Stevens G, Thompson JF, Firth I, O'Brien CJ, McCarthy WH, Quinn MJ. Locally advanced melanoma: results of postoperative hypofractionated radiation therapy. Cancer. 2000;88(1):88-94. Epub 2000/01/05.

[46] Aloia TA, Grubbs E, Onaitis M, Mosca PJ, Cheng TY, Seigler H, et al. Predictors of outcome after hyperthermic isolated limb perfusion: role of tumor response. Archives of surgery (Chicago, Ill : 1960). 2005;140(11):1115-20. Epub 2005/11/23.

[47] Kroon HM, Moncrieff M, Kam PC, Thompson JF. Outcomes following isolated limb infusion for melanoma. A 14-year experience. Annals of surgical oncology. 2008;15(11):3003-13. Epub 2008/05/30.

[48] Sanki A, Kam PC, Thompson JF. Long-term results of hyperthermic, isolated limb perfusion for melanoma: a reflection of tumor biology. Annals of surgery. 2007;245(4):591-6. Epub 2007/04/07.

[49] Wile AG, Guilmette E, Friedberg H, Mason GR. A model of experimental isolation perfusion using cis-platinum. Journal of surgical oncology. 1982;21(1):37-41. Epub 1982/09/01.

[50] Aigner K, Hild P, Henneking K, Paul E, Hundeiker M. Regional perfusion with cisplatinum and dacarbazine. Recent results in cancer research Fortschritte der Krebsforschung Progres dans les recherches sur le cancer. 1983;86:239-45. Epub 1983/01/01.

[51] Roseman JM. Effective management of extremity cancers using cisplatin and etoposide in isolated limb perfusions. Journal of surgical oncology. 1987;35(3):170-2. Epub 1987/07/01.

[52] Santinami M, Belli F, Cascinelli N, Rovini D, Vaglini M. Seven years experience with hyperthermic perfusions in extracorporeal circulation for melanoma of the extremities. Journal of surgical oncology. 1989;42(3):201-8. Epub 1989/11/01.

[53] Thompson JF, Gianoutsos MP. Isolated limb perfusion for melanoma: effectiveness and toxicity of cisplatin compared with that of melphalan and other drugs. World journal of surgery. 1992;16(2):227-33. Epub 1992/03/01.

[54] Fraker DL, Alexander HR, Andrich M, Rosenberg SA. Treatment of patients with melanoma of the extremity using hyperthermic isolated limb perfusion with melphalan, tumor necrosis factor, and interferon gamma: results of a tumor necrosis factor dose-escalation study. Journal of clinical oncology : official journal of the American Society of Clinical Oncology. 1996;14(2):479-89. Epub 1996/02/01.

[55] Cornett WR, McCall LM, Petersen RP, Ross MI, Briele HA, Noyes RD, et al. Randomized multicenter trial of hyperthermic isolated limb perfusion with melphalan alone compared with melphalan plus tumor necrosis factor: American College of Surgeons

Oncology Group Trial Z0020. Journal of clinical oncology : official journal of the American Society of Clinical Oncology. 2006;24(25):4196-201. Epub 2006/09/01.

[56] Ueno T, Ko SH, Grubbs E, Yoshimoto Y, Augustine C, Abdel-Wahab Z, et al. Modulation of chemotherapy resistance in regional therapy: a novel therapeutic approach to advanced extremity melanoma using intra-arterial temozolomide in combination with systemic O6-benzylguanine. Molecular cancer therapeutics. 2006;5(3):732-8. Epub 2006/03/21.

[57] Creech O, Jr., Krementz ET, Ryan RF, Winblad JN. Chemotherapy of cancer: regional perfusion utilizing an extracorporeal circuit. Annals of surgery. 1958;148(4):616-32. Epub 1958/10/01.

[58] Stehlin JS, Jr. Hyperthermic perfusion with chemotherapy for cancers of the extremities. Surgery, gynecology & obstetrics. 1969;129(2):305-8. Epub 1969/08/01.

[59] Di Filippo F, Calabro A, Giannarelli D, Carlini S, Cavaliere F, Moscarelli F, et al. Prognostic variables in recurrent limb melanoma treated with hyperthermic antiblastic perfusion. Cancer. 1989;63(12):2551-61. Epub 1989/06/15.

[60] Minor DR, Allen RE, Alberts D, Peng YM, Tardelli G, Hutchinson J. A clinical and pharmacokinetic study of isolated limb perfusion with heat and melphalan for melanoma. Cancer. 1985;55(11):2638-44. Epub 1985/06/01.

[61] Raymond AK, Beasley GM, Broadwater G, Augustine CK, Padussis JC, Turley R, et al. Current trends in regional therapy for melanoma: lessons learned from 225 regional chemotherapy treatments between 1995 and 2010 at a single institution. Journal of the American College of Surgeons. 2011;213(2):306-16. Epub 2011/04/16.

[62] Storm FK, Morton DL. Value of therapeutic hyperthermic limb perfusion in advanced recurrent melanoma of the lower extremity. American journal of surgery. 1985;150(1):32-5. Epub 1985/07/01.

[63] Grunhagen DJ, Brunstein F, Graveland WJ, van Geel AN, de Wilt JH, Eggermont AM. One hundred consecutive isolated limb perfusions with TNF-alpha and melphalan in melanoma patients with multiple in-transit metastases. Annals of surgery. 2004;240(6):939-47; discussion 47-8. Epub 2004/12/01.

[64] Siemann DW, Chapman M, Beikirch A. Effects of oxygenation and pH on tumor cell response to alkylating chemotherapy. International journal of radiation oncology, biology, physics. 1991;20(2):287-9. Epub 1991/02/01.

[65] Beasley GM, Petersen RP, Yoo J, McMahon N, Aloia T, Petros W, et al. Isolated limb infusion for in-transit malignant melanoma of the extremity: a well-tolerated but less effective alternative to hyperthermic isolated limb perfusion. Annals of surgical oncology. 2008;15(8):2195-205. Epub 2008/06/06.

[66] Lindner P, Doubrovsky A, Kam PC, Thompson JF. Prognostic factors after isolated limb infusion with cytotoxic agents for melanoma. Annals of surgical oncology. 2002;9(2):127-36. Epub 2002/03/13.

[67] Lindner P, Thompson JF, De Wilt JH, Colman M, Kam PC. Double isolated limb infusion with cytotoxic agents for recurrent and metastatic limb melanoma. European journal of surgical oncology : the journal of the European Society of Surgical Oncology and the British Association of Surgical Oncology. 2004;30(4):433-9. Epub 2004/04/06.

[68] Beasley GM, Caudle A, Petersen RP, McMahon NS, Padussis J, Mosca PJ, et al. A multi-institutional experience of isolated limb infusion: defining response and toxicity in the US. Journal of the American College of Surgeons. 2009;208(5):706-15; discussion 15-7. Epub 2009/05/30.

[69] Brady MS, Brown K, Patel A, Fisher C, Marx W. A phase II trial of isolated limb infusion with melphalan and dactinomycin for regional melanoma and soft tissue sarcoma of the extremity. Annals of surgical oncology. 2006;13(8):1123-9. Epub 2006/06/23.

[70] Mian R, Henderson MA, Speakman D, Finkelde D, Ainslie J, McKenzie A. Isolated limb infusion for melanoma: a simple alternative to isolated limb perfusion. Can J Surg. 2001;44(3):189-92. Epub 2001/06/16.

[71] Sharma K, Beasley G, Turley R, Raymond AK, Broadwater G, Peterson B, et al. Patterns of Recurrence Following Complete Response to Regional Chemotherapy for In-Transit Melanoma. Annals of surgical oncology. 2012. Epub 2012/04/06.

[72] Wieberdink J, Benckhuysen C, Braat RP, van Slooten EA, Olthuis GA. Dosimetry in isolation perfusion of the limbs by assessment of perfused tissue volume and grading of toxic tissue reactions. European journal of cancer & clinical oncology. 1982;18(10): 905-10. Epub 1982/10/01.

[73] Klaase JM, Kroon BB, van Geel BN, Eggermont AM, Franklin HR, Hart GA. Patient- and treatment-related factors associated with acute regional toxicity after isolated perfusion for melanoma of the extremities. American journal of surgery. 1994;167(6): 618-20. Epub 1994/06/01.

[74] Li Y, McClay EF. Systemic chemotherapy for the treatment of metastatic melanoma. Seminars in oncology. 2002;29(5):413-26. Epub 2002/10/31.

[75] Korn EL, Liu PY, Lee SJ, Chapman JA, Niedzwiecki D, Suman VJ, et al. Meta-analysis of phase II cooperative group trials in metastatic stage IV melanoma to determine progression-free and overall survival benchmarks for future phase II trials. Journal of clinical oncology : official journal of the American Society of Clinical Oncology. 2008;26(4):527-34. Epub 2008/02/01.

[76] Hodi FS, O'Day SJ, McDermott DF, Weber RW, Sosman JA, Haanen JB, et al. Improved survival with ipilimumab in patients with metastatic melanoma. The New England journal of medicine. 2010;363(8):711-23. Epub 2010/06/08.

[77] Sosman JA, Kim KB, Schuchter L, Gonzalez R, Pavlick AC, Weber JS, et al. Survival in BRAF V600-mutant advanced melanoma treated with vemurafenib. The New England journal of medicine. 2012;366(8):707-14. Epub 2012/02/24.

[78] Turley RS, Fontanella AN, Padussis JC, Toshimitsu H, Tokuhisa Y, Cho EH, et al. Bevacizumab-induced alterations in vascular permeability and drug delivery: a novel approach to augment regional chemotherapy for in-transit melanoma. Clinical cancer research : an official journal of the American Association for Cancer Research. 2012;18(12):3328-39. Epub 2012/04/13.

[79] Qi J, Chen N, Wang J, Siu CH. Transendothelial migration of melanoma cells involves N-cadherin-mediated adhesion and activation of the beta-catenin signaling pathway. Molecular biology of the cell. 2005;16(9):4386-97. Epub 2005/07/01.

[80] Hsu MY, Meier FE, Nesbit M, Hsu JY, Van Belle P, Elder DE, et al. E-cadherin expression in melanoma cells restores keratinocyte-mediated growth control and down-regulates expression of invasion-related adhesion receptors. The American journal of pathology. 2000;156(5):1515-25. Epub 2000/05/04.

[81] Augustine CK, Yoshimoto Y, Gupta M, Zipfel PA, Selim MA, Febbo P, et al. Targeting N-cadherin enhances antitumor activity of cytotoxic therapies in melanoma treatment. Cancer research. 2008;68(10):3777-84. Epub 2008/05/17.

[82] Beasley GM, Riboh JC, Augustine CK, Zager JS, Hochwald SN, Grobmyer SR, et al. Prospective multicenter phase II trial of systemic ADH-1 in combination with melphalan via isolated limb infusion in patients with advanced extremity melanoma. Journal of clinical oncology : official journal of the American Society of Clinical Oncology. 2011;29(9):1210-5. Epub 2011/02/24.

Chapter 11

Management of Brain Metastasis in Melanoma Patients

Sherif S. Morgan*, Joanne M. Jeter, Evan M. Hersh,
Sun K. Yi and Lee D. Cranmer*

Additional information is available at the end of the chapter

http://dx.doi.org/10.5772/55175

1. Introduction

The American Cancer Society estimates that 76,250 Americans will be diagnosed with malignant melanoma and 9,180 will die from the disease in 2012 [1]. The incidence is increasing both in the United States and worldwide [2]. Brain metastasis is a common problem in this population with 45-60% of those with metastatic melanoma developing brain metastases during the course of their illness [3]. Post-mortem studies demonstrate that brain lesions are present in 70-90% of patients who die of melanoma [3]. Development of brain metastases may have adverse impact both on a patient's prognosis and, if symptomatic, severe effects on quality-of-life (QOL) [4]. If left untreated, symptomatic brain lesions may be fatal within several weeks [3].

The literature pertaining to the treatment of brain metastasis from melanoma is scant when compared to brain metastases from more common solid tumors. In particular, brain metastases from non-small cell lung cancer (NSCLC) and breast cancer have been the subject of a larger number of investigative efforts. This chapter will extrapolate relevant results from other common solid tumors to the treatment of melanoma. In addition, systemic treatment approaches that may be useful in managing intracranial disease will be presented. Leptomeningeal involvement of the central nervous system, a less common form of central nervous system (CNS) invasion by melanoma, will not be discussed.

2. Treatment modalities

2.1. Surgery

Three randomized trials have investigated treatment of a single brain metastasis with whole brain radiation therapy (WBRT) alone or combined with surgical resection (Table 1) [5-7]. In all three, overall survival (OS) was the primary endpoint. In one study, the addition of surgery to WBRT achieved better control at the target lesion site than did WBRT alone [7]. Two of the trials indicated a survival benefit conferred by surgical treatment when added to WBRT, compared to WBRT alone. Differences in the proportion of patients with NSCLC, percentages of patients with extracranial disease, treatment of patients with non-metastatic intracranial disease, and cross-over from one treatment arm to the other may explain why the study of Mintz and co-workers did not indicate a survival benefit [6]. Extent of extracranial disease status was a consistent predictor of survival.

Study	**Centers (#)**	**Patients (#)**	**Disease Types # (%)**	**Median Survival**	**Recurrence/ Progression in CNS**		**Comments**
					Treated Site	**Distant**	
Patchell *et al.*, 1990 [7]	1	48 25-S 23-R	37 NSCLC (77%) 3 Mel. (6%)	40 w-S 15 w-R P<0.01	20%-S 52%-R P<0.02	20%-S 13%-R P=0.52	37% of enrolled patients with metastatic disease at enrollment. Extracranial disease and older age predicted decreased survival in multivariate analysis.
Noordijk *et al.*, 1994 [5]	5	63 32-S 31-R	33 NSCLC (52%) 6 Mel. (10%)	10 m-S 6 m-R P=0.04	NR	NR	Survival benefit in those with stable extra-cranial disease (12 m-S vs. 7 m-R, p=0.02) and patients younger than 61 y (19 m-S vs. 9 m-R, p=0.003). No survival benefit for surgery in patients with progressive extracranial disease or age"/>60.
Mintz *et al.*, 1996 [6]	8	84 41-S 43-R	45 NSCLC (53%)	5.6 m-S 6.3 m-R P=0.24	NR	NR	45% of enrolled patients with metastatic disease at enrollment. Only extracranial disease status predicted survival in multivariate analysis.

KPS: Karnofsky performance status; Mel: Melanoma patients; NR: Not reported; NSCLC: Non-small cell lung cancer; OS: Overall survival; QOL: Quality of life; R: Refers to treatment arm receiving WBRT alone; S: Refers to treatment arm combining surgery and WBRT

Table 1. Randomized trials of surgical resection of a single brain metastasis combined with WBRT versus WBRT alone

Since these studies primarily enrolled patients with primary NSCLC or breast cancer, their applicability to melanoma is uncertain. No prospective trials of surgery for melanoma patients with brain metastases have been published to date. However, a number of large retrospective studies have been reported (Table 2) [8-13]. Surgical treatment is consistently reported as a factor strongly associated with prolonged survival over those treated with WBRT alone. Selection biases are inherent in retrospective studies. Indeed, two of the studies specifically identified factors predicting patient selection for more or less aggressive treatment and follow-up based on the presumed severity of CNS involvement [10, 12]. Given that these retrospective reports in melanoma concur with the randomized trials of surgical therapy in non-melanoma brain metastases, similar randomized trials of surgery for melanoma brain metastases are probably unnecessary.

Traditionally, surgical management of brain metastases was restricted to individuals with a single accessible lesion. Bindal and co-workers found that individuals with a variety of primary solid tumors (n=56; melanoma=25/45%) undergoing resection of 2-3 brain metastases had survival rates equivalent to those undergoing resection of a single lesion [14]. In patients with complete resection of all known lesions, median survival was 14 months, equivalent to that for patients treated surgically for a single CNS lesion. Patients who could not undergo complete resection of CNS disease demonstrated inferior median overall survival of 6 months. Thus, presence of multiple CNS metastases is not a contra-indication to surgical treatment, although the advent of stereotactic radiosurgery (SRS) has made this approach less common.

2.2. Stereotactic Radiosurgery (SRS)

Stereotactic radiosurgery (SRS) has become a major modality in the local treatment of brain metastases. When compared to conventional techniques, SRS allows for safe and effective dose escalation. This is achieved through use of multiple modulated beamlets from a variety of angles, allowing optimized conformality and avoidance of normal tissues. SRS is minimally or non-invasive and allows targeting multiple CNS lesions including those that may be surgically accessible. Treatment is often performed on an outpatient basis and over a short time duration. Retreatment of the same or of new lesions is possible.

The Radiation Therapy Oncology Group (RTOG) conducted a large randomized study of SRS combined with WBRT (n=164) versus WBRT alone (n=167) (Table 3) [15]. The study enrolled patients with a variety of tumor types, although NSCLC patients comprised the largest proportion. The addition of SRS to WBRT resulted in a survival benefit for patients with a single brain lesion (6.5 months for combination therapy versus 4.9 months for WBRT alone, p=0.0393), but not for patients with multiple lesions (5.8 months for combination therapy versus 6.7 months for WBRT alone, p=0.9776) or all patients combined (6.5 months for the combination versus 5.7 months for WBRT alone, p=0.1356). At 6 months, SRS-treated patients required lower doses of corticosteroids and were more likely to discontinue steroid use altogether (52% in SRS+WBRT decreased their dose compared to 33% in the WBRT only group, p<0.0158). Patients receiving SRS also were more likely to improve their performance status (13% improved vs. 4% improved in WBRT group, p=0.0331). Local control of targeted tumors was better with SRS. Disease control at distant sites within the brain was equivalent.

Study	Dates, Patient Source Population, Institution	Melanoma Patients Studied and Treatment	Median Survival	CNS Recurrence Rates Based on Therapy Received	QOL
Raizer *et al.*, 2008 [13]	1991-2001 All metastatic melanoma patients (n=1114) at a single center	355 total 12 S/R +SRS 20 S + SRS 58 S/R 20 R + SRS 36 S 26 SRS 100 R 83 Supp.	Surgery (9 m) vs. no surgery (4 m), p<0.0001 R 4.0 m Supp. 2.0 m	NR	NR
Fife *et al.*, 2004 [12]	1985-2000 All patients with brain metastasis from melanoma (n=1137) at a single center	686 total 158 S/R 47 S 236 R 210 Supp.	All pts. 4.1 m S/R 8.9 m S 8.7 m R 3.4 m Supp. 2.1 m S= S/R, p=0.21 S or S/R >R > Supp., p<0.001	NR	NR
Buchsbaum *et al.*, 2002 [10]	1984-1998 All brain metastasis patients (n=1154) at a single center	74 total 14 S/R 19 R + SRS 3 S/R + SRS 10 S or SRS 25 R 3 Supp.	All pts. 5.5m (S or SRS) + R 8.8 m S or SRS 4.8 m R 2.3 m Supp. 1.1 m (S or SRS) + R vs. other groups, p<0.0001 S/R =R + SRS, p=0.5128	49% Local + R 17% R 20% S or SRS	NR
Zacest *et al.*, 2002 [11]	1979-1999 All surgically treated melanoma patients with brain metastasis at a single center	147 total 9 S 102 S/R 33 S/R/C 3 S/C	All pts. 8.5 m	50% overall recurrence rate	Neurological symptoms after treatment: Resolved 52% Improved 26% Unchanged 9% N/A 13%
Wronski and Arbit, 2000 [9]	1974-1994	91 total 49 S/R	All pts. 6.7 m	56% S/R vs. 46% S, p=NR	NR

Study	Dates, Patient Source Population, Institution	Melanoma Patients Studied and Treatment	Median Survival	CNS Recurrence Rates Based on Therapy Received	QOL
	All surgically treated brain metastasis patients (n=702) at a single center	29 S 13 died within 62 d of surgery	S/R (9.5 m) vs. S (8.3 m), p=0.67		
Sampson *et al.*, 1998 [8]	~1978-1998 All melanoma patients (n=6953) treated at a single center	524 total 87 S/R 52 S 180 R 205 C	Surgical therapy (NR) vs. R (120 d), p<0.0001 S/R (268 d) vs. S (195 d), p=0.9998 R (120 d) vs. C (39 d), p<0.0006	NR	No sig. difference in symptomatic results between patients treated with surgery and those treated with radiation (p=0.138)
Skibber *et al.*, 1996 [53]	1979-1991 All surgically treated melanoma patients with a single brain metastasis at two centers. No active non-CNS metastases present.	34 total 22 S/R 12 S	S/R (18 m) vs. S(6 m), p=0.002	Overall CNS relapse rate: 30% S/R vs. 90% S, p=0.02	NR
Hagen *et al.*, 1990 [54]	1972-1987 All surgically treated melanoma patients with a single brain metastasis at a single center	35 total 16 S 19 S/R	S (8.3 m) vs. S/R (6.4 m), p=NS	Median time to CNS relapse: S/R (26.6 m) vs. S (5.7 m), p<0.05	NR

C: Chemotherapy; Local Therapy: Treatment of CNS lesions with either surgery or stereotactic radiosurgery; KPS: Karnofsky performance status; NR: Not reported; NS: not significant; OS: Overall survival; QOL: Quality of life; R: Whole brain radiotherapy; S: Refers to treatment arm using surgery alone; Sig: Statistically significant; S/R: Surgery combined with whole brain radiotherapy; SRS: Stereotactic radiosurgery; Supp: Supportive care;

Table 2. Retrospective case series of surgery as treatment for brain metastasis in melanoma

A smaller study used the same design, but its primary endpoint was local disease control in patients with 2-4 brain lesions (Table 3) [16]. The study was halted at 60% of planned accrual due to meeting its primary endpoint (27 patients; 5 with melanoma). SRS-treated patients had significantly improved local disease control (p=0.0016). Median time-to-progression at SRS-treated sites was 6 months in patients treated with WBRT alone, versus 36 months in those treated with SRS and WBRT (p=0.0005). Extracranial disease status was the major survival determinant in a *post hoc* analysis.

Only two relatively small, single-arm prospective studies of SRS in melanoma have been published. One of these studies enrolled 31 patients, including 14 (45%) with melanoma (Table 3) [17]. Patients received only SRS as CNS therapy. Overall intracranial failure rate was 50% at 6 months. About one-third of patients failed within the SRS-treated tumor volume. The second study enrolled 45 melanoma patients receiving SRS at one of two treatment centers (Table 3) [18]. Up to 6 metastases were treated. Use of WBRT in conjunction with this therapy was not reported. Median survival of all patients was 4.2 months. The local control rate with SRS was 86%, although the follow-up period was not defined. Follow-up imaging was available for only 71 out of 86 treated lesions.

Numerous retrospective studies have reported the results of SRS therapy in melanoma (Table 4) [19-41]. These are quite variable in design. While some studied melanoma patients exclusively, others enrolled patients with other tumor types. Several studies appear to include the same set of patients treated at a given institution during overlapping time periods (noted in Table 4). Treatment and follow-up plans were not pre-specified or standardized. Although all patients received SRS, they often received a wide array of other therapies, including immediate or delayed WBRT, concurrent or delayed surgery, and partial brain irradiation. Patients received SRS both as primary brain metastasis therapy and as salvage therapy after failure of prior treatment. Some patients received therapy for a single metastasis, while others were treated for multiple brain metastases. Several studies specifically identify selection bias in the treated population, with more aggressive therapy being reserved for patients with more severe CNS disease [37, 38]. Collectively, the study heterogeneity limits the conclusions that can be reached from these retrospective analyses.

Reported median survival of melanoma patients in these series ranged from 4.4 to 11.1 months. These values approximate ranges reported in patients with brain metastases from other primary tumor types, in which median survival is estimated to be 6.5 to 10.5 months [10, 42, 43]. Several factors predicted shorter survival in multiple studies: decreased performance status or its surrogate indicators, multiple CNS lesions, greater intracranial tumor volume, infratentorial lesion location, and active extracranial disease.

Some studies did not find that the initial number of lesions predicted survival [28, 29, 34, 37, 39]. This contradicts the results of the only randomized trial of SRS with survival as the primary endpoint, in which a survival benefit was observed only in patients with a single CNS lesion (OS was 6.5 months in patients with SRS+WRBT compared to 4.9 months in the WBRT group alone; p=0.0393) [15]. This may be due to inadequate statistical power in the retrospective studies, given the heterogeneity of the populations under study.

CNS disease control was reported in most of these retrospective studies as 1-year actuarial control rates. At SRS-treated sites, reported in most of the studies, this was 47-87%. One-year control at non-SRS treated sites was 24-57%. The overall CNS control at one year was only 24-38%.

Study	Study Design	Patient Numbers & Tumor Types	Treatment	Median Survival	CNS Recurrence
Andrews *et al.*, 2004 [15]	Randomized Multi-institution, cooperative group study 1996-2001 Primary endpoint: median survival	331 total 64% Lung 10% Breast 5% Melanoma 21% Other 1-3 CNS metastases	164 SRS+R 167 R	Overall 6.5 m S+R vs. 5.7 m R, p=0.14 Single met. 6.5 m SRS+R vs. 4.9 m R, p=0.39 Multiple met. 5.8 m SRS+R vs. 6.7 m R, p=0.98	Time to intra-cranial progression SRS+R=R, p=0.13 Local control at 1 yr 82% SRS+R vs. 71% R, p=0.01
Kondziolka *et al.*, 1999 [16]	Randomized Single institution Primary endpoint: local control at SRS-treated site	27 total: 44% Lung 19% Melanoma 15% Renal 15% Breast 7% Other 2-4 CNS metastases	13 SRS+R 14 R	11 m SRS+R vs. 7.5 m R, p=0.22.	Median time to CNS failure: Local: 36 m SRS+R vs. 6 m R, p=0.0005 Any: 34 m SRS+R vs. 5 m R, p=0.002
Manon *et al.*, 2005 [17]	Single-arm Multi-institution, cooperative group study 1998-2003 Primary endpoint: 3m and 6m intracranial progression rate	31 total 45% Melanoma 45% Renal 10% Sarcoma 1-3 CNS metastases	31 SRS	8.3 m	Intra-cranial Failure Rates 3 m: Any 25.8% SRS-treated 19.3% Outside SRS 16.2% 6 m: Any 48.3% SRS-treated 32.2% Outside SRS field32.2%
Friehs *et al.*, 1998 [18]	Single-arm Multi-institution 1998-2003 Primary endpoint: Overall survival	45 total 100% Mel. 1-6 CNS metastases	45 SRS	4.2 m	86% of SRS-treated tumors controlled at follow-up. 13 (29%) with known distant failure in CNS.

KPS: Karnofsky performance status; Mel: Melanoma; Met: Metastasis/metastases; MMSE: Mini-Mental Status Examination; NR: Not reported; QOL: Quality of life; R: Whole brain radiotherapy; SRS+R: Stereotactic radiosurgery combined with whole brain radiotherapy; SRS: Stereotactic radiosurgery

Table 3. Prospective trials of stereotactic radiosurgery as treatment for brain metastases in melanoma

Study	**Study Design**	**Patient Numbers & Tumor Types**	**Treatment**	**Median Survival**	**CNS Control Rates (1-yr actuarial unless otherwise stated)**	**Comments (Prognostic factors multivariate unless otherwise noted)**
Liew *et al.*, 2011 [31]	1987-2008 Single institution All patients with mel. receiving GK	344 total 100% mel.	163 SRS 118 SRS+R 63 SRS + other	5.6 m after SRS 8.3 m from diagnosis of brain met	SRS treated sites 63% Distant 33%	R not sig. for survival or recurrence. Population may overlap with that of Mori et al., 1998 and Somoza et al., 1993.
Hara *et al.*, 2009 [27]	1999-2005 Single institution All pts. receiving Cyberknife therapy for mel. or renal cancer	62 total 44 mel. 18 renal	33 SRS 17 SRS sal. 5 SRS+R 7 SRS + Surg.	8.3 m 5.6 m for mel.	SRS-treated sites 87% Local and distant 38%	
Powell *et al.*, 2008 [34]	1998-2007 Single institution All patients receiving GK	76 total 50 mel. 23 renal 3 sarcoma	39 SRS 37 SRS+R	5.1 m Histology does not predict outcome	SRS-treated sites 78% Distant 37% Local and distant 26%	Local control higher for renal than mel . (94% vs. 63%, p=0.001)
Redmond *et al.*, 2008 [36]	1998-2006 Single institution All mel. pts. receiving GK	59 total 100% mel.	32 SRS 27 SRS+R	4.4 m	NR	Timing between SRS and R undefined.
Samlowski *et al.*, 2007 [37]	1999-2004 Single institution All mel. patients receiving LA-SRS	44 total 100% mel.	19 SRS 4 SRS +partial R 14 SRS+R 16% SRS with salvage R	11.1 m from brain metastasis diagnosis 48% 1-yr survival 18% 2-yr survival	SRS-treated sites 47%	Patients receiving SRS+R had a higher mean number of presented metastases (3.8) than those receiving salvage R after SRS failure (1.6). 22 (50%) treated with surgery at some point. Multiple lesions treated in 22 (50%).
Christopoulou *et al.*, 2006 [22]	1998-2004 Single institution All mel. patients receiving GK	29 total 100% mel.	All SRS 4 with prior R 2 with prior surg.	5.7 m	NR	
Gaudy-Marqueste *et al.*, 2006 [23]	1997-2003 Single institution All mel. patients receiving GK	106 total 100% mel.	106 SRS	5.1 m 13% 1-yr survival	SRS-treated sites 69%	No patients received planned R
Chang *et al.*, 2005 [20]	1991-2002 Single Institution	189 total 103 mel. 77 renal	130 SRS 16 SRS + R 43 SRS sal.	7.5 m	For mel. SRS-treated sites 47%	Inadequate patients treated with R to assess effects.

Study	Study Design	Patient Numbers & Tumor Types	Treatment	Median Survival	CNS Control Rates (1-yr actuarial unless otherwise stated)	Comments (Prognostic factors multivariate unless otherwise noted)
	All patients with mel., renal cancer or sarcoma receiving SRS as therapy	9 sarcoma		24% 1-y survival for mel.	Distant 24%	
Koc *et al.,* 2005 [29]	1999-2003 Single institution All mel. patients receiving GK as initial therapy	26 total 100% mel.	12 SRS 14 SRS+R	6 m 25% 1-yr survival	NR	
Radbill *et al.,* 2004 [35]	1996-2001 Single institution All mel. patients receiving GK	64 total 100% mel.	32 SRS 13 SRS sal. 8 SRS+R 8 SRS+surg. 2 SRS + R + surg. 1 NR	26 wk Single CNS met. (77 wk) vs. multiple (20 wk), p=0.003	SRS-treated sites 56% Distant 25%	Adjuvant R did not decrease distant failure, although small population receiving it.
Selek *et al.,* 2004 [38]	1991-2001 Single institution All mel. patients receiving LA-SRS	103 total 100% mel.	61 SRS 12 SRS + R 30 SRS sal.	Overall 6.7 m SRS 7.5 m SRS+R 3.7 m SRS sal. 5.4 m 25% 1-y survival	SRS-treated sites 48% SRS alone 60% SRS+R 0% SRS sal. 5% Distant 24% SRS alone 18% SRS+R 0% SRS sal. 51%	Patients with more aggressive disease were more likely to receive R after SRS.
Herfarth *et al.,* 2003 [28]	1986-2000 Two institutions All mel. patients treated with LA-SRS	64 total 100% mel.	All SRS	10.6 m	SRS-treated sites 81% Lesions ≥2 cm (64%) vs. <2 cm (88%), p=0.05 Distant CNS control NR	
Brown *et al.,* 2002 [19]	1990-2000 Single institution All patients with mel., renal cancer or sarcoma receiving SRS.	41 total 23 mel. 16 renal 2 sarcoma	20 SRS 4 R with SRS sal. 8 Surg. with SRS sal. 9 SRS + surg.	14.2 m No difference in survival SRS+R vs. SRS, p=0.54	6 m CNS control SRS-treated sites: SRS+R (100%) vs. SRS (85%), p=0.02 Distant: SRS+R (91%) vs. SRS (35%), p=0.004	
Gonzalez-Martinez *et al.,* 2002 [25]	1996-2002 Single institution All mel. patients receiving GK	24 total 100% mel.	10 SRS 14 SRS+R	5.5 m	NR	

Study	Study Design	Patient Numbers & Tumor Types	Treatment	Median Survival	CNS Control Rates (1-yr actuarial unless otherwise stated)	Comments (Prognostic factors multivariate unless otherwise noted)
Mingione *et al.*, 2002 [32]	1989-1999 Single institution All mel. patients receiving GK	45 total 100% mel.	29 SRS 16 SRS+R	10.4 m 31% 1-yr survival	NR	Adjuvant R had no impact on survival or CNS recurrence rate.
Yu *et al.*, 2002 [41]	1994-1999 Single institution All mel. patients receiving GK	122 total 100% mel.	83 SRS 12 SRS + R 10 SRS/R >1.5 m before SRS 17 SRS/R >1.5 m after SRS	7 m 26% 1-yr survival	SRS-treated sites 84% Distant 57%	Population may overlap with that of Lavine et al., 1999 and Chen et al., 1999.
Chen *et al.*, 1999 [21]	1994-1999 Single institution All patients receiving GK	199 total 88 mel. 40 NSCLC 5 SCLC 12 Renal 12 Breast 9 Colon 24 Other	199 SRS	8.5 m 7 m for mel.	89% of lesions with follow-up "controlled for the lifetime of the patient"	Use of R reported, but not defined. Population may overlap with that of Yu et al., 2002 and Lavine et al., 1999. Follow-up available for only 69% of lesions.
Lavine *et al.*, 1999 [30]	1994-1997 Single institution All mel. patients receiving GK	45 total 100% mel.	43 SRS. 2 SRS + R	8 m	3 m CNS control SRS-treated sites 97% Distant 81%	Population may overlap with that of Yu et al., 1999 and Chen et al., 1999. Other therapies in addition to SRS depending on clinical condition. Only 2 (4%) received SRS+R
Grob *et al.*, 1998 [26]	1993-1996 Single institution All mel. patients receiving GK	35 total 100% mel.	35 SRS	7 m	Actuarial control rate of evaluable, treated lesions: 3 m 98% 6 m 100% 9 m 95% 12 m 87% Distant CNS control not reported	
Mori *et al.*, 1998 [33]	1988-1996 Single institution All mel. patients receiving GK	60 total 100% mel.	12 SRS 36 SRS+R 12 SRS sal.	7 m median survival 21% 1-yr survival	Control in 46 pts. receiving SRS +/-R: SRS-treated sites: Overall 85%	Population may overlap with that of Mathieu et al., 2007 and Somoza et al., 1993.

Study	Study Design	Patient Numbers & Tumor Types	Treatment	Median Survival	CNS Control Rates (1-yr actuarial unless otherwise stated)	Comments (Prognostic factors multivariate unless otherwise noted)
					SRS+R 80% SRS 100% SRS sal. 86% Distant: Overall 70% SRS+R 77% SRS 56% SRS sal. 57%	
Seung *et al.*, 1998 [39]	1991-1995 Single institution (UCSF) All melanoma patients receiving GK	55 total 100% melanoma	28 SRS 11 SRS+ R 16 SRS sal.	35 wk	SRS-treated sites 77% Distant 36% Entire CNS 24%	
Gieger *et al.*, 1997 [24]	1992-1994 Single institution All mel. patients receiving LA-SRS	12 total 100% mel.	1 SRS 10 SRS+R 1 SRS sal.	8 m 36% 1-y survival	At least 6 patients with at least one SRS-treated lesions progressing. At least 3 (25%) developing new distant CNS lesions	Imaging follow-up not consistent.
Somoza *et al.*, 1993 [40]	1988-1992 Single institution All mel. patients receiving GK	23 total 100% mel.	19 SRS + R 4 SRS with R 3-12 m later	7 m 26% 1-y survival	NR	Population may overlap with that of Mathieu et al., 2007 and Mori *et al.*, 1998.

CNS: Central nervous system; GK: Gamma knife-based stereotactic radiosurgery; KPS: Karnofsky performance status; LA-SRS: Linear accelerator-based stereotactic radiosurgery; Mel: Melanoma; Met: Metastasis/metastases; NR: Not reported; QOL: Quality of life; Partial R: Partial brain irradiation; R: Whole brain radiotherapy; RPA: Recursive Partitioning Analysis; Sig: Statistically significant; SIR: Score Index for Radiosurgery; SRS: Stereotactic radiosurgery; SRS+R: Stereotactic radiosurgery combined with whole brain radiotherapy; SRS sal: Stereotactic radiosurgery salvage after failure of prior therapy; SRS+Surg: Combination therapy of stereotactic radiosurgery and conventional surgical resection; Surg: Surgical resection

Table 4. Retrospective studies of stereotactic radiosurgery for brain metastasis in melanoma

2.3. Comparative benefit of SRS versus surgery

The relative benefit of SRS versus surgery has not been tested in randomized clinical trials to date. One small randomized trial indirectly addressed this question, although not specifically for melanoma (Table 5) [44]. Sixty-four subjects with a single, surgically accessible brain lesion were randomly assigned to surgical excision and adjuvant WBRT or to SRS alone. A direct comparison of surgery and SRS is not possible due to the inclusion of adjuvant WBRT for all surgical patients and its omission in SRS-treated patients. Nine (14%) of the subjects had melanoma. No difference in overall survival was observed (9.5 months for surgery versus 10.3 months for SRS, p=0.8). A statistically non-significant improvement in local tumor control favored SRS (82% for surgery plus WBRT versus 97% for SRS, p=0.06). The one-year recurrence rate at distant CNS sites was significantly higher in the group receiving SRS alone (3% for surgery plus WBRT versus 26% for SRS alone, p<0.05). Thus, this study perhaps served to highlight the risks of omitting adjuvant treatment, rather than the relative merits of SRS versus surgery.

Two retrospective studies compared SRS to surgery [45, 46]. Melanoma patients were in the minority in both studies. O'Neill and co-workers analyzed patients seen from 1991-1999 at the Mayo Clinic who underwent either SRS or surgery for a solitary brain metastasis [45]. Eligible patients were candidates for either procedure: all had solitary lesions measuring less than 35 mm (maximum size conventionally treated with SRS), none of the lesions were surgically inaccessible, and none required immediate surgical decompression. Ninety-seven patients met these criteria, of whom only seven were melanoma patients. Seventy-four were treated surgically and twenty-three were treated with SRS. Although not achieving statistical significance, more SRS-treated patients received WBRT (96% SRS vs. 82% surgery, p=0.172). The treatment groups differed at baseline in performance status (worse in the SRS group, p=0.0016). Overall survival was similar between the two groups and was predicted by age, performance status, and systemic extracranial disease status rather than the type of brain metastasis treatment. Similar proportions of patients had CNS recurrence (29% SRS versus 30% surgery), but patients receiving surgery were more likely to have local recurrence at treated sites (58% of recurrences in 19 patients vs. 0% out of 6 recurrences in SRS-treated patients, p=0.02). Although this study suggests that local recurrences are more common after surgery, the retrospective nature of the study and the small number of patients limits its applicability.

In contrast, another single institution, retrospective study from a similar time period (1991-1994) suggested that SRS led to higher local recurrence rates than surgery [46]. Thirty-one patients were treated with SRS and sixty-two with surgery for brain metastases. Twenty-one patients (23%) had melanoma. Patients were matched with regard to histology, extracranial disease status, performance status, time from initial diagnosis to CNS metastasis, number of CNS metastases, age, and gender. Patients in the two groups were equally likely to have received WBRT. Patients receiving surgical treatment survived significantly longer than those treated with SRS (16.4 months surgery vs. 7.5 months SRS, p=0.0018). This improvement in survival was attributable to decreased rates of death from neurological causes in the surgical group (19% surgery vs. 50% SRS, p=0.037); deaths due to systemic disease were equivalent (p=0.28). Surgery yielded lower local tumor recurrence rates than SRS (8.1% surgery vs. 38.7% SRS). There was no statistically significant different in distant CNS recurrence rates between the two groups.

This retrospective study is subject to the biases inherent in such an undertaking. The authors matched patients for a variety of known relevant parameters, but the differences in local control may reflect the use of older SRS technology, high quality neurosurgical treatment at the referral center where the study was undertaken, or a combination of both. These discrepancies might explain the differences in results when contrasted with the results of the two other studies described [44, 45].

Collectively these studies do not indicate whether surgery or SRS is superior. There are no easily detectable differences in local control rates. Logistic differences therefore are important in selecting therapy. Unless a clinical situation arises in which surgery provides clear superiority (e.g. rapid control of symptomatic lesions; histological diagnosis), SRS will likely be the predominant modality employed to treat macroscopic melanoma lesions in the CNS.

2.4. Adjuvant Whole Brain Radiotherapy (WBRT)

Adjuvant therapy of the CNS is that which is administered in conjunction with definitive local therapy (surgery or SRS) of radiologically evident tumors to treat co-existing micrometastatic disease. This is distinguished from prophylactic cranial irradiation (PCI). PCI is administered in patients with systemic cancer after responses to systemic therapy, and has proven benefit in several conditions, such as small cell lung cancer (SCLC) [47, 48]. In melanoma, PCI has not been adequately assessed to recommend. Adjuvant CNS therapy has traditionally relied on WBRT. Although new systemic agents with proven anti-melanoma activity and CNS penetration may come to be used for this purpose as well, such use is experimental at present. Adjuvant WBRT is a controversial topic in metastatic brain tumor management, primarily due to questions of efficacy and of neurocognitive toxicity.

Three factors must be considered in determining whether or not to use adjuvant WBRT: (a) the effectiveness of WBRT in preventing emergence of new brain tumors; (b) the adverse effects of WBRT; and (c) the competing adverse effect of foregoing WBRT, namely an increased rate of CNS tumor progression. As new systemic therapies are proposed for this purpose, the same considerations apply. The relevant adverse effects relate to deterioration of neurocognitive function (NCF) and QOL, which could result from either WBRT itself or from progressive brain tumors. It is in balancing these factors that a rational decision regarding the use, or non-use, of adjuvant WBRT can be made.

2.4.1. Randomized trials of adjuvant WBRT in solid tumor patients

Despite the frequency of brain metastasis in melanoma patients, no prospective trials have been conducted to assess adjuvant WBRT in this population. Data from the treatment of brain metastases focusing on other tumor types must be reviewed to come to any conclusions (Table 5). Five randomized trials of adjuvant WBRT have been reported. Four of these are multi-institutional efforts, reflecting the difficulty in conducting this type of study [49-52]. A fifth study, discussed earlier, compared outcome in patients with a single brain metastasis treated with surgery and WBRT or with SRS alone [44]. The majority of patients in all of the studies were those with NSCLC primary tumors. Relatively few melanoma patients were enrolled.

Only one study used intracranial recurrence rate as the planned primary endpoint [52]. Ninety-five patients were enrolled after surgical resection of an isolated brain metastasis. Sixty percent had NSCLC. Forty-nine patients were randomized to receive adjuvant WBRT (50.4 Gy administered as 28-1.8 Gy fractions). The remaining forty-six patients were observed. Only

Study	Evaluable Patients (#)	Disease types #	Primary Endpoint	Median Survival	Recurrence/Progression in CNS		Comments
					S/SRS-site	Distant	
Patchell *et al.*, 1998 [52]	95 total 49 S+R 46 S	57 NSCLC 9 Breast 29 Other	CNS recurrence rate	S+R (48 wk) vs. S (43 wk), p=0.39	10% S+R 46% S P<0.001	14% S+R 37% S P<0.01	Single brain metastasis. Overall CNS recurrence rate (primary endpoint) significantly less in R-treated patients (18% S+R vs. 70% S, p<0.001). Decreased rate of neurological cause of death in group receiving R (14% S +R vs. 44% S, p=0.003)
Aoyama *et al.*, 2006 [49]	132 total 65 SRS+R 67 SRS	88 NSCLC 9 Breast 11 GI 10 Renal 14 Other	OS	SRS+R (7.5m) vs. SRS (8 .0 m), p=0.42	1-y rate 11% SRS +R 38% SRS P=0.002	1-y rate 42% SRS+R 64% SRS P=0.003	1-4 brain metastases. Overall CNS recurrence rate at 1-y: 47% SRS+R 76% SRS P<0.001 Salvage treatment required: 15% SRS+R 43% SRS P<0.001
Muacevic *et al.*, 2008 [44]	64 total 31 SRS 33 S+R	22 NSCLC 10 GU 11 Breast 9 Mel. 4 GI 8 Other	OS	9.5 m S+R 10.3 m SRS P=0.8	1-y rate 3% SRS 18% S+R P=0.06	1-y rate 26% SRS 3% S+R P=0.04	Single, surgically accessible brain metastasis. Study stopped early due to poor accrual.
Chang EL *et al.*, 2009 [50]	58 28 SRS+R 30 SRS	32 NSCLC 8 Breast 7 Mel. 4 Renal 7 Other	HVLT at 4 m vs. baseline	SRS+R (5.7 m) vs. SRS (15.2m), p=0.003	1-y rate 0% SRS+R 33% SRS P=0.01	1-y rate 27% SRS+R 55% SRS P=0.02	Up to 3 brain metastases. Decline in function at 4 m (primary endpoint): 48% SRS+R 24% SRS P=0.04 Study accrual stopped early due to achieving primary endpoint.
Kocher *et al.*, 2011 [51]	359 total SRS 100 SRS+R 99 S 79 S+R 81	190 NSCLC 29 Renal 42 Breast 18 Mel. 30 Colon 50 Other	Duration of functional independenc e (measured as deterioration of WHO PS to >2)	WBRT (10.7 m) vs. No WBRT (10.9 m), p=0.89	2-y rate S – 59% S+R – 27% (p < 0.001) SRS – 31% SRS+R – 19% (p = 0.040)	2-y rate S – 42% S+R – 23% (p = 0.008) SRS – 48% SRS+R – 33% (p = 0.023)	1-3 brain metastasis eligible. Either stable extracranial disease for 3 months or no extracranial metastases. Median Survival with WHO PS ≤2 (primary endpoint) 9.5m WBRT vs. 10.0 m no WBRT, p=0.709 Overall rate of CNS progression at 6 and 24 m: 15.2% and 31.4% WBRT vs. 39.7 and 54% no WBRT, p<0.0001 Neurological cause of death 25% WBRT vs. 43% no WBRT, p=NR

Table 5. Randomized trials of adjuvant WBRT with surgery or stereotactic radiosurgery for brain metastases

one patient in each group had melanoma. The CNS recurrence rate was 18% (9/49) in those receiving adjuvant WBRT. This contrasted sharply with a 70% (32/46) CNS recurrence rate in the observation group ($p<0.001$). The median time-to-CNS recurrence was markedly prolonged in those receiving adjuvant WBRT (220 weeks versus 26 weeks observation, $p<0.001$) due to decreased recurrence rates both at resection sites (10% WBRT versus 46% observation, $p<0.001$) and at distant sites within the brain (14% WBRT versus 37% observation, $p<0.01$). There was no difference in median survival (49 weeks WBRT versus 43 weeks observation, $p=0.39$) or in maintenance of independent function (maintenance of KPS >60%). A decreased rate of neurologic cause of death was evident in the WBRT-treated group (14% WBRT versus 44% observation, $p=0.003$), although the determination of this was less objective than determination of intracranial recurrence by imaging.

Another randomized trial tested adjuvant WBRT (30 Gy in 10 fractions) in conjunction with SRS [49]. The study enrolled 132 patients with one-to-four metastases measuring less than 3 cm in maximal dimension. Sixty-five patients received SRS and WBRT; sixty-seven received SRS alone. Two-thirds of those enrolled had NSCLC. The majority of the remainder had breast, colon or renal primary sites. The primary endpoint was overall survival. The researchers initially estimated that 89 evaluable patients per group would be required to detect a 30% difference in median survival time. A planned interim analysis, performed after 122 patients enrolled, led to early study termination. Four-to-five-fold more patients would have been required to detect a significant difference in the primary endpoint.

Although underpowered to detect a survival advantage, a number of secondary endpoints yielded significant results. CNS progression at 1 year was 47% in the combination therapy group and 76% in the SRS monotherapy group ($p<0.001$). WBRT improved control at one year for both SRS-treated sites (89% WBRT versus 72% without, $p=0.002$) and distant CNS sites (58% WBRT versus 36% without, $p=0.003$). No differences were observed in median survival, neurological cause of death, and acute or late neurological toxicity. Rates of systemic functional preservation (assessed by KPS), neurological preservation, and neurocognitive preservation (assessed by the Mini-Mental Status Examination, MMSE) were also not different.

A third trial randomized patients with 1-3 brain metastases to either SRS or SRS combined with adjuvant WBRT (30 Gy in 12 fractions) [50]. A novel endpoint for the study was chosen: change in performance on the Hopkins Verbal Learning Test-Revised (HVLT) at 4 months after primary therapy. The majority of enrolled patients were those with NSCLC primary tumors (55%), with melanoma in the minority (12%). The study was stopped early after accrual of 58 patients (28 SRS+WBRT, 30 SRS) due to its achieving the primary endpoint. Patients treated with the combination demonstrated a 52% decline in HVLT score at 4 months, versus a 24% decline in those receiving SRS only ($p=0.04$). This difference persisted at 6 months. Significant differences in performance on a panel of other neurocognitive tests were not detected. The study was stopped early and may have therefore been underpowered to detect other important differences in outcome. Decreased HVLT performance occurred despite decreased rates of CNS progression at one year in the combination therapy group (SRS-treated sites: 0% SRS +WBRT vs. 33% SRS, $p=0.01$; distant CNS: 27% vs. 55%, $p=0.02$). The authors also reported improved survival in the group treated with SRS alone (5.7 months SRS+WBRT vs. 15.2 months SRS, p=0.003).

Patients who were treated only with SRS required salvage therapy for intracranial progression in 87% of cases. Ten (33%) of the patients treated with SRS alone required craniotomy, ten (33%) received salvage WBRT and six (20%) received salvage SRS. In the group treated with SRS and adjuvant WBRT, two patients (7%) received salvage WBRT, and three (11%) progressed intracranially, but received no salvage therapy.

This study provides convincing evidence that the addition of adjuvant WBRT to SRS therapy for brain metastases impairs HVLT performance. This occurs despite a decreased rate of intracranial progression in those receiving WBRT. Salvage therapy for intracranial progression was required in the majority of patients treated with SRS alone, including salvage craniotomy in one-third of the patients. The clinical significance of HVLT deterioration due to adjuvant WBRT, vis a vis that of frequently needed salvage therapy for CNS disease was not addressed.

A fourth randomized trial assessing adjuvant WBRT enrolled patients with 1-3 brain metastases and stable or absent extracranial disease [51]. The majority of patients had NSCLC (53%); only 5% were melanoma patients. Patients received SRS or surgery as primary therapy and were then randomized to receive adjuvant WBRT (30 Gy in 10 fractions) or no additional therapy. The composite primary endpoint was median overall survival in patients with KPS of 0-2. In the intent-to-treat analysis, 180 patients were assigned to receive WBRT and 179 to observation. At the end of the study, per protocol, 164 patients received WBRT and 166 patients were on observation. Analysis was by intention-to-treat.

No differences were detected in the primary endpoint of survival with functional independence (9.5 months WBRT versus 10.0 months observation, p=0.709) or median overall survival (10.7 months WBRT versus 10.9 months observation, p=0.891). Intracranial recurrence rates were markedly suppressed by adjuvant WBRT. Overall intracranial progression occurred in 48% of WBRT-treated patients and in 78% of the observation group (p<0.001). This translated to improved progression-free survival (PFS) in the WBRT-treated group (4.6 months vs. 3.4 months observation, p=0.002). Two years after surgery, WBRT reduced the probability of relapse at intial site from 59% (observation) to 27% (p<0.001) and at distant CNS sites from 42% (observation) to 23% (p=0.008). Similarly, after SRS, WBRT reduced the probability of relapse at SRS-treated site from 31% (observation) to 19% (p=0.040) and at distant CNS sites from 48% (observation) to 33% (p=0.023). Neurological cause of death was suppressed by adjuvant WBRT (28% WBRT versus 44% observation; p<0.002). Extracranial disease progression rates at 24 months were identical (65% WBRT and 63% observation, p=0.73).

All four randomized trials showed decreased intracranial recurrence rates when adjuvant WBRT was administered, both at the site of treatment and at distant sites within the brain. Similar effects from adjuvant WBRT on distant CNS recurrence were reported by the trial of Muacevic and co-workers, in which patients were randomized to surgery with adjuvant WBRT versus SRS alone, discussed above [44]. The impact on the reduction in distant CNS recurrence with the use of adjuvant WBRT is likely from the eradication of subclinical microscopic disease present at the time of brain metastasis diagnosis. The effect of WBRT on CNS seeding from uncontrolled extracranial disease is unclear, but likely has a lesser effect. If seeding from extracranial disease was a dominant mechanism leading to CNS failure, adjuvant WBRT would not be predicted to decrease its occurrence.

No trial to date evaluating the omission of adjuvant WBRT after local therapy has demonstrated a survival benefit to WBRT. The study by Chang and co-workers indicated that the use of adjuvant WBRT after local therapy might be associated with a decrement in survival. It is difficult to draw firm conclusions about these data, as the study was stopped early, was not powered to detect a survival benefit, and contradicted the survival results of the other four larger randomized studies presented above. This includes the study by Aoyama and co-workers [50], which evaluated overall survival as its primary endpoint and was unable to detect a survival difference between its treatment arms, without a marked increase in sample size to over 800. The study by Kocher and co-workers demonstrated an improvement in PFS associated with adjuvant WBRT [51]. This study excluded patients with uncontrolled or progressive primary disease, mitigating extracranial disease burden as a competing risk for death

The studies presented here represent the best assessment of the efficacy of adjuvant WBRT therapy in treatment of solid tumor brain metastases. This therapy is clearly able to decrease intracranial recurrence rates, both at locally treated and distant sites within the CNS. The effect of this therapy on survival and the relative benefits versus the cognitive effects of the therapy are less clear. Melanoma patients formed a small fraction of the patients enrolled in these trials and one might therefore question whether these results even apply in the melanoma setting. To do so requires examination of the rather imperfect retrospective dataset regarding adjuvant WBRT specifically in melanoma.

2.4.2. Adjuvant WBRT in melanoma patients

The randomized studies discussed above primarily enrolled patients diagnosed with NSCLC. There have been no prospective studies evaluating the role of adjuvant WBRT specifically in the melanoma patient population. Many retrospective studies have been reported; unsurprisingly, these have indicated that adjuvant WBRT confers no survival benefit (see Tables 2, 4) [8-10, 12, 19, 29, 31, 32, 34, 35, 38, 39, 41, 53]. Since most melanoma patients with brain lesions present with active extracranial disease, any potential survival benefit due to adjuvant WBRT after local CNS therapy is probably undermined: extracranial disease serves as a competing cause of death, diluting any study's statistical power.

It is difficult to make firm conclusions based on the numerous melanoma case series on whether adjuvant WBRT actually decreases the rate of intracranial recurrence after local therapy. Selection and ascertainment biases are major concerns. Patients with clinically advanced disease are often selected for more aggressive therapy. Groups receiving aggressive therapy are likely to undergo more frequent and detailed surveillance for recurrence.

Several retrospective studies identify such biases. In the study of Buchsbaum and co-workers a paradoxically *higher* rate of CNS recurrence (49%) was identified in patients having received combined local CNS lesion therapy and adjuvant WBRT versus local therapy alone (20%) [10].

Follow-up scans were more frequent in the combined therapy group, possibly explaining the increased detection of progression and therefore higher documented recurrence rates. Samlowski and co-workers indicated that patients having received combined SRS and adjuvant WBRT had a higher mean number of CNS lesions at presentation than those selected for SRS alone [37]. Not surprisingly, more aggressive upfront therapy is apparently administered to patients with a greater initial disease burden.

Another study reported that patients receiving SRS with WBRT had 0% 1-year actuarial control within the CNS versus 60% for those treated with SRS alone (p=0.0005), strongly suggesting selection bias [38]. Those patients with initially more advanced disease were more likely to be treated with the combined modality technique. Advanced disease was found as a strong predictor for poorer outcomes. Therefore local control rates were likely confounded by the level of disease burden at presentation and not necessarily by the choice of treatment modality.

Other studies indicate similar paradoxical results in patients treated with adjuvant WBRT. Wronski and Arbit reported an increased risk of CNS recurrence (56%) in patients treated with surgery and WBRT versus 46% in those treated with surgery alone [9]. Another study reported a 20% failure rate at SRS-treated sites in patients receiving adjuvant WBRT versus 0% in those treated with SRS alone [33]. Perhaps indicative of a possible beneficial effect from adjuvant WBRT, failure at distant sites within the CNS was only 23% in the combination therapy group versus 44% in those treated with SRS alone. Those failing at the local site after combined modality treatment had larger initial volumes of disease compared with those treated with SRS alone. The additional fractionated dose contributed from WBRT at the site of failure may not have adequately addressed the increased tumor burden initially present. This was likely a significant confounder in local control outcomes.

Several studies concluded that WBRT does not significantly impact CNS recurrence rates. In one study of 333 melanoma patients, WBRT before or after SRS did not alter the intracranial recurrence rates [31]. The same study also showed that patient survival was significantly shorter with WBRT (4.5 months) compared to SRS alone (6.4 months, p=0.05). Again, selection bias for patients with more lesions or more aggressive disease could explain this result. Radbill *et al.* reported that adjuvant WBRT did not decrease the rate of failure at non-SRS-treated sites in the CNS (p=0.13) [35]. However, the number of patients treated with adjuvant WBRT (13%) was potentially too small to detect a benefit. Mingione *et al.*, studying 45 melanoma patients, of whom 16 received adjuvant WBRT, concluded that WBRT had no impact on outcomes [32]. Yu *et al.* also found that adjuvant WBRT did not decrease distant CNS recurrence; this conclusion was again limited by the small proportion of WBRT-treated patients (32/122 patients; 32%) [41].

Three studies have suggested a benefit from WBRT in preventing CNS recurrence in the melanoma population. One retrospective study of 35 melanoma patients undergoing resection of a single brain metastasis at a single institution from 1972 to 1987 documented a CNS recurrence rate of 37% in those treated with adjuvant WBRT, versus 69% in those not receiving this therapy (Table 2) [53]. Median time to CNS relapse was 26.6 months in the group receiving adjuvant WBRT, as compared to 5.7 months in those not receiving such therapy (p<0.05). Survival was predicted by the extracranial disease status, rather than receipt of adjuvant

WBRT. Death due to neurological causes was more common in the group that did not receive WBRT (24% WBRT versus 85% observation, p<0.01).

Another study during approximately the same time period (1979-1991) examined adjuvant WBRT after surgery in patients with a solitary CNS metastasis from melanoma (Table 2) [54]. Patients had no active extracranial disease and underwent resection of a single metastasis. Of the 34 subjects, 22 received WBRT. Median survival was improved in the combination therapy group (18 months versus 6 months with surgery alone, p=0.002), but CNS relapse rates were similar (30% surgery+WBRT *vs.* 22% surgery only; p=0.65). This study evaluated a highly selected patient group. This study and that of Hagen also suffer from being older studies, with more limited CNS imaging capabilities [53]. Nevertheless, the results tend to echo those of Patchell's randomized trial, suggesting a decreased CNS recurrence rate in CNS melanoma patients treated with adjuvant WBRT after local therapy [52].

Another report reviewed a single institution's experience with SRS in the treatment of 41 patients with radioresistant tumors, including 23 with melanoma [19]. Adjuvant WBRT improved local control (100% control with SRS and WBRT versus 85% with SRS alone at 6 months) and distant brain failure rates (17% failure with SRS and WBRT versus 64% failure with SRS alone). As might be predicted, adjuvant WBRT did not affect overall survival.

In summary, retrospective case series in melanoma indicate that adjuvant WBRT does not convey an overall survival benefit. This is consistent with the results of the randomized trials of WBRT primarily conducted in non-melanoma brain metastases. It is therefore reasonable to conclude that the addition of adjuvant WBRT does not improve the overall survival of the majority of melanoma patients with brain metastases.

As regards the effect of adjuvant WBRT on the prevention of CNS recurrence in melanoma, this collection of retrospective studies provides conflicting data. Some have shown no effect, others have shown decreased intracranial recurrence rates with the addition of WBRT, and still others have indicated that WBRT is associated with increased recurrence rates. Biases in treatment selection and ascertainment are strong confounders in many of the studies.

An ongoing randomized phase 3 trial is currently accruing for the comparison of distant intracranial control with the addition of adjuvant WBRT to observation following surgery and/or SRS in melanoma patients with 1-3 brain lesions (NCT01503827) [55]. Secondary endpoints will include the effects on OS, QOL, and NCF. This prospective, randomized, melanoma-specific trial will hopefully reconcile the contradictory observations reported in the retrospective studies discussed above. With improving systemic therapy, including agents able to penetrate the CNS at clinically relevant concentrations, even this randomized trial may not be able to answer its major questions about adjuvant WBRT in melanoma patient.

Salvage SRS: An alternative to WBRT?

An alternative strategy to managing CNS metastases involves the use of "salvage" SRS. After patients receive initial local therapy with SRS alone, WBRT is omitted to spare normal brain tissues from unnecessary radiation doses and avoid potential adverse neurocognitive effects. Patients undergo CNS imaging at planned intervals or if symptoms suggest progression. SRS is then used to treat new lesions.

This strategy has not yet been tested in a randomized trial for patients with brain metastases from melanoma. There are limited data that have included melanoma patients in the prospective evaluation of this treatment paradigm. For example, one prospective study assessed SRS as a single treatment modality in 41 patients with no more than 4 brain metastases [56]. Seven (16%) of the patients had melanoma primary tumors. Twenty-three of the enrolled patients (56%) experienced intracranial progression. Nine received salvage treatment with additional SRS and one with surgery and WBRT for persistent tumor. Eleven patients were treated with salvage WBRT due to an excessive number of new CNS lesions and two patients received non-radiotherapy palliative therapy. Intracranial recurrences were common in the absence of upfront WBRT; less than half of recurring patients (9/23) were eligible for salvage SRS therapy due to excessive number of new lesions, limited life expectancy or decreased performance status.

Data from a large, multi-institutional, retrospective study of 569 patients (16% with melanoma) support the feasibility of salvage SRS in replacement of upfront WBRT [57]. Of 268 patients treated initially with SRS alone, 98 received salvage therapy for CNS recurrence. Sixty-three (64%) of those needing salvage therapy received WBRT as part of the salvage regimen (which included SRS and/or surgery) and forty-seven (48%) received WBRT as the sole salvage therapy.

One retrospective study examined 45 patients (20 with melanoma, 44%) receiving SRS as salvage therapy [58]. Excellent local control at treated sites was achieved (92.4% at 52 weeks). Patients who received upfront WBRT were significantly less likely to require salvage therapy ($p=0.008$), although no survival benefit was reported.

A CNS metastasis management strategy in which SRS is used as sole initial therapy warrants continued evaluation, particularly for patients diagnosed with melanoma. The existing studies of this approach suggest that intracranial recurrence rates remain high with the omission of WBRT. Although salvage therapy with SRS may be planned initially, a large fraction of patients will require WBRT in the salvage setting to treat macroscopic recurrences, when WBRT is likely to be *least* effective

2.4.3. Neurocognitive effects of WBRT

A major argument against the use of adjuvant WBRT relates to its impact on NCF and higher executive neurologic functions, including learning, memory, calculation, and task planning. A variety of standardized neuropsychological tests measure global NCF, such as the MMSE. NCF impairment has a direct impact on overall QOL, affecting patients' ability to carry out activities of daily living, medical treatment compliance, and higher order planning and function [59].

One widely cited retrospective study examined patients treated at a single center for brain metastasis by either WBRT alone (n=370) or surgical metastectomy combined with WBRT (n=118) [60]. Radiation-associated dementia was reported at a rate of 1.9 (n=7) and 5.1% (n=5), respectively. Cases were defined as those patients treated for brain metastases with WBRT without evident CNS recurrence who subsequently developed "...a progressive dementing illness." Neither baseline neurocognitive data information for the identified cases nor information regarding the source populations was provided. Among the 12 cases identified, a variety of radiation dose and fractionation schemes were employed. The authors suggested that the incidence of radiation-related leukoencephalopathy might have been underestimated due to lack of sensitive tools for identifying neurocognitive dysfunction. Baseline neurocognitive dysfunction in patients with primary or secondary brain malignancy, however, is present in as many as 90% of patients prior to treatment [61] due to the general debility of patients with metastatic cancer, the neurocognitive effects of systemic chemotherapy and supportive therapies, and the age of the patients. Thus, the results of this relatively old study do not provide a clear picture of neurocognitive dysfunction associated with radiotherapeutic treatment of brain metastases.

Fairly good evidence shows that radiation therapy of the brain leads to neurocognitive dysfunction, which in some cases can be severe. A variety of patient-related factors play a role in the development of risk for developing radiation-associated neurocognitive dysfunction. These include patient age (children or those more than 50 years of age), other therapies received (chemotherapy and/or anti-convulsants), and length of survival post radiation therapy (as seen in survivors diagnosed with more favorable and indolent diseases, e.g., low-grade glioma) [62-68]. Factors related to radiation therapy delivery include total dose received, dose per fraction, and amount of cerebral volume irradiated [68-71].

More rigorous prospective assessments suggest that the neurocognitive impact of WBRT may be modest. Data from the study of primary brain tumor patients, in which extracranial disease and its treatment are not factors, may be relevant. For example, one study examined the dose-dependency of radiotherapy-associated neurocognitive dysfunction in patients treated for primary brain tumors [71]. Neuropsychological testing was undertaken up to 12 months after completion of radiotherapy. No dysfunction was observed in patients receiving up to 30 Gy, a typical dose used for adjuvant WBRT. Fraction size was not reported.

Another setting to examine the effects of WBRT is in diseases for which PCI is of proven benefit, such as SCLC. In two large studies evaluating the role of PCI for good responders with SCLC, there was no difference in NCF between those randomized to receive WBRT or not (24 Gy in 12 fractions-36 Gy in 18 fractions) [47, 48]. In the study by Gregor *et al.*, both groups of patients demonstrated baseline neurocognitive impairment versus normal controls, likely reflecting effects of prior treatment. Among those without baseline impairment, impairment in cognitive test performance was evident at 6 months and 1 year, but no obvious differences were seen when comparing PCI-treated and –untreated patients. The authors did not, however, describe rigorous statistical assessment of the longitudinal neurocognitive testing data [48].

Another prospective, non-randomized study showed no difference in cognitive function after 30-40 Gy of radiation therapy with 2-34 months of follow-up [72]. Again, a high degree of pre-existing neurocognitive deficit was already present. This may have been attributable to chemotherapy given prior to radiation therapy.

A non-randomized, prospective study of PCI was undertaken in NSCLC patients [73]. Seventy-five patients received induction radiochemotherapy for locally advanced NSCLC. Forty-seven received PCI (30 Gy over 3 weeks), while twenty-eight others did not. PCI reduced the overall rate of brain relapse from 54% to 13% at 3-4 years. In fifteen long-term survivors (10 PCI, 5 without PCI), no significant differences were noted in a battery of neuropsychological tests undertaken at a median of 47 (PCI) and 70 (no PCI) months.

A study recently presented short term follow-up of longitudinal NCF in patients having received PCI (small cell lung cancer; n=13), therapeutic cranial irradiation (TCI; brain metastases; n=16) or non-cranial irradiation (control: breast cancer; n=15) [74]. NCF was assessed prior to and during radiation treatment and 6-8 weeks after its completion. At 6-8 weeks after treatment, only verbal memory scores were lower in patients receiving cranial irradiation versus controls. Visual memory and attention were not affected. Pre-treatment verbal memory performance score was the major predictor of post-treatment outcome in univariate analysis, with a lesser contribution attributable to cranial irradiation. The data from this admittedly small study suggest that WBRT can have a negative impact on verbal memory, although other factors contributing to the baseline status seem dominant.

Aoyama and co-workers conducted a randomized trial of SRS with or without WBRT, discussed in detail above [75]. Baseline and follow-up MMSE scores were available for 110 and 92 of the 132 patients enrolled in the trial, respectively. Baseline MMSE scores were predicted by patient age, performance status, tumoral edema and total tumor volume, but not by the initial number of tumors.

Deterioration in MMSE occurred in equal proportions of each group (14/36 SRS + WBRT versus 12/46 SRS alone, p=0.21). Average time-to-deterioration was longer in the combined therapy group (13.6 months versus 6.8 months SRS alone, p=0.05). In the 14 members of the combined therapy group, the adjudged cause of deterioration was brain tumor progression in 3, toxic effects of radiotherapy in 5 and indeterminate in 6; in the group treated only with SRS, MMSE deterioration was due to brain tumor progression in 11 and indeterminate in 1 (combined vs. SRS, p<0.0001). The temporal trends in NCF between the two arms suggest that SRS-related cognitive decline may be associated with tumor recurrence, which may or may not be reversible with salvage therapy. Later dysfunction with WBRT is more variable in cause. Some may be attributable to CNS tumor recurrence, but other cases being attributable to late effects of radiation on normal brain tissue. Such treatment-associated damage would not be amenable to corrective therapy with further tumor-specific therapy.

The study of Chang and co-workers, discussed earlier, prospectively addressed NCF in the setting of adjuvant WBRT [50]. This study is notable in that the score on a specific neurocognitive test, HVLT, was the primary endpoint. Patients receiving adjuvant WBRT experienced greater rates of decline in their HVLT performance than those treated with SRS alone, despite decreased intracranial progression in the WBRT-treated patients.

The HVLT tests basic verbal learning capacity and is proposed as a screening test for mild dementia [76, 77]. The HVLT may have somewhat greater sensitivity for mild dementia than the MMSE, as well some logistical advantages [78]. In isolation, however, results from the HVLT must be judged cautiously, as it does not assess other more complex neurocognitive functions [79]. In studies of patients with brain metastases, the test is part of a battery of administered tests intended to develop a general overview of neurocognitive function [80, 81].

In the Chang study, a battery of neurocognitive function tests was administered, along with HVLT. Differences in performance on these other tests were not different between the two groups. The authors cautioned that the wide confidence intervals in the results of non-HVLT tests did not exclude a difference between the two test groups, but they also did not demonstrate a specific difference between the groups.

Studies of the effects of brain radiotherapy presented here vary in quality. They do not however give a clear picture suggesting severe adverse consequences of brain radiotherapy. Adverse effects are certainly identified in several studies, although their clinical significance is not certain and its cause is not clearly attributable to CNS radiotherapy. Intuitively, radiation therapy in and of itself is not beneficial for the nervous system. In the setting of brain metastasis treatment, however, the adverse effects of radiation therapy must be balanced against those of CNS tumor recurrence.

2.4.4. *Neurocognitive effects of brain tumor progression*

While little melanoma-specific data are available, the primary brain tumor literature reveals that there are significant negative cognitive effects from tumor progression. This literature is particularly useful, as cognitive deterioration in primary brain tumor patients is due entirely to incracranial disease and CNS treatment effects, as opposed to extracranial disease progression. Deterioration in MMSE was a strong predictor of impending intracranial tumor progression in a study of 1,244 glioma patients [82]. A change in MMSE score was seen even *prior* to radiographic progression. Decreased MMSE score also strongly correlated with performance status deterioration.

Another study in 445 brain metastasis patients (25 with melanoma) compared the drop in MMSE score before and after treatment with WBRT [83, 84]. The study was designed to assess the effect of the radiation fractionation schedules on survival, for which no effect was found. Tumor control was the primary factor in determining MMSE scores at 3 months. A 6.2 point drop (out of 30 possible) was seen in those with radiographic evidence of progression, compared to a 0.5 point drop in those with controlled tumors. In multivariate analysis, control of brain metastases was the only factor affecting MMSE score.

Another prospective brain metastasis study assessed a novel radiosensitizing agent combined with WBRT [85]. A detailed neurocognitive battery assessed NCF before and after therapy. Patients in the control arm, receiving WBRT alone, were subdivided into "good responders" (at least a 45% reduction in tumor size) and "poor responders" (less than a 45% reduction). Good responders had better NCF preservation rate, as well as a modest survival advantage (median survival 300 days versus 240 days; $p=0.03$).

These studies indicate that CNS tumor progression has adverse effects on neurocognitive status and QOL (reflected by performance status deterioration). While not melanoma-specific, there is no reason to believe that CNS progression of melanoma tumors would be any less adverse. These adverse effects of tumor progression must be balanced against those of adjuvant WBRT.

2.4.5. WBRT in advanced CNS melanoma

In some patients, disease in the CNS cannot reasonably be controlled using local treatment of brain metastases with surgery or SRS. At some point, lesion number becomes excessive, or lesions are present in locations that are not amenable to local treatment. Alternatively, a patient's extracranial disease may be so extensive that it is likely to be life-limiting, and the goal of CNS disease treatment is primarily symptom palliation. WBRT is often used in this circumstance, with the twin goals of improving survival and providing symptoms palliation.

No randomized, prospective studies are available to quantitate the benefit of WBRT, especially when compared to supportive care alone. A number of large retrospective case series have examined the questions specifically of survival, although these suffer from heterogeneous patient populations. In the study of Sampson and co-workers, 205 melanoma patients with brain metastases received systemic palliative chemotherapy, with median OS of 39 days, versus 120 days among the 180 patients treated only with whole brain radiotherapy (p=0.0006) [8]. Receipt of radiotherapy treatment was statistically significant in the multivariate analysis of another large retrospective study, with radiotherapy demonstrating median OS of 3.6 months, versus 1.3 months for those treated with corticosteroids alone (HR=0.38; p<0.001). In the study of Raizer and co-workers, 83 patients received no specific therapy for brain metastases, vesus 100 receiving WBRT alone [13]. Median OS was 2.0 and 4.0 months, respectively. The statistical significance of this difference was not reported.

The study of Fife and co-workers examined patients treated at a single center in Australia in the 1952-2000 date range [12]. For the 1985-2000 cohort, 210 patients received supportive care, versus 236 receiving radiotherapy alone. Median OS was 2.1 and 3.4 months in these two groups; in multi-variate Cox regression analysis, radiotherapy was associated with a decreased hazard ratio for death (HR-0.851; p=0.111). This may not have achieved statistical significance due to the heterogeneity of the patients in these two groups. In addition to treatment modality, other significant factors associated with survival were the presence of concurrent metastases at diagnosis, older age, and a longer time from initial melanoma diagnosis.

An older retrospective study identified 60 melanoma patients with cerebral melanoma metastases that were enrolled in two Radiation Therapy Oncology Group (RTOG) studies [86]. The study sought to determine the effects of WBRT on performance status, neurologic function, and neurologic symptoms. In the analysis, this study demonstrated that WBRT provided improvement of neurologic symptoms (including headache, motor loss, convulsion) in 76% of patients. Median survival in this uncontrolled report was 10-14 weeks, although the baseline clinical characteristics of the study population were quite variable.

Another retrospective study identified 87 patients who had received WBRT, of whom 46 (53%) had 3 or more metastases [87]. The majority of patients were already receiving dexamethasone before initiating radiation, and therefore it was difficult to isolate the effects of WBRT, since CNS signs and symptoms can be alleviated by corticosteroid treatment. The fraction of patients discontinuing corticosteroids due to symptom improvement served as a surrogate marker for palliative effects of WBRT. Upon completion of WBRT, 52% of all patients and 48% of symptomatic patients discontinued steroids. The same study demonstrated a small measurable response in tumor size following WBRT. Out of 87 patients, 65 had measurable disease at baseline; only 28 had at least one follow-up MRI scan to assess response. This may reflect a bias favoring follow-up scans being undertaken in those with responding disease. In these 28 patients at a median follow-up of 7 weeks, 75 tumors showed a median reduction in tumor size of 17%. The median OS of all patients evaluated in this study was 19 weeks. The median OS for patients who had undergone surgical resection prior to WBRT (22 patients) was 45 weeks, versus 16 weeks for those who did not undergo surgical resection ($p<0.0001$). Absence of extracranial disease (in 14 patients) was associated with higher median OS of 54 weeks, compared to 17 weeks in patients who had extracranial disease ($p<0.0001$).

Two prospective studies have combined WBRT with either temozolomide or fotemustine in melanoma patients with brain metastases [88, 89]. With temozolomide in a phase 2 study of 31 patients, only 3 (10%) demonstrated a response in the CNS, with median PFS in the CNS and OS of 2 and 6 months, respectively. In the phase 3 study of the combination with fotemustine, objective response rate (ORR) was 10% with median time-to-CNS-progression of 56 days and median OS of 105 days. These studies provide estimates of the clinical effect of WBRT, even though the relative contributions of WBRT and chemotherapy drug cannot be quantitated.

The use of WBRT in a patient with advanced CNS melanoma probably yields a modest survival benefit over supportive care alone. Symptom palliation is also probably a benefit of this therapy. There are many holes in the WBRT data set, many of which will never be answered definitively as melanoma treatment evolves. WBRT as a monotherapy has several signifcicant disadvantages, including its modest benefit at best, inability to undertake retreatment, and lack of effect on extracranial disease. These limitations will likely be overcome only with the design of systemic therapy regimens, to be administered concurrently with, or in lieu of, WBRT.

2.5. Systemic therapy

Until the recent approvals in 2011 of ipilimumab [90, 91] and vemurafenib [92], no therapy tested in a randomized trial demonstrated an improvement in overall survival for metastatic melanoma patients. Dacarbazine had been the standard first-line systemic treatment since it was approved in the United States in 1975. Metastatic melanoma patients with intracranial or meningeal metastases were generally excluded from clinical trial participation for three reasons: 1) brain metastases were thought to portend a poor prognosis; 2) systemic therapies that were tested were not very effective in intracranial disease; and 3) it was presumed that most agents would not cross the blood-brain barrier. In this section, we will cover efforts to use chemotherapy, molecularly-targeted therapy, and immunotherapy for the management of melanoma brain metastases (Table 6) [88, 89, 93-99].

2.5.1. Chemotherapy

Several chemotherapeutic regimens failed to demonstrate benefit in melanoma brain metastasis, including regimens containing platinum-based compounds, dacarbazine, etoposide, and others [87, 100-109]. This may be largely due to the low efficacy of many of the tested agents in melanoma generally. It is probably unreasonable to expect agents with limited activity against extracranial disease to have activity in the CNS, with the added barrier of CNS penetration. Three chemotherapy agents with defined CNS activity in non-melanoma neoplastic settings, namely temozolomide, thalidomide, and fotemustine have been investigated in some detail in melanoma [110, 111].

Temozolomide is metabolized to the same active metabolite as dacarbazine. It is orally bioavailable and penetrates the blood-brain barrier at clinically significant concentrations [111]. The drug is approved for the treatment of primary brain tumors, confirming its clinically significant penetration of the CNS. Since temozolomide is as effective as dacarbazine in treatment of metastatic melanoma and yields similar patient survival [112], several clinical trials evaluated its efficacy in melanoma patients with brain metastases.

A multicenter, open label, single-arm phase 2 study aimed to determine the efficacy and safety (both as primary endpoints) of temozolomide in metastatic melanoma patients who had developed brain metastasis [93]. The study enrolled 151 patients, comprising of 117 chemotherapy-naïve and 34 previously treated. The clinical condition of the enrollees did not require immediate surgery or radiation therapy, justifying chemotherapy as the sole therapy.

For chemotherapy-naïve patients, eight patients (7%) achieved response, including one complete (CR) and seven partial responses (PR); 34 patients (29%) achieved stable disease (SD) in brain lesions for at least 4 weeks. Median OS was 3.5 months. In previously treated patients, 1 patient (3%) achieved PR, 6 (18%) had SD, and the median OS was 2.2 months. Notably, 25% of the chemotherapy-naïve and 21% of previously treated patients had extensive intracranial disease, defined as more than 4 radiologically evident brain lesions. The authors concluded that further evaluation was warranted, particularly in combination with other treatment modalities, but activity as a single agent in this setting was limited.

The combination of temozolomide and WBRT has been evaluated. A prospective phase 2 trial evaluated the combination in patients with CNS melanoma [88]. In 31 evaluable patients, temozolomide and WBRT combination yielded an overall ORR of 9.7%, comprising of one CR in the CNS lasting 4.5 months and two PR in the CNS lasting 2 months and 7 months. Although the combination of temozolomide and WBRT could be safely administered, its efficacy was limited.

Thalidomide, an anti-angiogenic agent crossing the blood-brain barrier, has been tested in combination with temozolomide to treat melanoma patients with brain metastases. In a phase 2 study, the combination of temozolomide and thalidomide was tested in chemotherapy-naïve patients [96]. The primary endpoint was ORR in the brain assessed every 8 weeks. Of the 26 patients treated, 16 patients were symptomatic and 25 had extracranial metastases. Treatment-associated toxicity, especially hemorrhage and thromboembolism was a problem: eleven patients discontinued treatment before completing one cycle of treatment due to intracranial hemorrhage (n=7), pulmonary embolism (n=2), deep vein thrombosis (n=1), and grade 3 rash (n=1). Of 15 evaluable patients, 3 (12% of the intent-to-treat population) achieved CR or PR, while 7 patients had minor response or SD in the brain. Of the 10 patients who derived benefit, however, 5 patients progressed at extracranial sites. Overall OS was 5 months in all 26 patients, while it was 6 months in the 15 evaluable patients. Given the limited efficacy and the toxicity associated with the temozolomide/thalidomide combination, its use in melanoma is not warranted, outside the setting of a clinical trial.

Temozolomide has also been evaluated in the adjuvant setting. A multicenter phase 3 study compared temozolomide to dacarbazine in the time to develop CNS metastasis [94]. The study randomized 150 patients to receive either oral temozolomide or intravenous dacarbazine in combination with cisplatin and interleukin-2. Compared to dacarbazine, temozolomide reduced the 1-year CNS failure from 31.1% to 20.6%, but was not statistically significant (p=0.22). The median OS was not different between the two arms. Even though temozolomide penetrates the CNS, it did not delay incidence of CNS failure. Thus it appears that temozolomide may not be very effective in the adjuvant setting.

Fotemustine is a chloroethyl-nitrosurea approved in Europe for the treatment of metastatic melanoma. Fotemustine demonstrates high CNS penetration; its efficacy in melanoma patients with intracranial disease has been evaluated in three major studies. A French multicenter phase 2 study evaluated 153 metastatic melanoma patients for response to single-agent fotemustine [97]. Previously treated patients were allowed in the study. Since fotemustine crosses the blood brain barrier, patients with intracranial metastases were enrolled.

Out of the 153 evaluable patients, 36 (23.5%) had cerebral metastasis as the dominant disease site. In patients with cerebral metastases, the drug yielded an ORR of 25% in the CNS, similar to the 24.2% ORR observed in extracranial disease. The median OS of all patients was 85 weeks, but survival of the brain metastases patients was not reported. This study suggests that fotemustine has activity in melanoma, including CNS metastases. The magnitude of the benefit is similar in the CNS and at extracranial sites.

To confirm the observed activity, a phase 3 trial randomized 229 patients with metastatic melanoma to receive either fotemustine or dacarbazine [113]. Dacarbazine is a useful and interesting comparator in this study, as prior studies had failed to demonstrate any significant activity in the CNS [100, 102, 104]. This study enrolled patients with and without pre-existing brain metastases. Forty-three patients with brain metastases enrolled, of whom 22 received fotemustine, while 21 patients received dacarbazine.

Among all patients, fotemustine yielded an ORR of 15% versus dacarbazine's 7% (p=0.043). The authors reported a trend to improved survival among fotemustine-treated patients, with median OS of 7.3 months versus 5.6 months in the dacarbazine arm (p=0.067). In the brain metastases sub-group, fotemustine yielded a 6% ORR, while dacarbazine produced no responses. While myelosuppression was the most common adverse event observed in both arms, fotemustine-induced myelosuppression was more frequent and severe. In the fotemustine arm, 71% (vs. 14% with dacarbazine) of patients experienced neutropenia, and 51% (vs. 5% with dacarbazine) of patients experienced grade 3- 4 neutropenia. Similarly, thrombocytopenia was observed in 94% of patients receiving fotemustine (vs. 57% with dacarbazine) and grade 3- 4 occurred in 43% of patients (vs. 6% with dacarbazine).

The responses of patients who had brain metastases in this study were not as impressive as previously reported in the phase 2 study discussed above, although this might be expected in a more rigorous phase 3 study setting. Although not quite statistically significant, fotemustine delayed the median time-to-develop first brain metastasis among those without pre-existing brain lesions to 22.7 months, versus 7.2 months for patients treated with dacarbazine (p=0.059), suggesting that fotemustine might have activity as an adjuvant treatment after surgical management of CNS metastases. This has not been tested, as of 2012.

A multicenter phase 3 trial randomized 76 patients to receive fotemustine alone or in combination with WBRT in brain metastasis patients and sought to determine the cerebral response and time-to-cerebral-progression [89]. The primary endpoints of this study was to compare the CNS ORR (CR+PR), CNS control rate (CR+PR+SD), and the time to CNS progression. Compared to fotemustine alone, the combination did not significantly improve the ORR or the control rate. The addition of WBRT, however, delayed CNS progression; it was 49 days (range 11–539 days) in the fotemustine-only arm and 56 days (range 19–348 days) in patients treated with fotemustine and WBRT (Wilcoxon test, p=0.028). The combination did not, however, significantly improve the clinical CNS control rate (after 7 weeks) or OS. In regards to safety, myelosuppression was similar in both arms, but alopecia was much higher in the combination arm (40% compared to 2.6% in the fotemustine-only arm).

2.5.2. *Targeted agents*

Approximately 40 to 50% of all melanomas harbor a mutation in *BRAF* [114]. Notably, 95% of *BRAF* mutations are at the valine in the amino acid position 600, and over 90% of these are substitutions to aspartic acid (depicted as V600E). *In vitro*, the V600E mutation causes a 500-fold increase in the activity of B-Raf kinase; its expression is sufficient to cause tumor formation by normal melanocytes injected into nude mice [114].

Vemurafenib, a small molecule inhibitor of the V600E-mutant, was approved in the United States in 2011 for the treatment of metastatic melanoma in patients harboring the V600E mutation [92]. Clinical trials leading up to its approval excluded patients who had active intracranial disease. Thus, the efficacy of vemurafenib is not well studied in patients with pre-existing intracranial disease.

A single-arm, open-label, pilot study was conducted in metastatic melanoma patients with the V600E mutation and unresectable brain metastases, who failed previous treatments of temozolomide and/or WBRT. Four patients, with extensive disease (3 to 10+ brain metastases), were enrolled. At the time of the abstract presentation, the staging reports for two of the four patients were available. The first patient had a confirmed PR in both intracranial and extracranial lesions, while the second patient had minor responses in intracranial and extracranial metastases. Although very limited data, vemurafenib exhibits preliminary evidence of activity in melanoma patients with brain metastases who failed prior therapy [115]. Additional studies are in progress to demonstrate efficacy of vemurafenib in melanoma patients with intracranial disease. For example, NCT01378975 is an open-label single-arm phase 2 study enrolling metastatic melanoma patients with BRAF V600 and measurable brain metastases (symptomatic or asymptomatic). Patients are enrolled regardless of prior systemic treatment history for brain metastases (except for previous treatment with BRAF or MEK inhibitors). The high response rate of patients harboring V600E mutations in melanoma (~50% vs. ~5% for dacarbazine) suggests that vemurafenib, and potentially other BRAF-targeted therapies, might be useful in post-surgical/SRS adjuvant therapy as an alternative to WBRT. This hypothesis should be tested, especially if CNS activity is confirmed.

Dabrafenib is another potent and selective BRAF V600E inhibitor that inhibits growth of B-Raf mutant melanoma and mutant B-Raf colorectal xenografts in mice [116]. In a phase 1 study, 184 patients with metatastic melanoma, untreated brain metastases, or other solid tumors received dabrafenib [117]. Only three patients with wildtype B-Raf were evaluated, with no evidence of benefit; such patients were subsequently excluded. The study included 156 metastatic melanoma patients, of whom 10 had pre-existing brain metastases. For patients with intracranial disease due to melanoma, 9 out of the 10 patients had reductions in the size of their brain lesions as well as their extracranial disease, with 4 of them achieving complete resolution of the CNS lesions.

A phase 2 study specifically assessing the response to dabrafenib in melanoma patients with intracranial disease harboring a V600E or V600K mutation was recently published [98]. The study enrolled 172 patients, of whom 89 patients had not received previous local treatment for brain metastases (cohort A) and 83 patients who progressed following previous local treatment (cohort B). In cohort A, the overall intracranial response rate (OIRR), which is the primary endpoint of this study, was 39.2% (29/74) in patients with the V600E mutation and 6.7% (1/15) in patients with the V600K mutation. In cohort B, the OIRR was 30.8% (20/65) in patients with the V600E mutation and 22.2% (4/18) in patients harboring the V600K mutation. These data suggest clinical activity in melanoma brain metastases patients harboring the V600E mutation and some activity in V600K patients, whether or not they received prior therapy for their brain metastases.

Given the limited activity of agents available up to this time, such as temozolomide, findings of CNS activity may not require formal confirmation in a phase 3 randomized trial. It is difficult to imagine what the comparator agent of such a trial would be. However, a study of the combination of either WBRT or SRS with concurrent B-Raf inhibitors (vemurafenib or dabrafenib) or with B-Raf inhibitors following radiotherapy would be important in the development of optimal therapy for patients with CNS metastases of melanoma.

2.5.3. Immunotherapy of melanoma in the central nervous system

Following the success, and subsequent FDA approval, of ipilimumab in the management of metastatic melanoma [90, 91], several anecdotal case reports highlighted the activity of ipilimumab in melanoma patients with brain metastases [118, 119]. For example, a retrospective analysis assessing the activity of ipilimumab in melanoma patients with brain metastasis who were enrolled in a phase 2 trial [120] identified 12 patients, of whom 2 achieved PR and

3 had SD in brain metastases. The median OS of all 12 patients was 14 months (range was 2.7 to 56.4 months).

Another retrospective study evaluated the outcome of 77 patients who underwent radiosurgery between 2002 and 2010 for melanoma brain metastases, of whom 27 (35%) received ipilimumab [121]. Ipilimumab–treated patients displayed a median OS of 21.3 months, versus 4.9 months for those not treated with ipilimumab. Even when adjusted for performance status, ipilimumab treatment was associated with a higher survival probability (HR 0.48, p=0.03). The median survival of ipilimumab-treated patients with poor prognosis (11/27 patients), who had Diagnosis-Specific Graded Prognostic Assessment (DS-GPA; discussed in more detail below) score of 0-2 was 15.7 months, while those with better prognosis (16/27 patients), DS-GPA score of 3-4 had a median survival of 25.2 months. The survival of patients who received ipilimumab was similar whether they received ipilimumab before or after developing brain metastases.

To determine the efficacy of ipilimumab prospectively, Margolin and colleagues designed a phase 2 study to assess the activity of ipilimumab in melanoma patients with brain metastasis [99]. The study segregated patients into two cohorts; cohort A included 51 patients who were neurologically asymptomatic, while cohort B included 21 patients with symptoms requiring corticosteroids, which continued during the course of the study, if necessary. The overall ORR in cohort A was 18% (9/51) and 5% (1/21) in cohort B. When assessing response in brain lesions alone, the ORR in cohort A was 24% (12/51) and 10% (2/21) in cohort B. The ORR of extracranial disease was similar in each group to the intracranial response: ORR was 27% (14/51) and 5% (1/21) in cohorts A and B, respectively. The median OS was 7 months for cohort A and 3.7 months in cohort B. Since the study did not specifically address the cause of deaths for patients enrolled in the study, it is not clear whether the variation in OS between the two cohorts was due to progression of intracranial or extracranial disease, or additional complications associated with symptomatic intracranial disease.

A number of observations can be made from the results of this study: a) the response of brain lesions was similar to responses in extracranial metastases; and b) patients with asymptomatic intracranial disease, not on corticosteroid treatment, tended to respond better. The authors of the study present two hypotheses that may explain the difference in response between the two cohorts: i) as suggested by survival data, patients with symptomatic intracranial disease requiring corticosteroids have inherently poorer prognosis; or ii) corticosteroids may potentially interfere with the effector lymphocyte activation induced by ipilimumab. The authors did contend that corticosteroid use with ipilimumab did not entirely abrogate its efficacy.

A single-arm phase 2 study conducted in seven Italian centers assessed the combination of ipilimumab and fotemustine in patients with metastatic melanoma, including patients with asymptomatic brain metastases [95]. The open-label, single-arm phase 2 study enrolled 86 metastatic melanoma patients, of whom 20 had brain metastases at baseline. The overall study population disease control rate (defined as immune-related CR, PR, or SD) was 46.5% (40/86 patients). Similarly, ten of the brain metastasis patients (50%) achieved disease control. This study provides preliminary evidence that the combination of ipilimumab and fotemustine is active in patients with metastatic melanoma, including those with intracranial disease. To confirm the activity of the combination, a randomized phase 3 trial is planned and will compare the activity of the combination versus fotemustine alone in patients with advanced melanoma and brain metastases (NIBIT-M2; CA184-192).

Study	Treatment	Evaluable Patients	Primary Endpoint	Response	Median Survival	Comments
Agarwala *et al.*, 2004 [93]	TMZ	151 total 117 treatment naive 35 pts prior CTx	ORR in brain and toxicity	No prior CTx: ORR 7% SD 29% Prior CTx: PR 3% SD 18%	Treatment Naïve: 3.5m Prior CTx: 2.2m	
Margolin *et al.*, 2002 [88]	TMZ and WBRT	31 pts	ORR	CNS ORR 10% (1 CR and 2 PR)	PFS 2m OS 6m	
Hwu *et al.*, 2005 [96]	TMZ + Thalidomide	26 pts 16 symptomatic 25 extensive extracranial mets	ORR in CNS	15 evaluable pts 3 CR or PR (12% by intent-to-treat)	OS 5m OS 6m (for evaluable pts)	15 pts completed ≥ 1 cycle. 11 discontinued before completing 1 cycle: 7 for intracranial hemorrhage, 2 for pulmonary embolism, 1 deep vein thrombosis, and 1 for Grade 3 rash
Chiarion-Sileni *et al.*, 2011 [94]	CTI (TMZ + Cisplatin + IL2) vs. CDI (DTIC + Cisplatin + IL2 Phase 3	150 pts 118 evaluable (57 in CTI and 61 in CDI)	Time to CNS mets	CNS failure: CTI - 24/57 pts CDI 34/61 pts $P = 0.22$ 1y CNS failure rate CTI – 21% CDI – 31%	PFS CTI – 4.1m CDI – 3.9m $P=0.90$ OS CTI – 8.4m CDI – 8.7m 1y OS CTI – 31% CDI – 42%	
Jacquillat *et al.*, 1990 [97]	Fotemustine	153 evaluable pts; 36 (23.5%) had CNS disease	ORR	ORR 25% CNS	NR for CNS pts.	The overall ORR in all pts was 24%
Mornex *et al.*, 2003 [89]	Arm A: Fotemustine vs. Arm B: Fotemustine + WBRT Phase 3	76 pts Arm A: 39 pts Arm B: 37 pts	CNS ORR on day 50 CNS Control Rate (CR+PR +SD) on day 50	ORR 7.4% (arm A) 10.0% (arm B) $P = 0.73$ Control Rate 30% (arm A) 47% (arm B)	OS 86 days (arm A) 105 days (arm B). $P = 0.561$	

Study	Treatment	Evaluable Patients	Primary Endpoint	Response	Median Survival	Comments
			Time to objective CNS progression	$P = 0.19$ Time to CNS progression 49 days (arm A) 56 days (arm B) $P = 0.028$		
Long *et al.*, 2012 [98]	Dabrafenib	172 pts Cohort A: no prior CNS therapy, 89 pts Cohort B: Prior CNS therapy, 83 pts	OIRR	Cohort A V600E 39% V600K 6.7% Cohort B V600E 31% V600K 22%	At 6 months, Cohort A: 27% Cohort B: 41%	Study limited to V600E and V600K BRAF mutated melanoma
Margolin *et al.*, 2012 [99]	Ipilimumab	72 pts 51 Cohort A (no CNS symptoms) 21 Cohort B (CNS symptoms requiring corticosteroids) Phase 2	DCR (CR, PR, SD) at 12 wks	DCR Cohort A 18% Cohort B 5% DCR in CNS Cohort A – 24% Cohort B – 10%	OS Cohort A 7m Cohort B 3.7m	
Di Giacoma *et al.*, 2012 [95]	Fotemustine + Ipilimumab	86 pts total 20 CNS disease at baseline	Immune-related DCR (CR, PR, SD) at 24 weeks	DCR Overall 46.5% CNS 50%	CNS PFS 4.5m CNS OS 13.4m At 1-yr, 54% of CNS pts alive	Out of the 10 brain responses 5 PR or SD 5 CR

CNS: Central Nervous System; CR: Complete response; CTx: Chemotherapy; DC: Disease control; DCR: Disease control rate; DTIC: Dacarbazine; NR: Not reported; OIRR: Overall intracranial response rate; ORR: Objective response rate; OS: Overall survival; PFS: Progression-free survival; PR: Partial response; SD: Stable disease; TMZ: Temozolomide; WBRT: Whole-brain radiation therapy

Table 6. Prospective trials of systemic therapy treatments for melanoma brain metastases

3. Risk stratification

Several systems estimate risk of recurrence and death in patients with brain metastases, including some with melanoma-specific data (Table 7). Recursive Partitioning Analysis (RPA) is one such system [122-124]. This combines age, performance status, and extracranial disease status to assign a class from I to III that estimates survival. Its original intention was to stratify patients for enrollment in clinical trials. Its clinically available factors are useful to consider in a discussion of brain metastasis patients.

RPA's initial description included 1200 patients, 200 of whom were affected by melanoma. Histology and tissue of origin were significant prognostic factors, with melanoma being unfavorable. The validity of RPA has since been confirmed in the melanoma subgroup [10, 19, 35, 42, 43].

While originally intended for stratification of patients in radiation therapy trials, RPA class also stratifies risk in patients undergoing surgical metastectomy [125, 126]. In 2004, the RTOG study enrolled 333 patients between 1996 and 2001, of whom 167 were assigned to WBRT and SRS and 164 received WBRT alone [15]. Median survival was longer in patients with a single brain metastasis for patients receiving WBRT+SRS combination compared to patients who only received WBRT (6.5 months *vs.* 4.9 months, p=0.0393). This study shed light on a limitation of RPA: it does not take into account the number of brain metastases present.

The Diagnosis-Specific Graded Prognostic Assessment (DS-GPA) was developed by retrospective analysis of 4,259 patients newly diagnosed with brain metastases [127]. In addition to the factors in RPA, it includes number of brain metastases and the underlying disease giving rise to brain metastases. In the melanoma subset, the analysis identified two significant prognostic factors: performance status (represented by KPS) and number of radiologically evident brain metastases. For KPS, a score of 90-100 is 2 points, 70-80 is 1 point, and less than 70 is 0 points. A single brain metastasis is 2 points, 2 to 3 metastasis is 1 point, and more than 3 metastases is 0 points. The DS-GPA score, calculated by adding the point values from a patient's KPS score and number of metastases, ranges from 0 (worst prognosis) to 4 (best prognosis). Median OS for melanoma patients ranges from 3.4 months (GS-GPA score of 0 to 1.0) to 13.2 months (GS-GPA score of 3.5 to 4.0).

Several other systems have been developed for use in specific sub-populations. The Basic Score for Brain Metastases (BS-BM) was developed by analyzing results from 110 SRS-treated patients [128]. The system generates a score based on KPS, control of primary tumor site, and extracranial disease status. Only 19 patients (17%) of the initial group of patients had melanoma. The system has not yet been studied in melanoma patients specifically and focuses on SRS treatment. Its applicability to other treatment modalities remains to be established.

The Score Index for Radiosurgery (SIR) was developed from the study of 65 SRS-treated patients with brain metastases from a variety of primary tumor types [129]. SIR derives a score from patient age, performance status, systemic disease status, maximum CNS lesion volume, and number of CNS lesions. In the population initially studied, SIR was more accurate in predicting survival than RPA. A retrospective study confirmed its utility in melanoma patients [38].

The Malignant Melanoma-Gamma Knife Radiosurgery score (MM-GKR) also assesses outcomes in metastatic melanoma patients treated with SRS [23]. Scoring is based on performance status, age, and CNS lesion location. The authors claim greater prognostic accuracy than with either RPA or SIR, particularly in identifying patients with an especially poor prognosis.

The Prognostic Index (PI) score estimates prognosis in patients treated with palliative WBRT [43]. Factors used in this system include number of extracranial metastatic sites, RPA class,

CNS disease progression prior to WBRT, and the presence of meningeal disease. This system is focused on those with extensive disease, not amenable to local therapy with SRS or surgery.

Median survival times predicted by studies of brain metastasis patients generally are similar to those reported for melanoma patients with CNS involvement. With minor differences, the systems described utilize similar and easily available data to arrive at their risk estimations. RPA has probably been examined in the widest array of clinical trial settings. It also does not seem to be specific to a given treatment modality. Its components are fairly simple to derive from clinical parameters. It will therefore be used for further discussion.

System	**Prognostic Factors**	**Prognostic Classification**	**Median OS (all tumor types)**	**Median OS (melanoma)**	**Comments**	**References**
RPA	KPS, age, extra-cranial disease status, control of primary disease site	Class I: KPS≥70, age<65 y., controlled primary disease site, no extra-cranial disease Class II: Not Class I or III Class III: KPS<70	Class I: 7.1 m Class II: 4.2 m Class III: 2.3 m	Class I: 6.5-10.5 m Class II: 3.5-5.9 m Class III: 1.8-2.5 m	Validated for radiation therapy and surgery.	Gaspar *et al.*, 1997 [122] Gaspar *et al.*, 2000 [123] Buchsbaum *et al.*, 2002 [10] Lutterbach *et al.*, 2002 [124] Harrison *et al.*, 2003 [42] Morris *et al.*, 2004 [43] Radbill *et al.*, 2004 [35] Brown *et al.*, 2002 [19]
PI	Number of ECM, RPA class (see above), PD on imaging prior to WBRT, presence of LM	Index= Number of ECM sites + (2 x RPA class) + (2 if PD on pre-WBRT imaging) + (4 if LM present)	NR	Score: 2-4: 138 d 5-6: 80 d 7-8: 42 d 9-10: 18 d 11+: 15 d	To determine outcome following palliative WBRT.	Morris et al., 2004 [43]
SIR	Age, KPS, extra-cranial disease status, volume of largest CNS lesion, number of CNS lesions	Factor / 0 / 1 / 2: Age: ≥60 / 51-59 / ≤50 KPS: ≤50 / 60-70 / ≥70 Systemic disease status: PD / PR/SD / CR or NED Largest Lesion Volume (cm[3]): "/>13 / 5-13 / <5	Score: 0-3: 2.9 m 4-7: 7 m 8-10: 31 m	Score: ≤6: 4 m "/>6: 7 m	Point values for individual factors are added to derive score. Intended for assessment of outcome after SRS.	Weltman *et al.*, 2000 [129] Selek *et al.*, 2004 [38]

System	Prognostic Factors	Prognostic Classification					Median OS (all tumor types)		Median OS (melanoma)		Comments	References
		# of CNS lesions	≥3	2	2							
MM-GKR	Age, KPS, Adverse CNS lesion locations (brainstem, posterior fossa, nuclei, cerebellum)	Factor	0	1	1.5	2	NR		Score		Intended for assessment of outcome after SRS.	Gaudy-Marqueste *et al.*, 2006 [23]
		KPS	<80	-	-	≤80			0	7.1 m		
		Age	≤60	"/>60	-	-			1-2	5 m		
		Adverse Location	No	-	Yes	-			≥2.5	2.2 m		
BS-BM	KPS, control of primary tumor, presence of ECM	Factor	0		1		Score		NR		Not validated in melanoma, although study included 19 melanoma patients out of 110 total (17%). Score of 3 had OS not reaching median with 30 m of follow-up. Intended for assessment of outcome after SRS.	Lorenzoni *et al.*, 2004 [128]
		KPS	50-70		"/>70		0	1.9 m				
		Primary tumor control	No		Yes		1	3.3 m				
							2	13.1 m				
							3	ND				
		ECM	Yes		No							
DS-GPA	RPA factors (KPS, age, extra-cranial disease status, control of primary disease site) and number of brain mets	Factor	0	1	2		0.0-1.0	3.4m	0.0-1.0	3.4m	In melanoma, only 2 significant prognostic factors: KPS (p<0.0001) and number of brain mets (p<0.0001)	Sperduto *et al.*, 2010 [127]
		KPS	<70	70-80	90-100		1.5-2.5	6.4m	1.5-2.5	4.7m		
		# of brain mets	>3	2-3	1		3.0	11.6m	3.0	8.8m		
							3.5-4.0	14.8m	3.5-4.0	13.2m		

CNS: Central Nervous System; CR: Complete response; DS-GPA: Diagnosis-Specific Graded Prognostic Assessment; ECM: Extracranial metastases; KPS: Karnofsky performance status; LM: Leptomeningeal metastasis; MM-GKR: Malignant Melanoma-Gamma Knife Radiosurgery score; ND: Not defined; NED: No evidence of disease; NR: Not reported; OS: Overall survival; PD: Progressive disease; PI: Prognostic Index; PR: Partial Response; QOL: Quality of life; RPA: Recursive Partitioning Analysis; SD: Stable disease; SIR: Score Index for Radiosurgery

Table 7. Risk Stratification of Patients with Brain Metastases from Melanoma

An important caveat in discussing outcomes estimates derived using these risk stratification systems is that they all were first developed prior to 2011. Prior to that time, reliably effective and proven treatments for advanced melanoma were not available for general clinical use. Development of drugs with proven activity, such as ipilimumab and vemurafenib discussed above, are changing the outlook for melanoma patients. This includes patients with brain metastases. With these drugs, and more being developed with potentially even greater activity, the risk estimates of these systems will certainly change for the better. This is especially likely to be the case in patients with very high risk/poor prognosis disease. Treatment recommendations for the brain metastasis problem in melanoma will therefore likely be very fluid over the next several years, as new treatment paradigms for melanoma evolve.

4. Therapy of CNS disease

4.1. Unfavorable/poor risk

By definition, RPA class III patients have a KPS less than 70%. Often, they have multi-focal brain metastases, active extracranial disease, or both. Historically, their life expectancy was very limited. The PI prognostic system, intended to assess prognosis in this group as described above, uses days rather than months as the unit of time for its estimates [43].

Conventionally, surgery or SRS would only be used judiciously with palliative intent and well-defined goals. WBRT may be undertaken for symptom palliation and a very modest survival benefit [8, 12, 86, 130-132]. The anticipated duration of survival played an important part in designing any treatment approach, as even therapy of several weeks duration could consume a significant proportion of a patient's remaining lifespan. The burden of coming to repeated treatments (as might be the case with palliative WBRT, frequently administered as 10 treatments over 2 weeks) may lead to a significant QOL decrement in patients with poor performance status. By definition, RPA class III patients have such a poor performance status.

Prior to the approval in the United States of ipilimumab and vemurafenib in 2011, systemic therapy played a minimal role in this group. Exceptions included steroid therapy for tumor-associated edema and anti-convulsants for seizures. The low performance status and CNS disease in these patients excluded them from virtually all clinical trials. Activity of systemic agents with CNS penetration, such as temozolmide and fotemustine, was limited, with an onset of action too slow to benefit most patients with melanoma who were in this category.

As of 2011, BRAF mutational status serves as an important factor in making treatment decisions. This may be especially important in patients with RPA class III melanoma with CNS involvement. The BRAF inhibitors vemurafenib and dabrafenib, discussed above, have rapid onset of action, high response rates, preliminary evidence of CNS activity, oral administration and manageable toxicity profiles. As of November 2012, vemurafenib is approved in the United States and Europe, and debrafanib's approval is pending. For patients possessing an appropriate BRAF mutation, treatment with one of these agents would be reasonable to consider, even with RPA class III. Of course, the patient must be aware that information about this drug in the brain metastasis population is presently very limited. Data regarding combinations with radiotherapy is also very limited at this time. While a clinical trial would be the preferred setting to treat these patients, use of BRAF inhibition therapy would be reasonable to offer to BRAF-mutant melanoma patients with brain metastases and RPA class III.

For patients in whom a targetable BRAF mutation is not present, fewer options are available. Ipilimumab, discussed above, has a relatively slow onset of action, taking 3-4 months in phase 3 trials to confer a survival benefit versus controls [90, 91], with an overall low response rate.

For someone with a poor performance status unlikely to live that long, ipilimumab is unlikely to provide benefit, despite preliminary evidence of CNS activity. For these patients, further developments in melanoma therapy are awaited. Pallitative WBRT likely remains the standard therapy for these patients.

One peculiar circumstance remains: some patients present with RPA class III advanced disease, including brain metastases and poor performance status, but their BRAF mutational status is unknown. Given their overall condition and location of disease, obtaining a tumor specimen to determine BRAF mutation status may not be possible. A wait of 1-2 weeks for results of mutational testing may consume a significant portion of their remaining lifespan. In such patients, standard care would be supportive, potentially with the addition of WBRT. Given a frequency of BRAF mutations targeted by presently available drugs of about 50% and the lack of other proven options, a therapeutic trial of BRAF inhibition is unlikely to cause significant harm, and might lead to dramatic benefit if the patient possesses an appropriate mutation. Again, before embarking on such a treatment course, the patient must be aware of the limitations of our current dataset.

4.2. Favorable/good risk

Patients of RPA class I have a relatively good prognosis and warrant an aggressive treatment approach. Such patients are young, have a good performance status, and no active extracranial disease. However, among patients with metastatic melanoma, true RPA class I patients are infrequently encountered, especially those completely lacking detectable extracranial disease.

The major treatment decision for these patients relates to local therapy of existing brain lesions (Figure 1). The goal would be to treat all evident CNS disease by some form of definitive therapy (surgery or SRS). Traditionally, surgery was favored in cases involving one surgically accessible lesion, and benefit was reported in surgeries targeting up to 3 lesions [14, 133]. Surgery is also especially useful in specific situations where SRS is less favorable, such as large lesion size (> 3cm) or symptomatology (for example, bleeding). Surgery also yields a specimen to confirm the diagnosis and analyze for targetable alterations in the tumor, such as BRAF mutations status. In patients lacking any other evident disease, these data can be very important and only obtainable from a surgically resected CNS specimen. Otherwise, SRS is emerging as the preferred local therapy, both for its simpler administration and possibly for better local control [44]. SRS may also be able to provide definitive treatment at sites inaccessible to surgery. Surgery and SRS are not mutually exclusive: both may be necessary to provide definitive treatment of all lesions in multi-focal metastatic CNS disease.

SRS has been a remarkable addition to our armamentarium for treatment of brain metastases. Previously, surgery was the only approach to definitive treatment. If more than 3 lesions were present, or they were located in surgically inaccessible locations, surgery could not be used with the intention of long-term control. SRS allows treatment of multiple lesions, in sites inaccessible to surgery. It also offers the possibility of re-treatment. At some point, presumably, the number of lesions exceeds the ability of SRS to control the disease. The exact number is not defined, but some have advocated SRS to control up to five CNS lesions [37]. Beyond this, it may be unreasonable to expect a local treatment modality like SRS to control what is clinically widespread involvement in an organ system, even if limited to the CNS. Surgery and SRS may be able to control specific lesions that are symptomatic in such patients, but the overall treatment approach relies primarily on therapeutic WBRT and systemic therapy, discussed below under "Intermediate Risk."

In patients with RPA class I disease from melanoma, risk of failure in the CNS is high if treatment focuses solely on radiologically evident disease. This likely reflects the underlying biology, in which specific neurotropic sub-clones of melanoma develop that colonize the CNS, leading to brain metastases. Limiting treatment to surgery and/or SRS of only radiologically evident lesions ignores this biological reality. This observation is confirmed in the multiple randomized trials of adjuvant WBRT enrolling patients with multiple tumor types, including melanoma. Adjuvant WBRT decreases intracranial recurrence rates when combined with definitive local therapy. This effect is evident at both definitively treated macroscopic sites (treating residual contamination) and at distant sites within the CNS. At distant sites, adjuvant WBRT must accomplish this by either treating pre-existing radiologically undetectable micrometastatic disease or making the CNS less receptive to colonization from extracranial sites. The former is the more plausible biological explanation.

Approaches to address the problem of distant CNS recurrence have been discussed in detail earlier. Basically, these come down to either administering adjuvant WBRT up-front, or using an expectant management strategy, with regular imaging and re-treatment (primarily with SRS), at the time of CNS progression. Arguments against adjuvant WBRT include concern regarding its cognitive toxicity, its lack of clear survival benefit and inability to undertake re-treatment. As described earlier, cognitive effects of adjuvant WBRT, while not absent, are not unreasonable in the setting of CNS metastases, especially when balanced against the cognitive effects of tumor progression and those of re-treatment (as, for example, by SRS). Adjuvant WBRT is unlikely to be associated, in general, with an overall survival benefit overall due to extracranial disease as a competing cause of death. In the setting of RPA class I patients, who lack active extracranial disease, adjuvant WBRT may very well have a survival benefit [54, 134].

As noted above, the use of a salvage strategy, relying on SRS in the event of tumor progression, is associated with high rates of intracranial failure. The cognitive effects of such a strategy have not been assessed in detail, but the data regarding cognitive effects of allowing tumor progression have been reviewed and are clearly unfavorable. Whether the effects are better or worse than those due to adjuvant use of WBRT can only be answered by a randomized comparison of the two strategies.

We concede that the decision regarding use of adjuvant WBRT is not simple and clear-cut. To determine whether to recommend its use, the benefit of decreased intracranial progression rates must be balanced against its adverse effects. Overall, we believe that the published evidence generally supports the use of adjuvant WBRT in melanoma patients.

Systemic adjuvant therapy might be an alternative to adjuvant WBRT. Traditional cytotoxic therapy agents with known CNS activity, such as fotemustine or temozolomide, have not been shown clearly to impact the subsequent development of CNS disease in melanoma patients [113, 135]. In the setting of melanoma patients with CNS disease, their primary purpose was to treat extracranial disease, an important prognostic factor once CNS disease was controlled. By definition, true RPA class I patients have no active extracranial disease.

Newly developed agents, such as vemurafenib and ipilimumab, may have a role defined in the future for adjuvant therapy in patients with RPA class I CNS disease from melanoma. They may be able to affect both CNS recurrence rates and progression of extracranial disease. However, data supporting such use is not available at present. Their use as adjuvant therapies in this population is not warranted, outside the setting of a clinical trial.

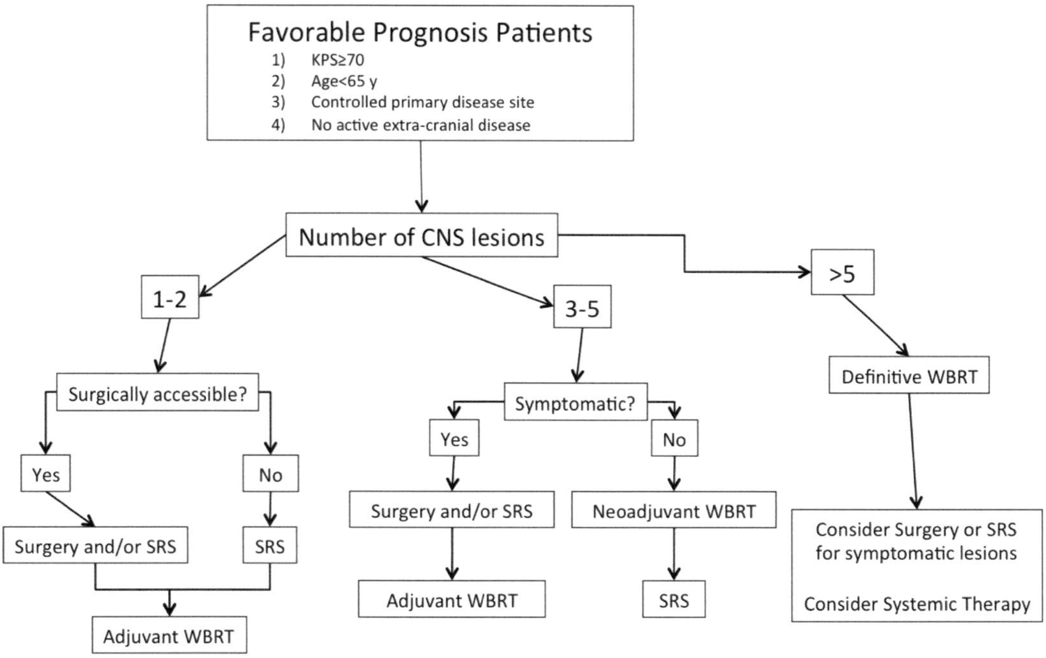

Figure 1. Treatment of melanoma patients with brain metastases with favorable risk profile, equivalent to RPA class I. In patients with more than one brain lesion who are to receive local therapy, it may be necessary to use both surgery and radiosurgery to treat all lesions. By definition, RPA class I patients have no active extracranial disease. Thus, systemic therapy is not indicated except in an experimental trial. CNS: central nervous system; KPS: Karnofsky performance status; RPA: Recursive Partitioning Analysis; SRS: stereotactic radiosurgery; WBRT: whole brain radiotherapy.

4.3. Intermediate risk

Treatment decisions in intermediate risk patients (equivalent to RPA class II) are probably most difficult of all (Figure 2). This relates to their variable clinical presentation. They have better performance status than those with unfavorable RPA class III. They are also of advanced age (according to RPA, anyone older than 65 years), have active extracranial disease, or both, conveying a negative prognosis relative to RPA class I. A logical way to divide this population is into those with CNS disease amenable to local definitive therapy and those with CNS disease too extensive for complete, definitive local therapy of all lesions.

Considerations regarding the use of adjuvant WBRT and the desirability for treatment in the context of a clinical trial are essentially the same as for favorable prognosis patients. The key differentiating question is whether local therapy of CNS lesions with surgery or SRS should be attempted at all. Several clinical situations argue against their use. Lesions may be inaccessible for surgery or too large for SRS or they may simply be too numerous. If definitive treatment of all CNS disease sites is possible, then it should be attempted. If CNS disease is not amenable to local therapy of all lesions, then treatment must rely on therapeutic WBRT and systemic therapy, with surgery or SRS reserved for large or symptomatic lesions.

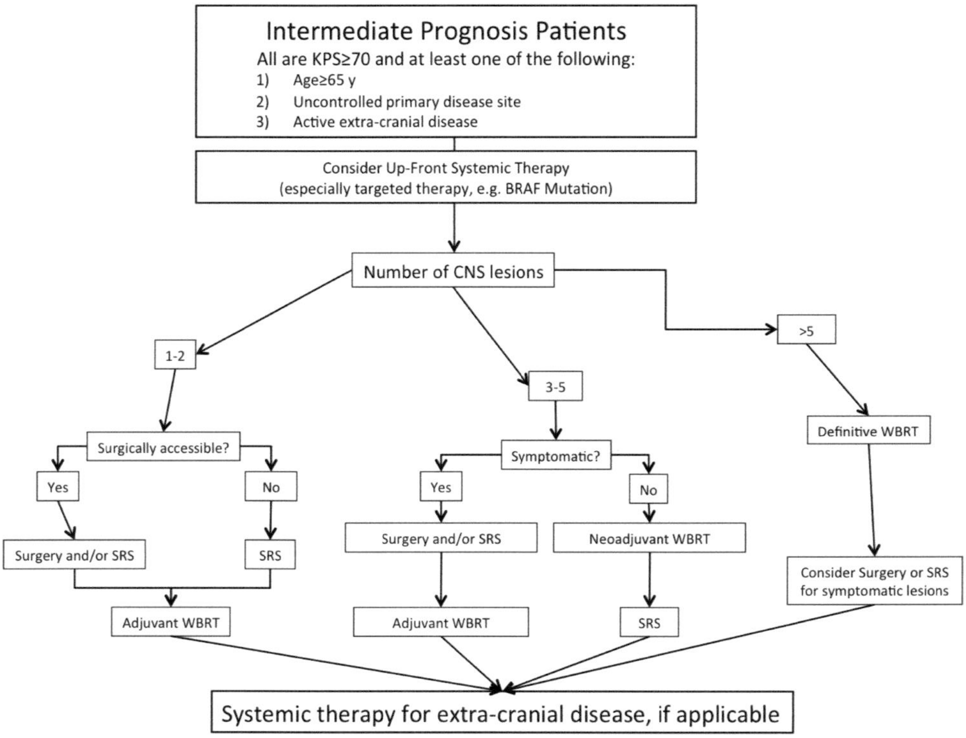

Figure 2. Treatment of melanoma patients with brain metastases with intermediate prognosis, equivalent to RPA class II. In patients with more than one brain lesion who are to receive local therapy, it may be necessary to use both surgery and radiosurgery to treat all lesions. Patients with active extracranial disease should be considered for systemic therapy. While in the past, few active systemic agents were available, newer therapies might have relevance early in the treatment of intermediate prognosis patients. For example, BRAF inhibition with vemurafenib has rapid onset of control, high response rates, and even preliminary evidence of CNS activity. Thus, early use of systemic therapy might be able to impact both CNS disease and extracranial disease. Extracranial disease activity is a consistent adverse prognostic factor in intermediate patients, once CNS disease is controlled. CNS: central nervous system; KPS: Karnofsky performance status; RPA: Recursive Partitioning Analysis; SRS: stereotactic radiosurgery; WBRT: whole brain radiotherapy.

In RPA class II patients with CNS melanoma, active extracranial disease status is a key prognostic factor. Disease outside the CNS represents a competing cause of death. Before the approval in 2011-2012 of agents with proven anti-melanoma activity (such as vemurafenib and ipilimumab), systemic therapy of the CNS was limited to temozolomide or fotemustine (in

Europe). Although these drugs treated extracranial disease as well, they were not highly active in either the CNS or extracranial compartments, and did not demonstrate clear or dramatic survival benefits.

Systemic therapy of melanoma in RPA class II patients is appearing brighter than it has in the past. Clinical trials are opening which permit these patients to enroll, and highly active agents, with CNS activity moreover, such as vemurafenib are available non-experimentally for patients with BRAF mutations. For patients lacking BRAF mutations, treatment with ipilimumab is a reasonable consideration, due to its survival benefit in a phase 3 trial, which included patients with pre-existing, treated brain metastases [90]. Most of these patients will live long enough to derive benefit from ipilimumab. As new agents are developed, their use in RPA class II melanoma patients is justified, even without demonstrable CNS activity, due to the active extracranial disease present in most of this population as a competing cause of death.

5. Directions for the future

Brain metastasis is part of the natural history of metastatic melanoma. It is a common problem and has a major adverse impact on treatment outcomes and QOL. The bulk of melanoma-specific research consists of retrospective analyses and single-center studies. Prospectively validated, comprehensive treatment paradigms do not yet exist. The preceding discussion suggests some important research questions for the future.

Optimal use of SRS technology remains undefined. One question relates to the treatment of multiple lesions. The only major randomized trial of SRS in brain metastasis therapy demonstrated a survival benefit in the presence of only a single brain metastasis [15]. No prospective data support a survival benefit from SRS when more than one lesion is present; retrospective data from several sources indicate that multiple CNS lesions are associated with worse survival [22, 26, 35].

At some point, the absolute number of CNS lesions poses a barrier to effective SRS therapy. Some argue that the presence of multiple lesions (up to about 5) should not preclude therapy, based on results indicating that the number of CNS melanoma lesions did not predict subsequent survival [39, 136]. Whether some threshold number of lesions exists is an unanswered question appropriate for investigation.

SRS itself is a generic term for a rapidly evolving technology. The relevance of even recently published results to current treatment technologies may be questioned. What is unlikely to change is the local nature of SRS therapy: SRS treats the radiated region, but not that which is unradiated. As discussed extensively, concurrent micrometastatic disease is not addressed by SRS, as it is also not by surgery. The use of adjuvant therapy after local treatment with surgery or SRS lacks melanoma-specific prospective data. Five randomized trials, described above, indicate that adjuvant WBRT can decrease intracranial recurrence rates, both at sites treated with surgery/SRS and at untreated sites. The adverse neurocognitive effects of WBRT and the efficacy of this modality in the metastatic melanoma population are valid questions. As noted above, such a study is in progress (NCT01503827) [55].

An alternative to the use of adjuvant WBRT is a planned radiosurgical salvage strategy. This presumably minimizes exposure of the CNS to WBRT and its adverse effects. Little data is available regarding this treatment approach. A randomized clinical trial would be most helpful, in which patients are randomized to receive immediate adjuvant WBRT after SRS therapy or undergo planned SRS salvage treatments, with WBRT only when SRS is not possible. This study would provide data to balance the neurocognitive consequences of immediate WBRT with those due to an increased rate of later macroscopic CNS progression. Further, some estimate of the neurocognitive cost of SRS re-treatment would be obtained.

SRS itself is used for adjuvant purposes after surgical metastectomy to treat residual disease at the resection site. The efficacy of this has not been defined. Additionally, such therapy does not treat occult disease at other sites within the CNS. A randomized trial comparing the efficacy of adjuvant SRS to either no adjuvant therapy or to adjuvant WBRT would be appropriate.

Finally, and perhaps most significantly, systemic therapy of melanoma is evolving rapidly, and those advances will have a major impact on treatment of CNS disease. Even now, convincing preliminary evidence of CNS activity of these several new agents has been presented. Previously, melanoma patients with CNS disease were excluded from clinical trials in the belief that the blood-brain barrier posed to great a hurdle to clinical efficacy. This no longer appears to be a valid assumption. As new agents emerge, their activity in the CNS should either be addressed in CNS-specific trials, or patients with CNS melanoma should be considered similar to any other melanoma patient, so long as their CNS disease is minimally or asymptomatic.

Much of this review has focused on the controversy of adjuvant therapy in the CNS. Adjuvant WBRT is not an optimal solution to this problem. It does not prevent CNS re-seeding from extracranial sites and cannot be used repeatedly. Adverse cognitive effects of WBRT are clearly demonstrable, even if their clinical impact is arguable. Critically, adjuvant WBRT also does not address the problem of extracranial disease, a major prognostic factor. Optimal adjuvant therapy to address these limitations is likely to be systemic. The development of highly active agents with CNS penetration opens the possibility of their use in melanoma patients after definitive treatment of brain metastases.

Several prior studies can provide necessary baseline data regarding rates of CNS progression for sample size calculations [113, 135]. Neurocognitive effects must be a secondary endpoint in any study, as it cannot be assumed that systemic agents are devoid of adverse neurocognitive effects. For example, case reports of melanoma patients treated with fotemustine reported toxic leukoencephalopathy with progressive dementia in several patients, [137, 138].

6. Conclusions

Brain metastasis is a frequent and serious problem for melanoma patients. New technologies, such as SRS and agents, such as vemurafenib and ipilimumab, are expanding our ability to treat this condition. Melanoma-specific studies guiding optimal employment of new technologies are limited. Most information regarding CNS treatment in melanoma is extrapolated from other conditions or is based on retrospective analyses from individual centers. Data from well-designed, prospective trials is lacking in many regards. This deficiency has been noted at least eight years previously by others [139]. At present, many of the same questions posed by those workers remain unanswered. Fortunately, melanoma treatment itself has not remained static, with new agents generating new questions regarding optimal treatment of the condition.

Well-designed, rigorous trials will allow our patients to receive the best and most cost-effective treatments available. Melanoma patients with brain metastases can look forward to a brighter future. We must, however, demand rigorous investigations to allow the best use possible of the arsenal being placed at our disposal to treat this challenging problem.

Abbreviations

BS-BM: Basic Score for Brain Metastases; CNS: Central Nervous System; CR: Complete Response; CT: Computed Tomography; DS-GPA: Diagnosis-Specific Graded Prognostic Assessment; Gy: Grey, unit of radiation dose; HVLT: Hopkin's Verbal Learning Test; KPS: Karnofsky Performance Status; MM-GKR: Malignant Melanoma-Gamma Knife Radiosurgery; MMSE: Mini-Mental Status Examination; MRI: Magnetic Resonance Imaging; NCF: Neurocognitive Function; NSCLC: Non Small Cell Lung Cancer; OIRR: Overall Intracranial Response Rate; ORR: Objective Response Rate; OS: Overall Survival; QOL: Quality-of-Life; PCI: Prophylactic Cranial Irradiation; PFS: Progression-Free Survival; PI: Prognostic Index; PR: Partial Response; RPA: Recursive Partitioning Analysis; RTOG: Radiation Therapy Oncology Group; SCLC: Small Cell Lung Cancer; SD: Stable Disease; SIR: Score Index for Radiosurgery; SRS: Stereotactic Radiosurgery; TCI: Therapeutic Cranial Irradiation; WBRT: Whole Brain Radiation Therapy

Author details

Sherif S. Morgan*[1], Joanne M. Jeter[1], Evan M. Hersh[1], Sun K. Yi[2] and Lee D. Cranmer*[1*]

*Address all correspondence to: lcranmer@azcc.arizona.edu

1 Section of Hematology and Oncology, Melanoma/Sarcoma Program, University of Arizona Cancer Center, University of Arizona, USA

2 Department of Radiation Oncology, College of Medicine, University of Arizona, USA

*Both of these authors contributed equally.

Conflict of Interest: The authors would like to disclose the following conflicts of interest:
Sherif Morgan: None to disclose.
Evan Hersh: GlaxoSmithKline, Bristol-Meyers Squibb, Pfizer, Genentech/Roche, Celgene.

Joanne Jeter: None to disclose.
Sun K Yi: None to disclose.
Lee Cranmer: Bristol-Meyers Squibb, Merck, Genentech/Roche, Celgene, Prometheus Laboratories.

References

[1] Siegel, R., D. Naishadham, and A. Jemal, *Cancer statistics, 2012.* CA Cancer J Clin, 2012. 62(1): p. 10-29.

[2] Little, E.G. and M.J. Eide, *Update on the current state of melanoma incidence.* Dermatol Clin, 2012. 30(3): p. 355-61.

[3] Fidler, I.J., et al., *The biology of melanoma brain metastasis.* Cancer and Metastasis Rev, 1999. 18(3): p. 387-400.

[4] Madajewicz, S., et al., *Malignant melanoma brain metastases. Review of Roswell Park Memorial Institute experience.* Cancer, 1984. 53(11): p. 2550-2.

[5] Noordijk, E.M., et al., *The choice of treatment of single brain metastasis should be based on extracranial tumor activity and age.* Int J Radiat Oncol Biol Phys, 1994. 29(4): p. 711-7.

[6] Mintz, A.H., et al., *A randomized trial to assess the efficacy of surgery in addition to radiotherapy in patients with a single cerebral metastasis.* Cancer, 1996. 78(7): p. 1470-6.

[7] Patchell, R.A., et al., *A randomized trial of surgery in the treatment of single metastases to the brain.* N Engl J Med, 1990. 322(8): p. 494-500.

[8] Sampson, J.H., et al., *Demographics, prognosis, and therapy in 702 patients with brain metastases from malignant melanoma.* J Neurosurg, 1998. 88(1): p. 11-20.

[9] Wronski, M. and E. Arbit, *Surgical treatment of brain metastases from melanoma: a retrospective study of 91 patients.* J Neurosurg, 2000. 93(1): p. 9-18.

[10] Buchsbaum, J.C., et al., *Survival by radiation therapy oncology group recursive partitioning analysis class and treatment modality in patients with brain metastases from malignant melanoma: a retrospective study.* Cancer, 2002. 94(8): p. 2265-72.

[11] Zacest, A.C., et al., *Surgical management of cerebral metastases from melanoma: outcome in 147 patients treated at a single institution over two decades.* J Neurosurg, 2002. 96(3): p. 552-8.

[12] Fife, K.M., et al., *Determinants of outcome in melanoma patients with cerebral metastases.* J Clin Oncol, 2004. 22(7): p. 1293-300.

[13] Raizer, J.J., et al., *Brain and leptomeningeal metastases from cutaneous melanoma: survival outcomes based on clinical features.* Neuro Oncol, 2008. 10(2): p. 199-207.

[14] Bindal, R.K., et al., *Surgical treatment of multiple brain metastases.* J Neurosurg, 1993. 79(2): p. 210-216.

[15] Andrews, D.W., et al., *Whole brain radiation therapy with or without stereotactic radiosurgery boost for patients with one to three brain metastases: Phase III results of the RTOG 9508 randomised trial.* Lancet, 2004. 363(9422): p. 1665-72.

[16] Kondziolka, D., et al., *Stereotactic radiosurgery plus whole brain radiotherapy versus radiotherapy alone for patients with multiple brain metastases.* Int J Radiat Oncol Biol Phys, 1999. 45(2): p. 427-34.

[17] Manon, R., et al., *Phase II trial of radiosurgery for one to three newly diagnosed brain metastases from renal cell carcinoma, melanoma, and sarcoma: an Eastern Cooperative Oncology Group study (E 6397).* J Clin Oncol, 2005. 23(34): p. 8870-6.

[18] Friehs, G.M., et al., *Outcomes in patients treated with gamma knife radiosurgery for brain metastases from malignant melanoma.* Neurosurg Focus, 1998. 4(6): p. e1.

[19] Brown, P.D., et al., *Stereotactic radiosurgery for patients with "radioresistant" brain metastases.* Neurosurgery, 2002. 51(3): p. 656-65; discussion 665-7.

[20] 20.Chang, E.L., et al., *Outcome variation among "radioresistant" brain metastases treated with stereotactic radiosurgery.* Neurosurgery, 2005. 56(5): p. 936-945.

[21] Chen, J.C.T., et al., *Stereotactic radiosurgery in the treatment of metastatic disease to the brain.* Stereotact Funct Neurosurg, 1999. 73(1-4): p. 60-3.

[22] Christopoulou, A., et al., *Integration of gamma knife surgery in the management of cerebral metastases from melanoma.* Melanoma Res, 2006. 16(1): p. 51-7.

[23] Gaudy-Marqueste, C., et al., *Gamma knife radiosurgery in the management of melanoma patients with brain metastases: a series of 106 patients without whole-brain radiotherapy.* Int J Radiat Oncol Biol Phys, 2006. 65(3): p. 809-16.

[24] Gieger, M., et al., *Response of intracranial melanoma metastases to stereotactic radiosurgery.* Radiat Oncol Investig, 1997. 5(2): p. 72-80.

[25] Gonzalez-Martinez, J., et al., *Gamma knife radiosurgery for intracranial metastatic melanoma: a 6-year experience.* J Neurosurg, 2002. 97(5 Suppl): p. 494-8.

[26] Grob, J.J., et al., *Radiosurgery without whole brain radiotherapy in melanoma brain metastases. Club de Cancerologie Cutanee.* Eur J Cancer, 1998. 34(8): p. 1187-92.

[27] Hara, W., et al., *Cyberknife for brain metastases of malignant melanoma and renal cell carcinoma.* Neurosurgery, 2009. 64(2)(SUPPLEMENT): p. A26-A32.

[28] Herfarth, K.K., et al., *Linac-based radiosurgery of cerebral melanoma metastases.* Strahlenther Onkol, 2003. 179(6): p. 366-371.

[29] Koc, M., et al., *Gamma knife radiosurgery for intracranial metastatic melanoma: an analysis of survival and prognostic factors.* J Neurooncol, 2005. 71(3): p. 307-313.

[30] Lavine, S.D., et al., *Gamma knife radiosurgery for metastatic melanoma: an analysis of survival, outcome, and complications.* Neurosurgery, 1999. 44(1): p. 59-64.

[31] Liew, D.N., et al., *Outcome predictors of Gamma Knife surgery for melanoma brain metastases. Clinical article.* J Neurosurg, 2011. 114(3): p. 769-79.

[32] Mingione, V., et al., *Gamma surgery for melanoma metastases in the brain.* J Neurosurg, 2002. 96(3): p. 544-51.

[33] Mori, Y., et al., *Stereotactic radiosurgery for cerebral metastatic melanoma: factors affecting local disease control and survival.* Int J Radiat Oncol Biol Phys, 1998. 42(3): p. 581-589.

[34] Powell, J.W., et al., *Gamma knife surgery in the management of radioresistant brain metastases in high-risk patients with melanoma, renal cell carcinoma, and sarcoma.* J Neurosurg (Special Supplements), 2008. 109(6): p. 122-128.

[35] Radbill, A.E., et al., *Initial treatment of melanoma brain metastases using gamma knife radiosurgery: an evaluation of efficacy and toxicity.* Cancer, 2004. 101(4): p. 825-33.

[36] Redmond, A.J., et al., *Gamma knife surgery for the treatment of melanoma metastases: the effect of intratumoral hemorrhage on survival.* J Neurosurg (Special Supplements), 2008. 109(6): p. 99-105.

[37] Samlowski, W.E., et al., *Multimodality treatment of melanoma brain metastases incorporating stereotactic radiosurgery (SRS).* Cancer, 2007. 109(9): p. 1855-1862.

[38] Selek, U., et al., *Stereotactic radiosurgical treatment in 103 patients for 153 cerebral melanoma metastases.* Int J Radiat Oncol Biol Phys, 2004. 59(4): p. 1097-106.

[39] Seung, S.K., et al., *Gamma knife radiosurgery for malignant melanoma brain metastases.* Cancer J Sci Am, 1998. 4(2): p. 103-9.

[40] Somaza, S., et al., *Stereotactic radiosurgery for cerebral metastatic melanoma.* J Neurosurg, 1993. 79(5): p. 661-6.

[41] Yu, C., et al., *Metastatic melanoma to the brain: prognostic factors after gamma knife radiosurgery.* Int J Radiat Oncol Biol Phys, 2002. 52(5): p. 1277-87.

[42] Harrison, B.E., et al., *Selection of patients with melanoma brain metastases for aggressive treatment.* Am J Clin Oncol, 2003. 26(4): p. 354-7.

[43] Morris, S.L., et al., *A prognostic index that predicts outcome following palliative whole brain radiotherapy for patients with metastatic malignant melanoma.* Br J Cancer, 2004. 91(5): p. 829-33.

[44] Muacevic, A., et al., *Microsurgery plus whole brain irradiation versus gamma knife surgery alone for treatment of single metastases to the brain: a randomized controlled multicentre Phase III trial.* J Neurooncol, 2008. 87(3): p. 299-307.

[45] O'Neill, B.P., et al., *A comparison of surgical resection and stereotactic radiosurgery in the treatment of solitary brain metastases.* Int J Radiat Oncol Biol Phys, 2003. 55(5): p. 1169-1176.

[46] Bindal, A.K., et al., *Surgery versus radiosurgery in the treatment of brain metastasis.* J Neurosurg, 1996. 84(5): p. 748-754.

[47] Arriagada, R., et al., *Prophylactic cranial irradiation for patients with small-cell lung cancer in complete remission.* J Natl Cancer Inst, 1995. 87(3): p. 183-90.

[48] Gregor, A., et al., *Prophylactic cranial irradiation is indicated following complete response to induction therapy in small cell lung cancer: results of a multicentre randomised trial. United Kingdom Coordinating Committee for Cancer Research (UKCCCR) and the European Organization for Research and Treatment of Cancer (EORTC).* Eur J Cancer, 1997. 33(11): p. 1752-8.

[49] Aoyama, H., et al., *Stereotactic radiosurgery plus whole-brain radiation therapy vs. stereotactic radiosurgery alone for treatment of brain metastases: a randomized controlled trial.* JAMA, 2006. 295(21): p. 2483-91.

[50] Chang, E.L., et al., *Neurocognition in patients with brain metastases treated with radiosurgery or radiosurgery plus whole-brain irradiation: a randomised controlled trial.* Lancet Oncol, 2009. 10(11): p. 1037-44.

[51] Kocher, M., et al., *Adjuvant whole-brain radiotherapy versus observation after radiosurgery or surgical resection of one to three cerebral metastases: results of the EORTC 22952-26001 study.* J Clin Oncol, 2011. 29(2): p. 134-41.

[52] Patchell, R.A., et al., *Postoperative radiotherapy in the treatment of single metastases to the brain: a randomized trial.* JAMA, 1998. 280(17): p. 1485-9.

[53] Hagen, N.A., et al., *The role of radiation therapy following resection of single brain metastasis from melanoma.* Neurology, 1990. 40(1): p. 158-60.

[54] Skibber, J., et al., *Cranial irradiation after surgical excision of brain metastases in melanoma patients.* Ann Surg Oncol, 1996. 3(2): p. 118-123.

[55] Fogarty, G., et al., *Whole brain radiotherapy after local treatment of brain metastases in melanoma patients--a randomised phase III trial.* BMC Cancer, 2011. 11: p. 142.

[56] Chitapanarux, I., et al., *Prospective study of stereotactic radiosurgery without whole brain radiotherapy in patients with four or less brain metastases: incidence of intracranial progression and salvage radiotherapy.* J Neurooncol, 2003. 61(2): p. 143-149.

[57] Sneed, P.K., et al., *A multi-institutional review of radiosurgery alone vs. radiosurgery with whole brain radiotherapy as the initial management of brain metastases.* Int J Radiat Oncol Biol Phys, 2002. 53(3): p. 519-526.

[58] Chen, J.C., et al., *Radiosurgical salvage therapy for patients presenting with recurrence of metastatic disease to the brain.* Neurosurgery, 2000. 46(4): p. 860-6; Discussion 866-7.

[59] Spreen, O. and E. Strauss, *A compendium of neuropsychological tests: administration, norms, and commentary*. 1998, New York: Oxford University Press.

[60] DeAngelis, L.M., J.Y. Delattre, and J.B. Posner, *Radiation-induced dementia in patients cured of brain metastases*. Neurology, 1989. 39(6): p. 789-96.

[61] Tucha, O., et al., *Cognitive deficits before treatment among patients with brain tumors*. Neurosurgery, 2000. 47(2): p. 324-33; discussion 333-4.

[62] Duffner, P.K., *Long-term effects of radiation therapy on cognitive and endocrine function in children with leukemia and brain tumors*. Neurologist, 2004. 10(6): p. 293-310.

[63] Vigliani, M.-C., et al., *A prospective study of cognitive functions following conventional radiotherapy for supratentorial gliomas in young adults: 4-year results*. Int J Radiat Oncol Biol Phys, 1996. 35(3): p. 527-533.

[64] Kieffer-Renaux, V., et al., *Patterns of neuropsychological deficits in children with medulloblastoma according to craniospatial irradiation doses*. Dev Med Child Neurol, 2000. 42(11): p. 741-745.

[65] Postma, T.J., et al., *Radiotherapy-induced cerebral abnormalities in patients with low-grade glioma*. Neurology, 2002. 59(1): p. 121-123.

[66] Brown, P.D., et al., *Effects of radiotherapy on cognitive function in patients with low-grade glioma measured by the Folstein Mini-Mental State Examination*. J Clin Oncol, 2003. 21(13): p. 2519-2524.

[67] van Breemen, M.S., E.B. Wilms, and C.J. Vecht, *Epilepsy in patients with brain tumours: epidemiology, mechanisms, and management*. Lancet Neurol, 2007. 6(5): p. 421-430.

[68] Klein, M., et al., *Effect of radiotherapy and other treatment-related factors on mid-term to long-term cognitive sequelae in low-grade gliomas: a comparative study*. Lancet, 2002. 360(9343): p. 1361-1368.

[69] Surma-aho, O., et al., *Adverse long-term effects of brain radiotherapy in adult low-grade glioma patients*. Neurology, 2001. 56(10): p. 1285-1290.

[70] Imperato, J.P., N.A. Paleologos, and N.A. Vick, *Effects of treatment on long-term survivors with malignant astrocytomas*. Ann Neurol, 1990. 28(6): p. 818-822.

[71] Moretti, R., et al., *Neuropsychological evaluation of late-onset post-radiotherapy encephalopathy: a comparison with vascular dementia*. J Neurol Sci, 2005. 229-230: p. 195-200.

[72] Penitzka, S., et al., *Assessment of cognitive function after preventive and therapeutic whole brain irradiation using neuropsychological testing*. Strahlenther Onkol, 2002. 178(5): p. 252-8.

[73] Stuschke, M., et al., *Prophylactic cranial irradiation in locally advanced non-small-cell lung cancer after multimodality treatment: long-term follow-up and investigations of late neuropsychologic effects*. J Clin Oncol, 1999. 17(9): p. 2700-9.

[74] Welzel, G., et al., *Memory function before and after whole brain radiotherapy in patients with and without brain metastases.* Int J Radiat Oncol Biol Phys, 2008. 72(5): p. 1311-1318.

[75] Aoyama, H., et al., *Neurocognitive function of patients with brain metastasis who received either whole brain radiotherapy plus stereotactic radiosurgery or radiosurgery alone.* Int J Radiat Oncol Biol Phys, 2007. 68(5): p. 1388-1395.

[76] Frank, R.M. and G.J. Byrne, *The clinical utility of the Hopkins Verbal Learning Test as a screening test for mild dementia.* Int J Geriatr Psychiatry, 2000. 15(4): p. 317-324.

[77] Kuslansky, G., et al., *Detecting dementia with the Hopkins Verbal Learning Test and the Mini-Mental State Examination.* Arch Clin Neuropsychol, 2004. 19(1): p. 89-104.

[78] Hogervorst E, C.M., Lapuerta P, Rue J, Swales K, Budge M., *The Hopkins Verbal Learning Test and screening for dementia.* Dement Geriatr Cogn Disord, 2002. 13(1): p. 13-20.

[79] Lacritz, L.H. and C.M. Cullum, *The Hopkins Verbal Learning Test and CVLT: a preliminary comparison.* Arch Clin Neuropsychol, 1998. 13(7): p. 623-628.

[80] Regine, W.F., et al., *Feasibility of neurocognitive outcome evaluations in patients with brain metastases in a multi-institutional cooperative group setting: results of Radiation Therapy Oncology Group Trial BR-0018.* Int J Radiat Oncol Biol Phys, 2004. 58(5): p. 1346-1352.

[81] Herman, M.A., et al., *Neurocognitive and functional assessment of patients with brain metastases: a pilot study.* Am J Clin Oncol, 2003. 26(3): p. 273-279.

[82] Brown, P.D., et al., *Detrimental effects of tumor progression on cognitive function of patients with high-grade glioma.* J Clin Oncol, 2006. 24(34): p. 5427-33.

[83] Regine, W.F., et al., *Neurocognitive outcome in brain metastases patients treated with accelerated-fractionation vs. accelerated-hyperfractionated radiotherapy: an analysis from Radiation Therapy Oncology Group Study 91-04.* Int J Radiat Oncol Biol Phys, 2001. 51(3): p. 711-7.

[84] Murray, K.J., et al., *A randomized Phase III study of accelerated hyperfractionation vs. standard in patients with unresected brain metastases: a report of the Radiation Therapy Oncology Group (RTOG) 9104.* Int J Radiat Oncol Biol Phys, 1997. 39(3): p. 571-574.

[85] Li, J., et al., *Regression after whole-brain radiation therapy for brain metastases correlates with survival and improved neurocognitive function.* J Clin Oncol, 2007. 25(10): p. 1260-6.

[86] Carella, R.J., et al., *Value of radiation therapy in the management of patients with cerebral metastases from malignant melanoma: Radiation Therapy Oncology Group Brain Metastases Study I and II.* Cancer, 1980. 45(4): p. 679-83.

[87] Franciosi, V., et al., *Front-line chemotherapy with cisplatin and etoposide for patients with brain metastases from breast carcinoma, nonsmall cell lung carcinoma, or malignant melanoma: a prospective study.* Cancer, 1999. 85(7): p. 1599-605.

[88] Margolin, K., et al., *Temozolomide and whole brain irradiation in melanoma metastatic to the brain: a phase II trial of the Cytokine Working Group.* J Cancer Res Clin Oncol, 2002. 128(4): p. 214-8.

[89] Mornex, F., et al., *A prospective randomized multicentre phase III trial of fotemustine plus whole brain irradiation versus fotemustine alone in cerebral metastases of malignant melanoma.* Melanoma Res, 2003. 13(1): p. 97-103.

[90] Hodi, F.S., et al., *Improved survival with ipilimumab in patients with metastatic melanoma.* N Engl J Med, 2010. 363(8): p. 711-23.

[91] Robert, C., et al., *Ipilimumab plus dacarbazine for previously untreated metastatic melanoma.* N Engl J Med, 2011. 364(26): p. 2517-26.

[92] Chapman, P.B., et al., *Improved survival with vemurafenib in melanoma with BRAF V600E mutation.* N Engl J Med, 2011. 364(26): p. 2507-16.

[93] Agarwala, S.S., et al., *Temozolomide for the treatment of brain metastases associated with metastatic melanoma: a phase II study.* J Clin Oncol, 2004. 22(11): p. 2101-7.

[94] Chiarion-Sileni, V., et al., *Central nervous system failure in melanoma patients: results of a randomised, multicentre phase 3 study of temozolomide- and dacarbazine- based regimens.* Br J Cancer, 2011. 104(12): p. 1816-21.

[95] Di Giacomo, A.M., et al., *Ipilimumab and fotemustine in patients with advanced melanoma (NIBIT-M1): an open-label, single-arm phase 2 trial.* Lancet Oncol, 2012.

[96] Hwu, W.J., et al., *Temozolomide plus thalidomide in patients with brain metastases from melanoma: a phase II study.* Cancer, 2005. 103(12): p. 2590-7.

[97] Jacquillat, C., et al., *Final report of the French multicenter phase II study of the nitrosourea fotemustine in 153 evaluable patients with disseminated malignant melanoma including patients with cerebral metastases.* Cancer, 1990. 66(9): p. 1873-8.

[98] Long, G.V., et al., *Dabrafenib in patients with Val600Glu or Val600Lys BRAF-mutant melanoma metastatic to the brain (BREAK-MB): a multicentre, open-label, phase 2 trial.* Lancet Oncol, 2012. 13(11): p. 1087-95.

[99] Margolin, K., et al., *Ipilimumab in patients with melanoma and brain metastases: an open-label, phase 2 trial.* Lancet Oncol, 2012. 13(5): p. 459-65.

[100] Beretta, G., et al., *Comparative evaluation of three combination regimens for advanced malignant melanoma: results of an international cooperative study.* Cancer Treat Rep, 1976. 60(1): p. 33-40.

[101] Christodoulou, C., et al., *Temozolomide (TMZ) combined with cisplatin (CDDP) in patients with brain metastases from solid tumors: a Hellenic Cooperative Oncology Group (HeCOG) Phase II study.* J Neurooncol, 2005. 71(1): p. 61-5.

[102] Costanza, M.E., et al., *Results with methyl-CCNU and DTIC in metastatic melanoma.* Cancer, 1977. 40(3): p. 1010-5.

[103] Daponte, A., et al., *Temozolomide and cisplatin in avdanced malignant melanoma.* Anticancer Res, 2005. 25(2B): p. 1441-7.

[104] Fletcher, W.S., et al., *Evaluation of cisplatin and DTIC in inoperable stage III and IV melanoma. A Southwest Oncology Group study.* Am J Clin Oncol, 1993. 16(4): p. 359-62.

[105] Kolaric, K., et al., *Phase II clinical trial of cis dichlorodiammine platinum (Cis DDP) in metastatic brain tumors.* J Cancer Res Clin Oncol, 1982. 104(3): p. 287-93.

[106] Krown, S.E., et al., *Phase II study of temozolomide and thalidomide in patients with metastatic melanoma in the brain: high rate of thromboembolic events (CALGB 500102).* Cancer, 2006. 107(8): p. 1883-90.

[107] Larkin, J.M., et al., *A phase I/II study of lomustine and temozolomide in patients with cerebral metastases from malignant melanoma.* Br J Cancer, 2007. 96(1): p. 44-8.

[108] Madajewicz, S., et al., *Phase II study--intra-arterial BCNU therapy for metastatic brain tumors.* Cancer, 1981. 47(4): p. 653-7.

[109] Reiriz, A.B., et al., *Phase II study of thalidomide in patients with metastatic malignant melanoma.* Melanoma Res, 2004. 14(6): p. 527-31.

[110] Carlino, M.S., G.B. Fogarty, and G.V. Long, *Treatment of melanoma brain metastases: a new paradigm.* Cancer J, 2012. 18(2): p. 208-12.

[111] Agarwala, S.S. and J.M. Kirkwood, *Temozolomide, a novel alkylating agent with activity in the central nervous system, may improve the treatment of advanced metastatic melanoma.* Oncologist, 2000. 5(2): p. 144-51.

[112] Middleton, M.R., et al., *Randomized phase III study of temozolomide versus dacarbazine in the treatment of patients with advanced metastatic malignant melanoma.* J Clin Oncol, 2000. 18(1): p. 158-66.

[113] Avril, M.F., et al., *Fotemustine compared with dacarbazine in patients with disseminated malignant melanoma: a Phase III study.* J Clin Oncol, 2004. 22(6): p. 1118-25.

[114] Dhomen, N. and R. Marais, *BRAF signaling and targeted therapies in melanoma.* Hematol Oncol Clin North Am, 2009. 23(3): p. 529-45, ix.

[115] Dummer, R., et al., *An open-label pilot study of vemurafenib in previously treated metastatic melanoma patients with brain metastases.* ASCO Meeting Abstracts, 2011. 29(15_suppl): p. 8548.

[116] Laquerre, S., et al., *A selective Raf kinase inhibitor induces cell death and tumor regression of human cancer cell lines encoding B-RafV600E mutation.* Molecular Cancer Therapeutics, 2009. 8(12 Suppl; abstract B88).

[117] Falchook, G.S., et al., *Dabrafenib in patients with melanoma, untreated brain metastases, and other solid tumours: a phase 1 dose-escalation trial.* Lancet, 2012. 379(9829): p. 1893-901.

[118] Schartz, N.E., et al., *Complete regression of a previously untreated melanoma brain metastasis with ipilimumab.* Melanoma Res, 2010. 20(3): p. 247-50.

[119] Hodi, F.S., et al., *CTLA-4 blockade with ipilimumab induces significant clinical benefit in a female with melanoma metastases to the CNS.* Nat Clin Pract Oncol, 2008. 5(9): p. 557-61.

[120] Weber, J.S., et al., *Safety and clinical activity of ipilimumab in melanoma patients with brain metastases: retrospective analysis of data from a phase 2 trial.* Melanoma Res, 2011. 21(6): p. 530-4.

[121] Knisely, J.P., et al., *Radiosurgery for melanoma brain metastases in the ipilimumab era and the possibility of longer survival.* J Neurosurg, 2012. 117(2): p. 227-33.

[122] Gaspar, L., et al., *Recursive partitioning analysis (RPA) of prognostic factors in three Radiation Therapy Oncology Group (RTOG) brain metastases trials.* Int J Radiat Oncol Biol Phys, 1997. 37(4): p. 745-51.

[123] Gaspar, L.E., et al., *Validation of the RTOG recursive partitioning analysis (RPA) classification for brain metastases.* Int J Radiat Oncol Biol Phys, 2000. 47(4): p. 1001-6.

[124] Lutterbach, J., et al., *Patients with brain metastases: hope for recursive partitioning analysis (RPA) Class 3.* Radiother Oncol, 2002. 63(3): p. 339-45.

[125] Agboola, O., et al., *Prognostic factors derived from recursive partition analysis (RPA) of Radiation Therapy Oncology Group (RTOG) brain metastases trials applied to surgically resected and irradiated brain metastatic cases.* Int J Radiat Oncol Biol Phys, 1998. 42(1): p. 155-9.

[126] Tendulkar, R.D., et al., *RPA classification has prognostic significance for surgically resected single brain metastasis.* Int J Radiat Oncol Biol Phys, 2006. 66(3): p. 810-7.

[127] Sperduto, P.W., et al., *Diagnosis-specific prognostic factors, indexes, and treatment outcomes for patients with newly diagnosed brain metastases: a multi-institutional analysis of 4,259 patients.* Int J Radiat Oncol Biol Phys, 2010. 77(3): p. 655-61.

[128] Lorenzoni, J., et al., *Radiosurgery for treatment of brain metastases: estimation of patient eligibility using three stratification systems.* Int J Radiat Oncol Biol Phys, 2004. 60(1): p. 218-224.

[129] Weltman, E., et al., *Radiosurgery for brain metastases: a score index for predicting prognosis.* Int J Radiat Oncol Biol Phys, 2000. 46(5): p. 1155-61.

[130] Broadbent, A.M., et al., *Survival following whole brain radiation treatment for cerebral metastases: an audit of 474 patients.* Radiother Oncol, 2004. 71(3): p. 259-65.

[131] Stone, A., et al., *A comparison of survival rates for treatment of melanoma metastatic to the brain.* Cancer Invest, 2004. 22(4): p. 492-7.

[132] Ellerhorst, J., et al., *Whole brain irradiation for patients with metastatic melanoma: a review of 87 cases.* Int J Radiat Oncol Biol Phys, 2001. 49(1): p. 93-7.

[133] Barker II, F.G., *Surgical and radiosurgical management of brain metastases.* Surg Clin North Am, 2005. 85(2): p. 329-45.

[134] Regine, W.F., et al., *Risk of symptomatic brain tumor recurrence and neurologic deficit after radiosurgery alone in patients with newly diagnosed brain metastases: results and implications.* Int J Radiat Oncol Biol Phys, 2002. 52(2): p. 333-8.

[135] Chiarion-Sileni, V., et al., *Temozolomide (TMZ) as prophylaxis for melanoma brain metastases (BrM): Results from a Phase III, multicenter study.* J Clin Oncol (Meeting Abstracts), 2008. 26(15_suppl): p. 20014.

[136] Samlowski, W.E., *Multimodality treatment of patients with metastatic melanoma with brain metastases*, in *American Society of Clinical Oncology Educational Book: 43rd Annual Meeting*, R. Govindan, Editor. 2007, American Society of Clinical Oncology: Alexandria, VA. p. 519-522.

[137] Gruss, C., et al., *Severe neurological disabilities after complete remission of advanced malignant melanoma following fotemustine therapy in combination with total brain irradiation.* Melanoma Res, 2002. 12(4): p. 403-4.

[138] Khalil, Z., et al., *Neurological toxicity during metastatic melanoma treatment with fotemustine.* Melanoma Res, 2005. 15(6): p. 563-4.

[139] Douglas, J. and V. Sondak, *RE: A comparison of survival rates for treatment of melanoma metastatic to the brain*, in *Cancer Invest*. 2004. p. 643-644.

Chapter 12

Surgical Treatment of Nevi and Melanoma in the Pediatric Age

Andrea Zangari, Federico Zangari,
Mercedes Romano, Elisabetta Cerigioni,
Maria Giovanna Grella, Anna Chiara Contini and
Martino Ascanio

Additional information is available at the end of the chapter

http://dx.doi.org/10.5772/54632

1. Introduction

Surgical care of children affected by melanocytic lesions is a complex area of pediatric surgery, where psychosocial aspects, involving parents and children of different ages, overlap with oncologic implications. In this challenging field results may be frustrating despite knowledge and experience.

Due to its rarity, the occurrence of malignant melanoma in children may be underestimated by involved professionals. Melanoma in children is rare, but it does exist and every effort should be done to assure proper treatment, which should be guaranteed in a pediatric tertiary care center by a multi-specialist approach.

The role of dermatologists is essential to achieve proper selection of indications to surgery, by clinical follow up and dermatoscopy techniques. On the other hand surgeon is expected to share a profound knowledge of indications and techniques of treatment. In fact, the awareness that simple excision of a nevus may represent the first and most important therapeutic intervention of a MM, before knowing the definitive diagnosis, is sometimes lacking even among pediatric care professionals and the occasional occurrence of a MM diagnosis may be confounding and cause of an incomplete care strategy.

Decisions about surgical treatment of congenital giant nevi in some cases may need psychological assessment because of complex relationships between patient's and parents' awareness and willingness.

Pediatric anesthesia offers a variety of techniques that can be personalized to suite patients from the newborn to the adolescent.

The intent of this chapter is to contribute to knowledge of this multifaceted field of pediatric surgery.

2. Nevomelanocytic lesions in the pediatric age

Current strategies for the treatment of nevomelanocytic lesions in children mostly derived from the more extensive experience in adults. Nevertheless, further knowledge and experience in this field have shown some peculiarities that require special considerations relevant to the pediatric age. In fact, due to the multifaceted field of congenital nevi, to the rarity of melanoma in children and to peculiar features of some nevic lesions in this age range, important implications related to treatment emerge.

2.1. Congenital nevi

Congenital nevi are present at birth and occur approximately in 1% of newborn infants. They result from a proliferation of benign melanocytes in the dermis, epidermis, or both. Occasionally, nevi that are histologically identical to congenital nevi may develop approximately during the first 2 years of life. These are referred to be considered tardive congenital nevi [1].

The etiology of congenital melanocytic nevi remains unclear. The melanocytes of the skin originate in the neuroectoderm, although the specific cell type from which they derive remains controversial [3, 4, 5].

One hypothesis is that pluripotential nerve sheath precursor cells migrate from the neural crest to the skin along paraspinal ganglia and peripheral nerve sheaths and differentiate into melanocytes upon reaching the skin [6]. There are many reports of familial aggregation of congenital nevi.

One study found that the MC1R (melanocortin-1-receptor) genotype, which corresponds to a red-haired genotype and a tendency to increased birthweight, was overrepresented in a cohort of congenital melanocytic nevi affected Northern European patients. How MC1R variants promote growth of congenital melanocytic nevi and the fetus itself is unknown as is the application of this finding to non-european and more darkly pigmented races [7].

Congenital nevi have been stratified into 3 groups according to size. Small nevi are less than 1.5 cm in greatest diameter, medium nevi are 1.5-19.9 cm in greatest diameter, and large or giant nevi are greater than 20 cm. Giant nevi are often surrounded by several smaller satellite nevi.

Large congenital nevi of the head or posterior midline may also be seen as a component of neurocutaneous disorder, with cranial and/or leptomeningeal melanosis. Neurocutaneous melanosis may result from an error in the morphogenesis of the neuroectoderm, which gives rise to the melanotic cells of both the skin and meninges. Clinically, patients may present with increased intracranial pressure due to hydrocephalus or a mass lesion. The prognosis of patients with symptomatic neurocutaneous melanosis is very poor, even in the absence of malignancy [8]. Significant association is between giant congenital nevi and neurofibromatosis, with development of neurofibromas [9]. The histology is characterized by the presence of melanocytes in the epidermis ordered in theques and/or malanocytes in the dermis as sheets, nests, cords and/or single cells [10].

The histology of large congenital nevus may be delivered into nevus cell, neuroid, epithelioid cell and/or spindle cell, dermal melanocytic and mixed [11].

In the *nevus cell type* histology may appear identical to acquired nevi, but in the congenital nevus melanocytes are more in the lower two-thirds of the reticular dermis or deeper and more associated with neurovascular structures in the reticular dermis. In the *neuroid type* of giant congenital nevi, the dermis imelanocyte cells appear to be arranged in palisaded around a cellular mass of homogeneous material (Varocay Body) and sheating of nerves by neuroid tissue (neuroid tubes). The neuroid type of giant congenital nevus may be associated with congenital anomalies of bone (club foot, spina bifida, atrophy). In the *Spindle cell and/or epithelioid cell type* of giant congenital nevus, the dermis is infiltrated in whole or in part by nests or sheets of epithelioid and/or spindle cells, but unlike acquired variety is involved deeper the reticular dermis, with neuroid elements. Sometime, in giant congenital nevi, architectural and cellular features may be so atypical making differentiation with melanoma very difficult. In the *dermal melanocytic type* of giant congenital nevi, appearance may be that of a giant blue nevus.

In large congenital nevi are occasionally present, within melanocytes, trace of other tissue like muscle, bone, placenta. Other tissues occasionally present intermixed with melanocytic elements are hemangiomas, increased numbers of mast cells, cartilage, calcificacion. Associated tumors include schwannoma, neuroid tumors, lipoma, rhabdomyosarcoma, neurofibroma, sebaceous nevus, blue nevus, hemangioma, lymphangioma and mastocytoma, nevi of Ota and Ito, Spitz nevus [12]. The etiology of congenital melanocytic nevi has not been elucidated. One possible cause is a mutation. An association between infantile hemangiomas and congenital melanocytic nevi has been suggested [13]. Future investigation may yield more definitive causative factors. A review of dermoscopy patterns in congenital nevi found that most nevi demonstrate a reticular, globular, or reticuloglobular pattern. The findings varied with age and the anatomic location of the nevus, with the globular pattern found more often in younger children and the reticular pattern found in patients aged 12 years or older [14]. The role of dermoscopy in congenital nevi is currently recruiting.

2.2. Association between congenital nevi and melanoma

The risk of melanoma development is proportional to to the size of congenital nevus., with a clear evidence of increased risk in patients with congenital nevi involving over 5% of the body surface. For giant congenital melanocytic nevi, the risk of developing melanoma has been reported to be as high as 5-7% [15]. Risk for the development of melanoma in smaller nevi has not been well quantified and the matter is still controversial (Fig.1). Also suggested is that melanoma developing within smaller congenital nevi usually occurs at puberty or later and develops more superficially in the skin, where it is easier to detect clinically. The lifetime risk of melanoma for patients with very large congenital nevi has benn estimated, approximately and considering variations in several countries and studies, at least 6%.

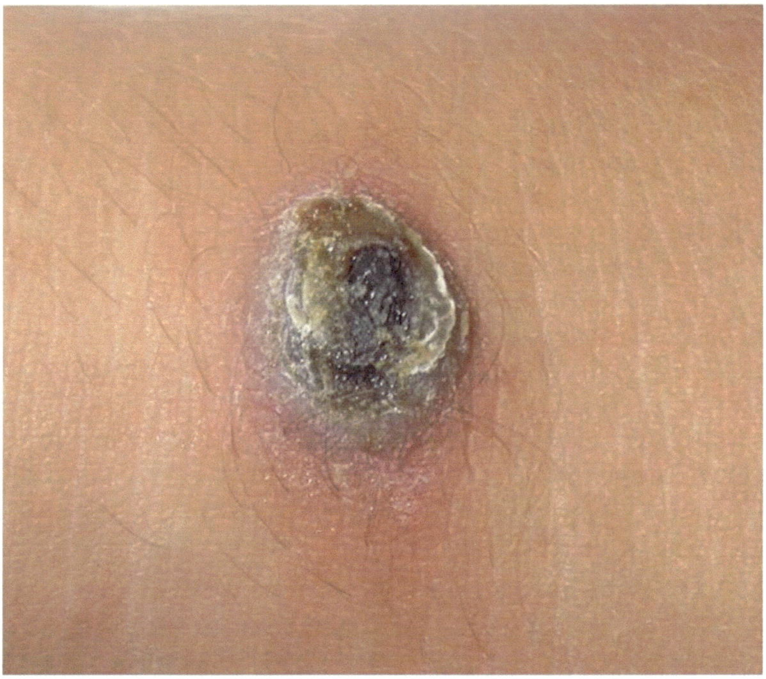

Figure 1. Malignant melanoma diagnosed in a small congenital lesion of the dorsal foot

2.3. Spitz nevus

It is also defined by other terms, including epithelioid cell and/or Spindle cell nevus, juvenile melanoma, benign juvenile melanoma. It occurs normally in children, but may appear in 15% of adolescents and adults. Spitz nevus is a unique, acquired, usually benign melanocytic tumor, so alarming in its clinical presentation and sometimes histologically confused with melanoma. It is possible that some lesions regress spontaneously. It can appear pink or tan, as a papule, often with teleangiectasies on the surface (Fig.2). A variety called Reed nevus, more frequent In adults, may also be confused with melanoma, but histologically is an acquired, predominantly spindle cells variety, darkly pigmented [16].

2.4. Common acquired melanocytic nevus

Acquired melanocytic nevus is a common disorder of melanocytes, occurring as a pigmented benign lesion, possibly localized in every part of the skin (palmoplantar areas included) and

http://dx.doi.org/10.5772/54632

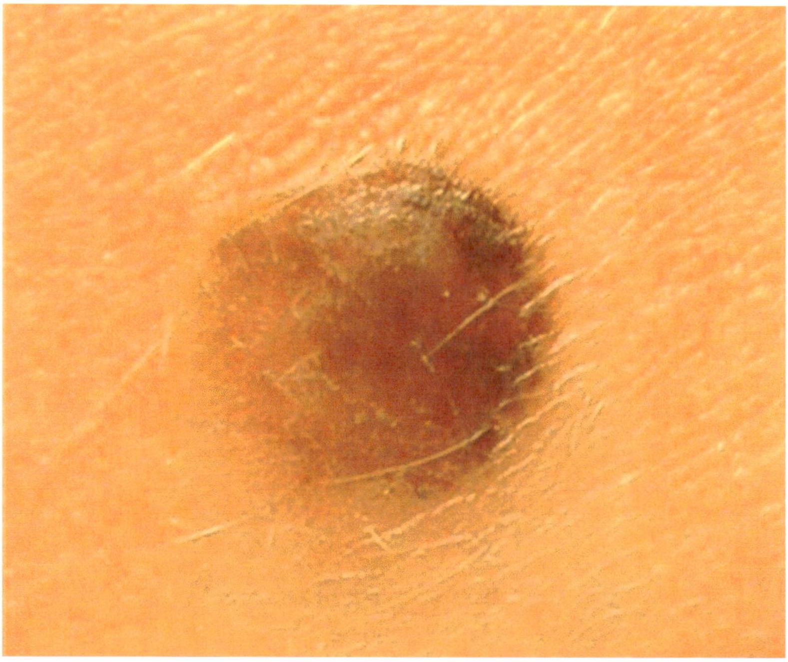

Figure 2. Spitz nevus

oral, ocular, genital mucosae. They first can appear after 6-12 months of life. Histology classifies acquired melanocytic nevi as a collection of melanocytic cells in the epidermis (Junctional), dermis (Intradermal), or both (Compound), disposed in isolated elements (epidermal variety, lentiginous pattern) or aggregated (junctional, intradermal and compound variety). There is evidence that number and size of common acquired nevi is associated with familiarity. Studies documented an increased number of nevi for pale skin, blond hair, blue or green eyes, tendency to sunburn. Typical acquired nevi usually have a round or oval, symmetric shape and relatively well-demarcated, smooth borders. The surface of nevi may be flat-topped, dome-shaped, papillomatous or peduncolated. More elevated acquired nevi tend to be more lightly pigmented, and flatter acquired nevi tend to be more darkly pigmented. More elevated and less pigmented lesions tend to have a prominent intradermal melanocytic component, whereas flatter and darker lesions have a more prominent junctional melanocytic component and a less prominent dermal component. Changes in acquired melanocytic nevi can be physiologic in puberty, pregnancy, corticosteroid administration and sun exposure; also changes may occur slowly during the years as normal evolution of nevi. Though most of times changes are benign, in presence of alterations of symmetry, color, borders, extension or regression, especially in a short time (months), a periodic monitoring of all nevi on the skin and mucosa is necessary, preferably with dermoscopy. When melanoma occurs on a melanocytic acquired nevi, changes may be global or, most of times, partial, that is the reason why asymmetry is a predominant parameter to be evaluated [17].

2.5. Blue nevus

The blue nevus consists of an acquired or congenital blue, blue-gray or blue-black papule, plaque or nodule, histologically composed by dermal dendritic, fibroblast-like cells containing melanin. Most of times it is localized on dorsa of hands and feet, usually singular. Common blue nevi remain unchanged or possibly regress. Particular types of blue nevi are:

- Cellular blue nevus is a blue-gray nodule or plaque 1 to 3 cm diameter mostly located on the buttock or sacrum.
- Combined blue nevus-melanocytic nevus, sometimes confused with atypical nevi or melanoma.

Malignant blue nevus, may develop in contiguity with cellular blue nevus, nevus of Ota, or de novo [18].

2.6. Dysplastic melanocytic nevi

Dysplastic nevus is an acquired, usually atypical-appearing melanocytic tumor, characterized histologically by epidermic and/or dermal melanocytic dysplasia. Dysplasia refers to abnormal tissue development. When applied to melanocytic tumors, dysplasia is referred to a disordered melanocytic proliferation in association with discontinuous and variable cellular atypia (mild, moderate and severe). About this spectrum of atypia, from slight to marked may be said that intraepidermal melanocytes in dysplastic melanocytic nevi occupy an intermediate position between typical and malignant, basing on nuclear and cytoplasmic features. Not all atypical-appearing melanocytic lesions have an atypical histology. It is generally believed that a melanocytic nevus appearing asymmetric, irregular in borders and pigmentation and with a diameter equal or more than 6 mm is considered dysplastic, but these characteristics are referred to "Atypical acquired Nevus", also called "Clark Nevus". Although the diagnosis of dysplastic nevus is suspected because of the atypical appearing, histological confirmation is required to establish the presence or not of dysplasia. It is important to define if atypical nevus is dysplastic, because it is a potential histogenic precursor of melanoma and marker of increased melanoma risk.

2.7. Halo nevi

Halo nevus, also referred as "Sutton's nevus" or "leukoderma acquisitum centrifugum", is a nevus surrounded by a macule of leukoderma (hypopigmented or apigmented area). It occurs in up to 1% of general population, with a peak of incidence in the second decade. It is commonly composed of a central pigmented nevus and an acquired surrounding depigmented halo. From 25 to 50% of patients have more than one halo nevi. Nevus regression can be complete and is caused by a lymphocytic aggression against nevus melanocytes with involvement of surrounding epidermal melanocytes. Association with vitiligo needs clinical and anamnestic analysis as a history for melanoma.

2.8. Nevus of Ota and Ito

Ota first described this nevus and called it "nevus fuscocaeruleus ophtalmomaxillaris. Nevus of Ota is usually congenital but may appear in early childhood or in puberty. It is usually characterized by unilateral, flat, blue-black macules in the skin innervated by the first and second branches of the trigeminal nerve. Oral, nasal and pharingeal mucosae, conjunctivae and tympanic membranes may be involved. More rarely pigmentation may extend to cornea, optic nerve, fundus oculi, retrobulbar fat and periosteum. Enlargement and darkening may be observed over time. Histology shows stellate melanocytes widely scattered in the reticular dermis. Overlying melanocytes may be reduced in size and contain increased melanin. Nevus of Ota does not improve with time. 66 cases of melanoma development in nevus of Ota have been reported. Effective treatment is photothermolysis with Q-Switched LASER needing multiple sessions, with good results. Nevus of Ito is analogous to nevus of Ota and may coexist in the same patient. The difference between the two types of nevi is that nevus of Ito involves the distribution of the lateral supraclavicular and brachial nerves.

2.9. Melanoma

Melanoma is a malignant tumor resulting from the trasformation of melanocytes of the skin and less frequently of mucosae. During embryonic life, melanoblasts migrate from neural crest to the basal-cell layer of epidermis and a minus part to skin appendages and dermis. Melanoma can arise from melanocytes located in these sites.

Risk for the development of melanoma remains low in pre-pubertal age, with an annual incidence of 0.7 cases per million children aged 0-9 years. Reaching adolescence the incidence of melanoma increases, with a rate of 13.2 cases per million children aged 15-19 years [2]. Prevention and early recognition of melanoma is mainly applied to adults through periodic clinical and dermoscopic controls. Only in recent years data documented alarm about increasing incidence of melanoma in adolescents. This increase, combined with other data about congenital nevi, allow physicians in the last years to play a crucial role in the identification of children at risk for melanoma, with particular regard to detection of risk factors in children and adolescents, and education about sun and artificial ultraviolet exposure.

3. Types of primary melanoma of the skin

3.1. Lentigo maligna

Lentigo maligna is a precursor lesion that may progress into invasive melanoma. It appears as a macular, freckled-like lesion of irregular shape, occurring most often in *elderly patients* (age over 60 years) in sun exposed and sun-damaged, atrophic skin. Lentigo maligna normally grows slowly for long periods (years) with a prolonged radial growth phase, before evolution in Lentigo Maligna Melanoma. Hstopathology reveals atrophic epidermis and increased numbers of atypical basilar melanocytes that may extend down the hair follicles and skin appendages.

3.2. Lentigo maligna melanoma

It is a melanoma in situ slow growing progressing to invasive melanoma with nests of malignant melanocytes invading the dermis. Lentigo Maligna Melanoma represents 4 to 15 % of all melanoma.

3.3. Superficial spreading melanoma

SSM is the most frequent type of melanocytic malignancy representing 70% of all melanomas.

Most commonly it occurs on the upper back of men and on the legs of women, although it can develop at any site, mucosa included. The usual history is that of slow change (months to 1-5 years) of a preexisting melanocytic lesion or can arise "de novo".

SSM most frequently presents as a macule asymmetric, variegated pigmentation (from brown to black, with variable presence of blue-gray, gray-white or pink areas as sign of regression along the borders or inside the lesion. Borders may present intact initially in presence of a precursor melanocytic nevus, but mostly are irregular. Dermoscopy can reveal better all these alterations, and more other parameters typical of SSM (salt-peppering areas, star-bust aspect, pseudopodes at borders, blue-white veil and so on). Diagnosis of SSM may be done from a macroscopic view, but dermoscopy helps much for *confirmation diagnosis* and for *early diagnosis*, when it is difficult to find macroscopically some alterations typical of melanoma.

Histopathology reveals a "pagetoid" distribution of atypical large melanocytes thruoughout the epidermis. The large cells may occur singularly or in nests and have a monomorphous appearance. In the dermis areas of invasion of atypical melanocytes are present.

3.4. Nodular melanoma

The second most common subtype of melanoma is nodular melanoma with a frequency of 15 to 30 percent of all types. NM is remarkable for its rapid evolution and may arise from melanocytic nevi or normal skin (de novo), but in lack of an apparent radial growth phase. NM is more common to arise "de novo" than from a preexisting nevus.

NM appears typically as a blue-black, blue-red or amelanotic nodule or papule. In certain cases it may be difficult to diagnose especially when it appears as an amelanotic reddish lesion.

Histopathology may demonstrates a little tendency for intraepidermal growth, but it typically arises at dermal-epidermal junction and from its onset with extention to the dermis, composed of large epithelioid cells, spindle cells, small cells, or a mix of these different cells.

3.5. Acral lentiginous melanoma

ALM is more common in darker skin individuals (60 to 72 percent in blacks, 29 to 46 percent in asians). In white skin people it represents only 2 to 8 percent of melanomas. ALM occurs on palms and more often on soles, or beneath the nail plate.

The biologic behavior of ALM is traditionally considered more aggressive with a poorer prognosis and this may be due to late diagnosis and/or to the different biologic origin of it.

3.6. Melanoma of the mucosa

It involves oral, nasal, vulva, anorectal, conjunctival mucosae and it may occur with or without a radial growth phase.

3.7. Desmoplastic melanoma

It is a rare subtype of melanoma, locally aggressive and with high rates of local recurrence. It may arise in association with LM, ALM and mucosal melanoma or "de novo". DM may appear as a pigmented macule, papule, nodule or reddish. Histologically it is caracterized by fibrous tissue and atypical spindle-shaped melanocytes that show a propensity to infiltrate cutaneous nerves.

The incidence of malignant melanoma is rapidly increasing in the last decades. The surveillance, epidemiology and results program (SEER) has documented a 32,7% increased in mortality rates over the period 1973 to 1995. on the other hand, the overall survival rate has been improving for melanoma in the last decades. Currently, cutaneous melanoma accounts for approximatively 1% of all cancer deaths [19, 20, 21, 22].

More recent studies indicate that the rate of increase in all age groups was 2.8% per year from 1981 to 2001 and in children (age < 20 years) was 1.1% per year from 1975 to 2001.1 The diagnosis is often delayed in children since melanoma is rare (300 to 420 new cases per year), and benign lesions, especially Spitz nevus, may mimic melanoma. The prognosis is good when there is prompt identification and wide local excision of early disease, but poor for those with advanced disease at presentation [23]. Case-control studies in adults have identified multiple host and environmental factors associated with increased risk of malignant melanoma. Host factors include fair skin, white race, blond or red hair, light eye color, tendency to burn with UV radiation exposure, increased number of benign nevi, dysplastic nevi, family history of melanoma, and xeroderma pigmentosum.6,7 Environmental factors include sunburns, often as a child, and increased exposure to UV radiation. Proposed risk factors for paediatric melanoma include congenital, dysplastic, or increased number of nevi; inability to tan; blue eyes; facial freckling; family history of melanoma; disorders of DNA excision repair like xeroderma pigmentosum; acquired or congenital immunosuppression and a previous history of malignancy [24, 25, 26].

Analysis regarding children and young adults with melanoma between 1973 and 2001 show how older age, more recent year of diagnosis, female sex, white race, and increased environmental UV radiation were all associated with a significant increase in the risk of melanoma. In the first year of life, the incidence of melanoma is similar by race, but it diverges by age 5 to 9 years and is more than 40-fold higher in white individuals by age 20 to 24 years.

The increase in incidence of melanoma in children, especially in adolescents, is similar to that seen in young adults. This may reflect increased cumulative UV exposure during childhood or adolescence, greater awareness and more frequent diagnosis of melanoma (eg, versus atypical Spitz nevus), differences in genetic predisposition, and/or other environmental factors. The increased risk of melanoma in girls, particularly on the lower extremities, may be a result of increased UV exposure. In adults, sun-related behaviours differ between men and women. [22] The increased rates of melanoma in adolescent and young women may reflect sunbathing or the widespread (> 25%) practice of indoor tanning [28].

Prognosis for young children, adolescents, and young adults with melanoma appears to be similar. Also increased is the risk of death in male children, those with regional or distant metastasis, primary sites other than the extremities or torso, increasing thickness of the primary lesion, earlier year of diagnosis, and previous cancer.

Melanoma-specific survival in children has improved by approximately 4% per year during the last 3 decades. It is difficult to explain this dramatic improvement. Although earlier diagnosis could be associated with improved survival, there has been no decrease in lesion thickness over the last decade. Furthermore, survival has improved for all stages of paediatric melanoma. The most notable improvement has been in the "unstaged" group, likely due to more complete staging. There are important differences in young children (age < 10 years) with melanoma compared with adolescents and young adults that may reflect distinct tumor biology and/or host characteristics.

Published large series of paediatric melanoma report 5-year survival rates of 74% to 80%. This is significantly worse than the 91% 5-year overall survival seen in recent analysis, after the exclusion of cases of melanoma in situ [29, 30]. Accepted prognostic factors in adult melanoma include primary lesion thickness, ulceration, and non-extremity site; increased age; regional lymph node involvement; satellite or in-transit metastases; elevated serum lactate dehydrogenase level; visceral or brain metastases.[4,9 However, prognosis and prognostic factors in children are less defined. In a recent review of more than 300 cases, the outcome for paediatric patients (5-year survival of 74%) was slightly worse than that of young adults, but these survival estimates have limitations. In a large European registry study of children, male sex, unfavorable site (lesions on the trunk), and/or second primary or regional or distant metastasis. [10] Advanced stage has been associated with poor prognosis in other paediatric studies [27].

In summary, paediatric melanoma is an important and increasing problem. Factors conferring risk of adult melanoma, including older age, white race (blue eyes, blond or red hair, freckling tendency, liability to tan and tendence to sunburn), family history of melanoma, elevate number of acquired melanocytic nevi (double risk in 50 to 99 of acquired melanocytic nevi), dysplastic nevi, environmental exposure to UV radiation, congenital or acquired immunosuppression are also important in paediatric melanoma.

4. Indications for excision of nevi

Indication for excision are usually assessed by dermatologists, paediatric surgeons, paediatrician and physicians.

Nevi can be divided into congenital and acquired. In turn congenital nevi can be small, intermediate and large (>20cm). Melanoma risk in small congenital nevi is debated, although in some reports it seems to be of importance [32] Some studies demonstrated an increased risk of malignant melanoma in small lesions as well as in intermediate lesions, but this is still a matter of controversy. In the lack of consensus about systematic removal of small congenital nevi, careful dermatologic monitoring and prompt excision after clinical changing is recommended [33] In the Literature there is a large agreement on the excision of large congenital nevi. In fact they show an increased risk for development of malignant melanoma, varying from 1% to 31%. Nonetheless malignancy is reported to occur despite complete excision and may be not preventable [34, 35]

Indications for surgical excision [36] of acquired nevi are mainly related to lesions resembling malignant melanoma, such as atypical nevi, Spitz nevi, and lesions presenting clinical signs and symptoms as diameter of more than 5 mm or increasing diameter, irregular margins, border notching, irregular pigmentation, asymmetry, rapid onset or increase in diameter, ulceration, bleeding, pain and itching. These last signs seem to represent the presentation symptoms of malignant melanoma in 85% of cases [37] Although the risk of malignant melanoma is higher in familial atypical nevi rather than in nonfamilial, features of atypical nevi have been reported to be the most frequent indication to surgery [38]

Some special consideration is given to Spitz nevus for possible misdiagnosis with MM. Most dermatologists and physicians recommend biopsy. In an interview with dermatologists, most responding specialists (93%) recommended the biopsy of suspected Spitz nevi. Sixty-nine percent of physicians would completely excise a lesion that was histologically diagnosed as an incompletely removed Spitz nevus. Seventy percent of general dermatologists and 80% of pediatric dermatologists would recommend excision with a 1- to 2-mm margin of normal-appearing skin around a Spitz nevus [39]. The lack of consensus about the nature and the ideal management of Spitz nevus reflects the uncertainty in histopathologic distinction between Spitz nevus and melanoma, and such a concern influences management. By some authors 2 mm margins excisional biopsy of clinically appearing Spitz nevus, as of any nevic lesion, is recommended

In some cases nevi located in sites of clinically difficult monitoring or placed in sites of exposure to frequent trauma are an indication for excision [38, 40]

5. Treatment of acquired nevi

Acquired melanocytic nevi begin to appear after the first 6 months of life and increase in number during childhood and adolescence, typically reaching a peak count in the third decade and then slowly regressing with age. They are classified as junctional nevi if the nests of melanocytes are in the dermal – epidermal junction, intradermal nevi if the nests are in dermis and compound nevi if the nests are located in both sites.

They usually have a diameter of less than 6 - 8 mm, a homogeneous surface, pigmentation, round or oval shape, regular outline, and demarcated border, sometimes with pigmentary stippling or perifollicular hypopigmentation.

These are rarely complicated by evolution in malignant melanoma so conservative treatment, that is clinical periodic control, is usually enough.

However, when removal of a naevus is necessary we have to do some considerations especially in order to the characteristics of the nevus and its position.

5.1. Anesthesia

Indications and surgical techniques of the excision of a skin lesion are similar to the adult and so the actual difference with children is the anesthetic management.

Analgesics are commonly administered prior to surgical procedure in children. The concept of preemptive analgesia is still controversial and its effectiveness may depend on the type of surgery. Nowadays the most commonly used medications are acetaminophen alone or with codeine, but also non – steroidal anti – inflammatory medications (ibuprofen) are effective analgesics for perioperative pain, but less used for the impact on bleeding.

In association with analgesics and anesthetic medicament the use of sedative is very common and useful also in children as in the adult. Midazolam is very convenient in children because not only alleviates the anxiety of surgery, but also induces an anterograde amnesia, useful for treatments requiring multiple visits. Furthermore, it can be administrated in various vehicles via the nasal, rectal, sublingual that are less traumatic than intramuscular injection in children.

Fentanyl is 100 times more potent than morphine and has less influence on GI motility than morphine, so reducing the effect of emesis and oxygen desaturation becoming more tolerable in children.

General anaesthesia is used in the excisional surgery of large lesions and occasionally in non – cooperative children. It is a very safe procedure, but the rate of complication increases in case of surgery in the first year of life and when the anesthesiologist has no pediatric experience.

In recent years the use of topical anesthetics, especially EMLA cream (eutectic mixture of local anesthetics), knows an important development in office procedures in children, although the incorrect use of EMLA causes failure in reducing pain of dermatologic procedure. In particular for an effective absorption of the anesthetic into the skin an occlusive dressing is useful.

5.2. Surgery

Any skin lesion presenting features of malignant melanoma are biopsied. Although melanoma in children is rare, the most frequent indication for excision of an acquired nevus is early diagnostic evaluation because of melanoma concern.

Excisional biopsy is the treatment of choice. It may be elliptical, wedge or circular, but the first is the most commonly used.

5.2.1. Simple excision

Skin incisions should be planned along or parallel to the relaxed skin tension lines (RSTLs). This allows, on one hand, a better wound healing, an easier matching of edge of the wound and lower tension of the sutures and, on the other hand, to hide the wound in a skin fold.

The elliptical excisional biopsy, as the other type of excisional biopsy, must include a portion of healthy tissue of 0,2 cm wideness from the perimeter of the lesion and the subcutaneous tissue. The possible exuberant tissue, called "dog - ear" can be corrected by extending the ellipse or removing the excess skin with a L or Y incision.

The wedge excisional biopsy is usually utilized for the lesions located on or close to the free margin of some particular structures as eyelid, lip, nose and ear. In the eyelids it is possible to make an incision along the edge and remove only the skin, although some lesions require excision of full thickness eyelid. 1/4 of eyelid or 1/3 of the lower lip can be completely excised and the defect closed with a simple suture without elaborated reconstructions.

The circular excisional biopsy is used when a skin limited incision is needed as in the case of nose or in the anterior region of the auricle. The defect can be closed with a skin graft or a skin flap.

When repairing the loss of substance by combination of skin edges is impossible, other techniques are necessary:

Grafts, rarely used for the excision of acquired nevi

5.2.2. Flaps

A flap is a portion of one or more tissues transferred from a donor site to a receiver maintaining a neurovascular connection ("pedicle").

The use of flap has many advantages including that of allow the repair of the defect by means of tissue similar or equal to those of the receiving site. It is very important for specialized tissues as lip or eyelid.

The skin flap, composed by skin only or including subcutaneous tissue, is transferred from one part of the body to another with its neurovascular pedicle or attached by just a margin to preserve vascular support.

There are two types of skin flap: those which rotate around a pivot point (rotation, transposition and interpolation flaps) and advancement flaps (single pedicle, V – Y, Y – V and bi – pedunculated.

The rotation flap is a semicircular flap that rotates from its pivot point to the receiving site (Fig.3). If tension is too high, the incision can be extended by a reverse incision from pivot point along the base of the flap (backcut).

The transposition flap is composed by a rectangle or square of skin and subcutaneous tissue that rotate around a pivot point close to lesion.

The advancement flap is brought forward on the lesion without rotation.

This can have only one pedicle, so feeding is maintained by exploiting the elasticity of the skin.

The advancement V – Y flap more than a flap is a V incision whose sides are closed in such a way that the final suture gives a Y.

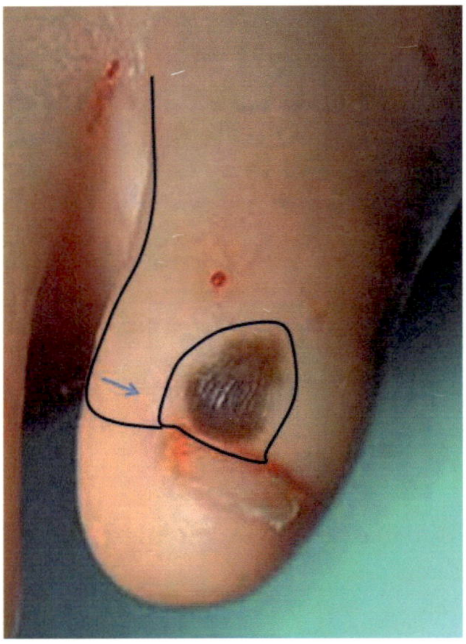

Figure 3. Rotational flap to excise a peliungueal nevus

6. Treatment of congenital nevi in the pediatric age

6.1. Indications and timing

Surgery of congenital nevi is predominantly indicated for preventive reasons, related to the risk of developing a malignant melanoma within the lesion during life. This indication has been discussed more extensively elsewhere in the chapter. Evaluation of all small and medium CNN for prophylactic excision should take place before the patient is aged 12 years. After this age, malignant potential rises sharply. Some authors advocate prophylactic excision of all CNN [35, 41, 42],

whereas others advocate clinical monitoring of small [38] or both small and medium nevi [43] The incidence of malignant melanoma appears higher in large congenital nevi, in the scalp, back, and buttocks and requires removal first. This increase in incidence is likely secondary to the total body surface area. The presence of an enlarging nodular mass indicates malignant change and requires immediate treatment. This mass may represent a rare neuroectodermal sarcoma.

The other important indication to treatment is the possible discomfort due to the presence of a visible difference or even disfigurement. Psychological implications of this condition can involve both parents and children, in a different manner for different ages. Parents feelings about their child's appearance are likely to influence the child's perception of his or her disfigurement, the developing body image and feelings of self-worth [44]. Parental strategies to deal with a physical difference vary considerably. Some discuss it openly, others may act as if it does not exist, parents may be over-protective or children may avoid issues related to their appearance for fear of upsetting their parents 45. Most children with a visible difference often experience appearance-related teasing and bullying during the course of their school career [46]. A link between appearance-related teasing, body dissatisfaction and general psychological disturbance has been discussed by Gilbert and Thompson [47]. The physical and psychological changes associated with adolescence increase the importance of physical appearance, and having a disfigurement during this period may present particular challenges. Image counts in the dating game, and joining an acceptable social grouping can be difficult if social confidence has been in some way weakened. Harter [48] reported that teenagers who believed their appearance determined their self-worth had lower self-esteem and greater depression than adolescents who believed their self-worth determined their feelings about their appearance.

Nonetheless, indications to surgical treatment should be carefully evaluated when the motivation of patient is doubtful. Treatment decisions made during childhood, adolescence and adulthood can be stressful. Deciding whether or not to undergo appearance-altering surgery may not be easily accepted, and those affected can question any motivation for putting themselves through the associated stress [49] Furthermore, expectations about outcomes may be unrealistic, and can generate disappointment when the aesthetic result becomes apparent. Given the multifaceted nature of surgical adjustment, the prevailing model of care needs to be expanded to offer psychosocial support and intervention as routine adjuncts or alternatives to surgical treatment. Interventions need to be carefully planned to take account of individual physical (e.g. growth) and social issues and the child with a visible difference or disfiguring lesion should receive continuing psychological support, preoperative assessment and follow up during the course of treatment.

Surgical excision with reconstruction, is the mainstay of treatment. If direct closure after complete excision is not possible, reconstruction may include excision with skin grafts, skin flaps, tissue expansion with subsequent flap rotation or full thickness skin grafting, autologous cultured human epithelium, artificial skin replacement, and free tissue transfer after tissue expansion [50, 51, 52] Chemical peels, dermabrasion, and laser treatments are adjunctive treatment choices, that have not been demonstrated to decrease the malignant potential, because of incomplete removal of cells in the treated area. If surgical excision is not feasible, management consists of examination and high-quality photographic documentation for life.

Serial excision of large congenital nevi by skin expansion should preferably start in early months of life, for their malignant potential and for their size, requiring many surgical stages. It is usually addressed at age 6 months, to decrease anesthetic and surgical risks [52, 53, 54]. Attempts to complete the treatment of particularly disfiguring lesions is preferably carried out before age 5, when possible, or at least in the pre-adolescent, to prevent important psychosocial implications linked to the different developmental stages of the child and to parental behavior [55]. The goals of treatment are to remove all or as much as feasible of the CNN and reconstruct the defect, preserving function and maintaining the aesthetic appearance. Each case requires tailoring of the operations to fit the anatomic defect and to respect anatomic units and relaxed skin tension lines when possible. Excision begins in the 6-9 month range, placing procedures 3-6 months apart.

6.2. Surgical techniques

Technical choices vary depending on nevus size and anatomical site and may be challenging in some cases of giant nevi.

General considerations, including anatomical and surgical principles, should be remembered.

Incisions are planned according to the orientation of the relaxed skin tension lines (RSTL) when possible, with attention to the most favorable and less visible site of the resulting scar, especially when the use of skin expanders is required.

A variable amount of subcutaneous tissue should be included in the excision, for its diagnostic value in the rare occasional finding of melanoma in the specimen. This amount is thinner in facial areas, to avoid nerve injuries, but enough to include hair follicles.

6.2.1. Small congenital nevi

Excision of small congenital nevi (diameter ≤1.5 cm) is usually performed with 2 mm margins of normally appearing skin, by simple excision. In special areas, as some parts of the nose, lip, eyelid or ear, serial excision or rotation, advancement or transposition flaps are often necessary.

6.2.2. Medium size congenital nevi

Excision of medium size nevi (diameter >1.5 <19 cm) can be achieved by serial excision or tissue expansion.

Serial excision

The efficacy of serial excision for the treatment of medium size congenital nevi has been reported by different authors [56] and it is the indication of choice when the procedure can be easily planned in 2 stages [57].

In children this indication can be extended to larger lesions, requiring more than 2 stages, when considering the possibility of avoiding morbidity related to tissue expansion, longer operating time of every stage, multiple expanding percutaneous injections and poor compliance by the patient. When surgical planning suggests too many operations to complete the removal of the lesion, tissue expansion should be seriously considered as an alternative.

Techniques of serial excision:

A symmetric, fusiform ellipse is drawn within the lesion, parallel to the RSTLs and the margins are undermined enough to obtain a tension free suture (Fig. 4)

In the subsequent period the surrounding skin is going to stretch and and adapt, releasing tension on the scar. After a minimum of 3 months a second excision is performed to complete nevus removal.

http://dx.doi.org/10.5772/54632

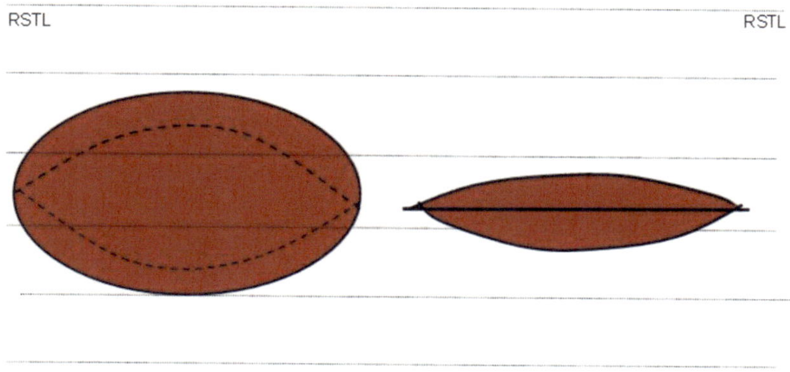

Figure 4. First stage of serial excision with the long axis of the lesion parallel tothe RSTL

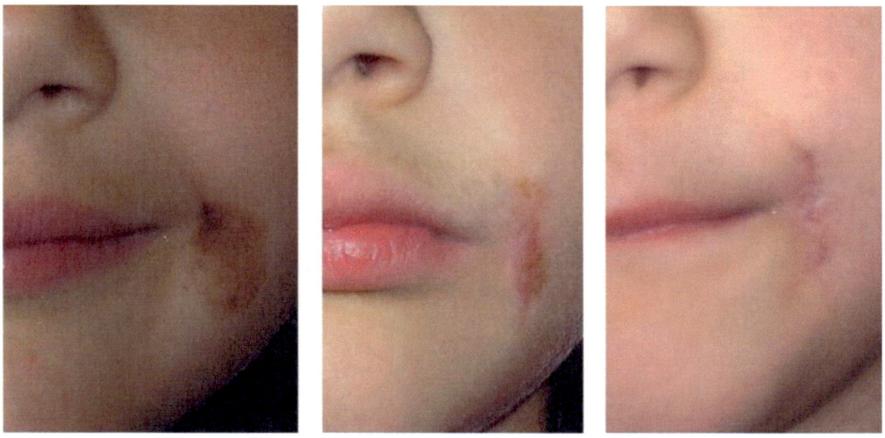

Figure 5. Serial excision of medium size congenital nevus, with final positioning of the scar in the nasogenien crease

When the resulting scar is desired to fall in a crease or for the treatment of particular anatomical sites, as nasal ala, oral commissure, lateral canthus, some modifications may be required. The fusiform excision may be planned to be eccentric and the skin undermined more on one side, to move the tissue in one direction rather than the opposite one. The direction of the prevalent movement can be towards a natural crease, the border of an aesthetic unit or an anatomical area not to be distorted, as nasal ala or oral commissure (Fig.5)

Flap surgery

In difficult anatomical sites and for wider intermediate sized lesions flap surgery is also indicated to obtain excision without tissue loss or distortion. An advancement flap may be used when its incision lines can be drawn along the borders of different aesthetic units. For example, in the case of a round nevus on the lateral aspect of nasal pyramid, incisions of an advancement flap could be outlined on the infraorbital and nasogenien folds to hide scars in

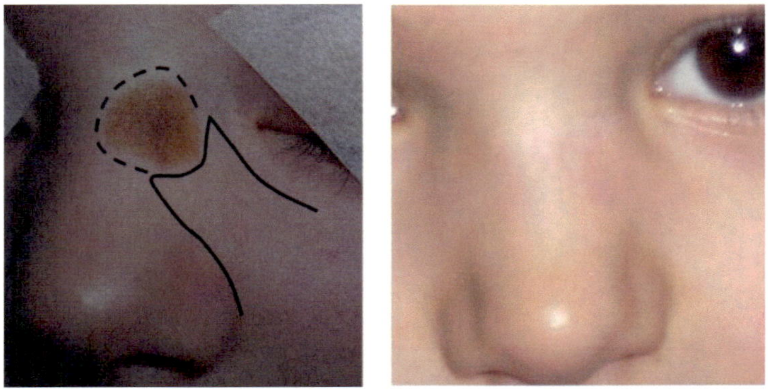

Figure 6. An advancement flap is drawn in the infraorbital area along infraorbital and nasogenien creases.

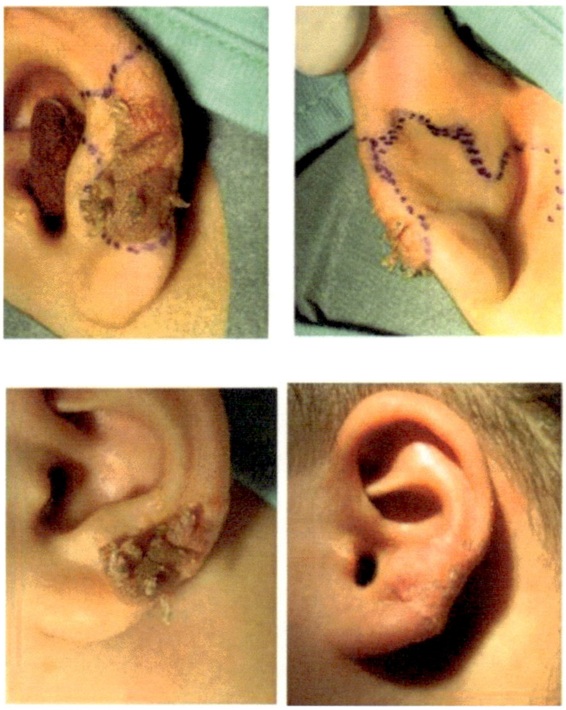

Figure 7. A bilobed flap is transposed from the retroauricular crease.

these creases (Fig.6). On the auricle, due to the adherence of local skin, a sufficient amount of tissue can be obtained from the retroauricular fold by a transposition flap (Fig.7).

6.2.3. Large or giant congenital nevi

Treatment of large or giant congenital melanocytic nevi (CGMN) (diameter>19 cm) always requires multiple surgical stages and complex strategies.

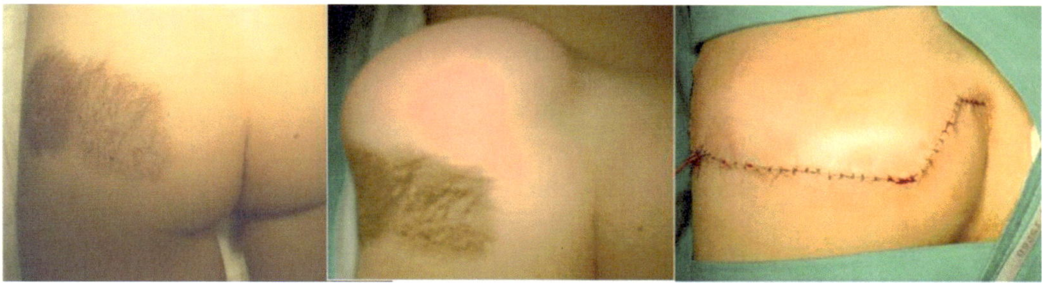

Figure 8. Skin expansion to excise a large congenital nevus of the gluteal region

6.2.4. Tissue expansion technique

Although multistaged direct excision, described elsewhere about medium size nevi, is sometimes feasible for the treatment of large lesions, skin expansion is the treatment of choice and will be discussed in more detail. In general terms, expansion of tissue is used to improve rotation, transposition or advancement of local or regional flaps, or to increase the harvest of full-thickness skin grafts. In adults, aside from their use in breast reconstruction, tissue expanders are used primarily for secondary burn and trauma reconstruction in the head and neck region. In the pediatric population, expanders have been used in a variety of reconstructive procedures. The most common indication in children is to reconstruct defects left by excision of giant congenital nevi (Fig.8).

Tissue expansion is contraindicated in infected skin. Although expansion is possible in radiated or scarred tissue, it is associated with a much higher complication rate and should be avoided whenever possible.

Surgical technique of skin expansion relies on the ability of skin and soft tissues to grow by generation of new tissue in response to tension. Tensive impulse is generated by implanting a subcutaneous device (expander) that is inflated over a period of weeks; new tissue is generated in response to the constant stretch caused by the progressive inflation. An increase in skin surface area after expansion is due to generation of new tissue rather than the stretching of existing skin, as supported by numerous studies. Fibroblast and epidermal hyperplasia induced by mechanical stress have been observed in culture. Histological response to expansion is similar in adult and pediatric skin. Within 1-3 weeks of expansion, the epidermis begins to thicken and the dermis thins while skin appendages do not change. The subcutaneous fat atrophy. Cellular proliferation reduces the resting tension of the skin over time, enabling further expansion to take place. Once the process is complete, the expanded skin eventually returns to its baseline thickness. The vessels of the skin and subcutaneous tissue also resume their pre-expanded size and number [58, 59].

Expanders are available in a variety of shapes and sizes, and there is no absolute ideal expander for a given site or condition. Expanders have different types of filling ports. These can be internal to the expander or remote and connected by a tube of various length, that is usually adjustable by the surgeon. Most experienced surgeons recommend using remote ports. These should be placed away from the expander. Internal ports have both a higher failure rate and a greater incidence of accidental expander rupture. In children, the use of internal ports is associated with a higher rate of exposure of the expander due to the pressure exerted on the skin by the port. As a rule, expansion proceeds best when the expander rests on a firm base like the ribs or skull. When placed within the abdominal wall, for example, expansion tends to be tess predictable. The incisions for expander placement and the remote port should be placed where they will not interfere with later advancement or compromise the blood supply to the expanded tissue. If possible the incisions for expander placement are placed in the proposed area to be excised. Incisions are never placed parallel to the edges of the expander. This creates a situation that increases implant exposure, additional scar tissue outside the lesion, possible stretching of the scar and a delay in inflation of expander. Incisions should be radial or almost perpendicular to the expander or in the form of a V or W

The broad base of the V or W should be directed toward the expander, thus facilitating implant insertion and inflation because the lines of tension are perpendicular to the wound. The open end of the V should be at least 2 to 3 cm from the pocket to accommodate expansion. In addition, a sigma (lazy S) incision can also be beneficial in instances where partial excision of some of the lesion might be helpful during the insertion phase. By this approach, partial excision can be done while an expander is placed. Once the wounds heal, the expander can then be inflated without worry because the end of the incision is almost radial to the expansion process [60]. The expander should be placed on top of the deep fascia (or subgaleal in the scalp), unless the plan is to incorporate muscle into the expanded flap. The pocket should always be larger than the base diameter of the expander. Blunt dissection in a single fascial plane is safest for preserving blood supply. Filling the expanders intraoperatively with sufficient saline to eliminate dead space can prevent postoperative bleeding and hematoma. An alternative to traditional prolonged expansion is immediate intraoperative expansion combined with broad undermining of the defect. In rapid expansion, the skin initially expands due to its elasticity and the displacement of interstitial fluid. Within minutes, the alignment of the collagen fibers changes due to the stretch. This process yields up to 20% more tissue for flap coverage. Intraoperative expansion is indicated for relatively small defects, such as in coverage of defects of the ear.

The rate of inflation is variable and largely based on surgeon preference. Patient comfort and signs of tissue perfusion, such as tension, color, and capillary refill, guide the filling rate. Filling is usually initiated 7-10 days postoperatively and performed once or twice a week, based on the above mentioned criteria and patient tolerance. The rate of expansion depends both on the body site as well as patient factors. Some skin is more amenable to expansion, and some patients can tolerate the discomfort better than others [61]. Tissue expansion should continue until the expanded area is larger than the defect, usually up to 2 months. As a general rule, the diameter of the expanded flap should be 2-3 times the diameter of the skin that is to be excised

Most surgeons overinflate tissue expanders beyond the manufacturer's recommended maximum capacity. Studies have demonstrated that significant overinflation is possible before weakening or rupturing.

The use of rotation and transposition flaps enables the transfer of tension from the tip of the flap more proximally to its base. A single or double back-cut can be performed prior to inset in order to gain extra length. The donor site should be closed in layers after the implant capsule is excised.

Scalp. Although tissue expansion does not increase the number of hair follicles, the size of the hair-bearing region can be doubled without a noticeable decrease in hair density. As such, tissue expansion may be used to reconstruct the scalp when removal of a medium or large nevus is needed. Expanders are most commonly placed in the occipital or posterior parietal regions. They are placed under the galea, superficial to the periosteum. It usually requires up to 12 weeks to complete the expansion in children. Radial scoring of the galea at the time of surgery can facilitate the process. Once the expansion is complete, flaps are advanced or transposed, based on named arteries of the scalp. It is important to orient flaps so that the correct direction of hair growth is maintained. Although galeal scoring or capuslotomy incisions can be useful, wide undermining is a safer method of recruiting tissue.

Forehead. The brow position is the most important structure to preserve during forehead expansion. When possible, two or more expanders are used with incisions hidden within the hairline.

Midforehead nevi are best treated using an expansion of bilateral normal forehead segments and medial advancement of the flaps, placing scars along the brow and at or posterior to the hairline. Hemiforehead nevi often require serial expansion of the uninvolved area of the forehead to reduce the need for a back-cut. Nevi of the supraorbital and temporal forehead can be treated with a transposition of the expanded normal skin medial to the nevus. When the temporal scalp is minimally involved with nevus, the parietal scalp can be expanded and advanced to create the new hairline. When the temporoparietal scalp is also involved with nevus, a combined advancement and transposition flap provides the proper hair direction for the temporal hairline and allows significantly greater movement of the expanded flap. Once the brow is significantly elevated on either the ipsilateral or contralateral side from the reconstruction, it can only be returned to the preoperative position with the interposition of additional, non–hair-bearing forehead skin. The largest expander possible beneath the uninvolved forehead skin should always be used, occasionally even carrying the expander under the lesion [62].

Face and Neck. The skin of the neck and face is relatively thin. Therefore, multiple expanders with smaller volumes are preferable to a single large expander. In general, however, a single larger expander is preferable to several smaller expanders. Careful planning is essential in determining where to place the expanders, and where incisions should be located in order to preserve aesthetic units, facial symmetry and matching skin color and to avoid distortion of the eyelids and oral commissure. The expander is usually placed above the platysma muscle to avoid risk of facial nerve injury and to keep the flap from being excessively bulky. The expanded flaps are positioned by advancement, rotation, or transposition. Incisions should be placed in skin creases such as the nasolabial fold or along the margins of aesthetic units. Expanding the hairless skin adjacent to the mastoid region can increase the available tissue for reconstructive procedures of the ear. The skin above the clavicle can be expanded to provide full-thickness skin grafts to the face.

Trunk. Unlike the head and neck, there are very few critical landmarks on the trunk that must be preserved. Aside from the breast and nipple-areola complex, distortion of the skin and soft tissues of the trunk is well-tolerated. For defects requiring excision, multiple expanders surrounding the defect are often employed. Expanders can also be used to expand the skin of the abdomen for use as a donor site of full-thickness skin grafts.

Extremities. Tissue expansion in the extremities has been reported to have a higher complication rate, in comparison to other regions and therefore, especially in children, should not be a first choice. Blood supply and drainage of the extremities is inferior to that of the trunk and head. This predisposes limbs, especially below the knee, to an increased rate of wound complications such as infection, dehiscence and prosthesis extrusion. Multiple expanders are usually required in the extremites.

Complications. Among all patients, the major complication rate is about 10% and includes implant exposure, deflation, and wound dehiscence. Minor complications also occur in about 10% of patients. These include filling port problems, seroma, hematoma, infection and delayed healing.

Patients under the age of 7 have the highest risk of complications. One explanation for this is that young children are more prone to expander rupture due to external pressure on the expanded skin. Expansion in the extremities caries twice the risk of complication compared to other regions. The use of tissue expansion in congenital nevi has a 5-7% complication rate. Tissue that has undergone serial expansion (two or more prior expansions) is at a higher risk for a major complication.

7. Surgery of primary melanoma

Pediatric melanoma is rare but increasing in incidence [63] limited options are possible for treatment. Early diagnosis and surgical management are the cornerstone of therapy and must adhere to the guidelines estabilished by the American Joint Committee on Cancer (AJCC) [64] Diagnosis of melanoma in children is more difficult than in adults, it relates to a number of variables, so many criteria used in adults are of limited value, for example the natural evolution of congenital and acquired nevi during childhood and adolescence [65] Historically, a wide excision with 5-cm margins with regional lymph node dissection was recommended for all melanomas. This indication, dating back 1907, was based on evaluations following a single necropsy, on a patient with advanced melanoma, assuming that in this way, all possible neoplastic foci would have been eliminated.

Furthermore, the indications suggested to extend the excision below the fascia, so as to also remove the superficial vascular and lymphatic structures.

This attitude has remained unchanged, until Breslow and Match described the treatment of melanoma with narrow margins [66]

Once decided to remove a suspicious lesion, it is recommended to perform a 1- to 2-mm circumferential margin. There are no prospective data to provide an evidence-based approach in this setting.

It has long been suggested that malignant cells may be shed into the bloodstream during any given surgical procedure for cancer. While there is no evidence to suggest that an incisional biopsy does cause local spread of melanoma, it is generally not advocated. [67]

There may be times that the incision is to big that the tissue are not able to cover the skin defect, in this case is possible to use a skin graft, or in order to avoid a graft, the surgical defect may be closed using a rotational or advancement flap

The orientation of the incision should follow the relaxed skin tension lines (RSTLs, also known as lines of Langer), however, at the level of the limbs incisions parallel to the major axis of the limb are used, not to alter the paths of lymphatic drainage.

In the setting of dysplastic changes or once the diagnosis of melanoma is established, in children, surgical excision should be performed with the same excision margins recommended for adults by the National Comprehensive Cancer Network (NCCN) in 2007, and depends on the Breslow depth of the primary lesion, Clark's level of tumor invasion may provide additional prognostic value for thin melanomas [68].

The basic oncologic criteria of surgery are: the resection margins and the depth of the skin excision.

When there is an in situ melanoma, excision should include 0,5 centimeter of normal skin surronding the tumor and takes off the skin layers down to the fat; in removing an invasive melanoma that is 2 mm thick the margins are extended to 1 cm and the excision goes through all skin layers and down to the fascia; margins are 2 cm for lesions greater than 2 mm in thickness. [69]

The depth of excision can reach muscolaris fascia, whose removal has no oncological meaning, furthermore the preservation of the fascia allows a better aesthetic result.

An exception is the localization to the face, in these cases also with melanomas more than 4 mm thick margins of 1 cm are used.

In recent years, great importance was served to sentinel lymph node biopsy (SLNB) for the detection of lymph node metastases, in fact in adult melanoma therapy, it has become a mandatory procedure in the current AJCC staging system; however its use in the pediatric population has been limited.

Lymph node are the most common site of initial metastases [70], the lack of disease in the sentinel lymph node should indicate the lack of dissemination.

SLNB will select, with a minimally invasive technique, patients who should undergo regional lymph node dissection for clinically occult loco-regional metastases, so as to avoid completion lymph node dissection if the sentinel node is negative.

SLNB was first described by Morton et al. in 1992 [71] The procedure is usually performed concurrent with re-excision of the primary lesion, and is advised for lesions thicker than 1 mm or for those between 0,76 mm and 1 mm with ulceration or reticular dermal invasion.

The procedure involves injection of the primary cutaneous lesion site with technectium-99m sulfur colloid followed by lymphoscintigraphy in the nuclear medicine suite. This is done on the morning of scheduled re-excision, and the patient is brought to the operating room in the afternoon. The lesion is injected with approximately 1 ml of 1% isosulfan blue dye. The dye is allowed to travel through lymphatics for several minutes, and a hand held gamma counter is used to determine the area of maximal radiolabeled tracer intensity for lymph node sampling. An incision is made over the area identified to have the most active uptake of radiolabeled tracer as determined by the handled gamma probe and the preoperative lymphoscintigraphy. Upon examination of the draining lymph node basin, all nodes that are blue, palpable, or show significant activity with the gamma probe are excised and sent fresh to pathology [72].

The incision must be oriented so as to allow an eventual loco-regional lymphadenectomy, the lymph node is identified with the gamma camera and visually with the blue dye; the lymph node is removed after ligation of the afferent and efferent lymphatic vessels, after the removal it is necessary to evaluate "ex vivo" the radioactivity of the lymph node and the possible presence of other involved nodes.

A small lymphocele may result in postoperative period, usually with the possibility of spontaneous regression.

Elective regional lymph node dissection is subsequently performed if the result of the SLNB is positive for metastases [38].

8. Treatment of metastatic disease

8.1. Congenital melanoma and transplacental metastases

Congenital melanoma as a result of placental transmission from a mother with metastatic melanoma is extremely rare, with only a few cases described in literature [73, 74, 75, 76, 77]

To date, metastatic disease transmission from fetus to mother has never been reported. [78, 79]

8.2. Lymph node metastases

8.2.1. Staging

After primary surgery and diagnosis of melanoma, staging of the disease is completed by pathologic detection of lymphatic involvement. Comprehensive staging guidelines for paediatric and adolescent melanoma have not been clearly established.

The American Joint Committee on Cancer (AJCC) provides a reproducible model on the natural history of melanoma and a detailed description of important prognostic variables. For localised disease, ulceration has been recognized as an important predictor of outcome and growing consideration is given to the significance of melanoma thickness. New importance has been recognized to the number of lymph nodes involved, the significance of in-transit or satellite metastases, the description of the sites of metastases and the prognostic value of serum lactic dehydrogenase [23].

Future trials including paediatric and adolescent melanoma patients should incorporate this new staging system to achieve a wider interpretation of results from institutions and patient populations. In addition, the routine use of sentinel node biopsy for the staging of paediatric and adolescent melanoma is mandatory, in order to determine the prognostic and therapeutic value of this procedure in young patients and to compare these results with those reported in the adult literature [80]

Although in adult patients the routine use of chest and abdomen computed tomography is not recommended in literature, in paediatric patients it has been found useful in about 25% of cases to identify clinically undetectable metastases from thick localised melanomas or patients with melanoma arising at an unknown primary site [81, 82]

The routine use of magnetic resonance imaging (MRI) to detect brain metastases is not advocated. For localised lesions under 1.5mm thick, investigations include a complete blood count, serum chemistries including liver function tests, and a chest radiograph.

Positron emission tomography (PET) is a very useful tool in adults, but its use in paediatric patients has not been validated [23]

8.2.2. Sentinel lymph nodes

Early primary excision of melanoma is the mainstay of definitive treatment of the tumour. With the introduction of sentinel lymph node biopsy (SLNB) the treatment of patients with melanoma has been revolutioned.

The adoption of SLNB has led to selection of patients who do not need elective lymph node dissection (ELND) and in which the morbidity linked to this procedure can be avoided. The techniques of preoperative lymphoscintigraphy and sentinel lymph node (SLN) biopsy have become the standard of care for staging adult patients after detection of a primary melanoma. SLNB is particularly important in intermediate-thickness (1.2-3.5 mm) primary melanomas in order to indicate elective lymphadenectomy and has also a prognostic value [83]. SLNB is a very promising technique also in paediatric patients [84, 85, 86]. However, due to paucity of available data, the role of SLNB in paediatric patients is still debated, as concerns both its prognostic [87] and therapeutic implications.

SLN biopsy should be included in the surgical management of children. The indications for SLN biopsy in paediatric and adolescent patients are based on the adult literature and include the presence of lesions thicker than 1 mm, the presence of ulceration or a Clark's level of invasion of IV or V in patients with lesion thickness of less than 1 mm. The technique is the same as in adults. Excision with 2 mm margins of normal skin is performed. After diagnosis of melanoma, the patient undergoes SLNB for tumour thickness ≥ 1 mm followed by wide excision of the tumour site with 2 cm margins and primary closure or skin graft. SLNB is performed using preoperative lymphoscintigraphy, intraoperative blue dye injection around the site of excision and hand-held gamma probe for radio-localization [38,88]. One day before the operation, between 18.5 and 40 MBq of Tc-99m microcolloid is injected intradermally around the scar. The drainage of the colloid is localized by detecting radiation, and the location of the SLN is marked on the skin. The position of the SLN is confirmed with a handheld gamma probe before starting the operation. At the author's center the procedure is performed under epidural anaesthesia and sedation or general anaesthesia. As reported by some authors, subcutaneous infusion anaesthesia (SIA) can be useful [89]. Patent blue is additionally injected intradermally around the scar as standard procedure. Sentinel lymph node biopsy is then accomplished with the help of repeated measurements with the handheld gamma probe. The SLN(s) is (are) removed, and the wound is closed.

A comparison between adults and patients younger than 21 years who underwent either lymph node dissection or SLNB showed a higher rate of lymph node metastasis in the paediatric age (44%) as compared to the adult (23.9%). However this finding had no statistical significance. In this series, paediatric patients either with Stage I or Stage II disease showed a 94.4% 10-year survival, while patients with Stage III melanoma had a 60.1% 10-year survival [90]

Recent data show that although the SLNB positivity rate is higher in paediatric and adolescent melanoma patients than in adults, non SLNB positivity and melanoma specific death rate are low [91]

8.2.3. Regional lymph nodes

In case of positive SLNB many surgeons would proceed to a completion lymph node dissection (CLND),

however survival advantage of this procedure is unclear, and is currently being investigated [92, 93, 94]

In a large series of paediatric melanoma cases 18 patients underwent SNLB, and 7 proceeded to undergo CLND because of findings of metastatic disease to the SLN; two of these had tumour-positive lymph nodes on pathologic analysis of the CLND specimen.

Similarly, the presence of metastases in regional lymph nodes after CLND has been diagnosed in 1 of 3 patients by some authors and in 1 of 4 patients by others [38, 92]

8.2.4. Adjuvant therapy

Consideration of systemic therapy after regional lymph nodes involvement by melanoma cells is under investigation. Treatment plans for children must be extrapolated from adult studies.

Interferon alfa-2b is currently used for adjuvant therapy in high-risk melanoma after surgery in adult patients and can also be used in paediatric melanoma patients with acceptable toxicity [95]

8.3. Distant metastases

The incidence of metastatic melanoma has increased over the last three decades, and the death rate continues to climb faster than that of most other cancers. According to the American Cancer Society, there were approximately 68,000 new cases of melanoma in the United States in 2009, and 8,700 melanoma-related deaths. Melanoma is difficult to treat once it has spread beyond the skin to other parts of the body (metastasized). Very few treatment options exist for people with metastatic melanoma.

8.3.1. Treatment of disseminated disease

Most reports describing the treatment of paediatric melanoma are from single institutions in which diagnostic criteria, staging and pathological evaluation of the primary tumour have varied significantly. Dacarbazine, which is the most active agent in adult melanoma, showed encouraging activity in four children with melanoma treated between 1975 and 1984 [96] Other traditional chemotherapeutic regimens have shown some efficacy in metastatic melanoma [23]. The availability of investigational therapies, such as interleukin-2, interferon alfa-2b and vaccines, has been generally restricted to patients who are older than 18 years of age and no prospective trials in adolescents have been performed. Collaborative efforts, now under discussion between paediatric and adult cooperative groups, should help facilitate the enrollment of younger patients onto trials that use experimental therapies.

8.3.2. Radiotherapy

Radiotherapy is rarely indicated in the management of primary paediatric melanoma. However, it should be considered in patients with head and neck melanomas at high risk for parotid or cervical metastases and in those who develop brain metastases. Brain metastases have been reported to occur during the course of the disease in up to 18% of children with melanoma [23]. Ultimately, as in adults, there is no effective therapy for metastatic melanoma in children. Therefore, the main focus of the parent, the paediatrician, and the dermatologist should be risk reduction and early detection of melanoma. The former consists primarily of avoiding intense sunlight exposure, using protective clothing and broad-spectrum sunblock, and educating children. Early detection requires a high index of clinical suspicion, especially by the paediatrician, who sees children with much more regularity than a dermatologist, of any rapidly growing or otherwise atypical pigmented lesion. In addition, the physician should recognize the elevated risk of any child with a family history of melanoma, GCMN, or dysplastic nevi. Again, prevention and early clinical diagnosis are the only current effective cure for cutaneous melanoma [97].

8.4. Prognosis

The outcome for children and adolescents with melanoma also appears to be similar to that reported for adults and is dependent on the initial stage of the tumour. Patients with localised disease have an excellent outcome, whereas those with nodal and distant metastases have estimated 10-year survivals of only 60 and 25%, respectively. Outcome is also stage-dependent and the thickness of the primary lesion correlates with the risk of nodal involvement and subsequent disease recurrence [23]

Melanomas arising on congenital nevi seem to have a better prognosis if they arise during early infancy than in childhood; moreover, metastatic melanoma associated with giant nevi have a worse prognosis than those associated with other skin lesions [32]

Melanoma has also reported to be more frequently metastatic in young children than in adolescents.This can be due to several causative factors but can also reflect a true biologic difference [98, 99]. There were significant differences in baseline characteristics of young children (age < 10 years) compared with adolescents and young adults: the former were more likely to be non-white, to have metastases, to have nodular or other histology, head, face, or neck primaries, thicker lesions and history of cancer.

Multivariate analysis for melanoma survival in children showed significantly worse survival for males, patients with regional or unstaged disease, nodular histology, increasing thickness of the primary tumor, primary disease in the head, face, neck, eye, orbit, central nervous system, genitals, or overlapping sites, earlier year of diagnosis and previous cancer. Five-year melanoma-specific survival for pediatric cases (age < 20 years) was 100% for in situ disease, 96.1% for localized disease, 77.2% for regional disease and 57.3% for distant disease. Five-year overall survival was 88.9% for young children (age < 10 years), 91.5% for adolescents (age 10 to 19 years) and 90.9% for young adults, but the latter data had not statistical significance [100]. Recent data confirm that paediatric melanoma patients in younger ages have an increased risk of lymph node metastasis and thicker tumors. This suggests that the younger paediatric patients may have a disease that differs biologically from that of the older ones [101].

Author details

Andrea Zangari[1], Federico Zangari[2], Mercedes Romano[2], Elisabetta Cerigioni[2], Maria Giovanna Grella[3], Anna Chiara Contini[3] and Martino Ascanio[2]

1 Pediatric Surgery Department San Camillo Hospital, Roma, Italy

2 Pediatric Surgery Department, University Hospital of Ancona, Italy

3 Catholic University of the Sacred Heart, Roma, Italy

References

[1] Clemmensen, O. J, & Kroon, S. The histology of "congenital features" in early acquired melanocytic nevi. *J Am Acad Dermatol*. Oct (1988). , 19(4), 742-6.

[2] Krengel, S, Hauschild, A, & Schafer, T. Melanoma risk in congenital melanocytic naevi: a systematic review. *Br J Dermatol*. Jul (2006). , 155(1), 1-8.

[3] Ansarin, H, Soltani-arabshahi, R, Mehregan, D, Shayanfar, N, & Soltanzadeh, P. Giant congenital melanocytic nevus with neurofibroma-like changes and spina bifida occulta. *Int J Dermatol*. Nov (2006). , 45(11), 1347-50.

[4] Cruz, M. A, Cho, E. S, Schwartz, R. A, & Janniger, C. K. Congenital neurocutaneous melanosis. *Cutis*. Oct (1997). , 60(4), 178-81.

[5] Silfen, R, Skoll, P. J, & Hudson, D. A. Congenital giant hairy nevi and neurofibromatosis: the significance of their common origin. *Plast Reconstr Surg*. Oct (2002). , 110(5), 1364-5.

[6] Cramer, S. F. The melanocytic differentiation pathway in congenital melanocytic nevi: theoretical considerations. *Pediatr Pathol*. (1988). , 8(3), 253-65.

[7] Kinsler, V. A, Abu-amero, S, Budd, P, Jackson, I. J, Ring, S. M, Northstone, K, et al. Germline Melanocortin-Receptor Genotype Is Associated with Severity of Cutaneous Phenotype in Congenital Melanocytic Nevi: A Role for MC1R in Human Fetal Development. *J Invest Dermatol*. May 10 (2012). , 1.

[8] Kadonaga, J. N, & Frieden, I. J. Neurocutaneous melanosis: definition and review of the literature. *J Am Acad Dermatol*. May (1991). Pt 1):747-55.

[9] Bousema, M. T, et al. Non-von Recklingausen's resembling a giant pigmented nevus. *J Am Acad Dermatol 20:358, 1989*

[10] Everett, M. A. Histopathology of congenital pigmented nevi. *Am J Dermatopathol*. Feb (1989). , 11(1), 11-2.

[11] Fitzpatrick, s, et al. Dermatology in General Medicine. Vol. I: 1028, (1999).

[12] Fitzpatrick, s, et al. Dermatology in General Medicine. Vol. I: 1030, (1999).

[13] Wu, P. A, Mancini, A. J, Marghoob, A. A, & Frieden, I. J. Simultaneous occurrence of infantile hemangioma and congenital melanocytic nevus: Coincidence or real association?. *J Am Acad Dermatol*. Feb (2008). Suppl):S , 16-22.

[14] Changchien, L, Dusza, S. W, Agero, A. L, et al. Age- and site-specific variation in the dermoscopic patterns of congenital melanocytic nevi: an aid to accurate classification and assessment of melanocytic nevi. *Arch Dermatol*. Aug (2007). , 143(8), 1007-14.

[15] Hale, E. K, Stein, J, Ben-porat, L, et al. Association of melanoma and neurocutaneous melanocytosis with large congenital melanocytic naevi--results from the NYU-LCMN registry. *Br J Dermatol*. Mar (2005). , 152(3), 512-7.

[16] Fitzpatrick, s, et al. Dermatology in General Medicine. Vol. I: 1034, (1999).

[17] Fitzpatrick, s, et al. Dermatology in General Medicine. Vol. I: 1018-1025, (1999).

[18] Fitzpatrick, s, et al. Dermatology in General Medicine. Vol. I: 1037-1041, (1999).

[19] Rigel, D. S, et al. The incidence of malignant melanoma in the United States:Issues As we approach the 21st century. *J Am Acad Dermatol* 34:839, (1996).

[20] Cosary, C. L, et al. SEER Cancer Statistics Review, 1973-1992: National Cancer Institute, NRH Pub. Bethesda, Maryland, (1995). (96-2789), 96-2789.

[21] Ries, L, Eisner, M, Kosary, C, et al. SEER Cancer Statistics Review Bethesda, MD, National Cancer Institute, (2004). http://seer.cancer.gov/csr/1975_2001/ , 1975-2000.

[22] Pappo, A. S. Ries LAG, Herzog C, et al: Malignant melanoma in the first three decades of life: A report from the U.S. Surveillance, Epidemiology and End Results (SEER) program. 23:721, (2004). abstr 7557)

[23] Pappo AS: Melanoma in children and adolescentsEur J Cancer 39:2651-2661, (2003).

[24] Kraemer, K. H, Lee, M. M, Andrews, A. D, et al. The role of sunlight and DNA repair in melanoma and nonmelanoma skin cancer: The xeroderma pigmentosum paradigm. Arch Dermatol 130:1018-1021, (1994).

[25] Tucker, M. A. Goldstein AM: Melanoma etiology: Where are we? Oncogene , 22, 3042-3052.

[26] Whiteman, D. C, Valery, P, Mcwhirter, W, et al. Risk factors for childhood melanoma in Queensland, Australia. Int J Cancer 70:26-31, (1997).

[27] Ahmed I: Malignant Melanoma: Prognostic IndicatorsMayo Clin Proc 72:356-361, (1997).

[28] Kaskel, P, Sander, S, Kron, M, et al. Outdoor activities in childhood: A protective factor for cutaneous melanoma? Results of a case-control study in 271 matched pairs. Br J Dermatol 145:602-609, (2001).

[29] Saenz, N. C, Saenz-badillos, J, Busam, K, et al. Childhood melanoma survival. Cancer 85:750-754, (1999).

[30] Milton, G. W, Shaw, H. M, Thompson, J. F, et al. Cutaneous melanoma in childhood: Incidence and prognosis. Australas J Dermatol 38:SS48, (1997). suppl 1), 44.

[31] Fears, T. R, Bird, C. C, Guerry, D I. V, et al. Average midrange ultraviolet radiation flux and time outdoors predict melanoma risk. Cancer Res , 62, 3992-3996.

[32] Tannous, Z. S. Mihm Jr MC, Sober AJ, et al Congenital melanocitic nevi: clinical and istopathologic features, risk of melanoma, and clinical management. J Am Acad Dermatol (2005). , 52(2), 197-203.

[33] Michel, J. L, Chalencon, F, Gentil-perret, A, et al. Congenital pigmented nevus: prognosis and therapeutic possibilities. Arch Pediatr (1999). , 6(2), 211-7.

[34] Ruiz-maldonado, R, Tamayo, L, Laterza, A. M, et al. Giant pigmented naevi: clinical histopatologic and therapeutic considerations. J Pediatr (1992).

[35] Zaal, L. H, & Mooi, W. J. Sillevis Smith JH, et al. Classification of congenital melanocytic naevi and malignant transformation: a review of the literature. Br J Plast Surg (2004). , 57(8), 707-19.

[36] Yesudian, P. D. Parslew RAG. A guide to the management of pigmented skin naevi in children. Curr Paediatr (2003). , 13, 407-12.

[37] Saenz, N. C, Saenz-badillos, J, Busam, K, et al. Childhood melanoma survival. Cancer (1999). , 85, 750-4.

[38] Zangari, A, Bernardini, M. L, Tallarico, R, Ilari, M, Giangiacomi, M, & Offidani, A. M. Martino A: Indications for excision of nevi and melanoma diagnosed in a pediatric surgical unit. J Pediatr Surg. (2007). Aug; , 42(8), 1412-6.

[39] Gelbard, S. N, Tripp, J. M, Marghoob, A. A, et al. Management of Spitz nevi: a survey of dermatologists in the United States. J Am Acad Dermatol (2002). , 47(2), 224-30.

[40] Dyon GCTMSnels MD, Elysèe TM, et al. Risk of cutaneous malignant melanoma in patients with nonfamilial atypical nevi from a pigmented lesions clinic. Leiden, The Netherlands. J Am Acad Dermatol (1999). , 40, 686-93.

[41] Zaal, L. H, Mooi, W. J, Klip, H, et al. Risk of malignant transformation of congenital melanocytic nevi: a retrospective nationwide study from The Netherlands. *Plast Reconstr Surg*. Dec (2005). , 116(7), 1902-9.

[42] Rhodes, A. R, & Melski, J. W. Small congenital nevocellular nevi and the risk of cutaneous melanoma. *J Pediatr*. Feb (1982). , 100(2), 219-24.

[43] Sahin, S, Levin, L, Kopf, A. W, et al. Risk of melanoma in medium-sized congenital melanocytic nevi: a follow-up study. J Am Acad Dermatol. Sep (1998). , 39(3), 428-33.

[44] Kearney-cooke, A. (2002). Familial influences on body image development. In T. F. Cash & T. Pruzinsky (Eds.), Body image: A handbook of theory, and clinical practice (New York: Guilford., 99-107.

[45] Bradbury, E. (1997). Understanding the problems. In R. Lansdown, N. Rumsey, E. Bradbury, A. Carr, & J. Partridge (Eds.), Visibly different: Coping with disfigurement (Oxford: Butterworth-Heinemann., 180-193.

[46] Turner, S, Thomas, P, Dowell, T, Rumsey, N, & Sandy, J. (1997). Psychological outcomes amongst cleft patients and their families. British Journal of Plastic Surgery, , 50, 1-9.

[47] Gilbert, S, & Thompson, J. (2002). Body shame in childhood & adolescence. In P. Gilbert & J. Miles (Eds.), Body Shame (Hove: Brunner-Routledge., 55-74.

[48] Harter, S. (1999). *The construction of the self: A developmental perspective*. New York: Guilford.

[49] Hearst, D, & Middleton, J. (1997). Psychological intervention and models of current working practice. In R. Lansdown, N. Rumsey, E. Bradbury, A. Carr, & J. Partridge (Eds.), *Visibly different: Coping with disfigurement* (Oxford: Butterworth-Heinemann., 158-171.

[50] Bauer, B. S, & Corcoran, J. Treatment of large and giant nevi. *Clin Plast Surg*. Jan (2005). vii., 32(1), 11-8.

[51] Margulis, A, Bauer, B. S, & Fine, N. A. Large and giant congenital pigmented nevi of the upper extremity: an algorithm to surgical management. *Ann Plast Surg*. Feb (2004). , 52(2), 158-67.

[52] Arneja, J. S, & Gosain, A. K. Giant congenital melanocytic nevi. *Plast Reconstr Surg*. Aug (2007). e-40e.

[53] Bauer, B. S, & Corcoran, J. Treatment of large and giant nevi. *Clin Plast Surg*. Jan (2005). vii., 32(1), 11-8.

[54] Pearson, G. D, Goodman, M, & Sadove, A. M. Congenital nevus: the Indiana University's approach to treatment. *J Craniofac Surg*. Sep (2005). , 16(5), 915-20.

[55] Rumsey, N, & Harcourt, D. Body image and disfigurement: issues and interventions. Body Image (2004). , 1(2004), 83-97.

[56] Vinod K JainMahendra K Singhi, and Rajiv Goyal: Serial Excision of Congenital Melanocytic Nevi. J Cutan Aesthet Surg. (2008). January; , 1(1), 17-18.

[57] Gosain, A. K, Santoro, T. D, & Larson, D. L. Gingrass RP Giant congenital nevi: a 20-year experience and an algorithm for their management. Plast Reconstr Surg. (2001). Sep 1; , 108(3), 622-36.

[58] Pasyk, K. A, Argenta, L. C, & Hassett, C. Quantitative analysis of the thickness of human skin and subcutaneous tissue following controlled expansion with a silicone implant. Plast Reconstr Surg. Apr (1988). , 81(4), 516-23.

[59] Timothy, M. Johnson, Md Lori Lowe, Md Marc D. Brown, Md Michael J. Sullivan, Md Bruce R. Nelson, Md: Histology and Physiology of Tissue Expansion. J Dermatol Surg Oncol (1993). , 19, 1074-1078.

[60] Chao, J. J, Longaker, M. T, & Zide, B. M. Expanding horizons in head and neck expansion. Copyright (1998). by W.B. Saunders Company

[61] Farhad HafeziBijan Naghibzadeh, Mohammad Pegahmehr, Amirhossein Nouhi: Use of overinflated tissue expanders in the surgical repair of head and neck scars Journal of Plastic, Reconstructive & Aesthetic Surgery ((2008). xx, 1e8

[62] BauerBruce S. M.D.; Few, Julius W. M.D.; Chavez, C. D. M.D., and; Galiano, R. D. B.A.: The Role of Tissue Expansion in the Management of Large Congenital Pigment-

ed Nevi of the Forehead in the Pediatric Patient. Plastic & Reconstructive Surgery: March (2001). Articles(3-pp), 668-675.

[63] Lange, J. R, Palis, B. E, Chang, D. C, Soong, S-J, & Balch, C. M. melanoma in children and teenagers: an analysis of patients from the national cancer data base. J Clin Oncol (2007). , 25(11), 2007-1363.

[64] Balch, C. M, Buzaid, A. C, Soong, S-J, Atkins, M. B, & Cascinelli, N. et alii Final Version of the American Joint Committee on Cancer Staging System for Cutaneous Melanoma. J Clin Oncol, 19, (16) (2001).

[65] Huynh, P. M, Grant-kels, J. M, & Grin, C. M. Childhood melanoma: update and treatment. Int J Dermatol (2005).

[66] Eedy, D. J. Surgical treatment of melanoma. Brit J Dermatol 149, (2003).

[67] Swanson, N. A. Lee Kl, Gorman A, Lee HN. Biopsy techniques: diagnosis of melanoma. Dermatol Clin 20, (2002).

[68] NCCNNCCN clinical practice guidelines in oncology: melanoma (Washington, DC: NCCN (2008). , 2

[69] Swetter, S. M. Malignant melanoma. eMedicine.com, Inc.(2004).

[70] Faries, M. B, & Morton, D. L. Surgery and sentinel lymph node biopsy. Semin Oncol (2007). December; , 34(6), 498-508.

[71] Morton, D. L, Wen, D. R, & Wong, J. H. Technical details of intraoperative lymphatic mapping for early stage melanoma. Arch Surg (1992). , 127, 392-399.

[72] Downard, C. D, Rapkin, L. B, & Gow, K. W. Melanoma in children and adolescents. Surgical Oncol ((2007).

[73] Wiggins, C. L, Berwick, M, et al. Malignant Melanoma in Pregnancy Newton Bishop Obstet Gynecol Clin N Am (2005). , 32(2005), 559-568.

[74] Richardson, S. K, & Tannous, Z. S. Mihm Jr MC. Congenital and infantile melanoma: review of theliterature and report of an uncommon variant, pigment-synthesizing melanoma. J Am AcadDermatol (2002). , 47, 77-90.

[75] Alexander, A, Samlowski, W. E, Grossman, D, et al. Metastatic melanoma in pregnancy: risk oftransplacental metastases in the infant. J Clin Oncol (2003). Baergen RN, Johnson D, Moore T, et al. Maternal melanoma metastatic to the placenta: a case report and review of the literature. Arch Pathol Lab Med 1997;121:508-11;, 21, 2179-86.

[76] Dildy III GAMoise Jr KJ, Carpenter Jr RJ, et al. Maternal malignancy metastatic to the products of conception: a review. Obstet Gynecol Surv (1989). Dargeon HW, Eversole J, Del Duca V. Malignant melanoma in an infant. Cancer 1950;3:299-306;, 44, 535-40.

[77] Brodsky, I, Baren, M, & Kahn, S. B. Lewis G Jr, Tellem M. Metastatic malignant melanoma from mother to fetus. Cancer (1965). , 18, 1048-54.

[78] Richardson, S. K, & Tannous, Z. S. Mihm Jr MC. Congenital and infantile melanoma: review of the literature and report of an uncommon variant, pigment-synthesizing melanoma. J Am Acad Dermatol (2002). , 47, 77-90.

[79] Brenn, T. Phillip H McKee P: Melanoma in children and adolescents Diagnostic Histopathology, January (2008). , 14(1), 18-27.

[80] Kogut, K. A, Fleming, M, Pappo, A. S, et al. Sentinel lymph node biopsy for melanoma in young children. J Pediatr Surg (2000). , 35, 965-6.

[81] Buzaid, A. C, Sandler, A. B, Mani, S, et al. Role of computed tomography in the staging of primary melanoma. J Clin Oncol (1993). , 1993(11), 638-643.

[82] Kaste, S. C, & Pappo, A. S. Jenkins III JJ, Pratt CB. Malignant melanoma in children: imaging spectrum. Pediatr Radiol (1996). , 1996(26), 800-805.

[83] Morton, D. L, Thompson, J. F, Cochran, A. J, et al. MSLT Group. Sentinel node biopsy or nodal observation in melanoma. N Engl J Med (2006). , 355, 1307-17.

[84] Roaten, J. B, Partrick, D. A, Pearlman, N, et al. Sentinel lymph node biopsy for melanoma and other melanocytic tumors in adolescents. J Pediatr Surg (2005). , 40, 232-5.

[85] Toro, J, Ranieri, J. M, Havlik, R. J, et al. Sentinel lymph node biopsy in children and adolescents with malignant melanoma. J Pediatr Surg (2003). , 38, 1063-75.

[86] Pacella, S. J, Lowe, L, Bradford, C, et al. The utility of sentinel lymph node biopsy in head and neck melanoma in the pediatric population. Plast Reconstr Surg (2003). , 112, 1257-65.

[87] Roka, F, Kittler, H, Cauzig, P, et al. Sentinel node status in melanoma patients is not predictive for overall survival upon multivariate analysis. Br J Cancer (2005). , 92, 662-7.

[88] Butter AndreanaHuib Tom, Chapdelaine Joyaube, Beaunoyer Mona, Flageole Helene, Bouchard Sarah: Melanoma in children and the use of sentinel lymph node biopsy. Journal of Pediatric Surgery ((2005).

[89] Topar GerdaZelger Bernhard: Assessment of value of the sentinel lymph node biopsy in melanoma in children and adolescents and applicability of subcutaneous infusion anestesia Journal of Pediatric Surgery ((2007).

[90] Livestro, D. P, Kaine, E. M, Michaelson, J. S, et al. Melanoma in the young: differences and similarities with adult melanoma: a case-matched controlled analysis. Cancer (2007). , 110, 614-24.

[91] Robert Howman-GilesMD et Al. Sentinel Lymph Node Biopsy in Pediatric and Adolescent Cutaneous Melanoma Patients. Ann Surg Oncol ((2010).

[92] Gow, K. W, Rapkin, L. B, Olson, T. A, Durham, M. M, & Wyly, B. Shehata BM: Sentinel lymph node biopsy in the pediatric population. Journal of Pediatric Surgery ((2008).

[93] Sabel, M. S, & Arora, A. The role of the surgeon in the management of melanoma. Minerva Chir (2006). , 61, 54-141.

[94] Mcmasters, K. M, Reintgen, D. S, Ross, M. I, et al. Sentinel lymph node biopsy for melanoma: controversy despite widespread agreement. Journal of Clinical Oncology (2001). , 19, 2851-5.

[95] Shah, N. C, Gerstle, J. T, Stuart, M, et al. Use of sentinel lymph node biopsy and high-dose interferon in pediatric patients with high-risk melanoma: the Hospital for Sick Children experience. J Pediatr Hematol Oncol (2006). , 28, 496-500.

[96] Boddie AW JrCangir A. Adjuvant and neoadjuvant chemotherapy with dacarbazine in high-risk childhood melanoma. Cancer. (1987). Oct 15; , 60(8), 1720-3.

[97] Fishman, C, & Mihm, M. C. Sober AJ: Diagnosis and Management of Nevi And Cutaneous Melanoma in Infants And Children. Clinics in Dermatology Y (2002). , 20, 44-50.

[98] Bressac-de-paillerets, B, Avril, M. F, Chompret, A, & Demenais, F. Genetic and environmental factors in cutaneous malignant melanoma. Biochimie. (2002). , 84, 67-74.

[99] Brenn, T. McKee PH: Melanoma in children and adolescents Diagnostic Histopathology, January (2008). , 14(1), 18-27.

[100] Strouse, J. J, Fears, T. R, & Tucker, M. A. Wayne AS: Pediatric Melanoma: Risk Factor and Survival Analysis of the Surveillance, Epidemiology and End Results Database *Journal of Clinical Oncology*, July 20), (2005). , 23(21), 4735-4741.

[101] Moore-olufemi, S, Herzog, C, & Warneke, C. Gershenwald Jerry E, Mansfield P, Ross M, Prieto V, Lally KP and Hayes-Jordan A: Outcomes in Pediatric Melanoma. Comparing Prepubertal to Adolescent Pediatric Patients. Annals of Surgery (2011). , 253(6), 1211-15.

Chapter 13

Adoptive Cell Therapy of Melanoma: The Challenges of Targeting the Beating Heart

Jennifer Makalowski and Hinrich Abken

Additional information is available at the end of the chapter

http://dx.doi.org/10.5772/53619

1. Introduction

The identification of melanoma-associated antigens, the isolation of tumor infiltrating T cells from melanoma lesions, and the significant progress in engineering redirected T cells has favored the development of various strategies in the adoptive immunotherapy of melanoma. Recent trials in adoptive cell therapy (ACT) have achieved spectacular results in inducing remission in advanced stages of the disease, although produced on-target off-tumor toxicities, emphasizing the tremendous potential benefit of harnessing the immune system for fighting the disease. Moreover, the identification of so-called melanoma stem cells along with strategies for selectively eliminating subsets of melanoma cells implies that there is a need for redefining therapeutic targets in melanoma. This review discusses current challenges in the rational design of adoptive cell therapy to target "the beating heart" of melanoma.

1.1. Advanced stages of melanoma resist conventional therapeutic regimens

Surgical resection of tumor lesions in early stages of the disease is the curative option for combating melanoma; a 10-year-survival rate of 75 - 85% can be achieved for melanoma in stage I or II. However, melanoma in stage III or IV is still associated with low survival rates of less than 1 year upon diagnosis [1]. Despite the development of novel drugs and major improvements in therapeutic regimens, significant responses were only achieved in predefined groups and of short duration. Treatment with the chemotherapeutic drug dacarbazine (DTIC) and vemurafenib, an inhibitor of mutated BRAF, produced a median progression-free survival of 64% with dacarbazine, respectively 84% with vemurafenib of approximately 6 months [2-4]. The biology of melanoma and the heterogeneity of malignant cells are thought to be responsible for this unsatisfactory situation. First, melanoma cells can persist for long periods of time in a "dormant" stage without any progression in tumor formation [5]. Second, melanoma cells can disseminate early into distant organs including the brain forming micro-metastases, which are small in cell numbers and frequently beyond the detection limit of current imaging procedures [6, 7]. Third, many melanoma cells are notoriously resistant to chemo- and radiation therapy [8-10], making alternative strategies in tumor cell elimination necessary.

Therefore, in more progressed stages of the disease the recruitment of the cellular immune defense to eliminate cancer cells is thought to be an alternative. Administration of high dose interleukin-2 (IL-2) [11] and anti-cytotoxic T-lymphocyte-associated antigen-4 (CTLA-4) antibody [12] as well as interferon (IFN) α-2b prolongs the disease-free survival although at a relatively low response rate and without being curative over time [13, 14]. However, these and other observations imply that activation or modulation of the patient's immune response may be effective in the treatment of melanoma. A number of approaches for enhancing the immune cell response against melanoma are currently explored with some success. In particular, the adoptive transfer of autologous T cells isolated from melanoma lesions and expanded to large numbers ex vivo has produced encouraging phase II results [15, 16]. The administration of patient's blood T cells engineered with defined specificity for melanoma-associated antigens are additionally being explored in a number of trials. In this review, we summarize evidence for the potency of adoptive T cell therapy in the treatment of melanoma and discuss current challenges in achieving long-term remission. Upcoming strategies in selective targeting cancer stem cells are also discussed.

2. Adoptive cell therapy can successfully fight melanoma

Melanoma can trigger a curative immune response; this conclusion is drawn from the clinical observation of spontaneous and complete melanoma regressions and of the higher frequency of melanomas among immune compromised patients [17, 18]. More direct evidence for the immune cell control of melanoma growth was obtained by the treatment with high dose IL-2, which produces an objective response rate of 16%. Indeed, some of the patients receiving thus treatment exhibit a long-term complete response for years [11, 19]. These observations are remarkable in light of the low and short-lived response rates after chemotherapy and currently drive the development of adoptive T cell therapy for treatment of late stage melanoma.

The development of adoptive cell therapy (ACT) was further strengthened by upcoming technologies in isolating tumor infiltrating lymphocytes (TIL's) from melanoma biopsies (Figure 1). First described in 1969 [20], TIL's from melanoma lesions consisted of both effector and helper T cell subsets and can be expanded *ex vivo* in the presence of IL-2. The expanded cells are then selected for melanoma reactivity. A strong rationale for using these T cells in adoptive therapy is provided by the observation that the infusion of high TIL numbers correlates with better clinical outcome [21, 22] although

http://dx.doi.org/10.5772/53619

the prevalence of TIL's in primary melanoma lesions and metastases is not a prognostic factor itself.

Protocols according to GMP standards have been established in several centers to isolate and amplify TIL's to numbers appropriate for adoptive therapy. Melanoma reactive T cells are expanded in the presence of IL-2 by culture on feeder cells expressing melanoma antigens [23]. Subsequent to TIL re-infusions, metastases regressed in the majority of patients and a stable disease phase followed. However, only few patients remained in complete remission [21]. The disappointing therapeutic efficacy, despite high numbers of infused TIL's is thought to be due to low responsiveness of highly expanded T cells which are unable to execute a productive anti-melanoma attack after administration to the patient. Current TIL protocols therefore attempt to administer so-called "young TIL's" (Figure 1), i.e. melanoma infiltrating T cells which underwent short-term culture expansions and therefore passed through fewer cell division cycles prior to re-infusion and thereby exhibit a less differentiated phenotype [24]. Another change in protocols is that TIL's are not selected for melanoma reactivity; the rationale behind this is that re-infusion of *ex vivo* IFN-γ secreting TIL's exhibited no major benefit compared to non-responding TIL's [16]. Early phase I trials showed improved persistence of young TIL's [25] and 50% response rates in a cohort of 20 patients [26], which is just as effective as traditionally grown TIL's [27]. Different non-randomized phase II trials at the NCI and at Sheba Medical Center confirmed these early observations (Table 1) [28, 29]. A roadmap describing critical steps for comparative testing the TIL strategy in a randomized multi-center setting was recently published in a White Paper on adoptive cell therapy [30].

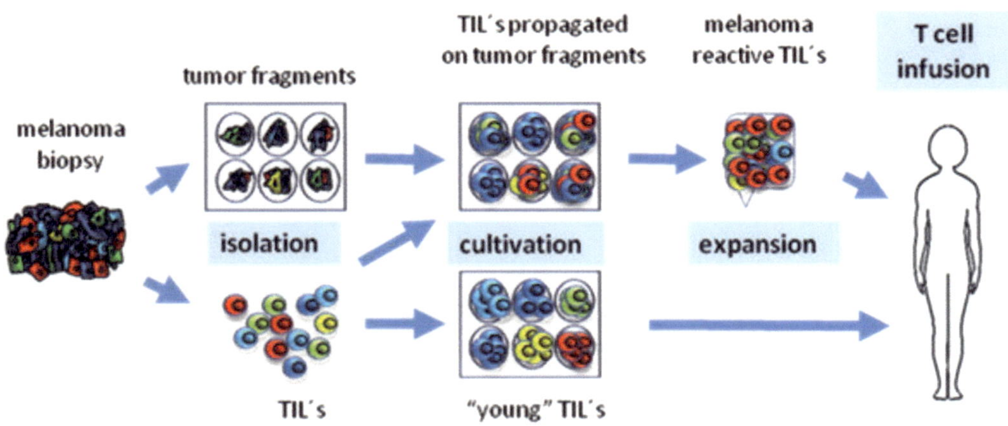

Figure 1. Adoptive cell therapy for metastatic melanoma. Adoptive cell therapy with tumor infiltrating lymphocytes (TIL´s) makes use of melanoma-specific TIL´s which are isolated from a melanoma biopsy, amplified *ex vivo* by stimulation with melanoma biopsy cells and propagated to high numbers in the presence of IL-2. In more recent trials, TIL´s are propagated short-term ex vivo without stimulation by melanoma cells and administered as "young" TIL´s.

Target antigen	Adoptively transferred T cells	NCT ID / Reference	Center
	melanoma specific CD8+ T cells	[118]	FHCRC
	melanoma specific T cells	[119]	LUMC
MART-1	MART-1 specific CD8+ T cells	[113]	DFCI
MART-1	MART-1 specific CD8+ T cells	NCT00512889	DFCI
MART-1	MART-1 specific CD8+ T cells	[87]	UR
MART-1	MART-1 specific CD8+ T cells	[33]	UNH
MART-1	MART-1 specific CD8+ T cells	NCT00324623	CHUV
MART-1	MART-1 specific CD8+ T cells	NCT01106235	FHCRC
NY-ESO-1	NY-ESO-1 specific CD8+ T cells and anti-CTLA-4 antibody	NCT00871481	FHCRC
	TILs	[114]	NIH
	TIL	[120]	NIH
	TILs	[27]	NIH
	TILs	[29]	NIH
	TILs	[115]	NIH
	TILs	NCT00287131	SMC
	TILs	NCT000604136	HMO
	TILs	NCT01005745	MOFFITT
	TILs and IFN-γ	NCT01082887	NUH
	"young" TILs	[116]	NIH
	"young" TILs	[28]	SMC
	"young" TILs	NCT01118091	NIH
	"young" TILs	NCT01319565	NIH
	"young" TILs	NCT01369888	MIH
	"young" TILs	NCT01468818	NIH
	"young" TILs	NCT00513604	NIH
MART-1	MART-1 specific TILs	NCT00720031	NUH
MART-1	MART-1 specific TILs (DMF5)	NCT00924001	CC
	IL-2 engineered TILs	[117]	NIH
	IL-2 engineered TIL	NCT00062036	NIH
	IL-12 engineered TIL	NCT01236573	NIH
	CXCR2 engineered TIL	[86]	MDACC
NY-ESO-1	anti-NY-ESO-1 TCR	[121]	NIH
NY-ESO-1	anti-NY-ESO-1 TCR	NCT00670748	NIH
MART-1	anti-MART-1 TCR (low-affinity)	[49]	NIH
MART-1	anti-MART-1 TCR	NCT00910650	UC
MART-1	anti-MART-1 TCR (high-affinity)	[38]	NIH
gp-100	anti-gp-100 TCR	[38]	NIH
MART-1	anti-MART-1 TCR	[114]	NIH
gp-100	anti-gp-100 TCR	[114]	NIH
MART-1	anti-MART-1 TCR	NCT00612222	NIH
gp-100	anti-gp-100 TCR	NCT00610311	NIH
MART-1	anti-MART-1 TCR plus MART-1 vaccination	NCT00923195	NIH
gp-100	anti-gp-100 TCR plus gp-100 vaccination	NCT00923195	NIH
p53	anti-p53 TCR	NCT00393029	NIH
VEGFR2	anti-VEGFR2 CAR engineered CD8+ T cells	NCT01218867	NIH
Ganglioside GD-3	anti-GD-3 CAR	PI: M. Davies	MDACC

CHUV, Centre Hospitalier Universitaire Vaudois; **DFCI**, Dana-Farber Cancer Institute; **FHCRC**, Fred Hutchinson Cancer Research Center; **HMO**, Hadassah Medical Organization; **LUMC**, Leiden University Medical Center; **MDACC**, M.D. Anderson Cancer Center; **MOFFITT**, H. Lee Moffitt Cancer Center and Research Institute; **NIH**, National Institutes of Health; **NUH**, Nantes University Hospital; **PI**, principal investigator; **SMC**, Sheba Medical Center; **UC**, University of California; **UR**, University of Regensburg

Table 1. Adoptive cell therapy trials in patients with metastatic melanoma

3. Adoptive cell therapy with antigen-specific T cells

The rationale for using melanoma antigen-specific T cells is based on the observation that the success of TIL therapy in some patients correlates with the presence of melanoma-reactive T cells, in particular with those cells specific for Melan-A, MART-1 or gp100 [23, 31]. The median survival of patients treated with Melan-A specific TIL's was 53.5 months compared to 3.5 months for patients who received TIL's without Melan-A specificity [32]. These observations together with a number of technical obstacles in obtaining TIL's from biopsies strengthened efforts to derive melanoma-specific T cell clones from peripheral blood lymphocytes for the use in adoptive cell therapy. The strategy was corroborated by a 50% response rate obtained after transfer of MART-1 or gp100 specific T cell clones isolated and propagated *ex vivo* from peripheral blood lymphocytes (Table 1) [33]. Melanoma reactive T cell clones in peripheral blood are rare, TIL therapy increases the otherwise low magnitude of the tumor-reactive T cell compartment *in vivo*, which matches the reactivity in the TIL product [34]. Interestingly, individual TIL products from different patients contain unique patterns of reactivity against shared melanoma-associated antigens [34]. TIL isolation and expansion *in vitro*, however, is extremely laborious. This limit leads to attempts to engineer patient's blood T cells with pre-defined specificity for more specifically redirecting the cytotoxic response toward melanoma. It is therefore assumed that the clinical efficacy of TIL therapy can be improved by application of T cells with more defined tumor-reactivity.

To engineer specificity for melanoma, T cell receptors (TCR's) were cloned from TIL's of responding melanoma patients and transferred to peripheral blood T cells of the same patient (Figure 2) [35-38]. The gp100 specific TCR was one of the first TCR's, cloned from melanoma TIL's and introduced *ex vivo* by retrovirus-mediated gene transfer into blood T cells, which thus obtained redirected specificity for gp100 positive cells. In contrast to their non-modified counterparts, TCR engineered T cells responded to $gp100^{+}$ melanoma cells by secreting pro-inflammatory cytokines including IFN-γ and by lysing the target cells [45, 46]. Similarly, blood T cells were engineered with recombinant TCR's with specificity for MART-1 or MAGE-A1. The functional avidity of cloned TCR's was improved and engineered T cells were successfully used in subsequent trials [47, 48]. About 30% of patients receiving ACT with MART-1 specific T cells responded with melanoma regression; 19% of patients treated with gp100 specific TCR T cells exhibited objective response, most responses were persistent [38]. TCR engineered T cells also showed efficacy towards brain metastases, which indicates that patients with otherwise incurable metastatic sites may benefit from ACT (Table 1) [115]. In patients with prolonged clinical remission, engineered T cells were present in the circulation for more than a year after initiation of treatment; this indicates that therapeutic efficacy and long-term anti-melanoma immunity may correlate with T cell persistence [49, 50].

However, the enthusiasm for adoptive cell therapy with TCR modified T cells has been dampened by several limitations. Tumor cells including those of the melanoma undergo clonal evolution, and some of these evolved cells evade T cell recognition, for instance, as a result of repression of their MHC complex [51], of mutations in their β2 microglobulin chain [52], and of deficiencies in their antigen processing machinery [51, 53]. Each of these altera-

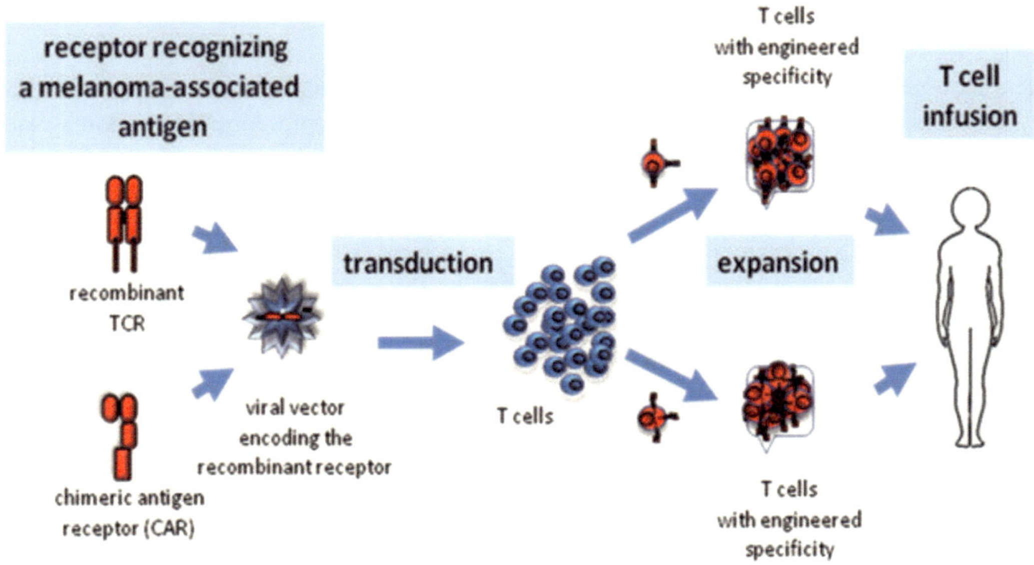

Figure 2. Adoptive cell therapy with redirected T cells. T cells from the peripheral blood of the patient are engineered *ex vivo* by retro- or lentiviral gene transfer with cDNA coding for a T cell receptor (TCR) with specificity for a melanoma-associated antigen. Alternatively, T cells are engineered with a chimeric antigen receptor (CAR) which recognizes a melanoma-associated antigen by an antibody-derived binding domain. Engineered T cells are expanded *ex vivo* prior to administration to the patient.

tions renders the melanoma cell invisible to a TCR-mediated T cell attack. A possible safety hazard moreover became apparent when analyzing in more detail the transgenic TCR, which is co-expressed with the physiological TCR in the same T cell. The transgenic TCR turned out to create new but unpredictable specificities by forming hetero-dimers of the recombinant α and β TCR chains with the respective chains of the physiological TCR. Undesirable mispairing of TCR chains may result in loss of specificity and may induce severe auto-reactivity [54, 55]. Tremendous efforts were subsequently made to solve the problem including replacement of TCR constant moieties by the homologous murine domains [56] and creation of additional cysteine bridges [57] to enforce preferential pairing of the recombinant $\alpha\beta$ TCR chains in the presence of the physiological TCR.

These and other technical difficulties promoted the development of an artificial "one-chain-receptor" molecule to redirect T cells in an antigen-restricted manner (Figure 3). In a seminal paper Zelig Eshhar of the Weizmann Institute of Science described a chimeric antigen receptor (CAR), also named immunoreceptor, which is composed in the extracellular part of a single chain antibody for antigen binding and in the intracellular part of the TCR/CD3ζ endodomain for provision of T cell activation [58]. The CAR modified T cell, also known as "T-body", becomes activated by binding to antigen, and secretes pro-inflammatory cytokines, amplifies and lyses target cells expressing the respective antigen. By using an antibody for binding, the CAR recognizes the target in a MHC-independent fashion and is therefore not affected by loss of HLA molecules, which frequently occurs during neoplastic progression. An additional advantage over transgenic TCR's is that CAR's can be used independently of the individual HLA subtype. However, the T-body strategy is restricted to antigens expressed on the surface of the target cell; intracellular antigens are not visible to CAR's. Due to the broad variety of antibodies available, a nearly unlimited panel of antigens can be targeted with high affinity and specificity, including those which are not classical T cell antigens, e.g. carbohydrates. High affinity CAR's activate engineered T cells even after binding to low amounts of target antigen; this not only makes the approach highly sensitive, but also makes the choice of the appropriate melanoma-selective antigen difficult.

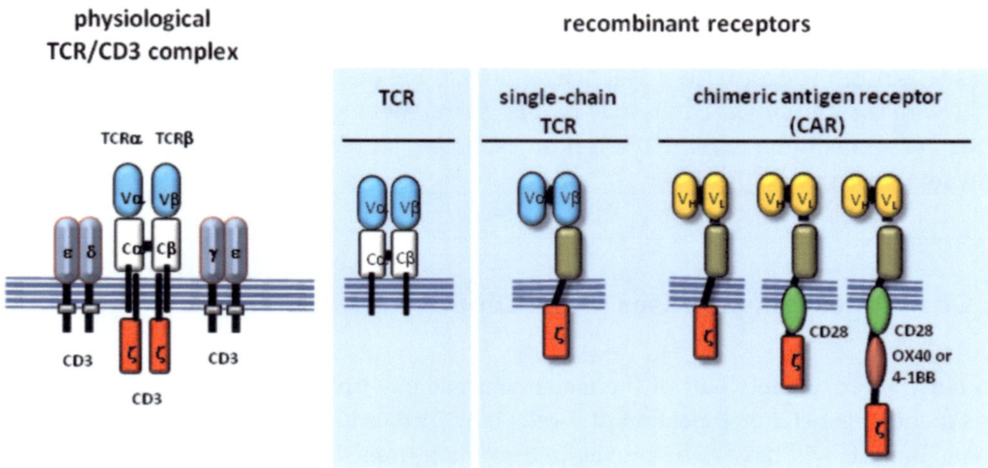

Figure 3. Recombinant receptors to redirect T cells for use in antigen-specific cell therapy. The physiologic T cell receptor (TCR)/CD3 complex consists of the α and β TCR chains, which recognize major histocompatibility complex (MHC)-presented antigen by binding through both variable regions Vα Vβ, and of the CD3 chains. Antigen engagement induces clustering of the TCR complex and the primary signal for T cell activation is generated by the intracellular CD3ζ chain. Recombinant TCR α and β chains can be engineered to T cells in order to provide a new specificity. Alternatively, the V regions of the TCR chains can be combined and fused to the intracellular CD3ζ chain to produce a T cell activation signal upon binding to antigen. The chimeric antigen receptor (CAR) makes use of an antibody binding domain for antigen recognition which is enigneered by fusing the variable (V) regions of the immunoglobulin heavy (H) and light (L) chain. The V_H-V_L single chain antibody is linked via a spacer to the intracellular CD3ζ chain to produce the primary T cell activation signal upon antigen binding. Intracellular signaling domains of costimulatory molecules like CD28 can be added to provide appropriate costimulation in addition to the primary CD3ζ signal.

T cells require two signals for full and lasting activation, one provided by the TCR and the other by costimulatory co-receptors; the prototype of which is CD28. The corresponding ligands are usually not present in the tumor micro-environment. Some effector functions including IL-2 secretion require CD28 costimulation along with the primary TCR/CD3ζ signal; this provides a rationale for combining the intracellular CD3ζ with the CD28 signaling domain in one polypeptide chain (Figure 3) [59]. Other costimulatory domains, such as 4-1BB (CD137) and OX40 (CD134), were also linked to CD3ζ; each domain has a different impact on T cell effector functions [60]. Costimulatory domains were furthermore combined in so-called 3rd generation CAR's, and a number of additional modifications have been introduced in the last years to improve T cell persistence and activation [61, 62]. CAR's with a costimulatory domain clearly demonstrated clinical benefit and improved T cell persistence compared to CAR's targeting the same antigen but with only the CD3ζ domain [63-65].

Various CARs were engineered for targeting melanoma-associated antigens, including HMW-MAA, also known as MCSP [67, 68], melanotransferrin [69], the ganglioside GD2 [70] and GD3 [71]. A clinical trial targeting melanoma cells with CAR engineered T cells is currently recruiting participants [66]. Recent phase I trials using CAR redirected T cells in the treatment of lymphoma/leukemia exhibited spectacular efficacy [72, 73]. However, the enthusiasm was dampened by reports on serious adverse events and even fatalities after CAR T cell therapy [74, 75]. Targeting ErbB2 produced a cytokine storm and respiratory failure in one case [76] which is thought to be due to low levels of antigen on a number of healthy cells which can trigger CAR T cell activation. On the one hand, this event points out that ACT with CAR modified T cells may be a powerful therapy; but, on the other hand, emphasizes the necessity for careful T cell dose escalation studies to balance anti-tumor efficacy and auto-immunity[61, 77, 78].

4. Challenges and premises in the adoptive cell therapy of melanoma

To date, approximately half of the melanoma patients treated with TIL ACT benefit from this therapy; genetic modification of T cells may further improve clinical response to melanoma, but this will have to be proven in upcoming trials. However, the strategy has potential challenges which need to be addressed.

A major challenge of redirected T cells is the tumor selectivity for the target antigen itself, which in most cases is not exclusively expressed on tumor cells but also on healthy cells [79], although almost always at lower levels: for instance MART-1, which is also expressed by melanocytes. When targeting these antigens, vitiligo and inner ear toxicity resulting in a certain degree of deafness are frequently observed side effects [38]. From this perspective it is reasonable to assume that off-target toxicities may be adverse reactions for clinical efficacy in an anti-melanoma response [80]. Since nearly all tumor-associated antigens are self-antigens, strategies will have to be developed to ensure that off-target toxicities are kept to a minimum. Whether T cells with low-avidity TCR or CAR are less prone to induce such undesirable side effects is currently under investigation.

Melanoma cells, like other cancer cells, down-regulate components of the MHC and become increasingly deficient in antigen processing. As a consequence, TCR engineered T cells can no longer bind to and destroy those melanoma cells. However, they may be visible to a CAR recognizing surface antigens in a MHC independent manner, because of the antibody-derived binding domain (Figure 3). TCR redirected T cells, on the one hand, may also recognize cross-presented targeted antigen, for instance by stroma cells, but this is not the case for CAR engineered T cells. Cross-presented antigen, on the other hand, may help to destroy stroma, which is required to eliminate large tumor lesions [39, 40].

To avoid mispairing of the recombinant TCR with the physiological TCR chains and the resulting unpredictable auto-immunity, TCR-like single chain antibodies were used as targeting domain in a CAR. Thus combining the MHC-restricted recognition of antigen with the T-body strategy. T cells with TCR-like CAR were redirected towards NY-ESO-1 and MAGE-A1, respectively [41, 42]. The possible advantages of these MHC restricted CAR's compared to the use of recombinant TCR's still has to be determined in trials.

The antibody-derived binding domain of a CAR displays extraordinary high affinity compared to a TCR. However, an increase in affinity, for instance, by affinity maturation, does not necessarily improve CAR redirected T cell activation above threshold [41, 43], which is not additionally modulated by CD28 costimulation [44]. A similar effect is also assumed for TCR mediated T cell activation. The TCR or CAR binding avidity probably affects the persistence of engineered T cells at the targeted tumor site. Strong binding to a target antigen may cause the T cells to be trapped and to become fully activated for a cytolytic attack, whereas low avidity interactions may not provide sufficiently long T cell – melanoma cell contacts. In addition to the binding avidity, the amount of target antigen on the cell surface also impacts on the selectivity of redirected T cell activation. In essence, low affinity binding directs the activity of engineered T cells preferentially toward target cells with abundant antigen levels; high affinity binding is likewise effective against low antigen levels on target cells. The optimized affinity to sustain a more selective T cell trafficking to the tumor and activation while avoiding targeting healthy cells that are expressing low quantities of the same antigen, however, still has to be determined.

A beneficial T cell-to-target cell ratio at the tumor site seems to be required for efficient tumor elimination. Higher numbers of engineered T cells applied per dose will probably increase clinical efficacy; the majority of recent trials have applied up to 10^{10} cells per dose [27]. These and higher numbers of engineered T cells can be generated by extended expansion protocols; however, cells with a "young" phenotype may not be generated for adoptive transfer under these conditions. Short-term amplification protocols are therefore envisioned for both TIL's and engineered blood T cells. However, the majority of recent trials targeting $CD19^+$ leukemia provided evidence for therapeutic efficacy at numbers less than or equal to 10^5 engineered T cells [73]. This once again raises the question of whether high T cell doses are required for a therapeutic effect.

The clinical outcome of adoptive cell therapy correlates with the persistence of adoptively transferred T cells [81]. As long as T cells engage their cognate antigen, T cells will expand and persist in detectable numbers; but when the antigen is no longer present, the T cell population will contract to potentially undetectable levels and disappear from circulation. To improve survival of CAR T cells, Epstein-Barr virus (EBV)-specific T cells were engineered with a tumor-specific CAR based on the rationale that T cells recognizing the low amounts of EBV antigens by their physiological TCR will be maintained in a sizable population in circulation and in the process providing enough CAR T cells to recognize and kill melanoma cells in the surrounding tissues. A clinical trial with EBV-specific T cells engineered with an anti-GD2 CAR thus showed benefit over non-virus-specific, CAR engineered T cells in the treatment of neuroblastoma [81].

Adoptively transferred $CD8^+$ T cell clones may be less persistent than $CD4^+$ T cell clones due to T cell exhaustion after extensive *ex vivo* amplification and multiple rounds of activation. In addition, $CD4^+$ T cell help is essential for $CD8^+$ T cell persistence *in vivo*; adoptively transferred pure $CD8^+$ T cell clones may fail to persist [82]. T cell therapy may be combined with antibody therapy to prolong the initiated immune response. For instance, CTLA-4 is upregulated on the surface of activated T cells, where it acts as negative regulator to return the T cell to a resting stage. Co-application of the anti-CTLA-4 blocking antibody, ipilimumab, may prolong the anti-tumor activation of transferred T cells, although it would also affect all the other T cells.

Besides maintaining a high number of T cells in circulation, another challenge is to accumulate significant numbers of effector T cells in the tumor lesion. A tightly controlled network of chemokines controls the migration of cells in the body; adoptively transferred T cells use these networks to accumulate at the tumor site. The expression of specific chemokine receptors controls how cells will migrate against the chemokine gradient into the targeted lesion. Melanoma cells secrete a number of chemokines including CXCL1. However, early imaging studies revealed that melanoma-specific T cells massively infiltrate the lungs, spleen and liver with some accumulation at the tumor site, which clearly represents a minority of the transferred cells, before the cells decline to undetectable levels in circulation [83-85]. Since those T cells do not express CXCR2, the receptor for melanoma secreted CXCL1, TIL's were engineered with CXCR2 which generated improved melanoma accumulation and anti-tumor activity in a mouse model [86]. The strategy is currently being explored in an early phase I trial (Table 1) [86].

One of the major hurdles of redirected immunotherapy of cancer in general is the tremendous heterogeneity of cancer cells with respect to the expression of the targeted antigen. Low or lack of antigen expression within the malignant lesions will negatively affect the long-term therapeutic efficacy of the approach. Several reports document relapse of antigen-loss tumor metastases after adoptive therapy with melanoma-reactive T cell clones [87-89] and argue for the use of polyclonal T cells with various melanoma specificities. Melanoma cells expressing the target antigen may successfully be eliminated by redirected T cells, whereas antigen-negative tumor cells will not be recognized. T cell populations modified with different CAR's recognizing different antigens expressed by the same tumor may be able to overcome these limitations. However, pro-inflammatory cytokines secreted by redirected T cells into the tumor micro-environment upon activation may attract a second wave of non-antigen restricted effector cells, which in turn may eradiate antigen-negative tumor cells. At least in an animal model, antigen-negative melanoma cells are indeed eliminated when co-inoculated with antibody-targeted cytokines [90]. Moreover, T cells engineered with induced expression of transgenic IL-12 attract innate immune cells including macrophages into the tumor tissue; they eliminate antigen-negative tumor cells in the same lesion [91].

Highly expanded T cells, such as TIL's, become hypo-responsive to CD28 costimulation and rapidly enter activation induced cell death, in particular upon IL-2 driven expansion [92].

This may be counteracted by expansion in the presence of IL-15 and IL-21 and/or by co-stimulation via 4-1BB by an agonistic antibody [93].

Metastatic melanoma patients with the B-raf activating mutation V600E transiently benefit from a small molecule drug, PLX4032 or vemurafenib, which inhibits the mitogen-activated protein kinase (MAPK) pathway. Treatment with vemurafenib is accompanied by increased T cell infiltrations in the melanoma lesions [94, 95]. Combination of B-raf inhibition with melanoma-specific ACT may provide an option to prolong the clinical response.

Although the TCR downstream signaling machinery is used by the prototype CAR, monocytes, macrophages as well as NK cells can also be redirected by CAR's in an antigen-specific fashion [96, 97]. Whether redirected non-T cells are advantageous in tumor elimination to cancer patients in general and to melanoma patients in particular has to be explored in clinical trials.

5. Does targeting "melanoma stem cells" provide hope for long-term remission from melanoma?

Observations that a number of malignant lesions display a tremendous cellular and phenotypic heterogeneity and contain pluripotent stem cells led to the hypothesis that cancer is initiated and maintained by so-called cancer stem cells (CSC's). Low abundance, induction of tumors upon transplantation under limiting conditions, radiation and chemo-resistance, self-renewal and a-symmetric differentiation into a variety of cell types are properties postulated for CSC's. The concept was sustained by deciphering the hierarchical organization in hematological malignancies [98], and subsequently in solid cancers including mammary, prostate, pancreatic, colon carcinoma and glioma [99-103]. Transplantation of melanoma cell subsets under limiting dilution conditions showed that a subset of cancer cells can induce tumors of the same histological phenotype as the parental tumor [99, 104, 105]. A first study using the limiting dilution transplantation assay identified a melanoma cell subset which exhibits stem-like capacities and expresses CD20 [106]. A conclusion drawn from these and other experiments was that melanoma is organized in a hierarchical manner originating from an initiator cell. In this context, several phenomena in melanoma biology which have been clinically observed but not well understood are described by the CSC model, for instance, metastatic relapse more than a decade after surgical treatment of the primary lesion. Residual CSC's are thought to drive cancer relapse even after years of "dormancy" [107]. Moreover, melanoma initiating cells were identified as expressing either the transporter protein ABCB5 [104] or the nerve growth factor receptor CD271; the latter occurs in melanoma in a frequency of approximately 1/2000 cells [108].

However, transplantation under more rigorous conditions, i.e., ideally of one isolated melanoma cell, revealed that nearly every fourth randomly taken melanoma cell (1/2 - 1/15) can induce tumors and raising the question of the validity the stem cell paradigm for melanoma [109, 110]. From these and subsequent studies, it has been concluded that the potential of melanoma induction is not closely associated with a particular phenotype and that the number of potential CSC's in melanoma may not necessarily be low. This resulted in a further conclusion that nearly every melanoma cell is capable to re-program to a tumor initiating cell under certain experimental conditions of xeno-transplantation irrespectively which particular marker phenotype the cell expressed at the time of isolation from a melanoma lesion.

Once the tumor is established, a minor subset seems to take over control of melanoma progression. Evidence is provided by recent observations from a pre-clinical model [69], which addressed the question of whether specific elimination of defined melanoma cells from an established xeno-transplanted lesion causes tumor regression by adoptive transfer of antigen-specific cytotoxic T cell. The rationale is that, if there is a clearly defined hierarchy of cancer cells in an established tumor, specific ablation of the melanoma sustaining cells from the established tumor tissue must inevitably lead to a decay of the tumor lesion independently of targeting the cancer cell mass. However, the melanoma sustaining cell may, but must not, be identical to CSC's identified by the transplantation assay. Targeted elimination of a minor subset of $CD20^+$ melanoma cells completely eradicated transplanted melanoma lesions, whereas targeted elimination of any random melanoma cell population in the same lesion did not. $CD20^+$ melanoma cells are rare, i.e. approximately 1-2%, in melanoma, independently of the histological type and the transplanted tumor tissue. A caveat is that in approximately 20% of melanoma samples, no $CD20^+$ melanoma cells could be detected by histological screening. When these tumors were transplanted, adoptive transfer of CD20-specific CAR T cells did not induce tumor regression. Interestingly, CD20 re-expression in a random subpopulation of those tumor cells did not render the tumor lesion sensitive for complete eradication with CD20-specific T cells. This indicates that CD20 expression *per se* is not dominant in maintaining melanoma progression. However, the phenotype of $CD20^+$ melanoma cells may be flexible and associated with additional capabilities which mediate the dominant effect.

The first clinical evidence confirming this concept was recently provided by a case report [111]. A patient with stage III/IV metastatic melanoma, which harbored $CD20^+$ melanoma cells at a frequency of 2%, received intra-lesional injections of the anti-CD20 therapeutic antibody rituximab and concomitant dacarbazine treatment. Dacarbazine as mono-therapy had already proved to be ineffective. This treatment produced lasting complete and partial remission accompanied by a decline of the melanoma serum marker S-100 to physiological levels, a switch of a T helper-2 to a more pro-inflammatory T helper-1 response, all without treatment related grade 3/4 toxicity. Although anecdotic, this data provides the first clinical evidence that targeting the subset of $CD20^+$ melanoma sustaining cells can produce regression of chemotherapy-refractory melanoma. Moreover, the report highlights the potency of selective cancer cell targeting in the treatment of melanoma.

These observations although so far based on a pre-clinical model and a clinical observation which will have to be reproduced in larger cohorts have major impact on the future development of melanoma therapy.

First, the melanoma maintaining cells may be more resistant to current therapy regimens than the bulk of melanoma cells. Standard therapy strategies attempt to eliminated all cancer cells in a tumor lesion; elimination of any other cancer cells than the tumor progressing cells will rapidly de-bulk the tumor lesion. The melanoma will inevitably relapse, driven by the remaining melanoma sustaining cells, which are extraordinary resistant to chemotherapeutics. This resistance is probably due to transporter molecules like ABCB5, which are highly expressed by a number of CSC's including melanoma [104] and therefore efficiently counteract chemotherapy. Melanoma maintaining cells like other CSC's are merely in a "dormant" state and replicate less frequently than the majority of cancer cells in the same lesion, which reduces the efficacy of anti-proliferative drugs. Low proliferative capacities together with the efficient export of chemotherapeutics contribute to CSC resistance toward a variety of therapeutic drugs. As a consequence, alternative strategies that specifically induce cell death of those cells are required. Moreover, the situation is exacerbated by the fact that the melanoma maintaining cells in the lesion are rare and unlikely to be eliminated by the random targeting provided by most therapeutic agents. Specific targeting by cytotoxic T cells redirected towards CD20 or by CD20-specific therapeutic antibodies like Rituxan™ (rituximab) or Arzerra™ (ofatumumab), probably as adjunct to a tumor de-bulking strategy, may improve the situation.

Second, whether the prevalence of $CD20^+$ melanoma maintaining cells in a tumor lesion may correlate with clinical progression or relapse has to be addressed. If so, the frequency of $CD20^+$ melanoma cells may serve as a surrogate marker for therapeutic efficacy and/or prognosis. Chemotherapy and/or radiation may induce amplification of these cells thus contributing to their accumulation during tumor progression and metastasis.

Third, melanoma maintaining cells may exhibit an extraordinary functional and phenotypic plasticity. As a consequence, continuous presence of targeting therapeutic agents will be required to eliminate those cells, which exhibit newly acquired melanoma initiating and/or maintaining capacities. In their pre-clinical model, Schmidt and colleagues [69] used CAR engineered T cells which penetrate tissues, scan for targets and persist for long-term acting as an antigen-specific guardian. These T cells are present in the targeted lesion as long as cells expressing the target antigen appear. Repetitive restimulation of these T cells, for instance by engaging their TCR with EBV-specific antigens [63, 81], may sustain persistence of CAR T cells in sufficient numbers over long periods of time. In this constellation, cellular therapy has a major advantage compared to pharmaceutical drugs, which are present in therapeutic levels for short periods; in the case of melanoma the required period for screening for re-appearance of such melanoma initiating cells may be many years. The development of an antigen-specific memory by adoptively transferred CAR T cells, as recently shown in a pre-clinical model [112], may be of benefit to patients in preventing a melanoma relapse.

Acknowledgements

Work in the author's laboratory was supported by the Deutsche Krebshilfe, Bonn and Ziel 2. NRW Programm of the Ministerium für Innovation, Wissenschaft, Forschung und Technologie des Landes Nordrhein-Westfalen and of the European Union.

Abbreviations

ACT, adoptive cell therapy; **CAR**, chimeric antigen receptor; **CTLA-4**, anti-cytotoxic T-lymphocyte-associated antigen-4; **CSC**, cancer stem cell; **EBV**, Epstein-Barr virus; **GMP**, Good Manufacturing Practice; **IFN**, interferon; **IL**, interleukin; **TCR**, T cell receptor; **TIL**, tumor infiltrating lymphocyte

Author details

Jennifer Makalowski[1,2] and Hinrich Abken[1,2*]

*Address all correspondence to: hinrich.abken@uk-koeln.de

1 Center for Molecular Medicine Cologne (CMMC), University of Cologne, Cologne, Germany

2 Dept. I Internal Medicine, University Hospital Cologne, Cologne, Germany

References

[1] Garbe C, Peris K, Hauschild A, Saiag P, Middleton M, Spatz A, Grob J-J, Malvehy J, Newton-Bishop J, Stratigos A, Pehamberger H, Eggermont A. Diagnosis and treatment of melanoma: European consensus-based interdisciplinary guideline. European Journal of Cancer 2010;46(2) 270-283.

[2] Chapman PB, Hauschild A, Robert C, Haanen JB, Ascierto P, Larkin J, Dummer R, Garbe C, Testori A, Maio M, Hogg D, Lorigan P, Lebbe C, Jouary T, Schadendorf D, Ribas A, O'Day SJ, Sosman JA, Kirkwood JM, Eggermont AM, Dreno B, Nolop K, Li J, Nelson B, Hou J, Lee RJ, Flaherty KT. Improved survival with vemurafenib in melanoma with BRAF V600E mutation. The New England Journal of Medicine 2011;364 (26) 2507-2516.

[3] Carter RD, Krementz ET, Hill GJ 2nd, Metter GE, Fletcher WS, Golomb FM, Grage TB, Minton JP, Sparks FC. DTIC (nsc-45388) and combination therapy for melanoma. I. Studies with DTIC, BCNU (NSC-409962), CCNU (NSC-79037), vincristine (NSC-67574), and hydroxyurea (NSC-32065). Cancer Treat Rep. 1976;60(5) 601-609.

[4] Flaherty KT, Puzanov I, Kim KB, Ribas A, McArthur GA, Sosman JA, O'Dwyer PJ, Lee RJ, Grippo JF, Nolop K, Chapman PB. Inhibition of mutated, activated BRAF in metastatic melanoma. The New England Journal of Medicine 2010;363(9) 809-819.

[5] Leiter U, Eigentler TK, Forschner A, Pflugfelder A, Weide B, Held L, Meier F, Garbe C. Excision guidelines and follow-up strategies in cutaneous melanoma: Facts and controversies. Clinics in Dermatology 2010;28(3) 311-315.

[6] Denninghoff VC, Kahn AG, Falco J, Curutchet HP, Elsner B. Sentinel lymph node: detection of micrometastases of melanoma in a molecular study. Molecular Diagnosis 2004;8(4) 253-258.

[7] Bedikian AY, Wei C, Detry M, Kim KB, Papadopoulos NE, Hwu WJ, Homsi J, Davies M, McIntyre S, Hwu P. Predictive Factors for the Development of Brain Metastasis in Advanced Unresectable Metastatic Melanoma. American Journal of Clinical Oncology 2010;34(6) 603-610.

[8] Bradbury PA, Middleton MR. DNA repair pathways in drug resistance in melanoma. Anti-cancer Drugs 2004;15(5) 421-426.

[9] Pak BJ, Chu W, Lu SJ, Kerbel RS, Ben-David Y. Lineage-specific mechanism of drug and radiation resistance in melanoma mediated by tyrosinase-related protein 2. Cancer Metastasis Reviews 2001;20(1-2) 27-32.

[10] Pak BJ, Lee J, Thai BL, Fuchs SY, Shaked Y, Ronai Z, Kerbel RS, Ben-David Y. Radiation resistance of human melanoma analysed by retroviral insertional mutagenesis reveals a possible role for dopachrome tautomerase. Oncogene 2004;23(1) 30-38.

[11] Atkins MB, Lotze MT, Dutcher JP, Fisher RI, Weiss G, Margolin K, Abrams J, Sznol M, Parkinson D, Hawkins M, Paradise C, Kunkel L, Rosenberg SA. High-dose recombinant interleukin 2 therapy for patients with metastatic melanoma: analysis of 270 patients treated between 1985 and 1993. Journal of Clinical Oncology 1999;17(7) 2105-2116.

[12] Hodi FS, O'Day SJ, McDermott DF, Weber RW, Sosman JA, Haanen JB, Gonzalez R, Robert C, Schadendorf D, Hassel JC, Akerley W, van den Eertwegh AJ, Lutzky J, Lorigan P, Vaubel JM, Linette GP, Hogg D, Ottensmeier CH, Lebbé C, Peschel C, Quirt I, Clark JI, Wolchok JD, Weber JS, Tian J, Yellin MJ, Nichol GM, Hoos A, Urba WJ. Improved survival with ipilimumab in patients with metastatic melanoma. The New England Journal of Medicine 2010;363(8) 711-723.

[13] Kirkwood JM, Ibrahim JG, Sondak VK, Richards J, Flaherty LE, Ernstoff MS, Smith TJ, Rao U, Steele M, Blum RH. High- and low-dose interferon alfa-2b in high-risk melanoma: first analysis of intergroup trial E1690/S9111/C9190. Journal of Clinical Oncology 2000;18(12) 2444-2458.

[14] Kirkwood JM, Strawderman MH, Ernstoff MS, Smith TJ, Borden EC, Blum RH. Interferon alfa-2b adjuvant therapy of high-risk resected cutaneous melanoma: the Eastern Cooperative Oncology Group Trial EST 1684. Journal of Clinical Oncology 1996;14(1) 7-17.

[15] Galluzzi L, Vacchelli E, Eggermont A, Fridman WH, Galon J, Sautès-Fridman C, Tartour E, Zitvogel L, Kroemer G. Trial Watch: Adoptive cell transfer immunotherapy. Oncoimmunology 2012;1(3) 306-315.

[16] Bernatchez C, Radvanyi LG, Hwu P. Advances in the treatment of metastatic melanoma: adoptive T-cell therapy. Seminars in Oncology 2012;39(2) 215-226.

[17] Grulich AE, van Leeuwen MT, Falster MO, Vajdic CM. Incidence of cancers in people with HIV/AIDS compared with immunosuppressed transplant recipients: a meta-analysis. Lancet 2007;370(9581) 59-67.

[18] Nathanson. Spontaneous regression of malignant melanoma: a review of the literature on incidence, clinical features, and possible mechanisms. National Cancer Institute Monograph 1976;44 67-76.

[19] Rosenberg SA, Yang JC, Topalian SL, Schwartzentruber DJ, Weber JS, Parkinson DR, Seipp CA, Einhorn JH, White DE. Treatment of 283 consecutive patients with metastatic melanoma or renal cell cancer using high-dose bolus interleukin 2. The journal of the American Medical Association 1994;271(12) 907-913.

[20] Clark WH Jr, From L, Bernardino EA, Mihm MC. The histogenesis and biologic behavior of primary human malignant melanomas of the skin. Cancer Research 1969;29(3) 705-727.

[21] Clemente CG, Mihm MC Jr, Bufalino R, Zurrida S, Collini P, Cascinelli N. Prognostic value of tumor infiltrating lymphocytes in the vertical growth phase of primary cutaneous melanoma. Cancer 1996;77(7) 1303-1310.

[22] Burton AL, Roach BA, Mays MP, Chen AF, Ginter BA, Vierling AM, Scoggins CR, Martin RC, Stromberg AJ, Hagendoorn L, McMasters KM. Prognostic significance of tumor infiltrating lymphocytes in melanoma. The American Surgeon 2011;77(2) 188-192.

[23] Vignard V, Lemercier B, Lim A, Pandolfino MC, Guilloux Y, Khammari A, Rabu C, Echasserieau K, Lang F, Gougeon ML, Dreno B, Jotereau F, Labarriere N. Adoptive transfer of tumor-reactive Melan-A-specific CTL clones in melanoma patients is followed by increased frequencies of additional Melan-A-specific T cells. Journal of Immunology 2005;175(7) 4797-4805.

[24] Itzhaki O, Hovav E, Ziporen Y, Levy D, Kubi A, Zikich D, Hershkovitz L, Treves AJ, Shalmon B, Zippel D, Markel G, Shapira-Frommer R, Schachter J, Besser MJ. Establishment and large-scale expansion of minimally cultured "young" tumor infiltrating lymphocytes for adoptive transfer therapy. Journal of Immunology 2011;34(2) 212-220.

[25] Shen X, Zhou J, Hathcock KS, Robbins P, Powell DJ Jr, Rosenberg SA, Hodes RJ. Persistence of tumor infiltrating lymphocytes in adoptive immunotherapy correlates with telomere length. Journal of Immunology 2007;30(1) 123-129.

[26] Besser MJ, Shapira-Frommer R, Treves AJ, Zippel D, Itzhaki O, Schallmach E, Kubi A, Shalmon B, Hardan I, Catane R, Segal E, Markel G, Apter S, Nun AB, Kuchuk I, Shimoni A, Nagler A, Schachter J. Minimally cultured or selected autologous tumor-infiltrating lymphocytes after a lympho-depleting chemotherapy regimen in metastatic melanoma patients. Journal of Immunotherapy 2009;32(4) 415-423.

[27] Dudley ME, Wunderlich JR, Yang JC, Sherry RM, Topalian SL, Restifo NP, Royal RE, Kammula U, White DE, Mavroukakis SA, Rogers LJ, Gracia GJ, Jones SA, Mangiameli DP, Pelletier MM, Gea-Banacloche J, Robinson MR, Berman DM, Filie AC, Abati A, Rosenberg SA. Adoptive cell transfer therapy following non-myeloablative but lymphodepleting chemotherapy for the treatment of patients with refractory metastatic melanoma. Journal of Clinical Oncology 2005;23(10) 2346-2357.

[28] Besser MJ, Shapira-Frommer R, Treves AJ, Zippel D, Itzhaki O, Hershkovitz L, Levy D, Kubi A, Hovav E, Chermoshniuk N, Shalmon B, Hardan I, Catane R, Markel G, Apter S, Ben-Nun A, Kuchuk I, Shimoni A, Nagler A, Schachter J. Clinical responses in a phase II study using adoptive transfer of short-term cultured tumor infiltration lymphocytes in metastatic melanoma patients. Clinical Cancer Research 2010;16(9) 2646-2655.

[29] Dudley ME, Yang JC, Sherry R, Hughes MS, Royal R, Kammula U, Robbins PF, Huang J, Citrin DE, Leitman SF, Wunderlich J, Restifo NP, Thomasian A, Downey SG, Smith FO, Klapper J, Morton K, Laurencot C, White DE, Rosenberg SA. Adoptive cell therapy for patients with metastatic melanoma: evaluation of intensive myeloablative chemoradiation preparative regimens. Journal of Clinical Oncology 2008;26(32) 5233-5239.

[30] Weber J, Atkins M, Hwu P, Radvanyi L, Sznol M, Yee C; Immunotherapy Task Force of the NCI Investigational Drug Steering Committee.

[31] Kawakami Y, Eliyahu S, Jennings C, Sakaguchi K, Kang X, Southwood S, Robbins PF, Sette A, Appella E, Rosenberg SA. Recognition of multiple epitopes in the human melanoma antigen gp100 by tumor-infiltrating T lymphocytes associated with in vivo tumor regression. Journal of Immunology 1995;154(8) 3961-39618.

[32] Benlalam H, Vignard V, Khammari A, Bonnin A, Godet Y, Pandolfino MC, Jotereau F, Dreno B, Labarrière N. Infusion of Melan-A/Mart-1 specific tumor-infiltrating lymphocytes enhanced relapse-free survival of melanoma patients. Cancer Immunology Immunotherapy 2007;56(4) 515-526.

[33] Khammari A, Labarrière N, Vignard V, Nguyen JM, Pandolfino MC, Knol AC, Quéreux G, Saiagh S, Brocard A, Jotereau F, Dreno B. Treatment of metastatic melanoma with autologous Melan-A/MART-1-specific cytotoxic T lymphocyte clones. The Journal of Investigative Dermatology 2009;129(12) 2835-2842.

[34] Kvistborg P, Shu CJ, Heemskerk B, Fankhauser M, Thrue CA, Toebes M, van Rooij N, Linnemann C, van Buuren MM, Urbanus JH, Beltman JB, Thor Straten P, Li YF, Robbins PF, Besser MJ, Schachter J, Kenter GG, Dudley ME, Rosenberg SA, Haanen JB, Hadrup SR, Schumacher TN. TIL therapy broadens the tumor-reactive CD8(+) T cell compartment in melanoma patients. Oncoimmunology 2012;1(4) 409-418.

[35] Johnson LA, Heemskerk B, Powell DJ Jr, Cohen CJ, Morgan RA, Dudley ME, Robbins PF, Rosenberg SA. Gene transfer of tumor-reactive TCR confers both high avidity

and tumor reactivity to nonreactive peripheral blood mononuclear cells and tumor-infiltrating lymphocytes. Journal of Immunology 2006;177(9) 6548-6559.

[36] Zhao Y, Zheng Z, Khong HT, Rosenberg SA, Morgan RA. Transduction of an HLA-DP4-restricted NY-ESO-1-specific TCR into primary human CD4+ lymphocytes. Journal of Immunology 2006;29(4) 398-406.

[37] Frankel TL, Burns WR, Peng PD, Yu Z, Chinnasamy D, Wargo JA, Zheng Z, Restifo NP, Rosenberg SA, Morgan RA. Both CD4 and CD8 T cells mediate equally effective in vivo tumor treatment when engineered with a highly avid TCR targeting tyrosinase. Journal of Immunology 2010;184(11) 5988-5998.

[38] Johnson LA, Morgan RA, Dudley ME, Cassard L, Yang JC, Hughes MS, Kammula US, Royal RE, Sherry RM, Wunderlich JR, Lee CC, Restifo NP, Schwarz SL, Cogdill AP, Bishop RJ, Kim H, Brewer CC, Rudy SF, VanWaes C, Davis JL, Mathur A, Ripley RT, Nathan DA, Laurencot CM, Rosenberg SA. Gene therapy with human and mouse T-cell receptors mediates cancer regression and targets normal tissues expressing cognate antigen. Blood 2009;114(3) 535-546.

[39] Spiotto MT, Rowley DA, and Schreiber H. "Bystander" elimination of antigen loss variants in established tumors. Nature Medicine 2004; 10(3) 294-298.

[40] Schüler T, Blankenstein T. Cutting edge: CD8+ effector T cells reject tumors by direct antigen recognition but indirect action on host cells. Journal of Immunology 2003;170(9) 4427-4431.

[41] Stewart-Jones G, Wadle A, Hombach A, Shenderov E, Held G, Fischer E, Kleber S, Nuber N, Stenner-Liewen F, Bauer S, McMichael A, Knuth A, Abken H, Hombach AA, Cerundolo V, Jones EY, Renner C. Rational development of high-affinity T-cell receptor-like antibodies. Proceedings of the National Academy of Sciences of the United States of America 2009;106(14) 5784-5788.

[42] Willemsen RA, Debets R, Hart E, Hoogenboom HR, Bolhuis RL, Chames P. A phage display selected fab fragment with MHC class I-restricted specificity for MAGE-A1 allows for retargeting of primary human T lymphocytes. Gene Therapy 2001;8(21) 1601-1608.

[43] Chmielewski M, Hombach A, Heuser C, Adams GP, Abken H.T cell activation by antibody-like immunoreceptors: increase in affinity of the single-chain fragment domain above threshold does not increase T cell activation against antigen-positive target cells but decreases selectivity. Journal of Immunology 2004; 173(12) 7647-7653.

[44] Chmielewski M, Hombach AA, Abken H. CD28 cosignalling does not affect the activation threshold in a chimeric antigen receptor-redirected T-cell attack. Gene Therapy 2011;18(1) 62-72.

[45] Schaft N, Willemsen RA, de Vries J, Lankiewicz B, Essers BW, Gratama JW, Figdor CG, Bolhuis RL, Debets R, Adema GJ. Peptide fine specificity of anti-glycoprotein 100

CTL is preserved following transfer of engineered TCR alpha beta genes into primary human T lymphocytes. Journal of Immunology 2003; 170(4) 2186-2194.

[46] Morgan RA, Dudley ME, Yu YY, Zheng Z, Robbins PF, Theoret MR, Wunderlich JR, Hughes MS, Restifo NP, Rosenberg SA. High efficiency TCR gene transfer into primary human lymphocytes affords avid recognition of melanoma tumor antigen glycoprotein 100 and does not alter the recognition of autologous melanoma antigens," Journal of Immunology 2003 ;171(6) 3287-3295.

[47] Hughes MS, Yu YY, Dudley ME, Zheng Z, Robbins PF, Li Y, Wunderlich J, Hawley RG, Moayeri M, Rosenberg SA, Morgan RA. Transfer of a TCR gene derived from a patient with a marked antitumor response conveys highly active T-cell effector functions. Human Gene Therapy 2005;16(4) 457-472.

[48] Willemsen R, Ronteltap C, Heuveling M, Debets R, Bolhuis R. Redirecting human CD4+ T lymphocytes to the MHC class I-restricted melanoma antigen MAGE-A1 by TCR alphabeta gene transfer requires CD8alpha. Gene Therapy 2005; 12(2) 140-146.

[49] Morgan RA, Dudley ME, Wunderlich JR, Hughes MS, Yang JC, Sherry RM, Royal RE, Topalian SL, Kammula US, Restifo NP, Zheng Z, Nahvi A, de Vries CR, Rogers-Freezer LJ, Mavroukakis SA, Rosenberg SA. Cancer Regression in Patients After Transfer of Genetically Engineered Lymphocytes. Science. 2006;314(5796) 126-129.

[50] Coccoris M, Swart E, de Witte MA, van Heijst JW, Haanen JB, Schepers K, Schumacher TN. Long-term functionality of TCR-transduced T cells in vivo. Journal of Immunology 2008; 180(10) 6536-6543.

[51] Seliger B. Molecular mechanisms of MHC class I abnormalities and APM components in human tumors. Cancer Immunology Immunotherapy 2008;57(11) 1719-1726.

[52] Sigalotti L, Fratta E, Coral S, Tanzarella S, Danielli R, Colizzi F, Fonsatti E, Traversari C, Altomonte M, Maio M. Intratumor heterogeneity of cancer/testis antigens expression in human cutaneous melanoma is methylation-regulated and functionally reverted by 5-aza-2'-deoxycytidine. Cancer Research 2004;64(24) 9167-9171.

[53] Vitale M, Pelusi G, Taroni B, Gobbi G, Micheloni C, Rezzani R, Donato F, Wang X, Ferrone S. HLA class I antigen down-regulation in primary ovary carcinoma lesions: association with disease stage. Clinical Cancer Research 2005;11(1) 67-72.

[54] Coccoris M, Straetemans T, Govers C, Lamers C, Sleijfer S, Debets R. T cell receptor (TCR) gene therapy to treat melanoma: lessons from clinical and preclinical studies. Expert Opinion on Biological Therapy 2010;10(4) 547-562.

[55] Bendle GM, Linnemann C, Hooijkaas AI, Bies L, de Witte MA, Jorritsma A, Kaiser AD, Pouw N, Debets R, Kieback E, Uckert W, Song JY, Haanen JB, Schumacher TN. Lethal graft-versus-host disease in mouse models of T cell receptor gene therapy. Nature Medicine 2010; 16(5) 565-570.

[56] Cohen CJ, Zhao Y, Zheng Z, Rosenberg SA, Morgan RA. Enhanced antitumor activity of murine-human hybrid T-cell receptor (TCR) in human lymphocytes is associat-

ed with improved pairing and TCR/CD3 stability. Cancer Research 2006;66(17) 8878-8886.

[57] Kuball J, Dossett ML, Wolfl M, Ho WY, Voss RH, Fowler C, Greenberg PD. Facilitating matched pairing and expression of TCR chains introduced into human T cells. Blood 2007;109(6) 2331-2338.

[58] Eshhar Z, Waks T, Gross G, Schindler DG. Specific activation and targeting of cytotoxic lymphocytes through chimeric single chains consisting of antibody-binding domains and the gamma or zeta subunits of the immunoglobulin and T-cell receptors. Proceedings of the National Academy of Sciences of the United States of America 1993;90(2) 720-724.

[59] Hombach A, Abken H. Costimulation tunes tumor-specific activation of redirected T cells in adoptive immunotherapy," Cancer Immunology Immunotherapy 2007;56(5) 731-737.

[60] Hombach AA, Abken H. Costimulation by chimeric antigen receptors revisited the T cell antitumor response benefits from combined CD28-OX40 signalling. International Journal of Cancer 2011;129(12) 2935-2944.

[61] Bridgeman JS, Hawkins RE, Hombach AA, Abken H, Gilham DE.Building better chimeric antigen receptors for adoptive T cell therapy. Current Gene Therapy 2010; 10(2) 77-90.

[62] Gilham DE, Debets R, Pule M, Hawkins RE, Abken H. CAR-T cells and solid tumors: tuning T cells to challenge an inveterate foe. Trends in Molecular Medicine 2012;18(7) 377-384.

[63] Savoldo B, Rooney CM, Di Stasi A, Abken H, Hombach A, Foster AE, Zhang L, Heslop HE, Brenner MK, Dotti G. Epstein Barr virus specific cytotoxic T lymphocytes expressing the anti-CD30zeta artificial chimeric T-cell receptor for immunotherapy of Hodgkin disease. Blood. 2007;110(7) 2620-2630.

[64] ClinicalTrials.gov A service of the U.S. National Institutes of Health. Trial ID: NCT00586391 http://clinicaltrials.gov/ct2/results?term=NCT+00586391

[65] ClinicalTrials.gov A service of the U.S. National Institutes of Health. Trial ID: NCT00709033 http://clinicaltrials.gov/ct2/results?term=NCT+00709033

[66] ClinicalTrials.gov A service of the U.S. National Institutes of Health. Trial ID: NCT01218867 http://clinicaltrials.gov/ct2/results?term=NCT01218867

[67] Reinhold U, Liu L, Lüdtke-Handjery HC, Heuser C, Hombach A, Wang X, Tilgen W, Ferrone S, Abken H. Specific lysis of melanoma cells by receptor grafted T cells is enhanced by anti-idiotypic monoclonal antibodies directed to the scFv domain of the receptor. The Journal of Investigative Dermatology 1999;112(5) 744-750.

[68] Burns WR, Zhao Y, Frankel TL, Hinrichs CS, Zheng Z, Xu H, Feldman SA, Ferrone S, Rosenberg SA, Morgan RA. A high molecular weight melanoma-associated antigen-

specific chimeric antigen receptor redirects lymphocytes to target human melanomas. Cancer Research 2010;70(8) 3027-3033.

[69] Schmidt P, Kopecky C, Hombach A, Zigrino P, Mauch C, Abken H. Eradication of melanomas by targeted elimination of a minor subset of tumor cells. Proceedings of the National Academy of Sciences of the United States of America 2011;108(6) 2474-2479.

[70] Yvon E, Del Vecchio M, Savoldo B, Hoyos V, Dutour A, Anichini A, Dotti G, Brenner MK. Immunotherapy of metastatic melanoma using genetically engineered GD2-specific T cells. Clinical Cancer Research 2009;15(18) 5852-5860.

[71] Lo AS, Ma Q, Liu DL, Junghans RP. Anti-GD3 chimeric sFv-CD28/T-cell receptor zeta designer T cells for treatment of metastatic melanoma and other neuroectodermal tumors. Clinical Cancer Research 2010;16(10) 2769-2780.

[72] Kalos M, Levine BL, Porter DL, Katz S, Grupp SA, Bagg A, June CH. T cells with chimeric antigen receptors have potent antitumor effects and can establish memory in patients with advanced leukemia. Science Translational Medicine 2011;3(95) 95ra73.

[73] Porter DL, Levine BL, Kalos M, Bagg A, June CH. Chimeric antigen receptor-modified T cells in chronic lymphoid leukemia. The New England Journal of Medicine 2011;365(8) 725-733.

[74] Lamers CH, Sleijfer S, Vulto AG, Kruit WH, Kliffen M, Debets R, Gratama JW, Stoter G, Oosterwijk E. Treatment of metastatic renal cell carcinoma with autologous T-lymphocytes genetically retargeted against carbonic anhydrase IX: first clinical experience. Journal of Clinical Oncology 2006; 24(3) 20-22.

[75] Brentjens R, Yeh R, Bernal Y, Riviere I, Sadelain M. Treatment of chronic lymphocytic leukemia with genetically targeted autologous T cells: case report of an unforeseen adverse event in a phase I clinical trial. Molecular Therapy 2010;18(4) 666-668.

[76] Morgan RA, Yang JC, Kitano M, Dudley ME, Laurencot CM, Rosenberg SA. Case report of a serious adverse event following the administration of T cells transduced with a chimeric antigen receptor recognizing ERBB2. Molecular Therapy 2010;8(4) 843-851.

[77] Hawkins RE, Gilham DE, Debets R, Eshhar Z, Taylor N, Abken H, Schumacher TN, ATTACK Consortium. Development of adoptive cell therapy for cancer: a clinical perspective. Human Gene Therapy 2010;21(6) 665-672.

[78] Büning H, Uckert W, Cichutek K, Hawkins RE, Abken H. Do CARs need a driver's license? Adoptive cell therapy with chimeric antigen receptor-redirected T cells has caused serious adverse events. Human Gene Therapy 2010;21(9) 1039-1042.

[79] Offringa R. Antigen choice in adoptive T-cell therapy of cancer. Current Opinion in Immunology 2009;21(2) 190-199.

[80] Overwijk WW, Theoret MR, Finkelstein SE, Surman DR, de Jong LA, Vyth-Dreese FA, Dellemijn TA, Antony PA, Spiess PJ, Palmer DC, Heimann DM, Klebanoff CA,

Yu Z, Hwang LN, Feigenbaum L, Kruisbeek AM, Rosenberg SA, Restifo NP. Tumor regression and autoimmunity after reversal of a functionally tolerant state of self-reactive CD8+ T cells. The Journal of Experimental Medicine 2003;198(4) 569-580.

[81] Pule MA, Savoldo B, Myers GD, Rossig C, Russell HV, Dotti G, Huls MH, Liu E, Gee AP, Mei Z, Yvon E, Weiss HL, Liu H, Rooney CM, Heslop HE, Brenner MK. Virus-specific T cells engineered to coexpress tumor-specific receptors: persistence and antitumor activity in individuals with neuroblastoma Nature Medicine 2008;14(11) 1264-1270.

[82] Antony PA, Piccirillo CA, Akpinarli A, Finkelstein SE, Speiss PJ, Surman DR, Palmer DC, Chan CC, Klebanoff CA, Overwijk WW, Rosenberg SA, Restifo NP. CD8+ T cell immunity against a tumor/self-antigen is augmented by CD4+ T helper cells and hindered by naturally occurring T regulatory cells. Journal of Immunology 2005;174(5) 2591-2601.

[83] Meidenbauer N, Marienhagen J, Laumer M, Vogl S, Heymann J, Andreesen R, Mackensen A. Survival and tumor localization of adoptively transferred Melan-A-specific T cells in melanoma patients. Journal of Immunology 2003;170(4) 2161-2169.

[84] Griffith KD, Read EJ, Carrasquillo JA, Carter CS, Yang JC, Fisher B, Aebersold P, Packard BS, Yu MY, Rosenberg SA. In vivo distribution of adoptively transferred indium-111-labeled tumor infiltrating lymphocytes and peripheral blood lymphocytes in patients with metastatic melanoma. Journal of the National Cancer Institute 1989;81(22) 1709-1717.

[85] Fisher B, Packard BS, Read EJ, Carrasquillo JA, Carter CS, Topalian SL, Yang JC, Yolles P, Larson SM, Rosenberg SA. Tumor localization of adoptively transferred indium-111 labeled tumor infiltrating lymphocytes in patients with metastatic melanoma. Journal of Clinical Oncology 1989;7(2) 250-261.

[86] Peng W, Ye Y, Rabinovich BA, Liu C, Lou Y, Zhang M, Whittington M, Yang Y, Overwijk WW, Lizée G, Hwu P. Transduction of tumor-specific T cells with CXCR2 chemokine receptor improves migration to tumor and antitumor immune responses. Clinical Cancer Research 2010;16(22) 5458-5468.

[87] Mackensen A, Meidenbauer N, Vogl S, Laumer M, Berger J, Andreesen R. Phase I study of adoptive T-cell therapy using antigen-specific CD8+ T cells for the treatment of patients with metastatic melanoma. Journal of Clinical Oncology 2006;24(31) 5060-5069.

[88] Yee C, Thompson JA, Byrd D, Riddell SR, Roche P, Celis E, Greenberg PD. Adoptive T cell therapy using antigen-specific CD8+ T cell clones for the treatment of patients with metastatic melanoma: in vivo persistence, migration, and antitumor effect of transferred T cells. Proceedings of the National Academy of Science of the United States of America 2002;99(25) 16168-16173.

[89] Lozupone F, Rivoltini L, Luciani F, Venditti M, Lugini L, Cova A, Squarcina P, Parmiani G, Belardelli F, Fais S. Adoptive transfer of an anti-MART-1(27-35)-specific

CD8+ T cell clone leads to immunoselection of human melanoma antigen-loss variants in SCID mice. European Journal of Immunology 2003;33(2) 556-566.

[90] Becker JC, Varki N, Gillies SD, Furukawa K, Reisfeld RA. An antibody-interleukin 2 fusion protein overcomes tumor heterogeneity by induction of a cellular immune response," Proceedings of the National Academy of Sciences of the United States of America 1996;93(15) 7826-7831.

[91] Chmielewski M, Kopecky C, Hombach AA, Abken H. IL-12 release by engineered T cells expressing chimeric antigen receptors can effectively Muster an antigen-independent macrophage response on tumor cells that have shut down tumor antigen expression. Cancer Research 2011;71(17) 5697-5706.

[92] Li Y, Liu S, Hernandez J, Vence L, Hwu P, Radvanyi L.MART-1-specific melanoma tumor-infiltrating lymphocytes maintaining CD28 expression have improved survival and expansion capability following antigenic restimulation in vitro. Journal of Immunology 2010;184(1) 452-465.

[93] Hernandez-Chacon JA, Li Y, Wu RC, Bernatchez C, Wang Y, Weber JS, Hwu P, Radvanyi LG. Costimulation through the CD137/4-1BB pathway protects human melanoma tumor-infiltrating lymphocytes from activation-induced cell death and enhances antitumor effector function. Journal of Immunology 2011;34(3) 236-250.

[94] Boni A, Cogdill AP, Dang P, Udayakumar D, Njauw CN, Sloss CM, Ferrone CR, Flaherty KT, Lawrence DP, Fisher DE, Tsao H, Wargo JA. Selective BRAFV600E inhibition enhances T-cell recognition of melanoma without affecting lymphocyte function. Cancer Research 2010;70(13) 5213-5219.

[95] Wilmott JS, Long GV, Howle JR, Haydu LE, Sharma RN, Thompson JF, Kefford RF, Hersey P, Scolyer RA. Selective BRAF inhibitors induce marked T-cell infiltration into human metastatic melanoma. Clinical Cancer Research 2012;18(5) 1386-1394.

[96] Pegram HJ, Jackson JT, Smyth MJ, Kershaw MH, Darcy PK. Adoptive transfer of gene-modified primary NK cells can specifically inhibit tumor progression in vivo. Journal of Immunology 2008;181(5) 3449-3455.

[97] Kruschinski A, Moosmann A, Poschke I, Norell H, Chmielewski M, Seliger B, Kiessling R, Blankenstein T, Abken H, Charo J. Engineering antigen-specific primary human NK cells against HER-2 positive carcinomas," Proceedings of the National Academy of Sciences of the United States of America 2008;105(45) 17481-17486.

[98] Bonnet D, Dick JE. Human acute myeloid leukemia is organized as a hierarchy that originates from a primitive hematopoietic cell. Nature Medicine 1997;3(7) 730-737.

[99] Al-Hajj M, Wicha MS, Benito-Hernandez A, Morrison SJ, Clarke MF. Prospective identification of tumorigenic breast cancer cells. Proceedings of the National Academy of Sciences of the United States of America 2003;100(7) 3983-3988.

[100] Dalerba P, Dylla SJ, Park IK, Liu R, Wang X, Cho RW, Hoey T, Gurney A, Huang EH, Simeone DM, Shelton AA, Parmiani G, Castelli C, Clarke MF. Phenotypic characteri-

zation of human colorectal cancer stem cells. Proceedings of the National Academy of Sciences of the United States of America 2007;104(24) 10158-10163.

[101] Singh SK, Clarke ID, Terasaki M, Bonn VE, Hawkins C, Squire J, Dirks PB. Identification of a cancer stem cell in human brain tumors. Cancer Research 2003;63(18) 5821-5828.

[102] Ricci-Vitiani L, Lombardi DG, Pilozzi E, Biffoni M, Todaro M, Peschle C, De Maria R. Identification and expansion of human colon-cancer-initiating cells. Nature 2007;445(7123) 111-115.

[103] Li C, Heidt DG, Dalerba P, Burant CF, Zhang L, Adsay V, Wicha M, Clarke MF, Simeone DM. Identification of pancreatic cancer stem cells. Cancer Research 2007;67(3) 1030-1037.

[104] Schatton T, Murphy GF, Frank NY, Yamaura K, Waaga-Gasser AM, Gasser M, Zhan Q, Jordan S, Duncan LM, Weishaupt C, Fuhlbrigge RC, Kupper TS, Sayegh MH, Frank MH. Identification of cells initiating human melanomas. Nature. 2008;451(7176) 345-349.

[105] Zabierowski SE, Herlyn M. Melanoma stem cells: the dark seed of melanoma. Journal of Clinical Oncology 2008;26(17) 2890-2894.

[106] Fang D, Nguyen TK, Leishear K, Finko R, Kulp AN, Hotz S, Van Belle PA, Xu X, Elder DE, Herlyn M. A tumorigenic subpopulation with stem cell properties in melanomas. Cancer Research 2005;65(20) 9328-9337.

[107] Zhou BB, Zhang H, Damelin M, Geles KG, Grindley JC, Dirks PB. Tumour-initiating cells: challenges and opportunities for anticancer drug discovery. Nature Reviews Drug Discovery 2009;8(10) 806-823.

[108] Boiko AD, Razorenova OV, van de Rijn M, Swetter SM, Johnson DL, Ly DP, Butler PD, Yang GP, Joshua B, Kaplan MJ, Longaker MT, Weissman IL. Human melanoma-initiating cells express neural crest nerve growth factor receptor CD271. Nature 2010;466(7302) 133-137.

[109] Quintana E, Shackleton M, Sabel MS, Fullen DR, Johnson TM, Morrison SJ. Efficient tumour formation by single human melanoma cells. Nature 2008;456(7222) 593-598.

[110] Quintana E, Shackleton M, Foster HR, Fullen DR, Sabel MS, Johnson TM, Morrison SJ. Phenotypic Heterogeneity among Tumorigenic Melanoma Cells from Patients that Is Reversible and Not Hierarchically Organized. Cancer Cell 2010;18(5) 510-523.

[111] Schlaak M, Schmidt P, Bangard C, Kurschat P, Mauch C, Abken H. Regression of metastatic melanoma in a patient by antibody targeting of cancer stem cells. Oncotarget 2012;3(1) 22-30.

[112] Chmielewski M, Rappl G, Hombach AA, Abken H. T cells redirected by a CD3ζ chimeric antigen receptor can establish self-antigen-specific tumour protection in the

long term. Gene therapy 2012;doi: 10.1038/gt.2012.21. http://www.nature.com/gt/journal/vaop/ncurrent/full/gt201221a.html

[113] Butler MO, Friedlander P, Milstein MI, Mooney MM, Metzler G, Murray AP, Tanaka M, Berezovskaya A, Imataki O, Drury L, Brennan L, Flavin M, Neuberg D, Stevenson K, Lawrence D, Hodi FS, Velazquez EF, Jaklitsch MT, Russell SE, Mihm M, Nadler LM, Hirano N. Establishment of antitumor memory in humans using in vitro-educated CD8+ T cells. Science Translational Medicine 2011;3(80) 80ra34.

[114] Hong JJ, Rosenberg SA, Dudley ME, Yang JC, White DE, Butman JA, Sherry RM. Successful treatment of melanoma brain metastases with adoptive cell therapy. Clinical Cancer Research 2010;16(19) 4892–4898.

[115] Rosenberg SA, Yannelli JR, Yang JC, Topalian SL, Schwartzentruber DJ, Weber JS, Parkinson DR, Seipp CA, Einhorn JH, White DE. Treatment of patients with metastatic melanoma with autologous tumor-infiltrating lymphocytes and interleukin 2. Journal of the National Cancer Institute 1994;86(15) 1159–1166.

[116] Dudley ME, Gross CA, Langhan MM, Garcia MR, Sherry RM, Yang JC, Phan GQ, Kammula US, Hughes MS, Citrin DE, Restifo NP, Wunderlich JR, Prieto PA, Hong JJ, Langan RC, Zlott DA, Morton KE, White DE, Laurencot CM, Rosenberg SA. CD8+ enriched "young" tumor infiltrating lymphocytes can mediate regression of metastatic melanoma. Clinical Cancer Research 2010;16(24) 6122-6131.

[117] Heemskerk B, Liu K, Dudley ME, Johnson LA, Kaiser A, Downey S, Zheng Z, Shelton TE, Matsuda K, Robbins PF, Morgan RA, Rosenberg SA. Adoptive cell therapy for patients with melanoma, using tumor-infiltrating lymphocytes genetically engineered to secrete interleukin-2. Human Gene Therapy 2008;19(5) 496-510.

[118] Wallen H, Thompson JA, Reilly JZ, Rodmyre RM, Cao J, Yee C. Fludarabine modulates immune response and extends in vivo survival of adoptively transferred CD8 T cells in patients with metastatic melanoma. PloS One 2009;4(3) e4749. http://www.plosone.org/article/info%3Adoi%2F10.1371%2Fjournal.pone.0004749

[119] Verdegaal EM, Visser M, Ramwadhdoebé TH, van der Minne CE, van Steijn JA, Kapiteijn E, Haanen JB, van der Burg SH, Nortier JW, Osanto S. Successful treatment of metastatic melanoma by adoptive transfer of blood-derived polyclonal tumor-specific CD4+ and CD8+ T cells in combination with low-dose interferon-alpha. Cancer Immunology Immunotherapy 2011;60(7) 953-963.

[120] Rosenberg SA, Yang JC, Sherry RM, Kammula US, Hughes MS, Phan GQ, Citrin DE, Restifo NP, Robbins PF, Wunderlich JR, Morton KE, Laurencot CM, Steinberg SM, White DE, Dudley ME. Durable complete responses in heavily pretreated patients with metastatic melanoma using T-cell transfer immunotherapy. Clinical Cancer Research 2011;17(13) 4550-4557.

[121] Robbins PF, Morgan RA, Feldman SA, Yang JC, Sherry RM, Dudley ME, Wunderlich JR, Nahvi AV, Helman LJ, Mackall CL, Kammula US, Hughes MS, Restifo NP, Raf-

feld M, Lee CC, Levy CL, Li YF, El-Gamil M, Schwarz SL, Laurencot C, Rosenberg SA. Tumor regression in patients with metastatic synovial cell sarcoma and melanoma using genetically engineered lymphocytes reactive with NY-ESO-1. Journal of Clinical Oncology 2011;29(7) 917-924.

Chapter 14

Cellular and Molecular Mechanisms of Methotrexate Resistance in Melanoma

Luis Sanchez del-Campo, Maria F. Montenegro,
Magali Saez-Ayala, María Piedad Fernández-Pérez,
Juan Cabezas-Herrera and
Jose Neptuno Rodriguez-Lopez

Additional information is available at the end of the chapter

http://dx.doi.org/10.5772/52414

1. Introduction

Melanoma is a cancer that develops in melanocytes, the pigment cells present in the skin. It can be more serious than the other forms of skin cancer because it may spread to other parts of the body (metastasize) and cause serious illness and death. For malignant melanomas standard treatment options have remained remarkably static over the past 30 years [1,2]. At present, the incidence of melanoma continues to increase despite public health initiatives that have promoted protection against the sun. Thus, during the past ten years, the incidence and annual mortality of melanoma has increased more rapidly than any other cancer and according to the American Cancer Society estimate, there will have been approximately 76,250 new cases of invasive melanoma diagnosed in 2012 in the United States, which resulted in approximately 9,180 deaths [3].

Unfortunately, the increase in incidence has not been paralleled by the development of new therapeutic agents with a significant impact on survival. Although many patients with melanoma localized to the skin are cured by surgical excision, increased time to diagnosis is associated with higher stage of disease, and those with regional lymphatic or metastatic disease respond poorly to conventional radiation and chemotherapy with 5-year survival rates ranging from 10 to 50% [4]. Currently, limited therapeutic options exist for patients with metastatic melanomas, and all standard combinations currently used in metastasis therapy have low efficacy and poor response rates. For instance, the only approved chemotherapy for metastatic melanoma, dacarbacine, has a response rate of about 10% and a median survival of 8-9 months.

The other approved agent for advanced melanoma is high dose interleukin-2, which can induce dramatic complete and durable responses [2]. However, only one patient in twenty derives lasting benefit. These data indicate the needed for alternative therapies for this disease and recent results indicated that combined therapies could became an attractive strategy to fight melanoma [2].

Other example of the complications involved in melanoma chemotherapy is the limited effectiveness of antifolates. Although methotrexate (MTX), the most frequently used antifolate, is an efficient drug for several types of cancer, it is not active against melanoma [5-7]. Undoubtedly, unravelling the mechanisms of melanoma resistance to MTX could yield important information on how to circumvent this resistance and could have important pharmacological implications for the design of novel combined therapies. Thus, although an old drug, MTX could become a valuable tool with which to improve melanoma therapy.

2. General mechanisms of resistance to classical antifolates

The antifolate methotrexate was rationally-designed nearly 70 years ago to potently block the folate-dependent enzyme dihydrofolate reductase (DHFR). DHFR (5,6,7,8-tetrahydrofolate: NADP+ oxidoreductase, EC 1.5.1.3) catalyses the reduction of 7,8-dihydrofolate (DHF) to 5,6,7,8-tetrahydrofolate (THF) in the presence of coenzyme NADPH as follows: DHF + NADPH + H+ → THF + NADP+. This enzyme is necessary for maintaining intracellular pools of THF and its derivatives which are essential cofactors in one-carbon metabolism. Coupled with thymidylate synthase (TS) [8], it is directly involved in thymidylate (dTMP) production through a *de novo* pathway. DHFR is therefore pivotal in providing purines and pyrimidine precursors for the biosynthesis of DNA, RNA and amino acids. In addition, it is the target enzyme [9] for antifolate drugs such as the antineoplastic drug MTX and the antibacterial drug trimethoprim (TMP). The mechanisms of resistance to MTX have been extensively studied, mainly in experimental tumours propagated *in vitro* and *in vivo* [5,10,11]; however, the specific basis for the resistance of melanoma cells to MTX is unclear. During decades the mechanism of resistance of melanoma to MTX was associated with general mechanisms of resistance detected in other epithelial cancer cell including reduced cellular uptake of this drug, high intracellular levels of DHFR and/or insufficient rate of MTX polyglutamylation, which diminishes long-chain MTX polyglutamates from being preferentially retained intracellularly [11]. However, recently, a melanoma-specific mechanism of resistance to cytotoxic drugs, including MTX, has been described [6,12,13].

Antifolate resistance in cancer cells is believed to be a multifactorial process in which dysregulation of apoptosis, insufficient rates of MTX polyglutamylation, and enhanced DNA repair play important roles [11,14]. In melanoma, another classical mechanism of resistance to MTX, the upregulation of endogenous dihydrofolate reductase (DHFR) activity, has been described [5]; however, the contribution of this mechanism to the overall resistance of melanoma to MTX as well as its possible impact on DNA damage response pathways in cells is unknown. 'Thymineless' death, which occurs upon the depletion of cellular dTTP pools, has been proposed as a mechanism by which antifolate drugs promote apoptosis in cancer cells [15,16]. Although the mechanism of dTTP depletion-induced apoptosis is yet to be determined, Pardee's group recently postulated that dTTP controls E2F1, which regulates both DNA synthesis and apoptosis. This hypothesis was based on the observation that MTX increased E2F1 levels in sensitive cancer cells, resulting in an increase in the E2F1-mediated apoptotic cascade.

Eukaryotic cells have developed complex checkpoint pathways that monitor DNA for damage or incomplete replication. Checkpoint pathways are amplified upon detection of aberrant DNA structures and lead to a delay in cell cycle progression during which damage can be repaired or replication be completed. Alternatively, in case of heavily damaged or seriously deregulated cells, checkpoint activation can result in apoptosis. As such, checkpoint mechanisms are essential for the maintenance of genomic integrity [17]. When vertebrate cells experience replication arrest or undergo DNA damage by UV irradiation, the ATR kinase [ataxia telangiectasia mutated (ATM)- and Rad3-related kinase] phosphorylates and activates the Chk1 protein kinase. Activated Chk1 inhibits Cdc25 phosphatases, which control inhibitory phosphorylation sites on cyclin-dependent kinases, the latter being critical regulators of cell cycle transitions [18,19]. Because the ability of cells to delay cell cycle progression and halt DNA synthesis represents a defensive mechanism that spares potential toxicity [20], the activation of Chk1 by MTX could constitute a key event in the resistance of melanoma to MTX.

In addition to these cellular mechanisms of resistance to MTX in melanoma, other mechanism that includes liver transformation of the drug has also been reported. A paradoxical response of malignant melanoma to MTX *in vivo* and *in vitro* has been described [21]. The authors observed that MTX showed consistent cytotoxicity for melanoma cells *in vitro* but was ineffective at equivalent concentrations *in vivo*. MTX undergoes oxidation to its primary metabolite 7-hydroxy-MTX (7-OH-MTX) in the liver by the enzyme aldehyde oxidase [11] and therefore, this transformation has been proposed as a novel mechanism of resistance to explain this paradox [11,21]. In contrast to the large body of literature available on the multiple modalities of MTX resistance, very little is known regarding the ability of 7-OH-MTX to provoke antifolate-resistance phenomena that may disrupt MTX activity. Recent studies seem to indicate that 7-OH-MTX which exceeds by far MTX in the plasma of MTX-treated patients can provoke distinct modalities of antifolate-resistance that severely compromise the efficacy of the parent drug MTX [22].

3. Melanoma-specific mechanisms of resistance to MTX

3.1. The critical role of alpha-folate receptor in the resistance of melanoma to MTX

Experiments from our laboratory and others provide evidence that melanosomes contribute to the refractory properties of melanoma cells by sequestering cytotoxic drugs and increasing melanosome-mediated drug export [6,12,13]. Concretely, we have described that folate receptor α (FRα)-endocytotic transport of MTX facilitates drug melanosomal sequestration and cellular exportation in melanoma cells, which ensures reduced accumulation of MTX in intracellular compartments [6]. An important observation in this study was that MTX was a cytostatic agent on melanoma cells. These cells were resistant to MTX-induced apoptosis but responded to the drug by arresting their growth. A similar response was observed when the murine B16/F10 melanoma cell line was grown in low folate. After 3 days in folate-deficient medium the cells had restricted proliferative activity and also increased their metastatic potential [23]. Taking this into consideration, the results indicate that MTX might also induce depletion of intracellular reduced folate coenzymes by reducing their transport though the FRα and/or competing with them for the reduced folate carrier (RFC). Melanoma cells may be highly sensitive to intracellular depletion of folate coenzymes, and in this situation may enter into a "latent" state. This form of melanoma should indeed be highly resistant to MTX, since antifolate drugs are more effective on fast-dividing cells, which require continuous DNA synthesis. Most likely, the high increases of DHFR expression in cells treated with MTX [5] would represent an adaptation mechanism that allows cells to survive with low intracellular concentrations of folate coenzymes. Increasing the recycling of folate molecules the cells would maintain other cellular functions that are dependent on folate coenzymes, such as the synthesis of purines, pyrimidines, amino acids and methylation reactions. The presence of this "latent" form of melanoma should be critical for the resistance to MTX during *in vivo* therapies. Although MTX chemotherapy could initially halt the development of the tumor, after clearance of the drug from the body the melanoma cells may reinitiate their progression, possibly with an increased metastatic potential [23].

A defect in intracellular folate retention is another recognized mechanism of drug resistance [5,10,11,21]. In addition to a decrease in antifolate polyglutamylation, melanoma cells may also export cytotoxic drugs by melanosome sequestration [12]. The results presented in this study indicated that drug exportation was an operative mechanism of resistance to MTX in melanoma cells. Although the mechanism by which cytotoxic drugs are sequestered into melanosomes remains unclear, we demonstrated that MTX-melanosome trapping may be a consequence of its FRα-endosomal transport [6]. To test the importance of this process on the resistance of melanoma to antifolates, we silenced the expression of the melanosomal structural protein gp100/Pmel17, which is known to play a critical role in melanosome biogenesis [24]. Recently, Xie and collaborators [13] provided the first direct evidence that disruption of the process of normal melanosome biogenesis, by mutation of gp100/Pmel17, increased sensitivity to cisplatin. We also observed that effective silencing of gp100/Pmel17 significantly increased the sensitivity of melanoma cells to MTX, favouring MTX-induced apoptosis. This observation strongly supports the hypothesis which indicates that melanosome biogenesis is a specialization of the endocytic pathway [25,26]; however, the exact mechanism by which MTX induces abnormal trafficking of early endosomes in melanoma cells, favoring the exportation of melanosomes, is still unclear. Whether MTX blocks the formation of carrier vesicles operating between early and late endosomes, inhibits the delivery of endocytosed material from endosomes to lysosomes, promoting, thus, the generation of exosomes [26] and/or induces a failure of lysosomal acidification, which is essential for normal endocytosis [27], remains to be determined.

http://dx.doi.org/10.5772/52414

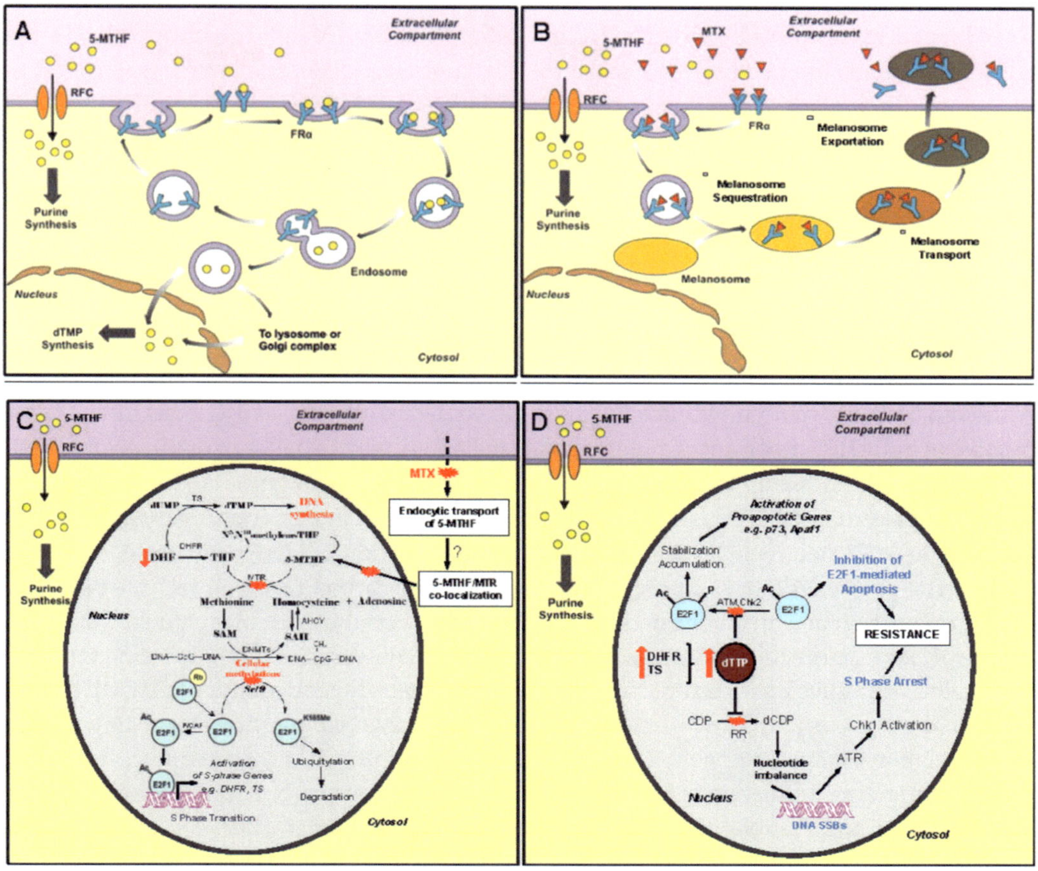

Figure 1. A) Possible mechanisms for transport and trafficking of folates in melanoma cells. (B) Mechanisms to explain the MTX-induced depletion of DHF in melanoma cells. (C) Folate deficiency induces DHF depletion and enhances the transactivational potential of E2F1. (D) Excess of dTTP inhibits E2F1-mediated apoptosis and activates Chk1 in melanoma cells. High levels of DHFR and TS could reactivate *de novo* dTMP biosynthesis impeding depletion of dTTP. Excess of dTTP would prevent apoptosis by several mechanisms. First, dTTP is an allosteric inhibitor of ribonucleotide reductase (RR), the enzyme which reduces cytidine diphosphate (CDP) and uridine diphosphate to dCDP and dUDP.

To explore the relationship between MTX exportation and melanosome trafficking, we studied the possible interaction of MTX with melanin [6]. Such interaction was confirmed by incubating this drug with synthetic 3,4-dihydroxyphenylalanine (DOPA)-melanin. Importantly, folic acid and 5-methyl-THF (5-MTHF), the natural source of cellular folates, did not appear to interact with synthetic DOPA-melanin. A comparison of the interaction of several folates (folic acid and 5-MTHF) and antifolates (MTX and aminopterin) with synthetic DOPA-melanin indicated that the double amino group of the pterin ring is an important molecular requirement for the drug-melanin interaction. Therefore, the physiological importance of the high affinity of melanin for antifolates, such as MTX and aminopterin, for drug melanosomal sequestration is also another important issue that remains to be addressed. Endocytic transport of molecules involves several processes, including the fusion of early and late endosomes and the dissociation of receptor-ligand complexes through the acidic pH of preformed vesicles [28]. After melanosome biogenesis from MTX-loaded endosomes, dissociated MTX could be trapped in the melanosomes by its interaction with melanins. In contrast, folate substrates would not be sequestered in melanosomes due to their low affinities for melanin; facilitated by the acidic pH of this organelle, uncharged reduced folates would leave the melanosome by passive diffusion and reach the cytosol, where they would become available for cellular functions. Therefore, elucidation of the molecular basis for the (anti)folate interaction with melanins could have important therapeutic implications, and this study might be used as a guide for the synthesis of new antifolates or for using existing antifolates in ways that escape melanin trapping.

3.2. MTX disrupts folate trafficking in melanoma cells

Although MTX is exported within a few hours in contact with cells, in this short time, MTX is capable of inducing important changes in folate metabolism by depleting dihydrofolate (DHF) early on and by inducing the expression of folate-dependent enzymes later on [7]. The increased expression of DHFR is a common occurrence in melanoma and other cancer cells in response to MTX treatment; however, the observed depletion of DHF was completely unexpected. The pathways that comprise folate-mediated one-carbon metabolism have been suggested to function in a metabolic network that interconnects the three biosynthetic pathways, namely *de novo* purine biosynthesis, *de novo* dTMP biosynthesis, and homocysteine remethylation. Recent studies provide direct evidence for cell cycle–dependent nuclear dTMP biosynthesis in the nucleus [29]. However, there are many unanswered questions regarding the role and regulation of nuclear *de novo* dTMP biosynthesis. Nothing is known about the transport, processing, and accumulation of folates into the nucleus, the one-carbon forms of folate present in the nucleus, and the relationship between cell cycle dependency of *de novo* dTMP biosynthesis and cell cycle-dependent accumulation of nuclear folate [29]. Although there is no data of how the homocysteine remethylation cycle is compartmentalized, the observation that MTX affected both DHF synthesis and E2F1 methylation (see below) seem to indicate that both the *de novo* dTMP biosynthesis and the homocysteine remethylation cycles might operate simultaneously in the nucleus.

Using HeLa and MCF-7 cells, Stover and coworkers observed that cytoplasmic serine hydroxymethyltransferase (SMTH), TS, and DHFR are all translocated into the nucleus during S and G_2/M phases following their modification by the small ubiquitin-like modifier (SUMO) [30,31]. This finding indicated that the folate cycle may be compartmentalized and that dTMP and DHF synthesis may occur in the nucleus during DNA synthesis. In a recent study, Wollack et al. [32] characterized 5-MTHF uptake and metabolism by primary rat choroid plexus epithelial cells *in vitro*. They distinguish two different processes for 5-MTHF transport, one that was FRα dependent and the other that was independent of this receptor and mediated by the proton couple folate transporter or reduced folate carrier (RFC). This investigation revealed that cellular metabolism of 5-MTHF depends on the route of folate entry into the cell. Thus, 5-MTHF taken up via a non-FRα–mediated process was rapidly metabolized to folylpolyglutamates, whereas 5-MTHF that accumulates via FRα remained non-metabolized and associated to endocytic compartments. The observation that MTX induces the overall depletion of FRα in melanoma cells [6] would suggest that MTX might also induce depletion of reduced folate coenzymes associated to endocytic compartments (Figure 1A and 1B). Therefore, a possible explanation for the depletion of DHF during MTX exposure could be that this drug diminishes the required supply of folates to the nucleus for the maintenance of both dTMP and DHF synthesis; however, how melanoma cells can control endocytic pathways to supply their own nucleus with folates is unknown. Recent studies have indicated that some endocytic proteins are also involved in direct signaling pathways from membranes to the nucleus, and mechanisms for the nuclear translocation of intact or fragmented endosome-localized proteins have been identified [33]. Another possibility is the existence of a late endosome-lysosome transport mechanism for folate [34]. The proximity of lysosomes to the nucleus suggests that folates could be released into the perinuclear region of the cytoplasm, perhaps facilitating their nuclear entry during cell division following the disassembly of the nuclear membrane [29].

Although the uptake of 5-MTHF into mammalian cells is mainly mediated by the RFC, the expression of FRα in several epithelial tissues and especially its overexpression in cancerous cells indicate that this receptor may confer a growth advantage to these cells [35]. The high affinity of FRα for 5-MTHF suggest that this GPI-anchored receptor may play an important role in maintaining nuclear folates even at low extracellular concentrations of this vitamin. This hypothesis is supported by the finding that induction of FRα expression in cells that normally do not express this receptor allows the cells to grow in low nanomolar folate concentrations [36]. On the other hand, the observation that methionine synthase was localized in the nucleus of melanoma cells could explain many of the unanswered questions on the role and regulation of the folate metabolism in the nucleus of these cancer cells. The methionine synthase -mediated catalysis of 5-MTHF would first supply THF and methionine to maintain both dTTP synthesis and the methylation reactions in the nucleus of the cells (Figure 1C) and second would prevent the nuclear accumulation of 5-MTHF, a potent inhibitor of SHMT [29]. Therefore, in melanoma, the existence of a specific folate transport pathway from the plasma membrane to the nucleus, mediated by FRα, is possible [37] and could shed light on the unknown function of overexpressed FRα in cancer cells [38].

4. Melanoma coordinates general and cell-specific mechanisms to promote MTX resistance

4.1. MTX induces E2F1 demethylation and prevents dTTP depletion in melanoma

MTX acts as a cytostatic agent in melanoma cells [6]. To discriminate between the mechanisms by which MTX could induce cell growth arrest without inducing apoptosis, the effect of this drug on the cell cycle of several melanoma cell lines was analysed [7]. The results indicated that, in all the tested melanoma cell lines, MTX conferred an arrest in early S phase; the G_1 peak shifted toward the G_1/S border, and cells were arrested with a minimal increase in their DNA content. Because S phase arrest has been recognized as a major mechanism of resistance in response to non-toxic concentrations of drugs that induce DNA replication stress, these preliminary results suggest that moderate DNA damage could be responsible for the cytostatic effect of MTX on melanoma cells.

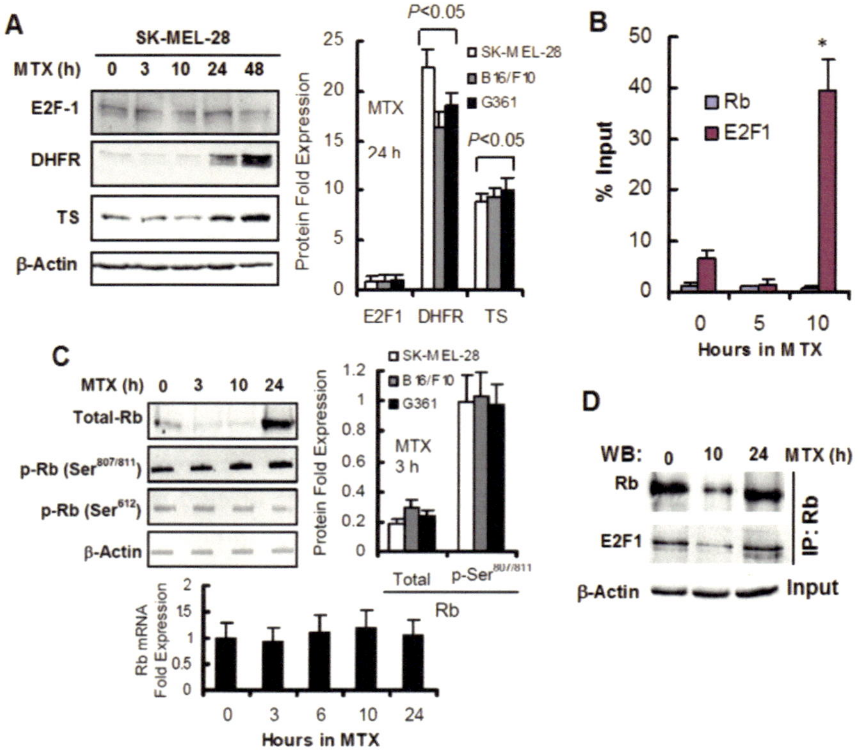

Figure 2. MTX enhances the transactivation potential of E2F1 in melanoma cells. (A) The time-dependent effect of MTX treatment (1 μM) on the expression of E2F1, DHFR, and TS proteins as assayed by western blot (WB). (B) ChIP experiments showing the occupancy of E2F1 and Rb on the DHFR promoter of B16/F10 melanoma cells (*$P < 0.05$). (C) The upper panels represent the time-dependent effects of MTX (1 μM) treatment on the expression and phosphorylation state of the Rb protein as assayed by WB. The lower panel depicts the Rb mRNA expression as assayed by qRT-PCR. The changes observed after MTX treatment were not statistically significant. (D) Co-immunoprecipitation assays were performed to test the interaction between Rb and E2F1.

To understand the mechanisms involved in G_1 cell cycle progression in MTX-treated melanoma cells, the effect of this drug on several G_1 cell cycle components was analysed. Although the protein levels of E2F1 were not affected by MTX (Figure 2A), this drug significantly increased the protein levels of DHFR and thymidylate synthase (TS), two E2F1-target genes involved in folate metabolism and required for G_1 progression and DNA synthesis (Figure 2A). Chromatin immunoprecipitation (ChIP) experiments that were designed to analyze the occupancy of E2F1 on the DHFR promoter of B16/F10 melanoma cells indicated that MTX stimulated the transcriptional activity of E2F1 (Figure 2B). First, we observed that MTX induced a transient decrease in the hypophosphorylated Rb protein in melanoma cells (Figure 2C) as evidenced by a noticeable lack of Rb co-immunoprecipitation with E2F1 in 10 h MTX-treated SK-MEL-28 cells when compared to untreated controls (Figure 2D). In addition, mass peptide analysis of immunoprecipitated E2F1, after trypsin digestion (Figure 3), indicated that MTX promoted the demethylation of E2F1 at Lys185 (Figures 3B and 3D). A negative crosstalk between methylation and other posttranslational modifications of E2F1, such as acetylation and phosphorylation, has been recently described [39]. We observed that MTX induced the transient co-immunoprecipitation of E2F1 with p300/CBP-associated factor (P/CAF) (Figure 3B), an interaction that has been associated with the transcriptionally active hyperacetylated form of this transcription factor [40]. The hyperacetylated status of E2F1 after MTX treatment was also confirmed by MALDI-TOF mass spectrometry (Figures 3B and 3D). In response to severe DNA damage, the E2F1 protein is stabilized through distinct mechanisms, including direct phosphorylation by Chk2 at Ser^{364} [41] or ATM kinase at Ser^{31} [42]. As we did not observe phosphorylation of E2F1 after MTX treatment (Figures 3C and 3D), these data further suggest that MTX induced moderate DNA damage without inducing double strand breaks (DSBs) [43].

MTX increased E2F1 levels in sensitive cancer cells [16]. However, we did not observe an MTX-mediated increase in E2F1 levels in melanoma cells (Figure 2A) [7], a result that could be explained, at least in part, by the results obtained after determination of dNTP pools in melanoma cells (Figure 4). Contrary to the effects of MTX in most cancer cells [16], this drug increased the levels of dTTP in melanoma. Increased levels of dTTP were accompanied by a decrease in dCTP levels, which resulted in a nucleotide imbalance that favored thymidine excess. The MTX-induced expression of DHFR and TS (Figure 2A) and the low levels of MTX accumulated in melanoma cells [6] could explain this paradoxical response of melanoma cells to a cytotoxic drug that typically depletes dTTP levels.

The data obtained in our study indicate that melanoma cells respond to the lack of folate coenzymes by enhancing the transactivational potential of E2F1. We observed that treatment of melanoma cells with MTX transiently affected the stability of Rb and the posttranslational state of E2F1 [7]. A crosstalk between the methylated and acetylated forms of E2F1 has been suggested [39]. Methylated E2F1 is prone to ubiquitination and degradation, whereas the demethylation of E2F1 favors its P/CAF-dependent acetylation. Together, the results suggest a model whereby the MTX-induced degradation of Rb and the demethylation of E2F1 would result in the accumulation of E2F1 in its 'free' state, and in the absence of DNA damage, free E2F1 would be acetylated, leading to the transcription of genes required for S phase (Figure 1C). The activation of E2F1 by MTX would allow S phase transition in melanoma cells, and importantly for melanoma survival, cells would recover an operative folate cycle, thereby restoring the original status of the Rb/E2F1 system. In the absence of exported MTX, high levels of TS and DHFR would impede the lethal depletion of dTTP and in turn, would produce a nucleotide imbalance that would favor a dTTP excess. Contrary to thymidine depletion, excess thymidine stops cells in S phase by blocking synthesis of DNA, an effect known as 'thymidine block' (Figure 1D) [15]. Recently, a mechanism by which dTTP allosterically feedback controls E2F1 has been proposed [15,16]. According to this mechanism, excess of dTTP inhibits E2F1 accumulation acting either upon production of E2F1 or its degradation. Because control of E2F1 is essential for cell survival, this mechanism would prevent E2F1 accumulation, which would result in activation of apoptosis through a process that involves p53 or p73, cytochrome c, and caspases (Figure 1D) [44].

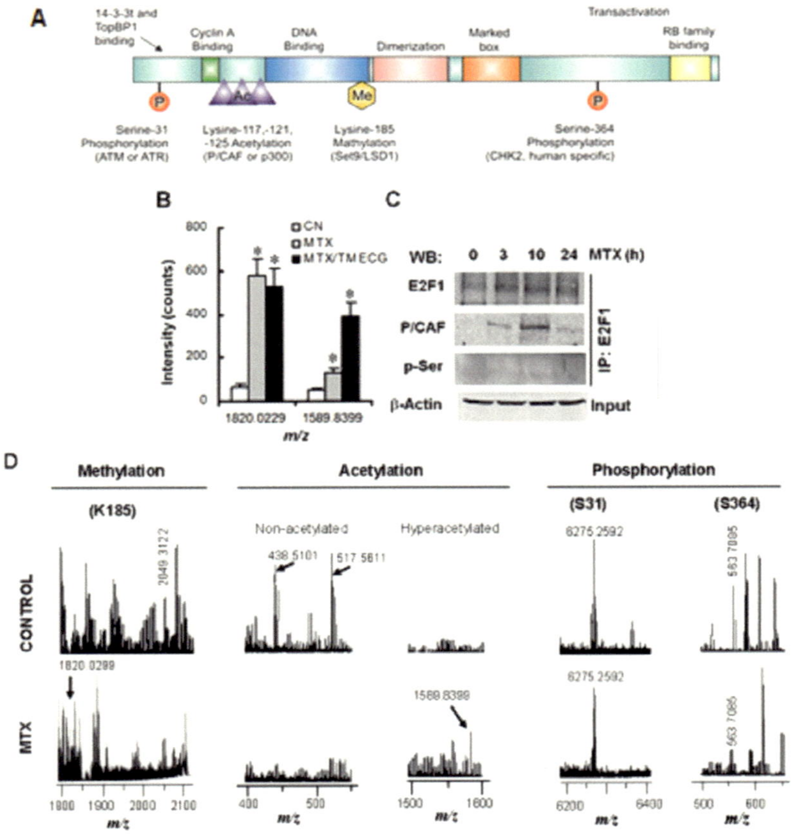

Modification	E2F1 Status	Peptide Sequence	Measured (m/z)	Theoretical (m/z)
Methylation (K185)	Non-methylated	(K)NHIQWLGSHTTVGVGGR(L)	1820.0299	1820.0331
	Methylated	(K)SK$_{Me}$NHIQWLGSHTTVGVGGR(L)	2049.3122	2049.3140
Acetylation (K117,120,125)	Non-acetylated	(R)HPGK(G)	438.5101	438.5097
		(K)SPGEK(S)	517.5611	517.5625
	Hyperacetylated	(R)HPGK$_{Ac}$GVK$_{Ac}$SPGEK$_{Ac}$SR(Y)	1589.8399	1589.8394
Phosphorylation (S31)	Non-phosphorylated	(R)LLDSSQIVIISAAQDASAPPAPTGPAAPAAGPC(Carbamidomethyl)DPDLLLFATPQAPRPTPSAPRPALGRPPVK(R)	6275.2592	6275.2600
	Phosphorylated	(R)LLDSS$_P$QIVIISAAQDASAPPAPTGPAAPAAGPC(Carbamidomethyl)DPDLLLFATPQAPRPTPSAPRPALGRPPVK(R)	6355.2361	6355.2398
Phosphorylation (S364)	Non-phosphorylated	(R)MGSLR(A)	563.7085	563.7006
	Phosphorylated	(R)MGS$_P$LR(A)	643.6799	643.6804

Figure 3. MTX induces demethylation and hyperacetylation of E2F1 in melanoma cells. (A) Schematic representation of the E2F1 protein. Residues susceptible to methylation (K185), acetylation (K117, K120, and K125), and phosphorylation (S31 and S364) are shown. (B) Relative intensity of unmethylated [(K)NHIQWLGSHTTVGVGGR(L); m/z 1820.0229] and hyperacetylated [(R)HPGKAcGVKAcSPGEKAcSR(Y); m/z 1589.8399] peptides in E2F1-trypsin digested samples. Peptides were analyzed in untreated SK-MEL-28 cells (CN) or treated for 10 h with 1 µM MTX (**P* < 0.05). Intensities were normalized with respect to an internal matrix control. (C) Cell lysates from SK-MEL-28 cells that had been treated with 1 µM MTX were used for IP assays with E2F1 to test the co-immunoprecipitation of E2F1 with P/CAF and the phosphorylated state of E2F1. (D) MALDI-TOF mass spectra of tryptic digests of immunoprecipitated E2F1. The characteristics peptides involving posttranslational modifications of E2F1 (methylation = Me, acetylation = Ac, and phosphorylation = P), as well as their measured and theoretical m/z are shown.

http://dx.doi.org/10.5772/52414

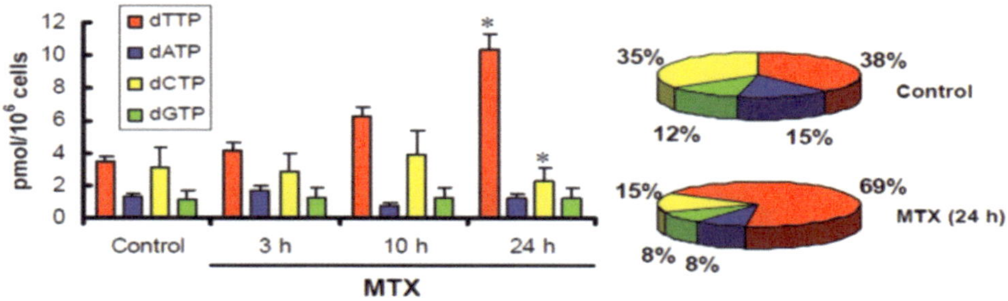

Figure 4. MTX does not deplete dTTP levels in melanoma cells. dNTP quantification in SK-MEL-28 control cells and cells subjected to MTX (1 μM) treatment (*$P < 0.05$). Data collected from the left panel was used to determine the total amounts of each dNTP at each time point. The percent contribution of each dNTP to the total pool after 24 h of treatment is represented.

4.2. Excess of dTTP favours Chk1 activation in melanoma after MTX treatment

Excess thymidine induces little detectable DNA damage in the form of DSBs. The ATR-mediated response appears to play a more prominent role under these cellular conditions [45]. As it is known that the central mechanism responsible for Chk1 activation upon DNA damage is the distribution of ATR into nuclear foci [46], the effects of MTX on the localization of ATR and the phosphorylation of Chk1 at Ser^{345} were analyzed by confocal microscopy and western blot, respectively (Figures 5A and 5B). Time- and dose-dependent experiments clearly indicated that MTX induced Chk1 phosphorylation in melanoma cells. Because Chk1 phosphorylation may not directly correspond to Chk1 activation, we next analyzed the dose-dependent effects of MTX on the stability of Cdc25A (Figure 5B). We found that Chk1 phosphorylation led to a corresponding decrease in Cdc25A abundance, indicating that MTX not only conferred Chk1 phosphorylation, but it also activated Chk1. Conversely, phosphorylation of Chk2 was not observed in melanoma cells that had been treated with MTX for as long as 48 h (Figure 5B), indicating that this drug specifically induced Chk1 activation in response to DNA single strand breaks (SSBs). To determine the extent to which Chk1 activation affected the resistance of melanoma to MTX, we took two independent experimental approaches. First, we silenced the expression of Chk1 in SK-MEL-28 (p53 mutant) cells and studied the sensitivity of the cells to MTX (Figure 5C). The results indicated that the downregulation of Chk1 increased the sensitivity of SK-MEL-28 cells to MTX and led to apoptosis. As a second approach, we evaluated the ability of Chk1 to protect B16/F10 murine cells (p53 wild-type) from MTX-induced apoptosis by first inducing an S phase arrest with MTX and then treating the S-arrested cells with a combination of MTX and 7-hydroxystaurosporine (UCN-01). We observed that B16/F10 S phase-arrested cells were sensitive to MTX treatment after the effective inhibition of Chk1 (Figure 5C).

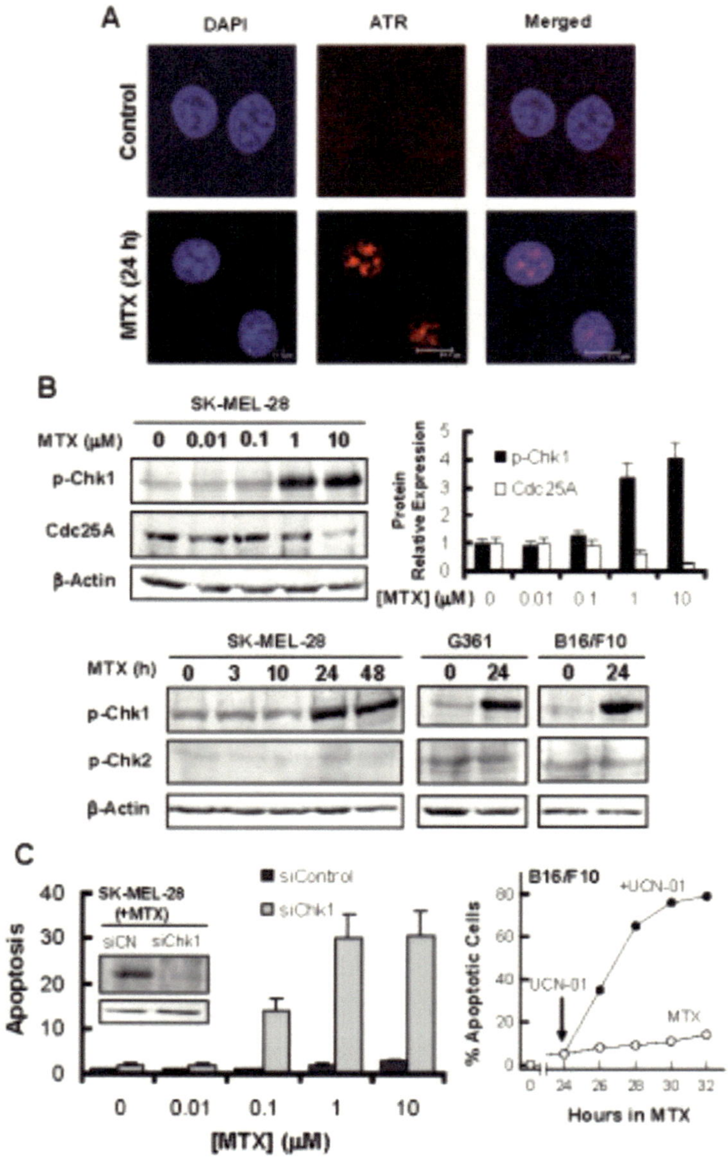

Figure 5. MTX activates Chk1 in melanoma cells. (A) SK-MEL-28 cells were treated with 1 μM MTX for 24 h and then examined for ATR nuclear foci. Nuclei were stained with DAPI. (B) The dose-dependent effects of MTX on Chk1 phosphorylation and Cdc25A degradation in SK-MEL-28 after 24 h of drug exposure (*$P < 0.05$). MTX (1 μM) induced the time-dependent phosphorylation of Chk1, but not Chk2, in different melanoma cell lines. (C) Chk1 siRNA sensitizes SK-MEL-28 cells to MTX-induced toxicity (left panel). siControl (siCN)- and siChk1-transfected cells were treated with increasing doses of MTX for 48 h (*$P < 0.05$). The effective silencing of Chk1 was tested by WB. The induction of the phosphorylated form of Chk1 was analyzed after 24 h of MTX treatment (1 μM). The induction of apoptosis by UCN-01 in MTX-arrested B16/F10 cells is shown in the right-side panel. Cells were incubated with 1 μM MTX continuously for 32 h, and 50 nM UCN-01 was added at 24 h to one group of cells following splitting of the culture. As a control experiment, SK-MEL-28 cells were treated with 50 nM UCN-01 only for 32 h.

Inhibitors of DNA synthesis, such as excess thymidine, hydroxyurea, and camptothecin, are normally poor inducers of apoptosis; however, these agents become potent inducers of death in S phase cells upon the small interfering RNA-mediated depletion of Chk1 [45]. Here, we observed that MTX activated Chk1 and induced an early S phase arrest in melanoma cells lines that were harboring either wild-type or mutant p53. The impact of MTX on the survival of Chk1-silenced melanoma cells and cells co-treated with UCN-01 indicates that MTX provokes a 'thymidine block'-like effect and that S phase arrest, as a result of Chk1 activation, might constitute a major and general p53-independent mechanism that is responsible for the resistance of melanomas to MTX. However, it would be difficult to understand this extreme resistance without taking into account the melanosome-mediated exportation of MTX. The activation of the DNA damage response pathway reflects the magnitude and extent of DNA damage that occurs in response to a specific genotoxic agent, and a dual role of Chk1, depending on the extent of DNA damage, has been proposed [45]. Thus, Chk1 may play an anti-apoptotic role in response to weaker replication fork stresses, whereas more catastrophic damage, such as the accumulation of DNA strand breaks, may result in the activation of apoptosis by Chk1. Together, the results indicate that low intracellular levels of MTX in melanoma induce moderate DNA damage that favors the anti-apoptotic role of Chk1 (Figure 1D).

5. Therapeutical implications

Although melanoma resistance to MTX was initially thought to be due to the classical mechanisms of resistance that have been observed in other epithelial cells, recent discoveries indicate that the resistance of melanoma to MTX might be due to the idiosyncrasies of these cancer cells [6,12] where drug melanosomal sequestration and its subsequent cellular exportation may have a marked protagonist. Unravelling the mechanisms of melanoma resistance to MTX could, therefore, yield important information on how to circumvent this resistance and could have important pharmacological implications for the design of novel combined therapies. Taking into account these observations, uses of combined treatments with MTX, to prevent melanosomal drug sequestration [6,12] or to avoid MTX-induced S phase arrest [19], are rational therapeutical approaches. The observation that MTX induces cellular depletion of DHF in melanoma [7] could generate novel combined therapies to efficiently inhibit DHFR with antifolates transported into the cells by FRα-independent processes. Also, of great interest is the observed effect of MTX on the posttranslational status of E2F1 in melanoma (Figure 3). Various studies have suggested that E2F1 plays dual roles in cell survival/apoptosis [47-50]. Therefore, the MTX-induced demethylation and acetylation of E2F1 could favour melanoma cell death when combined with E2F1-stabilizing drugs. In addition to E2F1 phosphorylation, acetylation has also been recognized to play a role in the activation and stabilization of the E2F1 protein during DNA damage and apoptosis [40]. A possible strategy to favour E2F1 apoptosis in melanoma by the combination of MTX with E2F1-stabilizing drugs is depicted in Figure 6.

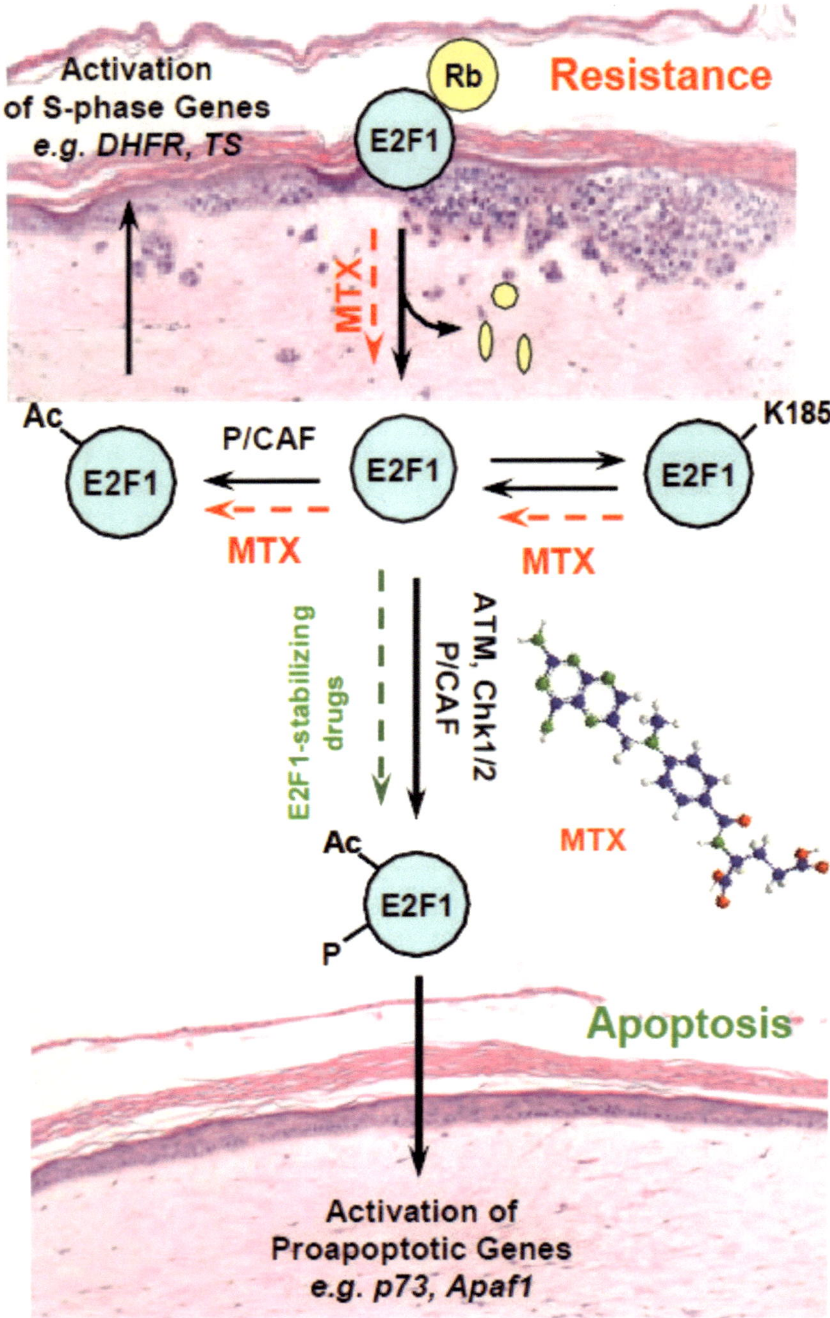

Figure 6. Proposed mechanism for the regulation of E2F1 by MTX. E2F1 is regulated by its interaction with Rb and by several posttranslational modifications, including methylation (Me), acetylation (Ac) and phosphorylation (P) [39]. The effects of MTX (red dashed line) on E2F1 status and that result in melanoma resistance are shown. A possible strategy to stabilize E2F1 (green dashed lines) to induce apoptosis in melanoma cells is also displayed.

6. Conclusions

Melanoma, the most aggressive form of skin cancer, is notoriously resistant to all current modalities of cancer therapy, including to the drug MTX. Melanosomal sequestration and cellular exportation of methotrexate have been proposed to be important melanoma-specific mechanisms that contribute to the resistance of melanoma to methotrexate. In addition, other mechanisms of resistance that are present in most epithelial cancer cells are also operative in melanoma. This chapter reviews how melanoma orchestrates these mechanisms to become extremely resistant to methotrexate, where both E2F1 and Chk1, two molecules with dual roles in survival/apoptosis, play prominent roles. The results indicated that MTX induced the depletion of DHF in melanoma cells, which stimulated the transcriptional activity of E2F1. The elevate expression of DHFR and TS, two E2F1-target genes involved in folate metabolism and required for G_1 progression, favoured dTTP accumulation, which promoted DNA single strand breaks and the subsequent activation of Chk1. Under these conditions, melanoma cells are protected from apoptosis by arresting their cell cycle in S phase. Excess of dTTP could also inhibit E2F1-mediated apoptosis in melanoma cells. In addition, these discoveries could open the way for the development of new combined and directed therapies against this elusive skin pathology.

Acknowledgements

Research described was supported in part by a grant from Ministerio de Ciencia e Innovación (MICINN) (Project SAF2009-12043-C02-01), Fundación Séneca, Región de Murcia (FS-RM) (15230/PI/10) and EU ERA293514. J.C-H is contracted by the Translational Cancer Research Group (Fundación para la Formación e Investigación Sanitarias). MPF-P has a fellowship from Ministerio de Educación, Cultura y Deporte. M.F.M is contracted by an agreement with the Fundación de la Asociación Española contra el Cáncer (FAECC). L.S-d-C has a postdoctoral fellowship from Fundación Séneca (Región de Murcia) for application in the Ludwig Institute for Cancer Research, Nuffield Department of Clinical Medicine, University of Oxford, Headington, Oxford, UK.

Author details

Luis Sanchez del-Campo[1], Maria F. Montenegro[1], Magali Saez-Ayala[1],
María Piedad Fernández-Pérez[1], Juan Cabezas-Herrera[2] and
Jose Neptuno Rodriguez-Lopez[1]

1 Department of Biochemistry & Molecular Biology A, University of Murcia, Spain

2 Research Unit of Clinical Analusis Service, University Hospital Virgen de la Arrixaca, Spain

References

[1] Sullivan, R. J, & Atkins, M. B. Molecular-targeted therapy in malignant melanoma. Expert Review of Anticancer Therapy (2009). , 9(5), 567-581.

[2] Ascierto, P. A, Streicher, H. Z, & Sznol, M. Melanoma: a model for testing new agents in combination therapies. J Transl Med (2010). , 8, 38.

[3] American Cancer SocietyCancer Facts & Figures 2011. Atlanta; 2011.

[4] Tawbi, H. A, & Buch, S. C. Chemotherapy resistance abrogation in metastatic melanoma. Clinical Advances in Hematology & Oncology (2010). , 8(4), 259-266.

[5] Kufe, D. W, Wick, M. M, & Abelson, H. T. Natural resistance to methotrexate in human melanomas. Journal of Investigative Dermatology (1980). , 75(4), 357-359.

[6] Sánchez-del-campo, L, Montenegro, M. F, Cabezas-herrera, J, & Rodríguez-lópez, J. N. The critical role of alpha-folate receptor in the resistance of melanoma to methotrexate. Pigment Cell & Melanoma Research (2009). , 22(5), 588-600.

[7] Saez-ayala, M, Fernandez-perez, M, Montenegro, M. F, Sánchez-del-campo, L, Chazarra, S, Piñero-madrona, A, Cabezas-herrera, J, & Rodríguez-lópez, J. N. Melanoma coordinates general and cell-specific mechanisms to promote methotrexate resistance. Experimental Cell Research (2012). , 318(10), 1146-1159.

[8] Lockshin, A, Moran, R. G, & Danenberg, P. V. Thymidylate synthetase purified to homogeneity from human leukemic cells. Proceedings of the National Academy of Sciences USA (1979). , 76(2), 750-754.

[9] Blakley, R. L. The Biochemistry of Folic Acid and Related Pteridines, Elsevier, New York; (1969).

[10] Zhao, R, & Goldman, I. D. Resistance to antifolates. Oncogene (2003). , 22(47), 7431-7457.

[11] Assaraf, Y. G. Molecular basis of antifolate resistance. Cancer & Metastasis Reviews (2007). , 26(1), 153-181.

[12] Chen, K. G, Valencia, J. C, Lai, B, Zhang, G, Paterson, J. K, Rouzaud, F, Berens, W, Wincovitch, S. M, Garfield, S. H, & Leapman, R. D. Hearing VJ Gottesman MM. Melanosomal sequestration of cytotoxic drugs contributes to the intractability of malignant melanomas. Proceedings of the National Academy of Sciences USA (2006). , 103(26), 9903-9907.

[13] Xie, T, Nguyen, T, Hupe, M, & Wei, M. L. Multidrug resistance decreases with mutations of melanosomal regulatory genes. Cancer Research (2009). , 69(3), 992-999.

[14] De Anta, J. M, Pérez-castro, A. J, Freire, R, & Mayol, X. The DNA damage checkpoint is activated during residual tumour cell survival to methotrexate treatment as an initial step of acquired drug resistance. Anticancer Drugs (2006). , 17(10), 1171-1177.

[15] Pardee, A. B, Li, C. J, & Reddy, G. P. Regulation in S phase by E2F. Cell Cycle (2004)., 3(9), 1091-1094.

[16] Wang, A, Li, C. J, Reddy, P. V, & Pardee, A. B. Cancer chemotherapy by deoxynucleotide depletion and E2F-1 elevation. Cancer Research (2005)., 65(17), 7809-7814.

[17] Bartek, J, & Lukas, J. Chk1 and Chk2 kinases in checkpoint control and cancer. Cancer Cell (2003)., 3(5), 421-429.

[18] Xiao, Z, Xue, J, Sowin, T. J, Rosenberg, S. H, & Zhang, H. A novel mechanism of checkpoint abrogation conferred by Chk1 downregulation. Oncogene (2005). , 24(8), 1403-1411.

[19] Tse, A. N, Carvajal, R, & Schwartz, G. K. Targeting checkpoint kinase 1 in cancer therapeutics. Clinical Cancer Research (2007)., 13(7), 1955-1960.

[20] Shi, Z, Azuma, A, Sampath, D, Li, Y. X, & Huang, P. Plunkett W. S-Phase arrest by nucleoside analogues and abrogation of survival without cell cycle progression by 7-hydroxystaurosporine. Cancer Research (2001)., 61(3), 1065-1072.

[21] Gaukroger J, Wilson L, Stewart M, Farid Y, Habeshaw T, Harding N, Mackie R. Paradoxical response of malignant melanoma to methotrexate in vivo and in vitro. British Journal of Cancer, 1983; 47(5) 671-679.

[22] Joerger, M, & Huitema, A. D. van den Bongard HJ, Baas P, Schornagel JH, Schellens JH, Beijnen JH. Determinants of the elimination of methotrexate and 7-hydroxy-methotrexate following high-dose infusional therapy to cancer patients. British Journal of Clinical Pharmacology (2006)., 62(1), 71-80.

[23] Branda, R. F, Mccormack, J. J, Perlmutter, C. A, Mathews, L. A, & Robison, S. H. Effects of folate deficiency on the metastatic potential of murine melanoma cells. Cancer Research (1988).

[24] Theos, A. C, Truschel, S. T, Raposo, G, & Marks, M. S. The Silver locus product Pmel17/ gp100/ Silv/ME20: controversial in name and in function. Pigment Cell Research (2005)., 18(5), 322-336.

[25] Raposo, G, & Marks, M. S. The dark side of lysosome-related organelles: specialization of the endocytic pathway for melanosome biogenesis. Traffic (2002)., 3(4), 237-248.

[26] Raposo, G, & Marks, M. S. Melanosomes-dark organelles enlighten endosomal membrane transport. Nature Reviews Molecular Cell Biology (2007)., 8(10), 786-797.

[27] Branda, R. F, Mccormack, J. J, Perlmutter, C. A, Mathews, L. A, & Robison, S. H. Effects of folate deficiency on the metastatic potential of murine melanoma cells. Cancer Research (1988)., 48(16), 4529-4534.

[28] Sabharanjak, S, & Mayor, S. Folate receptor endocytosis and trafficking. Advanced Drug Delivery Reviews (2004)., 56(8), 1099-1109.

[29] Stover, P. J, & Field, M. S. Trafficking of Intracellular Folates. Advances in Nutrition (2011). , 2(4), 325-331.

[30] Anderson, D. D, & Stover, P. J. SHMT1 and SHMT2 are functionally redundant in nuclear de novo thymidylate biosynthesis. PLoS ONE (2009). e5839.

[31] Anderson, D. D, Woeller, C. F, & Stover, P. J. Small ubiquitin-like modifier-1 (SUMO-1) modification of thymidylate synthase and dihydrofolate reductase. Clinical Chemistry and Laboratory Medicine (2007). , 45(12), 1760-1763.

[32] Wollack, J. B, Makori, B, Ahlawat, S, Koneru, R, Picinich, S. C, Smith, A, Goldman, I. D, Qiu, A, Cole, P. D, Glod, J, & Kamen, B. Characterization of folate uptake by choroid plexus epithelial cells in a rat primary culture model. Journal of Neurochemestry (2008). , 104(6), 1494-1503.

[33] Mosesson, Y, Mills, G. B, & Yarden, Y. Derailed endocytosis: an emerging feature of cancer. Nature Reviews Cancer (2008). , 8(11), 835-850.

[34] Wong AW, Scales SJ, Reilly DE. DNA internalized via caveolae requires microtubule-dependent, Rab7-independent transport to the late endocytic pathway for delivery to the nucleus. The Journal of Biological Chemestry 2007; 282(31) 22953-22963.

[35] Antony, A. C. Folate receptors. Annual Review of Nutrition (1996). , 16-501.

[36] Luhrs, C. A, Raskin, C. A, Durbin, R, Wu, B, Sadasivan, E, Mcallister, W, & Rothenberg, S. P. Transfection of a glycosylated phosphatidylinositol-anchored folate-binding protein complementary DNA provides cells with the ability to survive in low folate medium. The Journal of Clinical Investigation (1992). , 90(3), 840-847.

[37] Markert, S, Lassmann, S, Gabriel, B, Klar, M, Werner, M, Gitsch, G, Kratz, F, & Hasenburg, A. Alpha-folate receptor expression in epithelial ovarian carcinoma and non-neoplastic ovarian tissue. Anticancer Research (2008). A) , 3567-3572.

[38] Kelemen, L. E. The role of folate receptor alpha in cancer development, progression and treatment: cause, consequence or innocent bystander? International Journal of Cancer (2006). , 119(2), 243-250.

[39] Kontaki, H, & Talianidis, I. Lysine methylation regulates E2F1-induced cell death. Molecular Cell (2010). , 39(1), 152-160.

[40] Martínez-balbás, M. A, Bauer, U. M, Nielsen, S. J, Brehm, A, & Kouzarides, T. Regulation of E2F1 activity by acetylation. The EMBO Journal (2000). , 19(4), 662-671.

[41] Urist, M, Tanaka, T, Poyurovsky, M. V, & Prives, C. p. induction after DNA damage is regulated by checkpoint kinases Chk1 and Chk2. Genes & Development (2004). , 18(24), 3041-3054.

[42] Lin, W. C, Lin, F. T, & Nevins, J. R. Selective induction of E2F1 in response to DNA damage, mediated by ATM-dependent phosphorylation. Genes & Development (2001). , 15(14), 1833-1844.

[43] Chen, J, Zhu, F, Weaks, R. L, Biswas, A. K, Guo, R, Li, Y, & Johnson, D. G. E. F1 promotes the recruitment of DNA repair factors to sites of DNA double-strand breaks. Cell Cycle (2011). , 10(8), 1287-1294.

[44] Phillips, A. C, & Vousden, K. H. E. F-1 induced apoptosis. Apoptosis (2001). , 6(3), 173-182.

[45] Rodriguez, R, Meuth, M, & Chk, p. cooperate to prevent apoptosis during DNA replication fork stress. Molecular Biology of the Cell (2006). , 17(1), 402-412.

[46] Flynn, R. L, & Zou, L. ATR: a master conductor of cellular responses to DNA replication stress. Trends in Biochemical Sciences (2011). , 36(3), 133-140.

[47] Hallstrom, T. C, Mori, S, Nevins, J. R, & An, E. F1-dependent gene expression program that determines the balance between proliferation and cell death. Cancer Cell (2008). , 13(1), 11-22.

[48] Dynlacht, B. D. Live or let die: E2F1 and PI3K pathways intersect to make life or death decisions. Cancer Cell (2008). , 13(1), 1-2.

[49] Rogoff, H. A, & Kowalik, T. F. Life, death and E2F: linking proliferation control and DNA damage signaling via E2F1. Cell Cycle (2004). , 3(7), 845-846.

[50] Rogoff, H. A, Pickering, M. T, Frame, F. M, Debatis, M. E, Sanchez, Y, Jones, S, & Kowalik, T. F. Apoptosis associated with deregulated E2F activity is dependent on E2F1 and Atm/Nbs1/Chk2. Molecular and Cellular Biology (2004). , 24(7), 2968-2977.

Chapter 15

Surgery and the Staging of Melanoma

Z. Al-Hilli, D. Evoy, J.G. Geraghty,
E.W. McDermott and R.S. Prichard

Additional information is available at the end of the chapter

http://dx.doi.org/10.5772/53626

1. Introduction

An estimated 166,900 patients were diagnosed with malignant melanoma in developed countries last year [1]. The reported incidence of malignant melanoma continues to rise despite increasing understanding of its aetiology. In the United States 76,250 new cases are expected in 2012 with melanoma far outstripping other skin cancers in terms of mortality [2]. Similarly, in the UK, 12,818 new cases of malignant melanoma were diagnosed in 2010 [3]. Approximately, 85% percent of patients with cutaneous melanoma are diagnosed at a localized stage, while 10% have associated regional lymph node involvement and 5% of patients will have distant metastatic disease at presentation. The corresponding 5-year overall survival rates are 98.2% for localized disease, 62.4% for regional lymph node involvement and 15.1% for distant melanomas [4, 5].

Advances in the understanding of the molecular mechanisms and immunology of melanoma have lead to the development of promising novel therapeutic agents. Surgery, however, remains the mainstay of treatment and changes in the surgical approach have been guided by the greater understanding of melanoma pathogenesis. The management of the primary tumour has become more conservative, with acceptance of narrower excision margins. In addition, there has been a move away from the routine performance of elective regional lymph node dissection towards sentinel lymph node biopsy which is associated with less morbidity [6].

The new American Joint Committee on Cancer (AJCC) guidelines for the staging of melanoma were introduced into clinical practice in 2010 [7]. The two most important distinctions with previous guidelines are the incorporation of the mitotic rate of the primary tumor and the key role of the sentinel lymph node, including methods of analysis, in accurately staging clinically occult nodal disease [8].

The purpose of this chapter is twofold. Firstly, this chapter describes the appropriate surgical management of the primary tumour, the associated regional lymph node basin and distant metastatic disease. Secondly, the updated and revised AJCC staging system will be discussed and current controversies addressed.

2. Risk factors

The worldwide incidence of melanoma doubles every ten to fifteen years [9]. Risk factors associated with the development of malignant melanoma are varied and include genetic susceptibility, exposure to ultraviolet radiation, and immunologic factors. The most important of these is ultraviolet exposure where intermittent, unaccustomed sun exposure and sunburn were found to have considerable roles as risk factors for melanoma. However, despite the increase in public awareness, the practice of ultraviolet radiation protection behaviour is low. Also worryingly a survey performed in the US in 2005 documented that up to 14% of adults, primarily women and young adults used an indoor tanning device on at least one occasion [10].

Epidemiological studies have found that blue, green or grey eyes, blonde or red hair, light complexion, freckles, sun sensitivity, and an inability to tan, are risk factors for the development of melanoma [11, 12]. Countries with close proximity to the equator with predominantly fair-skinned populations have shown a higher preponderance to developing melanoma. Risk factors for melanoma also include a positive family history or personal history of melanoma/non-melanoma cancer or in-situ skin carcinomas, large numbers of melanocitic naevi in childhood, and xeroderma pigmentosum [13].

It is suggested that minimising radiation, and the adoption of photo-protective measures, can significantly reduce the risk of developing melanoma [13-15].

3. Surgery

3.1. Initial surgical biopsy

Melanoma can develop either in a pre-existing pigmented lesion or de novo. Features raising suspicion of melanoma in a pre-existing pigmented lesion include a change in size, irregular shape, irregular colour, diameter 7 mm or more, inflammation, oozing or a change in sensation [5,16]. The ABCD system of diagnosis (Asymmetry, Border irregularity, Colour change, and a Diameter greater than 6 mm) has also been advocated to assist early clinical diagnosis, to which 'E' (Evolving or Elevation) has been added [5,17,18]. Table 1 illustrates the seven point checklist and ABCDE system for the assessment of pigmented lesions.

http://dx.doi.org/10.5772/53626

Seven point checklist	The ABCDE lesion system
Major features	
Change in size	A Geometrical Asymmetry in 2 axes
Irregular shape	B Irregular Border
Irregular colour	C At least 2 different Colours in lesion
Minor features	D Maximum Diameter >6mm
Largest diameter 7mm or more	E Elevation
Inflammation	
Oozing	
Itch/ change in sensation	

Table 1. Seven point checklist and ABCDE system for assessment of pigmented lesions [19]

An excision biopsy is indicated for lesions suspected of being a melanoma. An excision biopsy is the recommended method for suspected malignant melanoma as it enables diagnosis and staging of the tumour and may determine future treatment and prognosis [20, 21]. The whole lesion should be excised with a 1-3 mm margin of normal skin including sub-dermal fat. It is crucial to plan this excision carefully with a view towards definitive treatment. Knowledge of lymphatic drainage and subsequent need for sentinel node biopsy should lead to narrow margin excision potentially avoiding interference with subsequent lymphatic mapping. In addition, a longitudinal orientation is preferred in the extremities and incision orientation should be along Langer's lines on the trunk. This allows for subsequent closure of a wide local excision and reduces the need for skin grafting if primary closure is to be achieved.

In certain areas (such as the face, palm of hand, sole of foot, ears, digits and subungal lesions) an excision biopsy may not be appropriate. In these cases, an incisional or punch biopsy of the thickest portion of the lesion may be performed [21]. Shave biopsy is avoided as it makes characterising the lesion difficult by underestimating tumour thickness, which is important in determining further treatment [21]. It also risks leaving residual tumour at the radial and deep margins.

Obtaining an adequate biopsy specimen is crucial for histopathological diagnosis and tumour staging. The tumour thickness, which remains the most powerful prognostic parameter, provides a guide to the margin clearance required for delayed wide excision and need for adjuvant therapy [20, 22]. Pathological examination should evaluate macroscopic features of the tumour such as width, symmetry, and circumscription, and microscopic features such as ulceration, microsatellitosis, angiolymphatic invasion and mitotic rate [22].

3.2. Management of the primary tumour

The surgical management of the primary tumour has shifted from extensive surgical resection, which was not only debilitating but also disfiguring, to a more conservative approach. A multidisciplinary team in a tertiary referral centre should ideally manage patients with malignant melanoma. This team should include: a surgeon, dermatologist,,medical oncologist, pathologist, radiologist, counsellor, specialist nurse and palliative care specialist [23].

Pathological assessment of the surgically excised biopsy specimen allows for staging of the tumour while the thickness of the melanoma at initial biopsy serves as a guide to the subsequent resection. The Breslow thickness, which is the most important prognostic indicator of localised disease, is defined as the distance of invasion and is measured from the granular layer of the epidermis to the point of deepest invasion by tumour cells [5, 24, 25].

Large randomised controlled trials have been performed in an attempt to elucidate the optimal resection margin in melanoma of various thickness (thin, intermediate, and thick melanomas) [26-31]. The trials reported data with not only differing lengths of follow-up but also differing margin excision widths. Therefore interpretation of the results is largely restricted to survival outcomes as a result of this heterogeneity.

The management of lentigo maligna and in situ melanoma present unique problems because of the characteristic, yet unpredictable, subclinical extension of atypical junctional melanocytic hyperplasia, which may extend several centimeters beyond the visible margins [33]. There are no randomized trials looking at the optimal resection margin in these lesions. Guidelines from the American Academy of Dermatology in 2011 recommend a resection margin of 0.5 to 1.0 cm for melanoma in situ [34]. The NCCN recommends a margin of 0.5 cm around the visible lesion. For large in-situ lentigo maligna melanoma, it is felt that surgical margins greater than 0.5 cm may be necessary to achieve a histologically negative margin [33]. More recently, topical imiquimod has been used in lentigo melanoma treatment prior to definitive surgical resection. In a study that included 40 patients, 33 of these were found to have a complete clinical response after the use of imiquimod 5% cream. On histological review, 30 of the patients had no evidence of melanoma. While studies have shown a limited role for this treatment, it does not replace surgery [35].

Three main trials (The World Health Organisation Trial, Swedish Melanoma Study and the French Cooperative Group) looked at the optimal resection margin for T1 and T2 melanomas. The World Health Organisation (WHO) trial included 612 patients with melanomas less than 2.0mm with patients being randomly assigned to a wide local excision with a either a 3cm margin or 1cm margin. At 12 years of follow up, similar survival rates between the groups were noted (87% and 85% respectively) with no statistically significant difference in recurrence dependent upon margin width. As a consequence of this trial recommendations were made that a 1cm margin be used for melanomas ≤1mm. Similarly, the Swedish Melanoma Study Group studied 989 patients with melanomas 0.8 to 2mm thick who were randomly assigned to either a 2cm or 5cm resection margin. At a median follow-up of 11 years the local recurrence rate for all groups was less than 1%. Again there was no significant difference noted in the overall or disease-free survival between the two groups. A third trial, the French Cooperative Group, included 362 patients with melanomas ≤2mm in thickness. Patients were randomly assigned to a wide local excision with either a 2cm or 5cm resection margin. No difference was noted between the groups in terms of local recurrence or overall survival. Therefore at present, a resection margin of 1cm is recommended for melanomas <1mm and 2cm for melanomas 1 - 2mm thick [26-28].

Melanomas between 2 - 4mm are considered intermediate thickness melanomas. Once again, there are a number of trials looking specifically at this cohort of patients which failed to show a benefit of greater than a 2cm excision margin. The Melanoma Intergroup Trial included 468 patients with melanomas of 1 to 4mm thickness. Patients were randomly assigned to an excision margin of either 2cm or 4cm. Forty two percent of patients in the group undergoing 2cm excision had a melanoma thickness >2.0mm, while 46% of patients in the 4cm resection group had melanomas >2.0mm. At mean follow up, a 2cm margin was shown to be as effective as a 4cm margin in both the local control and overall survival for patients with intermediate thickness melanomas. Local recurrence however, was primarily determined by the thickness of the primary lesion and the presence or absence of ulceration [29, 30]. A multi-centre European trial was also performed to tease out the need for wider margins in deeper, intermediate thickness melanomas. In total, 936 patients were included who were assigned randomly to have either a 2cm or 4cm resection margin. At a follow-up of almost 7 years there was no statistically significant difference noted for recurrence or survival between the two groups [31]. Finally a British trial was performed which recruited 900 patients with lesions greater than 2mm to a wide local excision with either a 1cm or 3 cm margin Interestingly, this study demonstrated a higher local recurrence rate when a 1cm margin was used. However, there was no statistically significant difference noted in overall survival. The authors therefore concluded that a margin of 1cm should be restricted to patients with a melanoma thickness of less than 2mm [32]. Therefore, at present a 2cm excision margin is recommended for intermediate (2 – 4mm) thickness melanomas.

There is unfortunately limited evidence or published data on the optimal resection margin for melanomas with a thickness of 4mm or greater. The British Trial included 243 patients with melanomas of > 4mm thickness and the results showed a higher local recurrence rate associated with a margin of 1cm [32]. However, the local recurrence rates with a 3cm margin appeared similar to other trials with only a 2cm margin of excision. In a retrospective review from MD Anderson which assessed patients with melanomas of greater than 6mm thickness, excision margins greater than 2 cm were not found to effect overall survival when compared to margins of 2cm or less. The 5-year overall and disease free survival rates were 55% and 30% in node negative compared to node positive patients which were included in the study. Nodal status, thickness, and ulceration were significantly associated with overall survival by multivariate analysis. However, the neither the disease free nor overall survival was effected by the presence of a local recurrence or the original excision margin in this study [36]. The study authors therefore concluded that a 2 cm margin of excision is adequate for patients with thick melanoma [36].However, overall there is insufficient data to support the preferred use of either a 2cm or 3cm margin, and consequently, it may be reasonable to allow the patient to decide, following an informed discussion of surgical options. The use of the larger 3cm margin may be recommended in patients with deep tumours (> 4mm depth), due to the higher risk of loco-regional recurrence [32]. In selected cases, however, margin size may be modified to accommodate individual anatomic or cosmetic considerations [23].

Although radial excision margins remain somewhat controversial, the depth of excision in clinical practice is defined as an excision down to but not including the deep fascia [37]. This definition has been internationally accepted and forms the basis of the current gold-standard management of melanoma. Unfortunately in facial areas where the 'deep fascia' is less clearly defined (for example, on the ear, nose, or eyelid), or other anatomic sites such as over the breast, existing studies provide no clear guidelines for optimal depth of excision [5].

Margins	
Tis	Histologically clear margins are adequate
T1	1cm margin is recommended
T2	1-2cm margin recommended
T3	2-3cm margin recommended

Table 2. Recommended excision margins based on tumor size [23]

Despite all the evidence discussed above, controversy still remains regarding the optimal width of the surgical excision margins in malignant melanoma and current evidence is not sufficient to address the optimal surgical management for all melanomas. Indeed a Cochrane review which has been recently published attempted to address this complex question [5]. Overall, there was no statistically significant difference in overall survival between either a narrow or wide excision, but this meta-analysis was confounded by the fact that excision margins were not standardized between studies within the overall analysis. Therefore the dilemma regarding surgical margin remains. However, guidelines regarding margin width have been published and should be adhered to where feasible. Further studies are required to determine the appropriate local treatment for thick melanoma which has not been comprehensively addressed in trials thus far.

3.3. In-transit metastasis

The treatment of advanced or recurrent melanoma remains controversial. Around 10% of patients develop in-transit or multiple cutaneous metastases but at least half will survive for two years without developing distant disease [38, 39]. Unfortunately, the 5-year survival has been reported as 12% with a median survival of 19 months [39].

In-transit metastases are defined as cutaneous or subcutaneous deposits of melanoma between the site of the primary disease and regional lymph nodes [40]. These deposits may be found localized around the primary tumour or may be widespread throughout the affected limb or on the head and neck or trunk, depending on the primary site [40] (Figure 1). It is thought that these metastases arise from dissemination of melanoma cells via the lymphatics to tissues located between the primary tumor and the regional lymph node basin. Other theories include that of drift metastases within tissue fluid of the limb or the local implantation of circulating haematogenous melanoma cells [41, 42].

The presence of small in-transit metastatic melanoma presents specific surgical problems. Unlike nodal disease, which can be managed by regional lymph node dissection, in-transit disease is often widespread and may necessitate multiple surgeries as the disease progresses and new deposits become apparent. In its most severe form, in-transit metastasis may become severely disabling and may be refractory to treatment. Treatment is therefore, palliative, even if staging investigations fail to show evidence of distant metastatic disease [40]. Recent studies have recommended that treatment should be tailored to the extent of the disease, with treatments associated with significant morbidity being reserved for bulky advanced metastases [40].

Several therapies have been proposed for the management of in-transit metastasis including surgery, radiotherapy, and intra-lesional therapy. In-transit metastasis are sharply circumscribed with a clear line of demarcation from normal dermis and epidermis. This line does not contain any in-situ component. Therefore, wide excision margins are not recommended for these lesions and a complete macroscopic excision and primary closure is sufficient. If lesions are grouped closely together, an en bloc excision is acceptable [40].

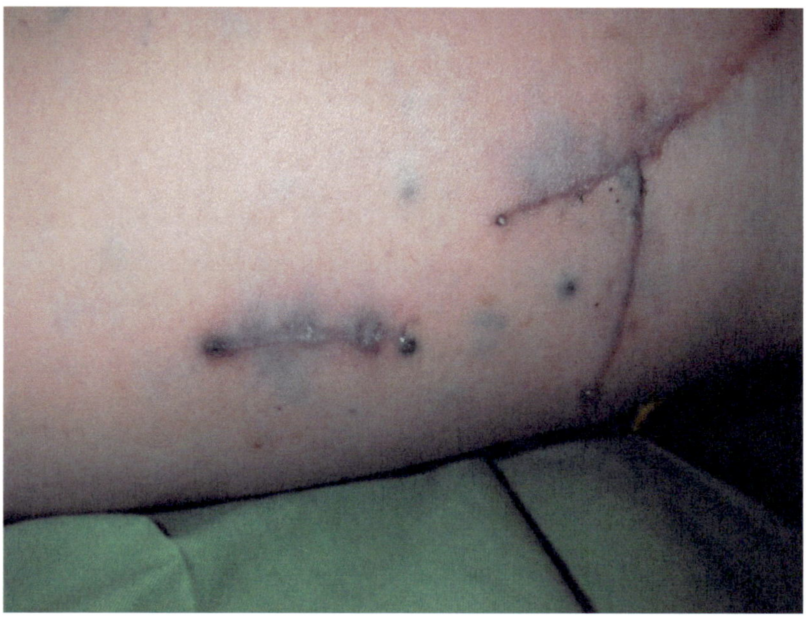

Figure 1. In-transit metastases on the left lower limb

There are numerous treatments available for the management of in-transit metastases that are not suitable for surgical treatment. Carbon dioxide laser therapy has been used in the management of small in-transit metastasis that are not amenable for surgical excision. This is performed as a day case under local anesthetic. Small lesions may be vaporized completely, while larger lesions are first circumscribed with the laser prior to excision of the central core. This well tolerated procedure is more suitable for smaller lesions.

In more advanced diseased, isolated limb perfusion has traditionally been the main method of treatment. This invasive procedure has been replaced by isolated limb infusion, which is simpler, minimally invasive, and a more economical alternative with comparable results [38, 39]. Isolated limb perfusion with chemotherapeutic agents was developed in New Orleans in the mid 1950s by Creech *et al* [38, 39, 43]. It is based on the principle of vascular isolation of the affected limb using a cardiopulmonary bypass circuit through open surgical cannulation of the major limb vessels. This procedure is technically difficult, expensive, and complications are common. Repeated limb perfusions are difficult to perform and morbidity rates increase from 28% to 51% [38]. A simpler alternative, isolated limb infusion was developed by Dr John Thompson in the Sydney Melanoma Unit [44]. It is a less invasive procedure, which involves percutaneous placement of venous and arterial catheters and the infusion of chemotherapeutic agents. This negates the need for a bypass circuit. As opposed to isolated limb perfusion, autologous blood or autologous transfusion of allogenic units is not required. The operating time is reduced from four hours to one hour, and the complication rates are documented to be lower, at only 1% [38, 43].

The presence of in-transit metastases indicates a poor prognosis. The development of in-transit disease may be rapidly followed by distant metastases [40]. The American Committee on Cancer Staging (AJCC) classify it as stage IIIB or IIIC disease, along with regional lymph node metastases. Five year survival rates in patients with stage III disease ranges from 18% to 60%. However, patients with in-transit metastasis have the worst prognosis, with 5 year survival of approximately 25%.

3.4. Reconstruction

The optimal treatment of patients undergoing melanoma excision is primary closure of the wound. Unfortunately, this is not always possible especially in patients with thick melanomas requiring wider excision margins. Therefore, in these cases reconstructive surgery must be considered and where feasible offered to the patient. This will usually depend on the site and extent of the excision to be performed. Skin grafting is the commonest technique employed to ensure skin cover of the anatomical defect. Traditionally, the graft is harvested from the contralateral limb, as melanoma was thought to metastasize primarily via lymphatic routes [15, 45, 46]. However, a recent study looking at the recurrence rates within skin graft donor sites, reported no difference in local recurrence rates when either the ipsilateral or contralateral limbs were used as graft sites. The authors of this study recommended that to improve patient recovery, harvesting the graft from the same limb as the primary tumor is both oncologically safe and technically superior to contralateral skin graft harvest [47]. In certain sites, such as the head and neck, the use of skin grafts may not always be ideal and may result in significant deformity. Local rotation flaps, such as rhomboid flaps, have been found to be safe, versatile, and more aesthetically pleasing when used in these areas [15, 48].

4. Management of the regional lymph node basin

The presence of regional lymph node metastatic disease is a significant predictor of outcome in melanoma and is associated with a 50% reduction in overall survival compared to that of patients without nodal involvement [23]. Indeed the regional lymph node status is thought to be the most powerful prognostic indicator in clinically localised melanoma. The risk of patients developing lymph node metastases increases exponentially with the increasing thickness of the primary melanoma. Melanomas less than 1mm rarely metastasise (less than 10%), while at least 25% of melanomas 1.5- 4.0mm and over 60% of melanomas greater than 4.0mm thick will have lymph node metastasis at presentation[49]. These data form the basis for the current guidelines on which patients should be offered a sentinel lymph node biopsy.

Patients with melanoma can present with either a clinically normal regional lymph node basin or palpable regional lymphadenopathy. Patients with stage III disease commonly have clinically negative lymph nodes but are found to have micro-metastatic disease on their sentinel lymph node biopsy. Such patients have been found to have a more favourable outcome than patients with clinically involved nodes at presentation [8]. The outcome of patients with stage III disease is determined by the number of metastatic nodes and the presence of either microscopic or macroscopic disease. The 5-year survival rate for patients with stage IIIA disease is 67%, and the 10-year survival is 60%. Patients with stage IIIB disease have survival rates estimated at 53%, while stage IIIC disease patients have the worst prognosis with a 5-year survival of approximately 26% [49]. The surgical management of the associated lymph node basin depends on the initial presentation of the patient.

4.1. The sentinel lymph node biopsy

Metastasis to regional lymph nodes is an important prognostic factor in patients with melanoma, upstaging patients to stage III disease and has been shown to occur in about 20% of patients with intermediate thickness melanoma [50]. A sentinel lymph node biopsy (SLNB) is a minimally invasive procedure that aims to identify patients with microscopic lymph node metastasis who would benefit from further lymph node dissection and adjuvant treatment. The sentinel node is defined as any lymph node that receives lymphatic drainage directly from a primary tumour site [51] (Figure 2).

The technical details of sentinel lymph node biopsy can be broken down into a number of steps. First, the patient undergoes preoperative lymphoscintigraphy which identifies the regional nodal basin and estimates the location of the sentinel node. Four intra-dermal injections of 0.1–0.2 ml of 10 MBq radio-colloid are performed around the melanoma or melanoma scar: the injection should raise a small wheal on the skin. The most commonly used radiotracers are 99mTc-labeled albumin (Europe), 99mTc-labeled sulphur colloid and

99mTc-antimony trisulphide colloid. Scintillation cameras are used to obtain dynamic images. These images allow identification of sentinel nodes within the regional nodal basin. They also allow discrimination of second-tier nodes, which may be falsely interpreted as sentinel nodes on delayed imaging. The surface location of the sentinel node may be marked on the skin preoperatively or, alternatively, a gamma probe can be use to locate the node intra-operatively. Intra-operative lymphatic mapping involves injection of vital blue dye (Isosulfan blue (Lymphazurin), Methylene Blue or Patent Blue V are used). A combination of radiotracers and blue dye has been shown to allow sentinel node identification in 99% of cases. The blue dye is injected intra-dermally in 2-4 locations at the site of the primary lesion, 10-15 minutes before skin incision. The dye is used to visualize the sentinel node intra-operatively. A gamma probe (covered in a sterile plastic sheath), which detects radiation, may be used to locate the sentinel node (Figure 3). Counts should be obtained over the skin before incision, to confirm the location of the sentinel node. A short skin incision is made, bearing in mind the potential need for complete lymph node dissection. The sentinel nodes are then identified using the blue dye and gamma probe as a guide, and they are removed with minimal dissection. An ex-vivo count should be obtained, by measuring the radioactivity of the sentinel node(s) after removal. A bed count is then also obtained following removal of the sentinel node(s), to ensure that no sentinel nodes remain [15, 52].

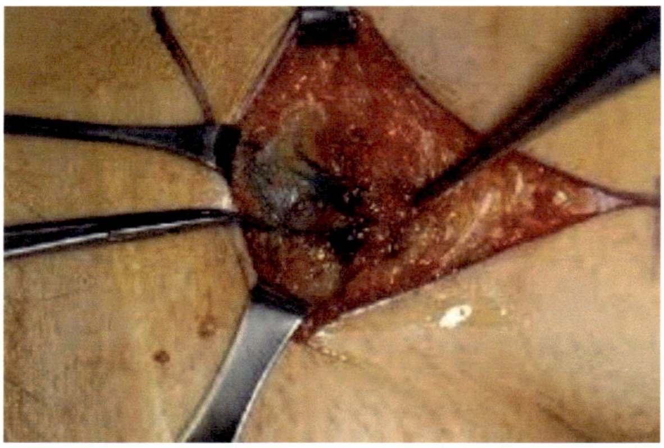

Figure 2. The Sentinel Lymph Node Biopsy

The Multicenter Selective Lymphadenectomy Trial-1 (MSLT-1) is the largest trial to address the role of lymphatic mapping with SLNB in determining prognosis and its impact on survival [53]. Patients with a primary cutaneous melanoma were randomly assigned to wide excision and postoperative observation of the regional lymph nodes with lymphadenectomy being performed only if nodal relapse was confirmed or to wide excision and sentinel-node biopsy with immediate lymphadenectomy if nodal micro-metastases were detected on biopsy [53]. The MSLT-1 trial confirmed the prognostic importance of SLN status, demonstrating that SLN status is the most statistically significant predictor of survival for clinically localized (stage I/II) intermediate thickness melanoma (1.2 to 3.5 mm). The 5-year disease-free

http://dx.doi.org/10.5772/53626

survival for patients with positive SLN status was 72.3%, compared to 90.2% in those with negative SLN status [53].

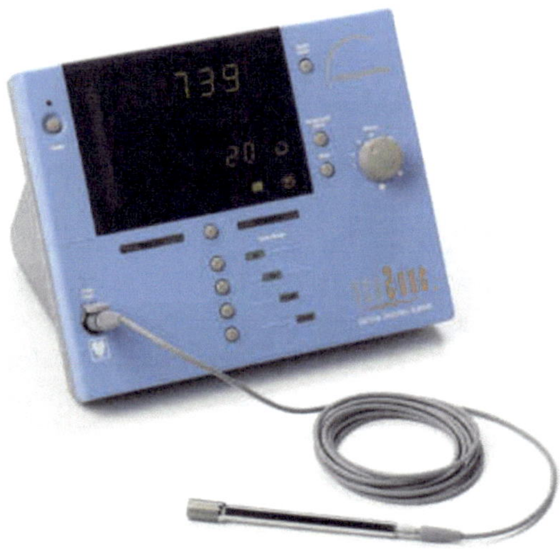

Figure 3. Gamma probe used to locate sentinel lymph node

The AJCC Melanoma Staging Committee recommends that a sentinel lymph node biopsy be performed as a staging procedure in patients for whom the information will be useful in planning subsequent treatments and follow-up regimens. Significant controversy surrounds the use of sentinel lymph node biopsy in thin, early melanomas. There are a number of reasons for this. Firstly, patients with a low-risk of nodal metastases are exposed to the morbidity of a potentially unnecessary procedure. Secondly, the routine use of sentinel lymph node biopsy is expensive: global application of sentinel lymph node biopsy in all patients is estimated to cost between $700,000 and $1,000,000 for every sentinel node metastasis detected [15, 54]. Therefore, for thin melanomas, the routine use of SLNB has not been advocated as the risk of positive nodes is around 5.1% [55]. Indeed, a rate of only 2.7% has been documented with melanomas thinner than 0.75mm [55]. SLNB may be considered, however, in patients with high risk features such as ulceration, a mitotic rate of greater than or equal to 1/mm^2 especially in patients with melanomas of ≥ 0.76 mm as they are associated with an approximately 10% risk of occult metastases in their sentinel lymph nodes [8]. SLNB is also recommended for patients with intermediate thickness melanoma (2 – 4mm). With regards to thick melanomas, it is expected that around 30% of patients will have evidence of lymph node involvement and the role for SLNB is less clear. It is, however, recommended that SLNB be performed in patients with no clinically evidence positive nodes as it allows for better chances at local disease control [50].

Recent editions of the AJCC melanoma guidelines have altered the criteria for the presence of regional lymph node disease. Originally, the 6th Edition of the AJCC melanoma guidelines recommended histological confirmation of all immunohistochemically (IHC) detected metastasis by routine H&E staining and only after this confirmation could metastatic disease be documented [56]. However, the more recently published guidelines state that positive nodes may be confirmed by either H&E staining or IHC staining with melanoma associated markers [7]. The three most commonly used IHC markers for melanoma are S-100, HMB-45, and Melan A/MART 1. Currently, S-100 remains the most sensitive marker for detection of melanoma, while HMB-45 and Melan A/MART 1 are used for their specificity [57].

More recently, reverse transcriptase polymerase chain reaction (RT-PCR) has been shown to be a promising staging tool used to identify patients with histologically unidentified micrometastatic disease. This technique relies on detection of distinct mRNA expressed by melanoma cells, such as tyrosinase, MAGE-3, MART-1, gp100 and other markers [58, 59]. There has been evidence suggesting the correlation between RT-PCR positive results in blood with stage of melanoma, tumor thickness and known prognostic indicators. The value of RT-PCR in regional lymph nodes is less clear. The number of false positives due to the presence of melanocytic naevi and Schwann cells has limited its use. However, there are results that show that positive results correlate with melanoma thickness [60]. Initial results from 30-month follow-up of the Sunbelt Melanoma Trial did not show any difference in disease-free or overall survival in RT-PCR positive and negative patients [61]. The results were subsequently included in meta-analysis where it has been suggested that RT-PCR may have valuable prognostic use in the prediction of overall and disease free survival [62]. The clinical relevance of the ability to detect micro-metastases by RT-PCR is still under investigation.

4.2. Elective regional lymph node dissection

Completion lymph node dissection (CLND) is recommended for patients with a positive SLN biopsy. It is performed with the intention of halting metastatic spread of melanoma in the early stages of the disease [15, 62, 64]. The five-year survival rate in patients with negative complete lymph node dissection stands at 62.5%, compared with 20.3% in patients with positive non-sentinel nodes [65]. However, the exact role of this and its reflection on overall survival in the setting of positive sentinel nodes has yet to be fully elucidated.

Currently, a complete lymph node dissection is carried out for all patients with a positive sentinel lymph node, irrespective of the type of metastases (micro or macro-metastasis) identified. The value of a complete lymph node dissection in this group of patients has not been extensively investigated and it must constantly be borne in mind that completion lymph node dissection is associated with significant patient morbidity [66]. Indeed, in the MSLT-1, no improvement in OS was seen in the total group randomized to receive SLNB followed by completion lymph node dissection (CLND) if the SLN was positive compared to those randomized to WLE and observation, with nearly identical 5-year melanoma specific-survival of 87.1% versus 86.6% ($P = 0.58$) [53]. Studies that looked at this difference did not show any statistical significant between the two groups. In addition, it is felt that micro-metastases will become evident if left untreated. Patients with nodal metastases were shown to have a survival advantage with early intervention compared with those who had a delayed lymphadenectomy only when they presented with clinically evident nodal metastasis [15, 53, 67].

However, a significant survival benefit has been noted in patients with a positive sentinel lymph node biopsy, who undergo a complete lymph node dissection, when compared with patients undergoing complete lymph node dissection after nodal metastases become apparent [68]. In a study conducted by Morton et al, a 5-year survival rate of 72% was seen in patients with positive sentinel lymph nodes, followed by immediate lymph node dissection, whereas patients undergoing a delayed lymph node dissection had a 5-year survival rate of only 52% [53]. Further positive non-sentinel lymph nodes are found in a relatively small proportion of patients: previously quoted figures ranged from 17%-24% [15, 69-71]. Interestingly a recent study has shown rates of further positive findings to be as low as 14.8% [15, 53].

Researchers have sought to identify factors which may increase a patient's likelihood of non-sentinel node metastases. Increasing Breslow depth has been associated with increased risk of non-sentinel node metastases, while a depth of less than 1mm has no association with any further positive nodes on completion lymph node dissection [15,65]. Studies have failed to show an association between specific tumour and patient characteristics with an increased rate of non-sentinel nodal metastasis [15, 71], However, a number of histopathological features have been shown to be associated with positive complete lymph node dissections. These include: nodular melanoma, ulceration, melanoma regression, and naevus association [15, 65]. Using a size/ulceration score, Reeves et al. showed ulceration to be an independent predictor of non-sentinel node deposits [72].

Recent studies have examined the association between the size of the sentinel lymph node deposits and the rate of positive complete lymph node dissection. Kunte et al. did not report any patients with micro-metastatic deposits on sentinel lymph node biopsy to have positive findings on complete lymph node dissection [15, 65, 73]. Another study showed a 3-year survival rate in patients with 1mm sentinel lymph node metastasis to be 100%, while 3-year survival in patients with deposits greater than 1mm was 80% [15, 74]. Ollila et al., however, found a significantly higher rate of recurrence in patients with sub-micrometastatic disease (ie. sentinel lymph node deposits less than 0.1mm), compared with node-negative patients [15, 75].

A significant number of these questions will be address by the publication of the results of The Multicenter Selective Lymphadenectomy Trial-II (MSTL-II) which are currently awaited [76, 77]. This trial aims to address the importance of SLN metastases, the relevance of molecular assessment of the SLN and to evaluate the therapeutic benefit of CLNB after SLNB. Within the trial, all patients with primary melanoma ≥1.2 mm or ≤1.2 mm with Clark level IV / V or ulceration undergo a SLNB. This will be analyzed by both H&E and IHC techniques. Patients with a negative SLNB by H&E and IHC will undergo RT-PCR. All SLN-positive patients identified by H&E/IHC or RT-PCR are randomized to one of two groups: observation of lymph node basin with clinical examination and repeated follow-up ultrasound scanning or to immediate CLND. Patients with negative SLN as determined by RT-PCR are assigned to routine follow-up. The primary endpoint of this study is to determine if

CLND will improve melanoma specific survival in patients with a positive SLNB. Secondary endpoints include assessing the predictive value of immune responses to melanoma- associated antigens, to analyze blood samples from patients for molecular markers of melanoma, both before and after surgery and to assess the quality of life of patients undergoing either CLND or observation after SLNB. Finally the study analyses the predictive value of certain DNA markers of the primary tumor in relation to disease outcome [76, 77].

In conclusion, in the setting of a negative sentinel lymph node biopsy, a completion lymph node dissection is clearly not indicated. The presence of positive nodes warrants consideration of complete lymph node dissection of the involved lymph node basin. Results of the MSLT-II trial are awaited and will give answers to the option of nodal observation.

5. Management of distant metastatic disease

The management of patients with metastatic melanoma remains challenging. Despite improved therapeutic options the prognosis remains poor. A complete surgical resection of metastatic disease in distant sites offers the best chance to improve survival. Patients with in-transit metastasis may be offered further surgical resection of the lesions. Favourable prognostic factors in patients with metastatic disease include a longer disease free survival, single site disease, complete resection and non-visceral metastases [78]. Patients that undergo resection of their non-visceral metastasis have been shown to have a medium survival of between 17 - 50 months, and a 5 - year survival of 9 - 35%. Patients with pulmonary metastasis, who have a complete resection, have a median survival of 8 - 20 months and a 5 year survival of 10 -25%. Brain and gastrointestinal tract metastasis confers a median survival of only 7-10 months [78]. Surgical resection in cases of advanced melanoma has been shown to give good palliation, if all the disease is completely removed. More recently, new systemic biological therapies have been developed, and when combined with surgery may be shown to aid in improved survival. These combinations, however, are still under review [79].

Chemotherapeutic agents have little role to play in the management of metastatic melanoma. Regimens that have previously been utilised include dacarbazine, temozolomide, high dose interleukin-2, paclitaxel and cisplatin or carboplatin. These show a response rate of less than 20% [33]. There is little evidence of its value in metastatic melanoma, however with combination treatments their role is yet to be fully examined.

In 2011, the FDA approved two newer therapies for metastasis melanoma. These include the highly selective BRAF inhibitor, vemurafenib, and ipilimumab, a fully human IgG1 monoclonal antibody. Around 40% to 60% of melanomas are shown to harbor a mutation in the gene encoding for the serine / threonine kinase protein kinase B-raf (BRAF) with 90% of the mutations resulting in a substitution of valine for glutamate at amino acid 600 (V600E) [80]. Mutated BRAF leads to constitutive activation of the mitogen-activated protein kinase pathway (MAPK) that in turn increases cellular proliferation and drives oncogenic activity. Sorafenib, the initial BRAF inhibitor failed to demonstrate significant response rates in melanoma and its use has been largely discontinued. Vemurafenib is a newer highly selective inhibitor with promising results. The main limitation of this novel agent is its limited response with an approximately 40% to 50% response rate in patients with a V600-mutated BRAF gene. Unfortunately, the median duration of response is only 5 to 6 months [33]. GSK2118436 is a newer highly selective inhibitor of BRAF that is still in pre-clinical trials [80].

Melanoma is an immunogenic tumor. Ipilimumab is a monoclonal antibody directed to the cytotoxic T lymphocyte antigen-4 (CTLA-4). Results of two randomized phase III trial of patients with unresectable metastatic disease that progressed during systemic therapy showed an overall improvement in survival in patients randomized to the ipilimumab arm [33,81,82]). In another phase III study looking at the role of ipilumumab and dacarbazine in patients with previously untreated metastatic melanoma, ipilumumab and dacarbazine was shown to have improved patient survival in comparison to the group receiving dacarbazine alone [83[. The limitation of ipilimumab is its association with autoimmune toxicity. In addition, clinical responses may take months to become apparent, and the overall response rate is less than 20% [33]. Research is ongoing in this area. The EORTC18071 trial is ongoing and compares adjuvant treatment with ipilimumab with observation in patients with high risk lymph node positive disease [84].

The role of biochemotherapy has also been studied. This involves using a combination of chemotherapy and biologic agents [33]. The results, however, show no additional survival benefit with this treatment. Finally, palliative radiotherapy may have a role in the setting of metastatic melanoma and has been shown to have good palliation of symptomatic disease [85-87].

6. Staging

An updated Cancer Staging Manual was recently published by the AJCC [7]. Modifications of the melanoma staging guidelines, which have been used since 2002, were based on a multivariate analysis on 38,918 patients [8]. In the revised guidelines melanoma patients have been categorised into 3 groups; those with localised disease with no evidence of metastases (stage I - II), patients with regional disease (stage III), and those with distant metastatic disease (stage IV). Primary tumour thickness remains the factor most associated with prognosis. Tumour thickness is defined in even integers (1.0, 2.0 and 4.0mm) with increasing thickness corresponding with worsening survival. Within each tumour thickness category, the presence of ulceration further upgrades the classification (Table 3).

Mitotic rate is an indicator of tumour proliferation and is measured as the number of mitoses per mm^2. Several studies have shown the mitotic rate to be an independent prognostic factor in patients with melanoma [88-91]. The AJCC guidelines now recommend the "hot spot" technique for calculating the mitotic rate, where the pathologist begins the mitotic count with the most active tumour focus. This is calculated as mitosis/mm^2 [8]. Multiple thresholds of mitotic rate were examined statistically, and the most significant correlation with survival was identified at a threshold of at least 1/mm^2, where a mitotic rate greater than or equal to 1/mm^2 was found to be independently associated with a poorer disease-specific survival in patients with T1 disease. For non-ulcerated, thin melanomas the 10-year survival was 95% if there were fewer than 1 mitosis per mm^2, compared with 88% 10-year survival if at least one mitosis per mm^2 was present. In addition, the level of invasion, as defined by Wallace Clark, was found to have no statistical significance in staging with the mitotic rate replacing it as an upstaging criterion from stages 1a to 1b [92].

T Classification	Thickness	Ulceration status/mitosis
Tx	Primary tumour cannot be assessed (for example, curettaged or severely regressed melanoma)	
T0	No evidence of primary tumor	
Tis	Melanoma in situ	
T1	Melanoma is 1.0mm or less in thickness	a: without ulceration and mitosis <1/mm2 b: with ulceration or mitoses ≥1/mm2
T2	Melanoma 1.01-2.0mm	a: without ulceration b: with ulceration
T3	Melanoma 2.01- 4.0mm	a: without ulceration b: with ulceration
T4	Melanoma more than 4.0mm	a: without ulceration b: with ulceration

Table 3. T Classification as recommended by the AJCC [7]

Stage III patients have documented lymph node metastasis (microscopic of macroscopic) (Table 4). S-100 is the most sensitive marker for melanocytic lesions while others such as HMB-45, MART-1/Melan-A, tyrosinase, and MITF are very specific but less sensitive [93]. In terms of documenting micro-metastasis, the AJCC accepts immunohistochemical staining of at least one melanoma specific marker to make the diagnosis. Around 5% to 40% of patients will be upstaged to stage III based on the presence of micro-metastatic disease. These patients have a better prognosis than those presenting with macro-metastatic disease as shown in several studies [8, 95]. The new AJCC guidelines reviewed the results of 3307 patients and make a clear distinction between each group. Staging of this group includes defining the number of nodes involved, the presence of microscopic versus macroscopic disease, as well as intra-lymphatic (in-transit or satellite) metastasis, the presence or absence of primary tumour ulceration, and the thickness of the primary melanoma. These factors were found to be predictive of survival on multivariate analysis. In the absence of nodal metastases, patients with intra-lymphatic metastases (N2c) have 5-year and 10-year survival rates of 69% and 52%, respectively while those with combined intra-lymphatic metastases and nodal metastases (N3) have survival rates of 46% and 33%, respectively [8].

N Classification	Nodes involved	Nodal metastatic mass
Nx	Regional nodes cannot be assessed (for example, previously removed for another reason)	
N0	No regional metastasis noted	
N1	1 node	a: micro-metastasis b: macro-metastasis
N2	2-3 nodes	a: micro-metastasis b: macro-metastasis c: in transit mets(s)/ satellite(s) without metastatic nodes
N3	4 or more metastatic nodes, or matted nodes, or in transit met(s)/ satellite(s) with metastatic node(s)	

Table 4. N Classification as recommended by the AJCC [7]

Finally, the database for stage IV patients was expanded to include 7972 patients and the new guidelines now incorporate the serum lactate dehydrogenase as a prognostic marker included in staging (Table 5). An elevated serum LDH was found to be an independent and a highly significant predictor of survival outcome. In a study that looked at the correlation between survival in advanced melanoma from two large trials (Oblimersen GM301 and EORTC 189510), the authors reported an elevated LDH in melanoma patients compared to the normal population. A relationship was found between LD and survival [95]. Patients with elevated serum LDH at diagnosis of melanoma are staged as M1c according to the AJCC guidelines.

M Classification	Site	Serum LDH
M0	No detectable evidence of distant metastases	
M1a	Metastases to skin, subcutaneous, or distant lymph nodes	Normal
M1b	Metastases to lung	Normal
M1c	Metastases to all other visceral sites or distant metastases to any site combined with an elevated serum LDH	Normal- visceral met(s) Elevated- Distant met(s)

Table 5. M Classification as recommended by the AJCC [7]

7. Follow-up

All patients with invasive melanoma should be followed up post-operatively, except for patients with melanoma in-situ. The aim of follow-up is to detect evidence of recurrent disease or a new primary melanoma early [97,98]. The primary site and adjacent skin should be examined for recurrence of new suspicious lesions, as well as the draining lymph node basins [23]. It is estimated that the lifetime risk of developing a second melanoma is around 4 - 6%. Furthermore, around 60 - 80% of recurrences are found at local and/or regional nodal sites. Around two thirds of these will occur within the first three years, 16% after the first five years. Recurrence after more than ten years is also recognised [23].

There is little evidence for the optimum protocol for follow-up. It appears reasonable that all patients with invasive melanoma should be followed up 6-monthly for 2 years. Thereafter, those with melanomas less than 1.0 mm in depth may be discharged from routine follow-up; other patients should be followed up for a further 3 years at 6-monthly intervals. Patients with stage III or IV disease require lifelong follow up [23].

8. Conclusion

The incidence of melanoma continues to rise steadily in the Western World. Despite increased awareness of the disease this does not appear to have a significant impact on its overall poor prognosis. Surgery remains the mainstay of treatment as there is little in the way of adjuvant systemic treatment. Adequate surgical margins with or without local reconstruction can improve local recurrence rates. The utilisation of the sentinel lymph node biopsy has allowed for accurate staging of the disease. The finding of positive sentinel lymph nodes requires patients to undergo further regional lymph node dissection to reduce the risk of loco-regional disease. The impact of this on overall survival has not yet been clearly elucidated. Increased understanding of the melanoma pathogenesis and molecular biology may lead to the development of novel promising therapeutic agents and individualised treatment plans for these patients..

Author details

Z. Al-Hilli, D. Evoy, J.G. Geraghty, E.W. McDermott and R.S. Prichard

St. Vincent's University Hospital, Elm Park, Dublin, Ireland

References

[1] Jemal A, Bray F, Center MM, Ferlay J, Ward E, Forman D. Global cancer statistics. CA: A Cancer Journal for Clinicians 2011; 61(2) 69–90

[2] American Cancer Society: Cancer Facts and Figures 2012. Atlanta, Ga: American Cancer Society, 2012. Last accessed Aug 3rd 2012

[3] Cancer Research UK. http://info.cancerresearchuk.org/cancerstats/types/skin/ (Accessed 6 Aug 2012)

[4] National Cancer Institute. http://seer.cancer.gov/statfacts/html/melan.html (Accessed 3rd Aug 2012)

[5] Sladden MJ, Balch C, Barzilai DA, Berg D, Freiman A, Handiside T, Hollis S, Lens MB, Thompson JF. Surgical excision margins for primary cutaneous melanoma. Cochrane Database of Systematic Reviews 2009, Issue 4. Art. No.: CD004835. DOI: 10.1002/14651858.CD004835.pub2

[6] Stebbins WG, Garibyan, Sober AJ. Sentinel lymph node biopsy and melanoma: 2010 Part I. Journal of the American Academy of Dermatology. 2010; 62(5) 723-734

[7] Edge SB, Byrd DR, Compton CC, Fritz AG, Greene FL, Trotti A (Eds.): AJCC Cancer Staging Manual. New York, NY, Springer, 2009

[8] Balch CM, Gershenwald JE, Soong SJ, Thompson JF, Atkins MB, Byrd DR, Buzaid AC, Cochran AJ, Coit DG, Ding S, Eggermont AM, Flaherty KT, Gimotty PA, Kirkwood JM, McMasters KM, Mihm Jr MC, Morton DL, Ross MI, Sober AJ, Sondak VK. Final Version of 2009 AJCC Melanoma Staging and Classification. Journal of Clinical Oncology. 2009; 27(36) 6199-206

[9] Cascinelli N, Marchesini R. Increasing incidence of cutaneous melanoma, ultraviolet radiation and the clinician. Photochemistry and Photobiology. 1989; 50 497-505

[10] The American Cancer Society. (2010). What are the key statistics about Melanoma?, In : The American Cancer Society, Available from http://www.cancer.org/Cancer/SkinCancerMelanoma/DetailedGuide/melanoma-skin-cancer-key-statistics (Accessed 8 Aug 2012)

[11] Evans RD, Kopf, Lew RA, Rigel DS, Bart RS, Friedman RJ, Rivers JK. Risk factors for the development of malignant melanoma: I. Review of case-control studies. The journal of Detmatologic Surgery and Oncology 1988; 14(4) 292-408

[12] Gellin GA, Kopf AW, Garfinkel L. Malignant melanoma: A controlled study of possibly associated factors. Archives of Dermatology 2008; 99(1) 61-67

[13] Friedman RJ, Rigel DS, Silverman MK, Kopf AW, Vissaert KA. Malignant melanoma in the 1990s: the continued importance of early detection and the role of physician examination and self-examination of the skin. CA A Cancer Journal for Clinicians 1991; 41(4) 201-206

[14] Brozena SJ, Fenske NA, Perez IR. Epidemiology of malignant melanoma, worldwirde incidence and etiologic factors. Seminars in Surgical Oncology 1993; 9(3) 165-167

[15] Joyce DP, Prichard RS, Hill ADK Current controversies in the surgical management of melanoma. Beaumont Hospital, Dublin, Ireland. In: Cao MY (ed.) Curreny management of malignant melanoma. In Tech. 2011 ISBN 978-953-307-264-7

[16] MacKie RM. Clinical recognition of early invasive malignant melanoma. British Medical Journal 1990; 301(6759)1005-1006

[17] Abbasi NR, Shaw HM, Rigel DS, Friedman RJ, McCarthy WH, Osman I, et al. Early diagnosis of cutaneous melanoma: revisiting the ABCD criteria. The Journal of the American Medical Association 2004; 292(22) 2771-6

[18] Friedman RJ, Rigel DS, Kopf AW. Early detection of malignant melanoma: the role of physician examination and self-examination of the skin. CA: A Cancer Journal for Clinicians 1985; 35(3) 130-51

[19] Whited JD, Grichnik JM. The rational clinical examination. Does the patient have a more of a melanoma? The journal of the American Medical Association 1998; 279(9) 696-701

[20] Swanson NA, Lee KK, Gorman A, Lee HN. Biopsy techniques: diagnosis of melanoma. Dermatologic Clinics 2002; 20(4) 677–80

[21] Newton-Bishop JA, Corrie PG, Evans J, Gore ME, Hall PN, Kirkham N, Roberts DL, Anstey AV, Barlow RJ, Cox NH. Melanoma Study Group; British Association of Dermatologists. UK Guidelines for the management of cutaneous melanoma. British Journal of Plastic Surgery 2002; 55(1): 46 - 54

[22] Herd RM, Hunter JAA, McLaren KM, Chetty U, Watson ACH, Gollock JM. Excision biopsy of malignant melanoma by general practitioners in south east Scotland 1982–91. British Medical Journal 1992; 305(6867) 1476–8

[23] Cahill R, Hill ADK, Redmond HP. Royal College of Surgeons in Ireland, Management of Cutaneous Melanoma Clinical Guidelines. 2006

[24] Balch CM, Soong SJ, Atkins MB, Buzaid AC, Cascinelli N, Coit DG, Fleming ID, Gershenwald JE, Houghton A Jr, Kirkwood JM, McMasters KM, Mihm MF, Morton DL, Reintgen DS, Ross MI, Sober A, Thompson JA, Thomson JF. An evidence-based staging system for cutaneous melanoma. CA: A Cancer Journal for Clinicians 2004; 54(3)131-49

[25] Balch CM, Buzaid AC, Soong SJ, Atkins MB, Cascinelli N, Coit DG, Fleming ID, Gershenwald JE, Houghton A Jr, Kirkwood JM, McMasters KM, Mihm MF, Morton DL, Reintgen DS, Ross MI, Sober A, Thompson JA, Thomson JF. New TNM melanoma staging system: linking biology and natural history to clinical outcomes. Seminars in Surgical Oncology 2003; 21(1) 43-52

[26] Cascinelli N, Belli F, Santinami M, Fait V, Testori A, Ruka W, Canaliere R, Mozzillo N, Rossi CR, MacKie RM, Nieweg O, Pace M, Kirov K. Sentinel lymph node biopsy in cutaneous melanoma: the WHO Melanoma Program experience. Annals of Surgical Oncology 2000; 7(6) 469–474

[27] Cohn-Cedermark G, Rutqvist LE, Andersson R, Breivald M, Ingvar C, Johansson H, Jönsson PE, Krysander L, Lindholm C, Ringborg U. Long term results of a randomized study by the Swedish Melanoma Study Group on 2-cm versus 5-cm resection margins for patients with cutaneous melanoma with a tumor thickness of 0.8-2.0 mm. Cancer. 2000; 89(7) 1495-1501

[28] Khayat D, Rixe O, Martin G, Soubrane C, Banzet M, Bazex JA, Lauret P, Vérola O, Auclerc G, Harper P, Banzet P, French Group of Research on Malignant Melanoma. Surgical margins in cutaneous melanoma (2 cm versus 5 cm for lesions measuring less than 2.1-mm thick).Cancer. 2003; 97(8) 1941-1946

[29] Balch CM, Soong S, Ross MI, Urist MM, Karakousis CP, Temple WJ, Mihm MC, Barnhill RL, Jewell WR, Wanebo HJ, Harrison R. Long-term results of a multi-institutional randomized trial comparing prognostic factors and surgical results for intermediate thickness melanomas (1.0 to 4.0 mm). Intergroup Melanoma Surgical Trial. Ann Surg Oncol. 2000; 7(2) 87-97

[30] Balch CM, Soong SJ, Smith T, Ross MI, Urist MM, Karakousis CP, Temple WJ, Mihm MC, Barnhill RL, Jewell WR, Wanebo HJ, Desmond R; Investigators from the Intergroup Melanoma Surgical Trial. Long-term results of a prospective surgical trial comparing 2 cm vs. 4 cm excision margins for 740 patients with 1-4 mm melanomas. Annals of Surgical Oncology. 2001 Mar;8(2):101-8

[31] Gillgren P, Drzewiecki KT, Niin M, Gullestad HP, Hellborg H, Månsson-Brahme E, Ingvar C, Ringborg U 2-cm versus 4-cm surgical excision margins for primary cutaneous melanoma thicker than 2 mm: a randomised, multicentre trial.. Lancet. 2011; 378(9803) 1635-1642

[32] Thomas JM, Newton-Bishop J, A'Hern R, Coombes G, Timmons M, Evans J, Cook M, Theaker J, Fallowfield M, O'Neill T, Ruka W, Bliss JM, United Kingdom Melanoma Study Group, British Association of Plastic Surgeons, Scottish Cancer Therapy Network. Excision margins in high-risk malignant melanoma. New England Journal of Medicine. 2004; 350(8) 757-766

[33] Coit DG, Andtbacka R, Anker CJ, Bichakjian CK, Carson WE 3rd, Daud A, Dilawari RA, Dimaio D, Guild V, Halpern AC, Hodi FS Jr, Kelley MC, Khushalani NI, Kudchadkar RR, Lange JR, Lind A, Martini MC, Olszanski AJ, Pruitt SK, Ross MI, Swetter SM, Tanabe KK, Thompson JA, Trisal V, Urist MM; National Comprehensive Cancer Network. Melanoma. Journal of the Nationall Comprehensive Cancer Network. 2012; 10(3) 366-400

[34] Bichakjian CK, Halpern AC, Johnson TM, Foote Hood A, Grichnik JM, Swetter SM, Tsao H, Barbosa VH, Chuang TY, Duvic M, Ho VC, Sober AJ, Beutner KR, Bhushan R, Smith Begolka W, American Academy of Dermatology Guidelines of care for the management of primary cutaneous melanoma. American Academy of Dermatology. Journal of the American Academy of Dermatology. 2011; 65(5) 1032-1047

[35] Cotter MA, McKenna JK, Bowen GM. Treatment of lentigo maligna with imiquimod before staged excision. Dermatologic Surgery 2008; 34(2) 147–151.

[36] Heaton KM, Sussman JJ, Gershenwald JE, Lee JE, Reintgen DS, Mansfield PF, Ross MI. Surgical margins and prognostic factors in patients with thick (>4mm) primary melanoma. Annals of Surgical Oncology. 1998; 5(4) 322-328

[37] Australian Cancer Network Melanoma Guidelines Revision Working Party. Clinical Practice Guidelines for the Management of Melanoma in Australia and New Zealand. Cancer Council Australia and Australian Cancer Network, Sydney and New Zealand Guidelines Group, Wellington 2008; 73-77

[38] Brady MS, Brown K, Patel A, Fisher C, Marx. A phase II trial of isolated limb infusion with melphalan and dactinomycin for regional melanoma and soft tissue sarcoma of the extremity. Annals of Surgical Oncology 2006; 13(8):1123-9

[39] Mian R, Henderson M, Speakman D, Finkelde D, Ainslie J, McKenzie A. Isolated limb infusion for melanoma: a simple alternative to isolated limb perfusion. Canadian Journal of Surgery. 2001; 44(3) 189-192

[40] Hayes AJ, Clarke MA, Harries M, Thomas JM. Management of in-transit metastases from cutaneous malignant melanoma. British Journal of Surgery. 2004; 91(6) 673-682

[41] McCarthy WH. Melanoma Margins for error-another view. ANZ Journal of Surgery 2002; 72(4) 304-306

[42] Heenan PJ, Ghasnawie M. The pathogenesis of local recurrence of melanoma at the primary excision site. British Journal of Plastic Surgery. 1999; 52(3) 209-213

[43] Al-Hilli Z, Waqar K, Hill ADK. Isolated limb infusion for melanoma. Surgeon. 2007 5(5) 310-312

[44] Thompson JF, Kam PC, Waugh RC, Harman R. Isolated limb infusion with cytotoxic agents: A simple alternative to isolated limb perfusion. Seminars in Surgical Oncology 1998; 14(3) 238-47

[45] Cade S. Malignant melanoma. Annals of the Royal College of Surgeons in England. 1961; 28: 331-366

[46] Roberts DL, Anstey AV, Barlow RJ, et al. U.K. guidelines for the management of cutaneous melanoma. British Journal of Dermatology. 2002; 146 7–17

[47] Schumacher HH, Chia HL, Simcock JW. Ipsilateral skin grafts for lower limb melanoma reconstruction are safe. Plastic and Reconstructive Surgery. 2010; 125(2) 89-91

[48] Lent WM, Ariyan S. Flap reconstruction following wide local excision for primary malignant melanoma of the head and neck region. Annals of Plastic Surgery. 1994; 33(1) 23-27

[49] Balch CM, Soong SJ, Gershenwald JE, et al. Prognostic factors analysis of 17,600 melanoma patients: validation of the American Joint Committee on Cancer melanoma staging system. Journal of Clinical Oncology 2001; 19(16) 3622–3634

[50] Wong SL, Balch CM, Hurley P, Agarwala SS, Akhurst TJ, Cochran A, Cormier JN, Gorman M, Kim TY, McMasters KM, Noyes RD, Schuchter LM, Valsecchi ME, Weaver DL, Lyman GH. Sentinel Lymph Node Biopsy for Melanoma: American Society of Clinical Oncology and Society of Surgical Oncology Joint Clinical Practice Guideline. Annals of Surgical Oncology 2012 July 6 [Epub ahead of print] PMID: 22766987

[51] Uren RF, Howman-Giles R, Thompson JF, Shaw HM, Quinn MJ, O'Brien CJ, McCarthy WH. Lymphoscintigraphy to identify sentinel lymph nodes in patients with melanoma. Melanoma Research 1994; 4(6)395–399

[52] Bagaria SP, Faries MB, Morton DL. Sentinel Node Biopsy in Melanoma: Technical Considerations of the Procedure as Performed at the John Wayne Cancer Institute. Journal Surgical Oncology. 2010; 101(8) 669–676

[53] Morton DL, Thompson JF, Cochran AJ, Mozzillo N, Elashoff R, Essner R, Nieweg OE, Roses DF, Hoekstra HJ, Karakousis CP, Reintgen DS, Coventry BJ, Glass EC, Wang HJ, MSLT Group. Sentinel-node biopsy or nodal observation in melanoma. New England Journal of Medicine. 2006; 355(13) 1307-1317

[54] Agnese DM, Abdessalam SF, Burak WE Jr, Magro CM, Pozderac RV, Walker MJ. Cost-effectiveness of sentinel lymph node biopsy in thin melanomas. Surgery. 2003;134(4):542-548

[55] Andtbacka RH, Gershenwald JE. Role of sentinel lymph node biopsy in patients with thin melanoma. Journal of the National Comprehensive Cancer Network. 2009; 7(3) 208-317

[56] AJCC cancer staging manual. 6th ed. Chicago, IL: Springer; 2002

[57] Spanknebel K, Coit DG, Bieligk SC, Gonen M, Rosai J, Klimst DS. Characterization of micrometastatic disease in melanoma sentinel lymph nodes by enhanced pathology: recommendations for standardizing pathologic analysis. American Journal of Surgical Pathology 2005; 29(3) 305-317

[58] Blaheta HJ, Ellwanger U, Schittek B, Sotlar K, MacZey E, Breuninger H, Thelen MH, Bueltmann B, Rassner G, Garbe C. Examination of regional lymph nodes by sentinel node biopsy and molecular analysis provides new staging facilities in primary cutaneous melanoma. The Journal of Investigative Dermatology 2000; 114(4) 637-642.

[59] Palmieri G, Ascierto PA, Cossu A, Mozzillo N, Motti ML, Satriano SM, Botti G, Caraco Cm Celentano E, Satriano RA, Lissia A, Tanda F, Pirastu M, Castello G; Melanoma Cooperative Group. Detection of occult melanoma cells in paraffin- embedded histologically negative sentinel lymph nodes using a reverse transcriptase polymerase chain reaction assay. Journal of Clinical Oncology 2001; 19(5) 1437-1443

[60] Prichard RS, Dijkstra B, McDermott EW, Hill AD, O'Higgins NJ. The role of molecular staging in malignant melanoma. European Journal of Surgical Oncology. 2003 May; 29(4) 306-14.

[61] Scoggins CR, Ross MI, Reintgen DS, Noyes RD, Goydos JS Beitsch PD, Urist MM, Ariyan S, Davidson BS, Sussman JJ, Edwards MJ, Martin RC, Lewis AM, Stromberg AJ, Conrad AJ, Hagendoorn L, Albrecht J, McMasters KM . Prospective multi-institutional study of reverse transcriptase polymerase chain reaction for molecular staging of melanoma. Journal of Clinical Oncology 2006; 24(18) 2849-2857

[62] Mocellin S, Hoon DS, Pilati P, Rossi CR, Nitti D. Sentinel lymph node molecular ultrastaging in patients with melanoma: a systematic review and meta-analysis of prognosis. Journal of Clinical Oncology 2007; 25(12) 1588-1595

[63] Callery C, Cochran AJ, Roe DJ, Rees W, Nathanson SD, Benedetti JK, Elashoff RM, Morton DL. Factors prognostic for survival in patients with malignant melanoma spread to regional lymph nodes. Annals of Surgery 1982;196:69–75

[64] Roses DF, Provet JA, Harris MN, Gumport SL, Dubin N. Prognosis of patients with pathologic stage II cutaneous malignant melanoma. Annals of Surgery 1985;201:103–7

[65] Kunte C, Geimer T, Baumert J, Konz B, Volkenandt M, Flaig M, Ruzicka T, Berking C, Schmid-Wendtner MH. Analysis of predictive factors for the outcome of complete lymph node dissection in melanoma patients with metastatic sentinel lymph nodes. Journal of the American Academy of Dermatology. 2011 Apr;64(4):655-662

[66] Garbe C, Hauschild A, Volkenandt M, Schadendorf D, Stolz W, Reinhold U, Kettelhack C, Frerich B, Keilholz U, Dummer R, Sebastian G, Tilgan W, Schuler G, Mackensen A, Kaufmann R. Evidence and interdisciplinary consensusbased German guidelines: surgical treatment and radiotherapy of melanoma. Melanoma Resarch 2008;18:61-67

[67] Wong SL, Brady MS, Busam KJ, Coit DG. Results of sentinel lymph node biopsy in patients with thin melanoma. Annals of Surgical Oncology. 2006;13(3) 302-309

[68] Kretschmer L, Hilgers R, Mohrle M, Balda BR, Breuninger H, Konz B, Kunte C, Marsch WC, Neumann C, Starz H. Patients with lymphatic metastasis of cutaneous malignant melanoma benefit from sentinel lymphonodectomy and early excision of their nodal disease. European Journal of Cancer 2004; 40: 212-218

[69] Ghaferi AA, Wong SL, Johnson TM, Lowe L, Chang AE, Cimmino VM, Bradford CR, Rees RS, Sabel MS. Prognostic significance of a positive nonsentinel lymph node in cutaneous melanoma. Annals of Surgical Oncology 2009; 16: 2978-84.

[70] Lee JH, Essner R, Torisu-Itakura H, Wanek L, Wang H, Morton DL. Factors predictive of tumour-positive non-sentinel lymph nodes after tumour-positive sentinel lymph node dissection for melanoma. Journal Clinical Oncology 2004; 22: 3677-84.

[71] Rossi CR, De Salvo GL, Bonandini E, Mocellin S, Foletto M, Pasquali S, Pilati P, Lise M, Nitto D, Rizzo E, Montesco MC. Factors predictive of non-sentinel lymph node involvement and clinical outcome in melanoma patients with metastatic sentinel lymph node. Annals of Surgical Oncology 2008;15 :1202-10

[72] Reeves ME, Delgado R, Busam KJ, Brady MS, Coit DG. Prediction of non-sentinel lymph node status in melanoma. Annals of Surgical Oncology 2003; 10: 27-31

[73] Glumac N, Hocevar M, Zadnik V, Snoj M. Sentinel lymph node micrometastasis may predict non-sentinel involvement in cutaneous melanoma patients. Journal of Surgical Oncology 2008;98 46-49

[74] van der Ploeg IM, Kroon BB, Antonini N, Valdes Olmos RA, Nieweg OE. Is completion lymph node dissection needed in case of minimal melanoma metastasis in the sentinel node? Annals of Surgery 2009;249:1003-7

[75] Ollila DW, Ashburn JH, Amos KD, Yeh JJ, Frank JS, Deal AM, Long P, Thomas ND, Meyers MO. Metastatic melanoma cells in the sentinel node cannot be ignored. Journal of the American College of Surgeons 2009; 208: 924-9, discussion 9-30

[76] Multicenter Selective Lymphadenectomy Trial II (MSLT-II) Clinical-Trials.gov identifier: NCT00297895

[77] Stebbins WG, Garibyan, Sober AJ. Sentinel lymph node biopsy and melanoma: 2010 Part II. Journal of the American Academy of Dermatology. 2010; 62(5) 737-748

[78] Coit DG. Role of Surgery in metastatic malignant melanoma: a review. Seminars in Surgical Oncology. 1993; 9(3) 239-245

[79] Leung AM, Hari DM, Morton DL. Surgery for distant melanoma metastasis. Cancer Journal. 2012; 18(2) 176-178

[80] Finn L, Markovic SN, Joseph RW. Therapy for metastatic melanoma: the past, present, and future. BMC Medicine. 2012; 2; 10: 23

[81] Hodi FS, O'Day SJ, McDermott DF, Weber RW, Sosman JA, Haanen JB, Gonzalez R, Robert C, Schadendorf D, Hassel JC, Akerley W, van den Eertwegh AJ, Lutzky J, Lorigan P, Vaubel JM, Linette GP, Hogg D, Ottensmeier CH, Lebbe C, Peschel C, Quirt I, Clark JI, Wolchock JD, Weber JS, Tian J, Yellin MJ, Nichol GM, Hoos A, Urba WJ. Improved survival with ipilimumab in patients with metastatic melanoma. The New England Journal of Medicine 2010; 363(8) 711-723

[82] Robert C, Thomas L, Bondarenko I, O'Day S, M DJ, Garbe C, Lebbe C, Baurain JF, Testori A, Grob JJ, Davidson N, Richards J, Maio M, Hauschild A, Miller WH Jr, Gascon P, Lotem M, Harmankaya K, Ibrahim R, Francis S, Chenn TTm Humphrey R, Hoos A, Wolchock JD. Ipilimumab plus dacarbazine for previously untreated metastatic melanoma. The New England journal of Medicine 2011; 364(26) 2517-2526

[83] Robert C, Thomas L, Bonderanko I, O'Day S, MD JW, Garbe C, Lebbe C, Baurin JF, Testori A, Grobb JJ, Davidson N, Richards J, Maio M, Hauschild A, Miller WH Jr,

Gascon P, Lotern M, Harmankaya K, Ibrahim R, Francis S, Chenn TT, Humphrey R, Hoos A, Wolchock JD. Ipilumumab plus dacarbazine for previously untreated metastatic melanoma. New England Journal of Medicine. 2011 264(26) 2517-2526

[84] Eggermont AM, Robert C. New drugs in melanoma: it's a whole new world. European Journal of Cancer. 2011 47(14) 2150-2157

[85] Seegenschmiedt MH, Keilholz L, Altendorf-Hofmann A, Urban A, Schell H, Hohenberger W, Sauer R. Palliative radiotherapy for recurrent and metastatic malignant melanoma: prognostic factors for tumor response and long-term outcome: a 20-year experience. International Journal of Radiation Oncology, Biology and Physics 1999; 44(3) 607–618

[86] Overgaard J, von der Maase H, Overgaard M. A randomized study comparing two high-dose per fraction radiation schedules in recurrent or metastatic malignant melanoma. International Journal of Radiation Oncology, Biology and Physics 1985; 11(10) 1837–1839

[87] Olivier KR, Schild SE, Morris CG, Brown PD, Markovic SN. A higher radiotherapy dose is associated with more durable palliation and longer survival in patients with metastatic melanoma. Cancer 2007; 110(8) 1791–1795

[88] Barnhill RL, Katzen J, Spatz A, Fine J, Berwick M. The importance of mitotic rate as a prognostic factor for localized cutaneous melanoma. Journal of Cutaneous Pathology 2005; 32(4) 268–273

[89] Azzola MF, Shaw HM, Thompson JF, Soong SJ, Scolyer RA, Watson GF, Colman MH, Zhang Y. Tumor mitotic rate is a more powerful prognostic indicator than ulceration in patients with primary cutaneous melanoma: an analysis of 3661 patients from a single center. Cancer 2003; 97(6)1488–1498

[90] Francken AB, Shaw HM, Thompson JF, Soong SJ, Accrott NA, Azzola MF, Scoyler RA, Milton GW, McCarthy WH, Colman MHm McGovern VJ. The prognostic importance of tumor mitotic rate confirmed in 1317 patients with primary cutaneous melanoma and long follow-up. Annals of Surgical Oncology 2004; 11(4) 426–433

[91] Gimotty PA, Elder DE, Fraker DL, Botbyl J, Sellers K, Elenitsas R, Ming ME, Schuchter L, Spitz FR, Czerniecki BJ, Geurry D. Identification of high-risk patients among those diagnosed with thin cutaneous melanomas. Journal of Clinical Oncology 2007; 25(9) 1129–1134

[92] Clark WH Jr, From L, Bernardino EA, Mihm MC. The histogenesis and biologic behavior of primary human malignant melanomas of the skin. Cancer Research 1969; 29(3) 705-727

[93] Ohsie SJ, Sarantopoulos GP, Cochran AJ, Binder SW. Immunohistochemical characteristics of melanoma. Journal of Cutaneous Pathology 2008; 35(5) 433–444

[94] Cascinelli N, Belli F, Santinami M, Fait V, Testori A, Ruka W, Canaliere R, Mozzillo N, Rossi CR, MacKie RM, Nieweg O, Pace M, Kirov K. Sentinel lymph node biopsy

in cutaneous melanoma: the WHO Melanoma Program experience. Annals of Surgical Oncology 2000; 7(6) 469–474

[95] Agarwala S, Keilholz U, Gilles E, Bedikian AY, Wu J, Kay R, Stein CA, Itri M, Suciu S, Eggermont AM, LDH correlation with survival in advanced melanoma from two large, randomized trials (Oblimersen GM301 and EORTC 18951). European Journal of Cancer 2009; 45(1) 1807-1814

[96] Martini L, Brandani P, Chiarugi C, Reali UM. First recurrence analysis of 840 cutaneous melanomas: a proposal for a follow-up schedule. Tumori 1994; 80(3) 188-197

[97] Poo-Wwu WJ, Ariyan S, Lambe L, Papac R, Zelterman D, Hu GL, Brown J, Fischer D, Bolognia J, Buzaid AC. Follow-up recommendations for patients with American Joint Committee on Cancer Stages I-III malignant melanoma. Cancer 1999; 86: 2252-2258.

Chapter 16

Melanoma: Treatments and Resistance

Jonathan Castillo Arias and
Miriam Galvonas Jasiulionis

Additional information is available at the end of the chapter

http://dx.doi.org/10.5772/54202

1. Introduction

In the past two decades, it has been observed an increased incidence of skin cancer around the world [1-4]. This increase is particularly important in melanoma [5]. Latin-American data have shown both an increase in incidence rates of skin cancer [6] and in mortality from malignant melanoma [7]. The number of melanoma cases worldwide is increasing faster than any other cancer. Although early detection, appropriate surgery, and adjuvant therapy have improved outcomes, the prognosis of metastatic melanoma remains very poor. Advanced melanoma is still associated with an extremely poor median survival, ranging from 2 to 8 months, with only 5% surviving more than 5 years and remains one of the most treatment-refractory malignancy [8]

2. Treatments

The only way to cure a malignant melanoma is early detection and appropriate surgical treatment, because once it reaches an advanced stage, is highly resistant to conventional radiotherapy and chemotherapy [9]. The median survival for patients with metastatic disease is approximately 8 months [10], and chemotherapy has so far failed to improve survival. Treatment options include radiation therapy, chemotherapy, immunotherapy and biochemotherapy which are summarized below.

2.1. Radiotherapy

The use of adjuvant radiotherapy (RT) in melanomas has been controversial. *In vitro* studies have shown that melanoma cells possess a broad shoulder on the cell survival curve and thus have a large capacity for DNA repair. As a result, hypofractionated RT schedules have been developed to counteract this perceived radioresistance, producing excellent locoregional control rates of 85% and higher [11,12]. Radiation Therapy Oncology Group (RTOG) Trial 83-05 was a prospective randomized study comparing hypofractionation to conventional fractionation. The results showed no difference in partial or complete response rates between the two schedules, and the overall response rates were approximately 70% [13]. The role of adjuvant radiation therapy (RT) following nodal surgery in malignant melanoma remains controversial. Despite the high incidence of distant metastases, loco-regional control remains an important goal in the management of melanoma. Surgery and adjuvant RT provides excellent loco-regional control, although distant metastases remain the major cause of mortality.[14]

2.2. Chemotherapy

Chemotherapeutic agents are cytotoxic anticancer drugs which aim is impair the cell division, resulting in the death of rapidly dividing cells. They are widely used in the treatment of malignancies; however, melanomas are resistant to many forms of traditional chemotherapy.

2.2.1. Chemotherapy with single drugs in melanoma

Several antitumoral drugs have been used to treat the melanoma. One of the most known is dacarbazine. In 1975, dacarbazine (DTIC) became the first US Food and Drug Administration (FDA) approved chemotherapeutic agent for the treatment of metastatic melanoma. The response rates with dacarbazine were 15–25%, with median response ranging from 5 to 6 months, but with less than 5% of complete responses [17-19]. Long-term follow-up of patients treated with DTIC alone shows that less than 2% of the patients could survive for 6 years [15,16]. In a meta-analysis comparing two or three-drugs combination regimens with DTIC alone, Huncharek et al. [20] concluded that there was no advantage for the combination in terms of response or survival. Since survival was not improved by the use of single or combination chemotherapy for metastatic melanoma, treatment decisions remain controversial, and quality of life and toxicity issues from treatment assume greater importance.

An orally analogue of DTIC is temozolomide whose activity has been tested in several clinical studies as single agent in metastatic malignant melanoma [18,21,22]. A randomized phase III trial comparing TMZ to DTIC on patients with advanced melanoma demonstrated a statistically significant increase in progression-free survival (1.9 months vs 1.5 months) when TMZ was administered [18].

Fotemustine (FTMU) is the most active nitrosourea used against the metastatic melanoma. It has been widely tested in Europe and has shown overall response of 20–25% including 5–8% of complete response rates and it was the first drug to show significant efficacy in brain metastases [23,24]. However, at conventional doses, little or no activity was observed against melanoma brain metastases [25].

Platinum-based drugs are widely used in the treatment of cancer. In patients with melanoma, cisplatin was shown to induce a 15% response rate with a short median duration of 3 months. Doses up to 150 mg/m^2 in combination with amifostine produced tumor responses in 53% of patients. However, all of those responses were partial, and the median response duration was only 4 months [26]. Regarding carboplatin, in a study on 26 chemotherapy-naive metastatic melanoma patients, a response rate of 19% with 5 partial responses was reported and thrombocytopenia was the dose-limiting toxicity [27].

The vinca alkaloids, especially vindesine and vinblastine, have induced responses in approximately 14% of melanoma patients and they are usually used in combination with other drugs [28]. Docetaxel or paclitaxel, do not have a significant activity in melanoma [29-32]. The role of tamoxifen (TAM) as single agent at standard or high-doses in the treatment of melanoma is negligible with a response rate ranging between 0% and 10%. Currently all of these drugs are rarely used as single agent therapy in metastatic melanoma.

2.2.2. Chemotheraphy with combined drugs in melanoma

In a phase II study, Lattanzi et al. [33] reported their experience with the addition of TAM to the three-drug combination regimen of cisplatin, carmustine and dacarbazine (the Dartmouth regimen) and showed high response rates (55%) with a 20% complete response. Since then several randomized clinical trials have been conducted to confirm the therapeutic benefit of TAM in combination with chemotherapy.

Cocconi et al. [34] published a small phase III trial demonstrating an improvement of response and survival with the addition of tamoxifen to dacarbazine compared to dacarbazine alone. However, two large randomized trials with low and high-dose tamoxifen in combination with either dacarbazine alone or the Dartmouth regimen failed to demonstrate an advantage to the addition of tamoxifen [35,36].

The efficacy of the combination of paclitaxel and carboplatin in the treatment of metastatic melanoma was reported some years ago. Although originally tested in two small phase II clinical trials and deemed not sufficiently clinically active, this evidence suggests that the combination of paclitaxel and carboplatin may be worth further consideration [37].

2.3. Immunotherapy

Immunotherapy in melanoma consists of various approaches leading to specific or non-specific immunomodulation. Immunotherapies are being used for melanoma patients in stage II–III patients in the adjuvant setting, where only a fraction of patients have widespread (microscopic) disease with the aim to prevent relapse of disease, prolong relapse-free survival and, ideally, prolong overall survival (OS). In patients with stage IV disease, there is a need for adequate systemic therapies as median OS for this patient group is only 6–9 months [38]. However, for the first time in >30 years, prospective randomized trials in patients with distant metastatic melanoma demonstrated an OS benefit [39].

Some agents used in the treatment against the melanoma are ipilimumab and tremelimumab, fully human IgG1 and IgG2 monoclonal antibodies, respectively. They block cytotoxic T-lymphocyte- associated antigen 4 (CTLA-4), a negative regulator of T cells, and thus augment T-cell activation and proliferation [40,41]. A phase-III trial was completed first and its results were reported in 2010 [39]. This trial compared ipilimumab alone or in combination with a gp100-peptide vaccine, compared to the vaccine alone in patients who had failed prior therapy or therapies. Melanoma patients receiving ipilimumab and ipilimumab + vaccination had a significantly better survival outcome than those receiving the vaccine alone. Ipilimumab was combined with high-dose IL-2 in 36 patients in the surgery branch of the NCI, with some remarkable observations. There were six patients (17%) with long-lasting complete response, all over 5 years, and none of the patients relapsed. Moreover, there was no increased toxicity as compared to high-dose IL-2 alone [42]. Other study showing a combination of tremelimumab with high-dose interferon yielded a high overall response rate of 30% in 33 melanoma patients, with three complete responses and seven partial responses, all long-lasting responses. Again, there was no increased toxicity compared to high-dose IFN therapy alone [43].

Interferon-α (IFN-α) has been approved in the adjuvant setting for the treatment of high-risk melanoma based on clinical trials in the early 1990s [44,45]. In a metastatic situation, melanoma patients treated with the single agent IFN-α showed approximately 15% of responses, with less than 5% of complete response rates and median response duration between 6 and 9 months with a maximum of 12 months for the best studies [46]. These response rates, while encouraging, were not significant enough to lead to its widespread use in the treatment of metastatic melanoma. However, observations that patients with non-visceral disease were more likely to respond suggested that the use of IFN-α may demonstrated a grater impact in patients with micrometastasis [46, 47]. Other combination studied was IL-2 with IFN-α. This association did not seem to achieve better results (median response rate of 18% with three complete responses) than if these agents were given alone [48-50]. By contrast, in a small randomized phase III trial comparing continuous infusion IL- 2 plus interferon vs. continuous infusion decreasing IL-2 plus interferon, Keilholtz and colleagues [51], demonstrated improved response rates and reduced toxicity with decreasing doses of IL-2.

2.4. Biochemotherapy

Because chemotherapy and cytokines have different and synergistic mechanisms of action and in order to improve response rates and durable remissions, several groups developed in the early 1990s the concept of biochemotherapy, a combination of chemotherapy and biologic response modifiers.

Dacarbazine/IFN-α is one of the most evaluated combinations in metastatic malignant melanoma. In a randomized phase II trial, Falkson et al. [52] reported that the association of IFN-α with dacarbazine resulted in an encouraging response rate (53% vs. 20% for dacarbazine alone) and a higher duration of response (8.9 months vs. 2.5 months) but IFN-α significantly increased the toxicity. However, a follow up of a large randomized trial demonstrated no benefit for the addition of IFN-α to dacarbazine and significantly more severe toxic events occurred with treatments containing IFN-α [36].

The other approaches of biochemotherapy have involved sequential chemotherapy (cisplatin, vinblastine, and dacarbazine, CVD) followed by biologic response modifiers (continuous infusion of 9 MIU/m2 of IL-2 + IFN-α) because of concern of toxicity when drugs were given simultaneously or concurrent with chemo-immunotherapy. Both approaches have produced promising results with overall response rates between 40% and 60% and a long-term remission rate of about 9%. The sequential approach was compared to chemotherapy alone in a randomized trial conducted at the MD Anderson Cancer Center. Although both response rate and time to progression were improved in the sequential biochemotherapy group, the survival difference was at borderline significance and the toxicity was very high [53]. The results of the largest phase III trial (ECOG/Intergroup E3695 trial) and most definitive test for biochemotherapy comparing concurrent CVD-Bio to CVD alone showed that biochemotherapy produced slightly higher response rates and significantly longer median progression-free survival than CVD alone, but once again failed to show any improvement in either overall survival or durable responses. Considering the extra toxicity and complexity, this concurrent biochemotherapy regimen should not be recommended for patients with metastatic melanoma [54].

2.5. Signal transduction inhibitors

In the past decades, no significant impact on survival has been made in spite of increased response rates achieved with combinations of chemotherapeutics or with the combination of chemotherapy and cytokines such as interferon (IFN) or interleukin-2 (IL-2). However, great advances have been made in a very short time, both in terms of targeted drugs that kill melanoma cells.

Sorafenib was designed to inhibit tyrosine kinase activity of CRAF, but this drug inhibits both the wild-type RAF protein as the V600E mutant protein. Subsequently, it was shown that sorafenib is actually a multikinase inhibitor, can inhibit many other molecules such as VEGFR2 and 3, PDGFR, p38 MAPK, FLT3, c-Kit and RET [55]. Although preclinical experiments, both *in vitro* and in animal models, seemed to be encouraging, the results of clinical trials have not confirmed the efficacy of sorafenib for the treatment of disseminated melanoma [56]

After the failure of sorafenib in melanoma, was synthesized a more specific BRAF inhibitors, in particular against the protein with the V600E mutation: PLX4032, a low molecular weight drug, for oral administration. In the first clinical trial published in 2010 [57], the objective response was observed in 81% of the $BRAF^{V600E}$ melanoma patients with 2 complete responses and 24 partial responses. Responses occurred in patients with visceral metastases in locations usually resistant to treatment such as liver, intestine and bone. However, despite having achieved a good response, relapses occur early, usually in a period of 8-12 months after treatment [58].

The possibility that c-Kit was a therapeutic target in melanoma has long since shuffled. In fact, c-Kit is a protein that acts as a receptor for a growth factor essential for epidermal melanocytes and has a role in the differentiation and migration of melanocytic cells during embryonic development [59]. In 2011, a phase-II study from China reported 20–30% response rates and prolongation of progression-free survival with imatinib treatment [60].

From 15 to 30% of melanomas have mutations of NRAS. RAS activation mutations stimulate MAP kinase pathway, but also the route of PI3K/AKT among others. A phase II trial using the RAS inhbitor Tipifarnib was performed; however, it was closed for lack of response. None of the patients was selected based on the presence of mutations of NRAS [61].

MEK is a protein of the MAP kinase pathway, located downstream BRAF. Several MEK inhibitors (PD0325901, AZD6244, GSK1120212, and E6201) have been synthesized. Bases on some results, it appears that these pharmacological agents may be effective as single agents in the treatment of melanoma. However, there are many preclinical studies suggesting that it would be a good alternative to the combined treatments, both to avoid resistance in the use of drugs directed against BRAF/V600E mutation, as for the treatment of BRAF mutations other than V600E or mutations of NRAS, especially if associated with inhibitors of PI3K/AKT pathway [62-65]

Different derivatives of rapamycin (CCI-779 or temsirolimus) have been used as inhibitors of the PI3K/AKT pathway. These inhibitors act on mTOR molecule downstream AKT/PKB. There are also dual inhibitors of PI3K and mTOR, PI3K and AKT [66]. Although clinical outcomes of these drugs in phase II trials have not been good, there are several authors proposing their use in combined therapies especially with drugs that inhibit the MAP kinase pathway [62, 63, 65, 67] or even, simultaneous inhibition via PI3K/AKT [68].

3. Resistance to the treatments in melanoma

Simultaneous resistance to several structurally unrelated drugs that do not necessarily have a common mechanism of action is called multidrug resistance phenomena. An important principle in multidrug resistance is that cancer cells are genetically heterogeneous. Although the process results in uncontrolled cell growth for clonal expansion of cancer, tumor cells exposed to chemotherapeutic agents will be selected by their ability to survive and grow in the presence of cytotoxic drugs. Therefore, in any population of cancer cells that are exposed to chemotherapy, more than one mechanism of multidrug resistance may be present [69]. Different types of multidrug resistance mechanisms have been described in cancer cells. Natural resistance to hydrophobic drugs sometimes known as classical multidrug resistance, usually results in the expression of efflux pumps with an ATP-dependent drug broad specificity. These pumps belong to a family of conveyors called ABC transporters (ATP-binding cassette) that show sequence and structural homology [70]. The resistance is caused by increased output by lowering the intracellular concentration of the drug. Resistance may also occur due to reduced entry of the drug. Water-soluble drugs, which are returned by carriers that are used to carry nutrients into the cell, or agents that enter through endocytosis, could fail without evidencing of increased output. Examples of this kind of drugs include the antifolate methotrexate, nucleotide analogues such as 5-fluorouracil and 8-azaguanine, and alkylating agents such as cisplatin [71,72]. Multidrug resistance can also result from the activation of coordinated systems of detoxification, such as DNA repair systems and cytochrome P-450 [73]. In another hand, resistance can also result from a defective apoptotic pathway. This can occur because of malignant transformation, such as in cancer, or as a result of non-functional mutant p53 [74]. Alternatively, cells may acquire apoptotic pathways changes during exposure to chemotherapy and changes in the levels of ceramides [75] or changes in the cell cycle machinery, which triggers checkpoints and prevent initiation of apoptosis. Below we present several mechanisms of resistance to the treatments that have been described in melanoma.

3.1. Antipoptotic characteristics in melanoma

Melanocytes and their stem cell precursors are activated to secrete melanin and protect neighboring keratinocytes and other epidermal cells from further damage [76]. Thus, melanocytes should be programmed to survive. Keratinocytes promote melanocyte expression of Bcl-2 by secreting neuronal growth factor (NGF) and stem cell grow factor (SCF). NGF binds to its receptors in the melanocyte membrane and increases the levels of Bcl-2 [77]. SCF interacts with its receptor c-KIT on the membrane and leads to the activation of transcription factor Mitf, which induces proliferation and differentiation of melanocyte precursors [78]. Tumorigenic melanoma cells may take advantage of high endogenous Bcl-2 levels to survive under adverse environmental conditions that they may encounter during metastatic progression and, given the connection between apoptosis and drug sensitivity, bypass the effects of chemotherapeutic drugs. Similarly, BclxL and Mcl-1, other anti-apoptotic members of the Bcl-2 family, are strongly expressed in normal melanocytes, benign nevi, primary melanoma and melanoma metastases, and may contribute to melanoma resistance to therapy [79,80]

In melanoma, two members of the IAP family, survivin and ML-IAP, have been associated with tumor progression, as they become detectable in melanocytic nevi and further overexpressed in invasive and metastatic melanomas [81,82]. Survivin is abundantly expressed, and its subcellular localization varies depending upon tumor thickness and invasiveness. Survivin overexpression has been shown in squamous cell carcinoma (SCC), and it is involved in UVB-induced carcinogenesis. The presence of survivin both in the nucleus and in the cytoplasm throughout the epidermal layers of psoriatic lesions suggests the involvement of this protein in the keratinocyte alterations typical of this disease [81]. Similarly, suppression of survivin can increase the sensitivity of melanoma cells to chemotherapeutic agents [83,84]. ML-IAP is also upregulated in melanoma cell lines and absent in normal melanocytes [85]. ML-IAP's effects on the mitochondrial pathways are considered to be related to a direct inhibition of the pro-apoptotic factor Smac/Diablo, and the caspases 9 and 3 [86]. The role of ML-IAP on melanoma chemoresistance has not been proven yet, but the overexpression of ML-IAP in breast cancer cell lines (MCF-7) or in HeLa cells protects against the drug Adriamycin and other apoptotic inducers, including TNF-α, FADD or BAX [86,87].

3.2. p53 pathway

p53 suppresses tumor development through multiple activities including induction of growth arrest, apoptosis, senescence, and autophagy [88,89]. Environmental agents such as UV that induce cellular damage activate the p53 tumor suppressor and p53 activation results in p53-dependent programmed cell death (apoptosis) in many cell types. Melanocytes are resistant to UV-induced apoptosis suggesting that p53 activity is somehow blocked (non-functional p53), a state shared with melanoma cells [90], which are resistant to conventional modes of chemotherapy that aim to stimulate p53-dependent apoptosis.

Melanoma is one of a number of tumor types where p53 is still wild type, indicating that other events are contributing to p53 inactivation, in fact p53 function could be disabled by lesions that disrupt other components of the pathway. Studies using mouse models of melanoma have shown that disruption of the upstream p53 regulator p14 ^{ARF} can functionally replace p53 loss during melanomagenesis [91]. Analogous to the human situation, tumors arising in these mouse models present wild type p53 [91]. Moreover, the abnormal phosphorylation of p53 by Chk2 kinase may contribute to the resistance of melanoma cells to radiotherapy [92]. Disruption of apoptosis downstream of p53 may alleviate pressure to mutate p53 and simultaneously decrease drug sensitivity [93]. For example, Apaf-1 and caspase 9 can be essential downstream effectors of p53-induced apoptosis and their disruption can facilitate oncogenic transformation of cultured fibroblasts [94]. In melanomas, Apaf-1 protein and mRNA expression are frequently downregulated in metastatic cell lines and tumor specimens [95]. Interestingly, Apaf-1 protein levels can be restored by addition of the methylation inhibitor 5-aza-2′-deoxycytidine (5azaCdR), suggesting that DNA methylation contributes to suppression of Apaf-1 levels. Whether methylation blocks Apaf-1 mRNA expression directly by interfering with the recruitment of transcription factors at the Apaf-1 promoter or by affecting a regulator of Apaf-1 expression remains an open question. In any case, Apaf-1 downregulation compromises the apoptotic response of melanoma cells in response to p53 activation [95] or E2F-1 [96]. Restoring physiological levels of Apaf-1 through gene transfer or 5aza2dC treatment enhances chemosensitivity, alleviating cell death defects associated with reduced Apaf-1 expression [95].

In tumor cells, the selective pressure to delete or inactivate p53 is very high. This primarily occurs through mutations in p53, amplification/overexpression of its inhibitors like Mdm2, Mdm4 (Mdm2 family member) [97]. The key molecule in the p53 regulatory network is Mdm2, an E3 ubiquitin ligase with potentially oncogenic activity. Dynamic fine-tuning of the Mdm2-centered network dictates the proper rapidity, intensity, and duration of a p53 response, resulting in the appropriate biological outcomes [98]. Although p53 is one of the most frequently mutated tumor suppressor genes in cancer, it is mutated in only about 13% of uncultured melanoma specimens [99-101]. The absence of p53 mutations in melanoma has been attributed to the epistatic loss of ARF [101] or amplification of HDM2 [102], both of which lead to a functionally debilitating interaction between HDM2 and p53. Ji et al. have provided important data that HDM2 antagonism can effectively restore p53 function, suppress melanoma growth, and synergize with MEK inhibition [103].

3.3. Signaling pathways in melanoma

In malignant melanoma, the PI3K/AKT signaling pathway is frequently constitutively activated [104]. Several studies indicate that only a combinatorial inhibition of PI3K/AKT and MAPK signalling induces apoptosis in melanoma cells efficiently [105,106]. On the other hand, inappropriate activation of survival signaling pathways such as those mediated by mitogen-activated protein kinase (MEK)/extracellular-regulated kinase (ERK) and phosphoinositide 3-kinase (PI3K)/AKT, either as consequences of genetic alterations or resulting from environmental stimulations, is known to play a central role in the resistance of melanoma to apoptosis [107,108].

One-third of primary melanomas and about 50% of metastatic melanoma cell lines showed reduced expression of PTEN as a result of allelic deletion, mutation or transcriptional silencing [109,110], suggesting that inactivation of PTEN is a late, but frequent, event on melanomagenesis [111,112]. Multiple lines of evidence point to the PI3K/AKT/PTEN pathway as a putative candidate for therapeutic intervention in melanoma because PTEN overexpression can revert the invasive phenotype of human and mouse melanoma cell lines [113,114] and elevated PTEN activity may sensitize cells to chemotherapeutic drugs [115].

Recent progress in the identification of genes relevant for melanomagenesis was made, revealing the importance of several signaling pathways. Sinnberg et al. [116] suggest that the oncogenic transcription factor Y-box binding protein-1 (YB-1) play a pivotal role in melanoma cells. YB-1 could be a key player, activated by the signalling pathways MAPK and PI3K/AKT. Indeed, was demostrated that both signaling pathways are able to increase S102-phosphorylation and nuclear translocation of YB-1. It is known that S102-phosphorylated YB-1 can induce the expression of the catalytic subunit of PI3K and by this increases PI3K activity [117].

In melanoma cells, the NF-kB pathway can be altered by upregulation of the NF-kB subunits p50 and RelA [118,119] and downregulation of the NF-kB inhibitor IkB [120,121]. Consequently, downstream NF-kB targets like c-myc, cyclin D1, the anti-apoptotic factor TRAF2, the invasion-associated proteins Mel-CAM or the pro-angiogenic chemokine GRO are also frequently upregulated in melanoma [122]. Recent studies have highlighted that some components of NF- kB family, such as p50 and p65/ RelA proteins, are overexpressed in the nuclei of dysplastic nevi and melanoma cells compared to those of normal nevi and healthy melanocytes, respectively [123]. Other data show that a hyperactivation of NF-kB can be also caused by an increased expression of other factors involved indirectly in NF-kB pathway. Recent studies on the gene expression profile of melanoma cells have shown an increased expression of Osteopontin (OPN) [124], a secreted glycophosphoprotein that induces NF-kB activation through enhancement of the IKK activity based on phosphorylation and degradation of IkBa [125]. Indeed, OPN induces AKT phosphorylation and, in turn, phosphorylated AKT binds to IKKa/b and activates IKK complex [125]. Mutational activation of BRAF, common in human melanomas, has been also associated with an enhanced IKK activity and a concomitant increase in the rate of IkBa ubiquitination and its subsequent degradation. This process overall entails a constitutive induction of NF-kB activity and an increased survival of melanoma cells [126]. Combination of these data with others reported in literature strongly suggests that the enhanced activation of NF-kB may be due to deregulations occurring in upstream signaling pathways such as RAS/RAF, PI3K/AKT and NIK [121].

Oncogenic mutations on Ras-family members, RAS and B-RAF, have been shown to impinge at multiple levels on AKT/NF-kB, RAF/MAPK and RAL/Rho signaling pathways [127] producing survival signals to disengage cell cycle checkpoint controls, favor metastasis and block pro-apoptotic stimuli. In support of this hypothesis, overexpression of N-RAS in human melanoma cells enhances Bcl-2 expression and contributes to a higher tumorigenicity and drug resistance in mouse xenotransplant models (i.e. subcutaneous injections) [128]. Chin and collaborators have generated melanomas in the context of a specific genetic background (INK4a/ARF deficiency) by conditional overexpression of H-RAS in melanocytes. Once the tumors were formed, downregulation of H-RAS expression led to a marked tumor regression by enhanced apoptosis of the tumor cells and also on the host-derived endothelial cells [129]. High-throughput analyses of genetic alterations in human cancers demonstrate that specifically, B-RAF, a RAS effector, was found to be mutated in 66% of human melanomas. Mutations are restricted to a few single amino-acid changes (primarily on V599) that render a constitutive active kinase with transforming properties in NIH3T3 cells [130]. Interestingly, previous studies indicate that wild-type B-RAF may inhibit programmed cell death downstream of cytocrome C release [131].

Although >50 mutations in BRAF have now been described, the most common BRAF mutation in melanoma, accounting for 80% of all of the BRAF mutations, is a valine to glutamic acid (V600E) substitution [130,132]. Acquisition of a V600E mutation in BRAF destabilizes the inactive kinase conformation switching the equilibrium towards the active form, leading to constitutive activity [132]. Mechanistically, mutated BRAF exerts most of its oncogenic effects through the activation of the MAPK pathway [133]. MAPK activity drives the uncontrolled growth of melanoma cells by upregulating the expression of cyclin D1 and through the suppression of the cyclin dependent kinase inhibitor $p27^{KIP1}$. Pre-clinical studies have shown that introduction of mutated BRAF into immortalized melanocytes leads to anchorage independent growth and tumor formation in immunocompromised mice [133]. Conversely, downregulation of mutated BRAF using RNAi causes cell cycle arrest and apoptosis in both *in vitro* and *in vivo* $BRAF^{V600E}$ mutant melanoma models [133]. Although it has been suggested that the acquisition of the $BRAF^{V600E}$ mutation is an early event in melanoma development, with 80% of all benign nevi showing to be BRAF mutant, the available evidence indicates that mutant BRAF alone cannot initiate melanoma [134,135].

3.4. DNA Mismatch Repair (MMR) proteins

Late et al. [136] determined that melanoma cells exhibiting resistance to cisplatin, etoposide and vindesine present a reduction of 30 to 70% in the nuclear content of each of the DNA mismatch repair (MMR) proteins hMLH1, hMSH2 and hMSH6. A decreased expression level of up to 80% of mRNAs encoding hMLH1 and hMSH2 was observed in drug-resistant melanoma cells selected for cisplatin, etoposide and fotemustine. In melanoma cells that acquired resistance to fotemustine, the activity of *O*6-methylguanine-DNA methyltransferase (MGMT) was considerably enhanced. The data of this group indicate that modulation of both MMR components and MGMT expression level may contribute to the drug-resistant phenotype of melanoma cells.

DNA mismatch repair (MMR) deficiency and increased *O*6-methylguanine-DNA methyltransferase (MGMT) activity have been related to resistance to *O*6-guanine methylating agents in tumour cell lines. However, the clinical relevance of MMR and MGMT as drug resistance factors is still unclear. In a retrospective study, the expression levels of the MMR proteins, hMSH2, hMSH6 and hMLH1, Ma et al. [137] analysed by immunohistochemistry in melanoma metastases from 64 patients, who had received dacarbazine (DTIC) based chemotherapy. All tumours showed positive nuclear staining for hMLH1. The response rates were similar in patients with hMSH2 and/or hMSH6 positive tumours to these in patients with negative tumours. In other retrospective study, Ma et al. [138] analysed the levels of the DNA repair protein *O*(6)-methylguanine-DNA methyltransferase (MGMT) in melanoma metastases from patients receiving dacarbazine (DTIC) either as a single drug or as part of combination chemotherapy regimens, and related the expression levels to the clinical response to treatment. DTIC as single agent was given to 44 patients, while 21 received combination chemotherapy. Objective responses to chemotherapy were seen in 12 patients, while 53 patients failed to respond to treatment. The expression of MGMT was determined according to the proportion of antibody-stained tumor cells, using a cut-off level of 50%. In 12 of the patients, more than one metastasis was analyzed, and in seven of these cases, the MGMT expression differed between tumours in the same individual. Among the responders a larger proportion (six out of 12, 50%) had tumors containing less than 50% MGMT-positive tumor cells than among the non-responders (12 out of 53, 23%). These data are consistent with the hypothesis that MGMT contributes to resistance to DTIC-based treatment. The conclusion that can be drawn from the fact that the development of drug resistance in melanoma cells is accompanied by down modulation of certain components of the MMR system and by an increase in MGMT activity when *O*6-alkylating agents are applied has several far-reaching implications regarding primary and acquired clinical resistance to these drugs. Furthermore, reduction or deficiency in MMR may increase the mutation rate in affected cells leading subsequently to an increased rate of development of resistance to other drugs having different targets. In addition, an enhanced mutation rate may contribute to increased phenotypic variation and therefore the clinical aggressiveness of melanomas and their metastases.

Recently, Li et al. [139] demonstrated the expression of DNA repair genes ERCC1 and XPF is induced by cisplatin in melanoma cells and that this induction is regulated by the MAPK pathway, with the role of DUSP6 phosphatase being particularly important. This induction contributes to increased drug resistance, which is one of the major obstacles to melanoma treatment, suggesting that ERCC1 or XPF inhibitors could be used to enhance the effectiveness of cisplatin treatment.

3.5. Multidrug Resistance Proteins (MRP)

The intrinsic multidrug resistance and sensitivity in melanomas and in pigment-producing cells involves multiple ABC transporters and melanosome biogenesis [140]. Melanoma cells express a group of ABC transporters, including ABCA9, ABCB1, ABCB5, ABCB8, ABCC1, ABCC2, and ABCD1 [140,141].

ABCC1 was shown to cooperate with glutathione S-transferase M1 to help melanoma cells escape the cytotoxicity of vincristine [141]. Have been described too that B16 melanoma

(B16M) cells presenting high ABCC1 and GSH content show high metastatic activity and high multidrug and radiation resistance [142]. Elevated expression of ABCC2 was shown to cause cisplatin resistance by reducing nuclear DNA damage, decreasing cell cycle G2-arrest, and increasing reentry into the cell cycle [4].

Has been reported that ABCB5 and ABCB8 mediate doxorubicin resistance in melanoma cells [143, 144]. ABCB5 shares 73% of sequence homology with the classic and the most studied multidrug resistance protein ABCB1 (P-gp, MDR1) [145,146] and was firstly detected in tissues derived from the neuroectodermal lineage including melanocyte progenitors [145], melanoma cell lines and patient specimens [143,146-148]. In melanoma, ABCB5-expressing cells are endowed with self-renewal, differentiation and tumorigenicity abilities [149,150]. Their abundance in clinical melanoma specimens correlates positively with the neoplasic progression suggesting that ABCB5 expression is associated with tumor aggressiveness. Moreover, the growth of melanoma xenografts in mice was delayed when the animals were treated with a monoclonal anti-ABCB5 antibody [149]. As a member of the ABC transporter family, ABCB5 is thought to play a role in drug efflux. This was supported by experiments measuring the intracellular accumulation of Rhodamine 123 [145]. These data suggest that ABC proteins may be important molecular targets for the reversal of multidrug resistance in melanoma cells.

4. Does oxidative stress contribute to the resistance in melanoma?

Free radicals are implicated in the pathogenesis of a multistage process of carcinogenesis. They can cause DNA base alterations, strand breaks, damage to tumor suppressor genes and enhanced expression of proto-oncogenes. The burst of reactive oxygen species (ROS) and the reactive nitrogen species (RNS) has been implicated in the development of cancer [151,152]. Excessive production of ROS can be harmful to both normal and cancer cells. High levels of ROS cause damage to lipids, DNA and cellular proteins, disrupting their normal function. However, some cancer cells can develop mechanisms that use ROS for purposes such as mitogenic upregulation of the expression of antioxidant enzymes [153-155]. Several studies have investigated the role of antioxidant enzymes in cancer and it has been shown that these enzymes play a significant role in regulating cancer growth and survival [156,157]. The carcinogenic effect of oxidative stress is attributed primarily to the genotoxicity of ROS in various cellular processes [158]. For example, hydroxyl radicals can react with purines andor pyrimidines as well as chromatin proteins, resulting in base modifications and genomic instability which can cause alterations in gene expression [159]. These data have suggested the accumulation of ROS as a common phenomenon in many cancer cells. Such accumulations can cause direct damage to DNA by increasing the cellular mutation and/or promoting and maintaining the tumorigenic phenotype by activating a second messenger in intracellular signaling cascades [160]. In addition, ROS have been determined to cause epigenetic alterations that affect the genome and play a major role in the development of carcinogenesis in humans [161]. More specifically, the production of ROS is associated with alterations in DNA methylation patterns [162, 163]. In particular, hydroxyl radicals that produce DNA lesions, such as 8-hydroxyl-2-deoxyguanosine, 8-hydroxyguanine, 8 -OHdG [164-166], and damage to the single strand of DNA [167] have been shown to decrease DNA methylation by means of interfering with the ability of DNA to function as a substrate for the DNA methyltransferases (DNMTs) and thus resulting in global hypomethylation [168].

Oxidative stress may play different roles in the pathogenesis of melanoma and non-melanoma skin cancer. It is likely that in non-melanoma skin cancers, a diminished antioxidant defense caused by chronic UV exposure contributes to the occurrence of mutations and carcinogenesis, whereas melanoma cells are equipped with a high antioxidant capacity and might use their ability to generate ROS for damaging surrounding tissue and thus supporting tumour progression and metastasis [169]. Gidanian et al. showed that melanosomes derived from melanoma cells in comparison to melanocytes actively produce excessive amounts of ROS [170]. Higher intracellular levels of ROS in melanoma cells were also detected by the studies by Meyskens et al. [171]. They furthermore showed that due to these elevated levels of ROS, melanin itself becomes progressively more oxidized and starts to function as a pro-oxidant [172]. They also showed that oxidation of melanin can be further increased by binding of metals, such as iron. These melanin-metal complexes can be converted by the Fenton reaction thereby producing even more ROS [173]. There is supportive evidence that sustained oxidative stress is related to oxidative DNA damage [174]. Atypical melanocytes have increased levels of oxidative stress and oxidative DNA damage [175, 176]. In line with these observations, Leikam et al. found that ROS production was accompanied by enhanced DNA damage [177].

4.1. Oxidative stress by antitumoral treatments

The cytotoxicity of some antitumoral drugs like actinomycin-D (AMD), adriamycin (ADR), cisplatin (Cis-Pt), vincristine (VCR), cytosine arabinoside (Ara-C) and dacarbazine (DTIC) are, to a greater or lesser extent, linked to the generation of free radicals and/or to the antioxidant defense of the cells. AMD and ADR are xenobiotics, which, in the cell, enter to cycles of oxidation and reduction, generating ROS [178,179]. Cis-Pt does not produce ROS; however, during its detoxification the level of glutathione (GSH) decreases [180]. In the case of DTIC, it has been shown that the resistance of melanoma cells to that drug is also partly linked to changes in the level of GSH [17,181]. ROS generated by mitochondria intensify the apoptosis induced by cytosine arabinoside [182].

Radiotherapy is a cornerstone in the treatment of several cancers. Ionic irradiation exposes all cells to high levels of oxidative stress, thus resulting in the formation of ROS, increasing DNA damage and ultimately leading to cell death. Another mechanism of the action of radiotherapy is to alter cellular homeostasis, thus modifying the signal transduction pathways and predisposing to apoptosis [183]. However, there are conflicting reports on the effect of radiotherapy on oxidative stress. Some studies have reported increased oxidative stress after radiotherapy [184], while others have reported decreased oxidative stress after radiotherapy in cancer patients [185, 186].

4.2. Transcription factors Nrf1 and Nrf2 are regulators of oxidative stress signaling

Nrf1 (NF-E2 related factor-1) and Nrf2 (NF-E2 related factor-2) nowadays are known as two oxidative stress sensitive transcription factors that belong to the CNC/bZIP family of transcription factors consisting of NF-E2, Nrf1, Nrf2, Nrf3, BACH1, and BACH2 [45–48]. Both Nrf1 and Nrf2 are responsible for regulating the expression of many antioxidant genes including peroxiredoxin-1 (Prx-1), thioredoxin-1 (Txn-1), GCLC (Glutamate cysteine ligase catalytic subunit - an enzyme responsible for catalyzing the formation of glutathione), glutathione peroxidase (GPX-1), drug metabolizing enzymes (cytochrome P-450s), and several ATP Binding Cassette (ABC) transporters that are responsible for drug efflux [187-190]. All of these genes are essential for the maintenance of oxidative homeostasis and contain an Electrophile Response Element (EpRE) to which Nrf1 and Nrf2 bind (also known as the Antioxidant Response Element). Both Nrf1 and Nrf2 are essential to the cellular response to oxidative stress and several studies have shown that knockdown of Nrf1 and/or Nrf2 expression sensitizes cells to oxidative stress [191-193]. It has also been suggested that Nrf2 responds to inducible oxidative stimuli and that Nrf1 regulates oxidative stress [194]. Increased oxidative stress has been shown to promote tumor proliferation and survival through deregulation of redox-sensitive pathways [153,195,196]. Nrf2 resides predominantly in the cytoplasm where it interacts with the actin-associated cytosolic protein INrf2, which is also known as Keap1 (Kelch-like ECH-associated protein 1). INrf2 functions as a substrate adaptor protein for a Cul3/Rbx1-dependent E3 ubiquitin ligase complex to ubiquitinate and degrade Nrf2, thus maintaining a steady-state level of Nrf2 [197].

Data from tumor cell lines isolated and profiled from human patients have indicated that many tumors have adapted to exploit the cytoprotective actions of Nrf2 both *in vivo* and *in vitro* through mutations of Keap1 and Nrf2, which lead to the constitutive upregulation and permanent activation of Nrf2-signaling to enhance the tolerance of the cancer cells to toxins and thereby limit the efficacy of chemotherapeutic agents. The loss of INrf2 (Keap1) function is shown to lead to nuclear accumulation of Nrf2, activation of metabolizing enzymes and drug resistance [198]. Studies have reported mutations resulting in dysfunctional Nrf2 in lung, breast and bladder cancers [199-203].

In a study carried out by Matundan et al. [204], they demonstrated the basal Nrf2 expression pattern in human melanoma was increased in 7 of 8 human melanoma cell lines. Immunoblots of Nrf2 showed over-expression in 6 of 8 metastatic melanoma cell lines and they determined that Nrf2's contribution was protective against redox stress in melanoma, and that decreased Nrf2 activation sensitizes melanoma cell lines to existing chemotherapeutics [204].

4.3. NRF2 are related with the expression of multidrug resistance proteins

Ogura and colleagues reported previously that Nrf2 binds within the *ABCB1* promoter's -126 and -102 regions, which contain the ATTCAGTCA motif. They have purified Nrf2 from the nuclear extract of K562/ADM cells, a multidrug-resistant cell line derived from human myelogenous leukemia K562 cells. This group determined that ATTCAGTCA motif is a positive regulatory element of MDR1 gene and that the motif is important for Nrf2 binding.

These results suggest that Nrf2 may be involved in the positive regulation of the *ABCB1* gene transcription [205].

Maher and collaborators examined the possibility that Nrf2 is also involved in the expression levels of ABCC1 in mouse embryo fibroblasts. The constitutive expression levels of Mrp1 mRNA and protein were significantly lower in Nrf2 (-/-) cells compared with those in wild type cells. In addition, significant induction by diethyl maleate was observed in wild type, but not in Nrf2 (-/-) cells, suggesting the involvement of Nrf2 in both the constitutive and inducible mRNA and protein expression of ABCC1. In addition, the uptake of [^{3}H]2,4-dinitrophenyl-S-glutathione, a typical substrate of ABCC1, into isolated membrane vesicles also demonstrated that Nrf2 regulates the transport activity of glutathione conjugates in mouse fibroblasts [206]. In another hand, Maher evaluated whether oxidative conditions (that is, the disruption of hepatic GSH synthesis) or the administration of nuclear factor-E2-related factor-2 (Nrf2) activators (oltipraz and butylated hydroxyanisole) can induce hepatic ABC transporters and whether that induction is through the NRF2 transcriptional pathway. Livers from hepatocyte-specific glutamate-cysteine ligase catalytic subunit-null mice had increased nuclear NRF2 levels, marked gene and protein induction of the Nrf2 target gene NAD(P)H: quinone oxidoreductase 1, as well as ABCC2, ABCC3, and ABCC4 expression. The treatment of wild type and Nrf2-null mice with oltipraz and butylated hydroxyanisole demonstrated that the induction of ABCC2, ABCC3, and ABCC4 is NRF2-dependent. In Hepa1c1c7 cells treated with the Nrf2 activator tert-butyl hydroquinone, chromatin immunoprecipitation with Nrf2 antibodies revealed the binding of NRF2 to antioxidant response elements in the promoter regions of mouse ABCC2 [-185 base pairs (bp)], ABCC3 (-9919 bp), and ABCC4 (-3767 bp). In this way, the activation of the Nrf2 regulatory pathway was shown to stimulate the coordinated induction of hepatic ABCs [190].

4.4. NRF2 represses the p53 pathway

You et al. [207] confirmed that Nrf2 is directly involved in the basal expression of Mdm2 through the antioxidant response element, which is located in the first intron of this gene. This linkage between Nrf2 and Mdm2 appears to cause the accumulation of p53 protein in Nrf2-deficent MEFs. They also showed that ovarian carcinoma A2780 cells silenced for Nrf2 by shRNA displayed higher levels of p53 activation in response to hydrogen peroxide treatment, leading to increased cell death. Collectively, those results suggest novel evidence that the inhibition of Nrf2 can suppress Mdm2 expression, which may result in p53 signaling modulation. Thus, forced inhibition of Nrf2 expression in cancer cells may be lead to activation of apoptosis response through the activation of p53 signaling.

4.5. Nrf2 and signalling pathways

The functional interaction between the Keap1-Nrf2 pathway and PTEN-PI3K-AKT pathway has been reported in several studies using cell lines. The pharmacological inhibition of the PI3K-AKT pathway represses the nuclear translocation of Nrf2 [208, 209]. In another hand, Beyer et al. showed that AKT phosphorylation was robustly augmented in the P/K-Alb mice in Nrf2-dependent manner, which is consistent with the previous report that Nrf2 positively regulates the activation of AKT [210]. Recently, Mitsuishi et al. [211] demonstrated a contribution of Nrf2 to cellular metabolic activities in proliferating cells, and the positive feedback loop between the PTEN-PI3K-AKT and Keap1-Nrf2 pathways, which appears to be one of the most substantial mechanisms for promoting the malignant evolution of cancers. It should be noted that Nrf2 accumulation, which is achieved by the functional impairment of Keap1 combined with the sustained activation of PI3K-AKT pathway, allows Nrf2 to get involved in the modulation of metabolism under pathological conditions. In contrast, temporary accumulation of Nrf2 at a low level is sufficient for Nrf2 to exert the cytoprotective function under physiological conditions [211].

Su et al. [212] reported the first evidence that Nrf2 is phosphorylated by MAPKs *in vivo*, however the nuclear accumulation of Nrf2 was slightly enhanced by its phosphorylation. This group concluded that direct phosphorylation of Nrf2 by MAPKs has a limited contribution in regulating the Nrf2-dependent antioxidant responses.

4.6. Nrf2 and anti-apoptotic features

Nrf2 resides predominantly in the cytoplasm where it interacts with the actin-associated cytosolic protein INrf2, which is also known as Keap1 (Kelch-like ECH-associated protein 1). INrf2 functions as a substrate adaptor protein for a Cul3/Rbx1-dependent E3 ubiquitin ligase complex to ubiquitinate and degrade Nrf2, thus maintaining a steady-state level of Nrf2 [197]. A study conducted by Niture et al. demonstrated that INrf2, in association with Cul3/Rbx1, ubiquitinates and degrades Bcl-2 [213]. However they recently demonstrated that Nrf2 binds to Bcl-2 ARE and regulates expression and induction of the Bcl-2 gene. Nrf2 mediated the up-regulation of Bcl-2, down regulated the activity of pro-apoptotic Bax protein and caspases 3/7, and protected cells from etoposide/radiation-mediated apoptosis that leads to drug resistance. Thus, they demonstrate that Nrf2-mediated up-regulation of Bcl-2 plays a significant role in preventing apoptosis, increasing cell survival, and drug resistance [214].

5. Conclusion

Melanoma continues to increase in incidence in many parts of the world, but there is currently no curative treatment once the disease has spread beyond the primary site because of the absence of effective therapies. This is believed to be largely due to the resistance of melanoma cells to induction of apoptosis by available chemotherapeutic drugs and biological reagents. Drug resistance is likely not only a primary consequence of acquired genetic alterations selected during or after therapy, but rather inherent to the malignant behavior of melanoma cells at diagnosis. Data support the existing hypothesis that talks about melanoma cells are "born to survive". Their aggressive behavior stems from intrinsic survival features of their paternal melanocytes nourished by additional alterations acquired during tumor progression. These inherent survival mechanisms may be partly caused by the oxidative stress to which melanoma cells are exposed. Nrf2 is a transcription factor that is considered a double-edged sword because it participates in the regulation of oxidative stress, however has been shown that overexpression of Nrf2 is a common phenomenon in several cancer types, participating in chemoresistance and tumor survival. We assume that this phenomenon also overlaps in melanoma, thus the intrinsic or extrinsic resistance produced in melanoma cells is partly due to overexpression of Nrf2, which can promote cell survival through mechanisms already reviewed in this chapter. Although these mechanisms presented in the last part of this chapter were not studied in melanoma, we believe that future studies endorse our theory. The knowledge about melanoma treatment has been widespread in recent years, but still is not enough, hence we must deepen in this area in order to improve the existing treatments and create effective targeted therapeutic target against this disease.

Acknowledgements

This work was supported by FAPESP (2011/12306-1).

Author details

Jonathan Castillo Arias[1] and Miriam Galvonas Jasiulionis[2]

*Address all correspondence to: mjasiulionis@gmail.com

1 Pharmacological Biochemistry Laboratory, Institute of Biochemistry, Faculty of Sciences, Universidad Austral de Chile, Valdivia, Chile

2 Pharmacology Department, Universidade Federal de São Paulo, São Paulo, Brazil

References

[1] Karagas MR, Greenberg ER, Spencer SK, Stukel TA, Mott LA. Increase in incidence rates of basal cell and squamous cell skin cancer in New Hampshire, USA. New Hampshire Skin Cancer Study Group. International journal of cancer Journal international du cancer. 1999;81(4):555-9. Epub 1999/05/04.

[2] Gloster HM, Jr., Brodland DG. The epidemiology of skin cancer. Dermatologic surgery : official publication for American Society for Dermatologic Surgery [et al]. 1996;22(3):217-26. Epub 1996/03/01.

[3] Plesko I, Severi G, Obsitnikova A, Boyle P. Trends in the incidence of non-melanoma skin cancer in Slovakia, 1978-1995. Neoplasma. 2000;47(3):137-42. Epub 2000/10/24.

[4] Liedert B, Materna V, Schadendorf D, Thomale J, Lage H. Overexpression of cMOAT (MRP2/ABCC2) is associated with decreased formation of platinum-DNA adducts

and decreased G2-arrest in melanoma cells resistant to cisplatin. The Journal of investigative dermatology. 2003;121(1):172-6. Epub 2003/07/04.

[5] Hughes BR, Altman DG, Newton JA. Melanoma and skin cancer: evaluation of a health education programme for secondary schools. The British journal of dermatology. 1993;128(4):412-7. Epub 1993/04/01.

[6] Zemelman V, Roa J, Tagle SR, Valenzuela CY. Malignant melanoma in Chile: an unusual distribution of primary sites in men from low socioeconomic strata. Clinical and experimental dermatology. 2006;31(3):335-8. Epub 2006/05/10.

[7] Zemelman V, Garmendia ML, Kirschbaum A. Malignant melanoma mortality rates in Chile (1988-98). International journal of dermatology. 2002;41(2):99-103. Epub 2002/05/02.

[8] Jemal A, Siegel R, Ward E, Hao Y, Xu J, Murray T, et al. Cancer statistics, 2008. CA: a cancer journal for clinicians. 2008;58(2):71-96. Epub 2008/02/22.

[9] Pawlik TM, Sondak VK. Malignant melanoma: current state of primary and adjuvant treatment. Critical reviews in oncology/hematology. 2003;45(3):245-64. Epub 2003/03/14.

[10] Lee ML, Tomsu K, Von Eschen KB. Duration of survival for disseminated malignant melanoma: results of a meta-analysis. Melanoma research. 2000;10(1):81-92. Epub 2000/03/11.

[11] Ang KK, Peters LJ, Weber RS, Morrison WH, Frankenthaler RA, Garden AS, et al. Postoperative radiotherapy for cutaneous melanoma of the head and neck region. International journal of radiation oncology, biology, physics. 1994;30(4):795-8. Epub 1994/11/15.

[12] Stevens G, Thompson JF, Firth I, O'Brien CJ, McCarthy WH, Quinn MJ. Locally advanced melanoma: results of postoperative hypofractionated radiation therapy. Cancer. 2000;88(1):88-94. Epub 2000/01/05.

[13] Sause WT, Cooper JS, Rush S, Ago CT, Cosmatos D, Coughlin CT, et al. Fraction size in external beam radiation therapy in the treatment of melanoma. International journal of radiation oncology, biology, physics. 1991;20(3):429-32. Epub 1991/03/01.

[14] Conill C, Valduvieco I, Domingo-Domenech J, Arguis P, Vidal-Sicart S, Vilalta A. Loco-regional control after postoperative radiotherapy for patients with regional nodal metastases from melanoma. Clinical & translational oncology : official publication of the Federation of Spanish Oncology Societies and of the National Cancer Institute of Mexico. 2009;11(10):688-93. Epub 2009/10/16.

[15] Comis RL. DTIC (NSC-45388) in malignant melanoma: a perspective. Cancer treatment reports. 1976;60(2):165-76. Epub 1976/02/01.

[16] Hill GJ, 2nd, Metter GE, Krementz ET, Fletcher WS, Golomb FM, Ramirez G, et al. DTIC and combination therapy for melanoma. II. Escalating schedules of DTIC with

BCNU, CCNU, and vincristine. Cancer treatment reports. 1979;63(11-12):1989-92. Epub 1979/11/01.

[17] Bedikian AY, Millward M, Pehamberger H, Conry R, Gore M, Trefzer U, et al. Bcl-2 antisense (oblimersen sodium) plus dacarbazine in patients with advanced melanoma: the Oblimersen Melanoma Study Group. Journal of clinical oncology : official journal of the American Society of Clinical Oncology. 2006;24(29):4738-45. Epub 2006/09/13.

[18] Middleton MR, Grob JJ, Aaronson N, Fierlbeck G, Tilgen W, Seiter S, et al. Randomized phase III study of temozolomide versus dacarbazine in the treatment of patients with advanced metastatic malignant melanoma. Journal of clinical oncology : official journal of the American Society of Clinical Oncology. 2000;18(1):158-66. Epub 2000/01/07.

[19] Chapman PB, Einhorn LH, Meyers ML, Saxman S, Destro AN, Panageas KS, et al. Phase III multicenter randomized trial of the Dartmouth regimen versus dacarbazine in patients with metastatic melanoma. Journal of clinical oncology : official journal of the American Society of Clinical Oncology. 1999;17(9):2745-51. Epub 1999/11/24.

[20] Huncharek M, Caubet JF, McGarry R. Single-agent DTIC versus combination chemotherapy with or without immunotherapy in metastatic melanoma: a meta-analysis of 3273 patients from 20 randomized trials. Melanoma research. 2001;11(1):75-81. Epub 2001/03/20.

[21] Bleehen NM, Newlands ES, Lee SM, Thatcher N, Selby P, Calvert AH, et al. Cancer Research Campaign phase II trial of temozolomide in metastatic melanoma. Journal of clinical oncology : official journal of the American Society of Clinical Oncology. 1995;13(4):910-3. Epub 1995/04/01.

[22] Newlands ES, Blackledge GR, Slack JA, Rustin GJ, Smith DB, Stuart NS, et al. Phase I trial of temozolomide (CCRG 81045: M&B 39831: NSC 362856). British journal of cancer. 1992;65(2):287-91. Epub 1992/02/01.

[23] Jacquillat C, Khayat D, Banzet P, Weil M, Fumoleau P, Avril MF, et al. Final report of the French multicenter phase II study of the nitrosourea fotemustine in 153 evaluable patients with disseminated malignant melanoma including patients with cerebral metastases. Cancer. 1990;66(9):1873-8. Epub 1990/11/01.

[24] Khayat D, Giroux B, Berille J, Cour V, Gerard B, Sarkany M, et al. Fotemustine in the treatment of brain primary tumors and metastases. Cancer investigation. 1994;12(4): 414-20. Epub 1994/01/01.

[25] Ahmann DL. Nitrosoureas in the management of disseminated malignant melanoma. Cancer treatment reports. 1976;60(6):747-51. Epub 1976/06/01.

[26] Glover D, Glick JH, Weiler C, Fox K, Guerry D. WR-2721 and high-dose cisplatin: an active combination in the treatment of metastatic melanoma. Journal of clinical oncol-

ogy : official journal of the American Society of Clinical Oncology. 1987;5(4):574-8. Epub 1987/04/01.

[27] Evans LM, Casper ES, Rosenbluth R. Phase II trial of carboplatin in advanced malignant melanoma. Cancer treatment reports. 1987;71(2):171-2. Epub 1987/02/01.

[28] Quagliana JM, Stephens RL, Baker LH, Costanzi JJ. Vindesine in patients with metastatic malignant melanoma: a Southwest Oncology Group study. Journal of clinical oncology : official journal of the American Society of Clinical Oncology. 1984;2(4): 316-9. Epub 1984/04/01.

[29] Aamdal S, Wolff I, Kaplan S, Paridaens R, Kerger J, Schachter J, et al. Docetaxel (Taxotere) in advanced malignant melanoma: a phase II study of the EORTC Early Clinical Trials Group. Eur J Cancer. 1994;30A(8):1061-4. Epub 1994/01/01.

[30] Bedikian AY, Weiss GR, Legha SS, Burris HA, 3rd, Eckardt JR, Jenkins J, et al. Phase II trial of docetaxel in patients with advanced cutaneous malignant melanoma previously untreated with chemotherapy. Journal of clinical oncology : official journal of the American Society of Clinical Oncology. 1995;13(12):2895-9. Epub 1995/12/01.

[31] Einzig AI, Hochster H, Wiernik PH, Trump DL, Dutcher JP, Garowski E, et al. A phase II study of taxol in patients with malignant melanoma. Investigational new drugs. 1991;9(1):59-64. Epub 1991/02/01.

[32] Agarwala SS, Glaspy J, O'Day SJ, Mitchell M, Gutheil J, Whitman E, et al. Results from a randomized phase III study comparing combined treatment with histamine dihydrochloride plus interleukin-2 versus interleukin-2 alone in patients with metastatic melanoma. Journal of clinical oncology : official journal of the American Society of Clinical Oncology. 2002;20(1):125-33. Epub 2002/01/05.

[33] Lattanzi SC, Tosteson T, Chertoff J, Maurer LH, O'Donnell J, LeMarbre PJ, et al. Dacarbazine, cisplatin and carmustine, with or without tamoxifen, for metastatic melanoma: 5-year follow-up. Melanoma research. 1995;5(5):365-9. Epub 1995/10/01.

[34] Cocconi G, Bella M, Calabresi F, Tonato M, Canaletti R, Boni C, et al. Treatment of metastatic malignant melanoma with dacarbazine plus tamoxifen. The New England journal of medicine. 1992;327(8):516-23. Epub 1992/08/20.

[35] Rusthoven JJ, Quirt IC, Iscoe NA, McCulloch PB, James KW, Lohmann RC, et al. Randomized, double-blind, placebo-controlled trial comparing the response rates of carmustine, dacarbazine, and cisplatin with and without tamoxifen in patients with metastatic melanoma. National Cancer Institute of Canada Clinical Trials Group. Journal of clinical oncology : official journal of the American Society of Clinical Oncology. 1996;14(7):2083-90. Epub 1996/07/01.

[36] Falkson CI, Ibrahim J, Kirkwood JM, Coates AS, Atkins MB, Blum RH. Phase III trial of dacarbazine versus dacarbazine with interferon alpha-2b versus dacarbazine with tamoxifen versus dacarbazine with interferon alpha-2b and tamoxifen in patients with metastatic malignant melanoma: an Eastern Cooperative Oncology Group

study. Journal of clinical oncology : official journal of the American Society of Clinical Oncology. 1998;16(5):1743-51. Epub 1998/05/20.

[37] Rao RD, Holtan SG, Ingle JN, Croghan GA, Kottschade LA, Creagan ET, et al. Combination of paclitaxel and carboplatin as second-line therapy for patients with metastatic melanoma. Cancer. 2006;106(2):375-82. Epub 2005/12/13.

[38] Garbe C, Eigentler TK, Keilholz U, Hauschild A, Kirkwood JM. Systematic review of medical treatment in melanoma: current status and future prospects. The oncologist. 2011;16(1):5-24. Epub 2011/01/08.

[39] Hodi FS, O'Day SJ, McDermott DF, Weber RW, Sosman JA, Haanen JB, et al. Improved survival with ipilimumab in patients with metastatic melanoma. The New England journal of medicine. 2010;363(8):711-23. Epub 2010/06/08.

[40] O'Day SJ, Hamid O, Urba WJ. Targeting cytotoxic T-lymphocyte antigen-4 (CTLA-4): a novel strategy for the treatment of melanoma and other malignancies. Cancer. 2007;110(12):2614-27. Epub 2007/11/16.

[41] Robert C, Ghiringhelli F. What is the role of cytotoxic T lymphocyte-associated antigen 4 blockade in patients with metastatic melanoma? The oncologist. 2009;14(8): 848-61. Epub 2009/08/04.

[42] Nancey S, Boschetti G, Cotte E, Ruel K, Almeras T, Chauvenet M, et al. Blockade of cytotoxic T-lymphocyte antigen-4 by ipilimumab is associated with a profound long-lasting depletion of Foxp3(+) regulatory T cells: A mechanistic explanation for ipilimumab-induced severe enterocolitis? Inflammatory bowel diseases. 2012;18(8):E1598-600. Epub 2011/11/10.

[43] Tarhini A, Lo E, Minor DR. Releasing the brake on the immune system: ipilimumab in melanoma and other tumors. Cancer biotherapy & radiopharmaceuticals. 2010;25(6):601-13. Epub 2011/01/06.

[44] Pehamberger H, Soyer HP, Steiner A, Kofler R, Binder M, Mischer P, et al. Adjuvant interferon alfa-2a treatment in resected primary stage II cutaneous melanoma. Austrian Malignant Melanoma Cooperative Group. Journal of clinical oncology : official journal of the American Society of Clinical Oncology. 1998;16(4):1425-9. Epub 1998/04/29.

[45] Grob JJ, Dreno B, de la Salmoniere P, Delaunay M, Cupissol D, Guillot B, et al. Randomised trial of interferon alpha-2a as adjuvant therapy in resected primary melanoma thicker than 1.5 mm without clinically detectable node metastases. French Cooperative Group on Melanoma. Lancet. 1998;351(9120):1905-10. Epub 1998/07/08.

[46] Agarwala SS, Kirkwood JM. Interferons in melanoma. Current opinion in oncology. 1996;8(2):167-74. Epub 1996/03/01.

[47] Agarwala SS, Kirkwood JM. Potential uses of interferon alpha 2 as adjuvant therapy in cancer. Annals of surgical oncology. 1995;2(4):365-71. Epub 1995/07/01.

[48] Rosenberg SA, Lotze MT, Yang JC, Linehan WM, Seipp C, Calabro S, et al. Combination therapy with interleukin-2 and alpha-interferon for the treatment of patients with advanced cancer. Journal of clinical oncology : official journal of the American Society of Clinical Oncology. 1989;7(12):1863-74. Epub 1989/12/01.

[49] Sparano JA, Fisher RI, Sunderland M, Margolin K, Ernest ML, Sznol M, et al. Randomized phase III trial of treatment with high-dose interleukin-2 either alone or in combination with interferon alfa-2a in patients with advanced melanoma. Journal of clinical oncology : official journal of the American Society of Clinical Oncology. 1993;11(10):1969-77. Epub 1993/10/01.

[50] Whitehead RP, Figlin R, Citron ML, Pfile J, Moldawer N, Patel D, et al. A phase II trial of concomitant human interleukin-2 and interferon-alpha-2a in patients with disseminated malignant melanoma. Journal of immunotherapy with emphasis on tumor immunology : official journal of the Society for Biological Therapy. 1993;13(2): 117-21. Epub 1993/02/01.

[51] Keilholz U, Goey SH, Punt CJ, Proebstle TM, Salzmann R, Scheibenbogen C, et al. Interferon alfa-2a and interleukin-2 with or without cisplatin in metastatic melanoma: a randomized trial of the European Organization for Research and Treatment of Cancer Melanoma Cooperative Group. Journal of clinical oncology : official journal of the American Society of Clinical Oncology. 1997;15(7):2579-88. Epub 1997/07/01.

[52] Falkson CI, Falkson G, Falkson HC. Improved results with the addition of interferon alfa-2b to dacarbazine in the treatment of patients with metastatic malignant melanoma. Journal of clinical oncology : official journal of the American Society of Clinical Oncology. 1991;9(8):1403-8. Epub 1991/08/01.

[53] Eton O, Legha SS, Bedikian AY, Lee JJ, Buzaid AC, Hodges C, et al. Sequential biochemotherapy versus chemotherapy for metastatic melanoma: results from a phase III randomized trial. Journal of clinical oncology : official journal of the American Society of Clinical Oncology. 2002;20(8):2045-52. Epub 2002/04/17.

[54] Atkins MB, Hsu J, Lee S, Cohen GI, Flaherty LE, Sosman JA, et al. Phase III trial comparing concurrent biochemotherapy with cisplatin, vinblastine, dacarbazine, interleukin-2, and interferon alfa-2b with cisplatin, vinblastine, and dacarbazine alone in patients with metastatic malignant melanoma (E3695): a trial coordinated by the Eastern Cooperative Oncology Group. Journal of clinical oncology : official journal of the American Society of Clinical Oncology. 2008;26(35):5748-54. Epub 2008/11/13.

[55] Wilhelm S, Carter C, Lynch M, Lowinger T, Dumas J, Smith RA, et al. Discovery and development of sorafenib: a multikinase inhibitor for treating cancer. Nature reviews Drug discovery. 2006;5(10):835-44. Epub 2006/10/04.

[56] Wellbrock C, Hurlstone A. BRAF as therapeutic target in melanoma. Biochemical pharmacology. 2010;80(5):561-7. Epub 2010/03/31.

[57] Flaherty KT, Puzanov I, Kim KB, Ribas A, McArthur GA, Sosman JA, et al. Inhibition of mutated, activated BRAF in metastatic melanoma. The New England journal of medicine. 2010;363(9):809-19. Epub 2010/09/08.

[58] Solit D, Sawyers CL. Drug discovery: How melanomas bypass new therapy. Nature. 2010;468(7326):902-3. Epub 2010/12/18.

[59] Yoshida H, Kunisada T, Grimm T, Nishimura EK, Nishioka E, Nishikawa SI. Review: melanocyte migration and survival controlled by SCF/c-kit expression. The journal of investigative dermatology Symposium proceedings / the Society for Investigative Dermatology, Inc [and] European Society for Dermatological Research. 2001;6(1):1-5. Epub 2002/01/05.

[60] Guo J, Si L, Kong Y, Flaherty KT, Xu X, Zhu Y, et al. Phase II, open-label, single-arm trial of imatinib mesylate in patients with metastatic melanoma harboring c-Kit mutation or amplification. Journal of clinical oncology : official journal of the American Society of Clinical Oncology. 2011;29(21):2904-9. Epub 2011/06/22.

[61] Flaherty KT, Hodi FS, Bastian BC. Mutation-driven drug development in melanoma. Current opinion in oncology. 2010;22(3):178-83. Epub 2010/04/20.

[62] Ko JM, Fisher DE. A new era: melanoma genetics and therapeutics. The Journal of pathology. 2011;223(2):241-50. Epub 2010/12/03.

[63] Davies MA, Samuels Y. Analysis of the genome to personalize therapy for melanoma. Oncogene. 2010;29(41):5545-55. Epub 2010/08/11.

[64] Friedlander P, Hodi FS. Advances in targeted therapy for melanoma. Clinical advances in hematology & oncology : H&O. 2010;8(9):619-27. Epub 2010/12/16.

[65] Tawbi H, Nimmagadda N. Targeted therapy in melanoma. Biologics : targets & therapy. 2009;3:475-84. Epub 2010/01/08.

[66] Courtney KD, Corcoran RB, Engelman JA. The PI3K pathway as drug target in human cancer. Journal of clinical oncology : official journal of the American Society of Clinical Oncology. 2010;28(6):1075-83. Epub 2010/01/21.

[67] Rother J, Jones D. Molecular markers of tumor progression in melanoma. Current genomics. 2009;10(4):231-9. Epub 2009/12/02.

[68] Werzowa J, Koehrer S, Strommer S, Cejka D, Fuereder T, Zebedin E, et al. Vertical inhibition of the mTORC1/mTORC2/PI3K pathway shows synergistic effects against melanoma in vitro and in vivo. The Journal of investigative dermatology. 2011;131(2):495-503. Epub 2010/11/05.

[69] Dean M, Fojo T, Bates S. Tumour stem cells and drug resistance. Nature reviews Cancer. 2005;5(4):275-84. Epub 2005/04/02.

[70] Dean M, Rzhetsky A, Allikmets R. The human ATP-binding cassette (ABC) transporter superfamily. Genome Res. 2001;11(7):1156-66. Epub 2001/07/04.

[71] Shen DW, Goldenberg S, Pastan I, Gottesman MM. Decreased accumulation of [14C]carboplatin in human cisplatin-resistant cells results from reduced energy-dependent uptake. Journal of cellular physiology. 2000;183(1):108-16. Epub 2000/03/04.

[72] Shen D, Pastan I, Gottesman MM. Cross-resistance to methotrexate and metals in human cisplatin-resistant cell lines results from a pleiotropic defect in accumulation of these compounds associated with reduced plasma membrane binding proteins. Cancer research. 1998;58(2):268-75. Epub 1998/01/27.

[73] Schuetz EG, Beck WT, Schuetz JD. Modulators and substrates of P-glycoprotein and cytochrome P4503A coordinately up-regulate these proteins in human colon carcinoma cells. Molecular pharmacology. 1996;49(2):311-8. Epub 1996/02/01.

[74] Lowe SW, Ruley HE, Jacks T, Housman DE. p53-dependent apoptosis modulates the cytotoxicity of anticancer agents. Cell. 1993;74(6):957-67. Epub 1993/09/24.

[75] Liu YY, Han TY, Giuliano AE, Cabot MC. Ceramide glycosylation potentiates cellular multidrug resistance. FASEB journal : official publication of the Federation of American Societies for Experimental Biology. 2001;15(3):719-30. Epub 2001/03/22.

[76] Matsumura Y, Ananthaswamy HN. Molecular mechanisms of photocarcinogenesis. Frontiers in bioscience : a journal and virtual library. 2002;7:d765-83. Epub 2002/03/19.

[77] Zhai S, Yaar M, Doyle SM, Gilchrest BA. Nerve growth factor rescues pigment cells from ultraviolet-induced apoptosis by upregulating BCL-2 levels. Experimental cell research. 1996;224(2):335-43. Epub 1996/05/01.

[78] Kawaguchi Y, Mori N, Nakayama A. Kit(+) melanocytes seem to contribute to melanocyte proliferation after UV exposure as precursor cells. The Journal of investigative dermatology. 2001;116(6):920-5. Epub 2001/06/16.

[79] Leiter U, Schmid RM, Kaskel P, Peter RU, Krahn G. Antiapoptotic bcl-2 and bcl-xL in advanced malignant melanoma. Archives of dermatological research. 2000;292(5): 225-32. Epub 2000/06/27.

[80] Tron VA, Krajewski S, Klein-Parker H, Li G, Ho VC, Reed JC. Immunohistochemical analysis of Bcl-2 protein regulation in cutaneous melanoma. The American journal of pathology. 1995;146(3):643-50. Epub 1995/03/01.

[81] Dallaglio K, Marconi A, Pincelli C. Survivin: a dual player in healthy and diseased skin. The Journal of investigative dermatology. 2012;132(1):18-27. Epub 2011/09/09.

[82] Oberoi-Khanuja TK, Karreman C, Larisch S, Rapp UR, Rajalingam K. Role of melanoma inhibitor of apoptosis (ML-IAP), a member of baculoviral IAP repeat (BIR) domain family in the regulation of C-RAF kinase and cell migration. The Journal of biological chemistry. 2012. Epub 2012/06/20.

[83] Pennati M, Colella G, Folini M, Citti L, Daidone MG, Zaffaroni N. Ribozyme-mediated attenuation of survivin expression sensitizes human melanoma cells to cisplatin-

induced apoptosis. The Journal of clinical investigation. 2002;109(2):285-6. Epub 2002/01/24.

[84] Mesri M, Wall NR, Li J, Kim RW, Altieri DC. Cancer gene therapy using a survivin mutant adenovirus. The Journal of clinical investigation. 2001;108(7):981-90. Epub 2001/10/03.

[85] Vucic D, Stennicke HR, Pisabarro MT, Salvesen GS, Dixit VM. ML-IAP, a novel inhibitor of apoptosis that is preferentially expressed in human melanomas. Current biology : CB. 2000;10(21):1359-66. Epub 2000/11/21.

[86] Vucic D, Deshayes K, Ackerly H, Pisabarro MT, Kadkhodayan S, Fairbrother WJ, et al. SMAC negatively regulates the anti-apoptotic activity of melanoma inhibitor of apoptosis (ML-IAP). The Journal of biological chemistry. 2002;277(14):12275-9. Epub 2002/01/22.

[87] Kasof GM, Gomes BC. Livin, a novel inhibitor of apoptosis protein family member. The Journal of biological chemistry. 2001;276(5):3238-46. Epub 2000/10/12.

[88] Vousden KH, Prives C. Blinded by the Light: The Growing Complexity of p53. Cell. 2009;137(3):413-31. Epub 2009/05/05.

[89] Donehower LA, Lozano G. 20 years studying p53 functions in genetically engineered mice. Nature reviews Cancer. 2009;9(11):831-41. Epub 2009/09/25.

[90] Perlis C, Herlyn M. Recent advances in melanoma biology. The oncologist. 2004;9(2): 182-7. Epub 2004/03/30.

[91] Chin L, Pomerantz J, Polsky D, Jacobson M, Cohen C, Cordon-Cardo C, et al. Cooperative effects of INK4a and ras in melanoma susceptibility in vivo. Genes & development. 1997;11(21):2822-34. Epub 1997/11/14.

[92] Satyamoorthy K, Chehab NH, Waterman MJ, Lien MC, El-Deiry WS, Herlyn M, et al. Aberrant regulation and function of wild-type p53 in radioresistant melanoma cells. Cell growth & differentiation : the molecular biology journal of the American Association for Cancer Research. 2000;11(9):467-74. Epub 2000/09/28.

[93] Schmitt CA, Fridman JS, Yang M, Baranov E, Hoffman RM, Lowe SW. Dissecting p53 tumor suppressor functions in vivo. Cancer cell. 2002;1(3):289-98. Epub 2002/06/28.

[94] Soengas MS, Alarcon RM, Yoshida H, Giaccia AJ, Hakem R, Mak TW, et al. Apaf-1 and caspase-9 in p53-dependent apoptosis and tumor inhibition. Science. 1999;284(5411):156-9. Epub 1999/04/02.

[95] Soengas MS, Capodieci P, Polsky D, Mora J, Esteller M, Opitz-Araya X, et al. Inactivation of the apoptosis effector Apaf-1 in malignant melanoma. Nature. 2001;409(6817):207-11. Epub 2001/02/24.

[96] Furukawa Y, Nishimura N, Furukawa Y, Satoh M, Endo H, Iwase S, et al. Apaf-1 is a mediator of E2F-1-induced apoptosis. The Journal of biological chemistry. 2002;277(42):39760-8. Epub 2002/08/01.

[97] Toledo F, Wahl GM. Regulating the p53 pathway: in vitro hypotheses, in vivo veritas. Nature reviews Cancer. 2006;6(12):909-23. Epub 2006/11/28.

[98] Wang X. p53 regulation: teamwork between RING domains of Mdm2 and MdmX. Cell Cycle. 2011;10(24):4225-9. Epub 2011/12/03.

[99] Castresana JS, Rubio MP, Vazquez JJ, Idoate M, Sober AJ, Seizinger BR, et al. Lack of allelic deletion and point mutation as mechanisms of p53 activation in human malignant melanoma. International journal of cancer Journal international du cancer. 1993;55(4):562-5. Epub 1993/10/21.

[100] Albino AP, Vidal MJ, McNutt NS, Shea CR, Prieto VG, Nanus DM, et al. Mutation and expression of the p53 gene in human malignant melanoma. Melanoma research. 1994;4(1):35-45. Epub 1994/02/01.

[101] Hocker T, Tsao H. Ultraviolet radiation and melanoma: a systematic review and analysis of reported sequence variants. Human mutation. 2007;28(6):578-88. Epub 2007/02/14.

[102] Muthusamy V, Hobbs C, Nogueira C, Cordon-Cardo C, McKee PH, Chin L, et al. Amplification of CDK4 and MDM2 in malignant melanoma. Genes, chromosomes & cancer. 2006;45(5):447-54. Epub 2006/01/19.

[103] Ji Z, Njauw CN, Taylor M, Neel V, Flaherty KT, Tsao H. p53 rescue through HDM2 antagonism suppresses melanoma growth and potentiates MEK inhibition. The Journal of investigative dermatology. 2012;132(2):356-64. Epub 2011/10/14.

[104] Meier F, Busch S, Lasithiotakis K, Kulms D, Garbe C, Maczey E, et al. Combined targeting of MAPK and AKT signalling pathways is a promising strategy for melanoma treatment. The British journal of dermatology. 2007;156(6):1204-13. Epub 2007/03/29.

[105] Lasithiotakis KG, Sinnberg TW, Schittek B, Flaherty KT, Kulms D, Maczey E, et al. Combined inhibition of MAPK and mTOR signaling inhibits growth, induces cell death, and abrogates invasive growth of melanoma cells. The Journal of investigative dermatology. 2008;128(8):2013-23. Epub 2008/03/08.

[106] Smalley KS, Haass NK, Brafford PA, Lioni M, Flaherty KT, Herlyn M. Multiple signaling pathways must be targeted to overcome drug resistance in cell lines derived from melanoma metastases. Molecular cancer therapeutics. 2006;5(5):1136-44. Epub 2006/05/30.

[107] Soengas MS, Lowe SW. Apoptosis and melanoma chemoresistance. Oncogene. 2003;22(20):3138-51. Epub 2003/06/06.

[108] Hersey P, Zhuang L, Zhang XD. Current strategies in overcoming resistance of cancer cells to apoptosis melanoma as a model. International review of cytology. 2006;251:131-58. Epub 2006/08/31.

[109] Birck A, Ahrenkiel V, Zeuthen J, Hou-Jensen K, Guldberg P. Mutation and allelic loss of the PTEN/MMAC1 gene in primary and metastatic melanoma biopsies. The Journal of investigative dermatology. 2000;114(2):277-80. Epub 2000/01/29.

[110] Zhou XP, Gimm O, Hampel H, Niemann T, Walker MJ, Eng C. Epigenetic PTEN silencing in malignant melanomas without PTEN mutation. The American journal of pathology. 2000;157(4):1123-8. Epub 2000/10/06.

[111] Poetsch M, Dittberner T, Woenckhaus C. PTEN/MMAC1 in malignant melanoma and its importance for tumor progression. Cancer genetics and cytogenetics. 2001;125(1):21-6. Epub 2001/04/12.

[112] Whiteman DC, Zhou XP, Cummings MC, Pavey S, Hayward NK, Eng C. Nuclear PTEN expression and clinicopathologic features in a population-based series of primary cutaneous melanoma. International journal of cancer Journal international du cancer. 2002;99(1):63-7. Epub 2002/04/12.

[113] Hwang PH, Yi HK, Kim DS, Nam SY, Kim JS, Lee DY. Suppression of tumorigenicity and metastasis in B16F10 cells by PTEN/MMAC1/TEP1 gene. Cancer letters. 2001;172(1):83-91. Epub 2001/10/12.

[114] Kotelevets L, van Hengel J, Bruyneel E, Mareel M, van Roy F, Chastre E. The lipid phosphatase activity of PTEN is critical for stabilizing intercellular junctions and reverting invasiveness. The Journal of cell biology. 2001;155(7):1129-35. Epub 2002/01/05.

[115] Mayo LD, Dixon JE, Durden DL, Tonks NK, Donner DB. PTEN protects p53 from Mdm2 and sensitizes cancer cells to chemotherapy. The Journal of biological chemistry. 2002;277(7):5484-9. Epub 2001/12/01.

[116] Sinnberg T, Sauer B, Holm P, Spangler B, Kuphal S, Bosserhoff A, et al. MAPK and PI3K/AKT mediated YB-1 activation promotes melanoma cell proliferation which is counteracted by an autoregulatory loop. Experimental dermatology. 2012;21(4): 265-70. Epub 2012/03/16.

[117] Astanehe A, Finkbeiner MR, Hojabrpour P, To K, Fotovati A, Shadeo A, et al. The transcriptional induction of PIK3CA in tumor cells is dependent on the oncoprotein Y-box binding protein-1. Oncogene. 2009;28(25):2406-18. Epub 2009/05/12.

[118] Meyskens FL, Jr., Buckmeier JA, McNulty SE, Tohidian NB. Activation of nuclear factor-kappa B in human metastatic melanomacells and the effect of oxidative stress. Clinical cancer research : an official journal of the American Association for Cancer Research. 1999;5(5):1197-202. Epub 1999/06/03.

[119] McNulty SE, Tohidian NB, Meyskens FL, Jr. RelA, p50 and inhibitor of kappa B alpha are elevated in human metastatic melanoma cells and respond aberrantly to ultraviolet light B. Pigment cell research / sponsored by the European Society for Pigment Cell Research and the International Pigment Cell Society. 2001;14(6):456-65. Epub 2002/01/05.

[120] Yang J, Richmond A. Constitutive IkappaB kinase activity correlates with nuclear factor-kappaB activation in human melanoma cells. Cancer research. 2001;61(12): 4901-9. Epub 2001/06/19.

[121] Dhawan P, Richmond A. A novel NF-kappa B-inducing kinase-MAPK signaling pathway up-regulates NF-kappa B activity in melanoma cells. The Journal of biological chemistry. 2002;277(10):7920-8. Epub 2002/01/05.

[122] Baldwin AS. Control of oncogenesis and cancer therapy resistance by the transcription factor NF-kappaB. The Journal of clinical investigation. 2001;107(3):241-6. Epub 2001/02/13.

[123] McNulty SE, del Rosario R, Cen D, Meyskens FL, Jr., Yang S. Comparative expression of NFkappaB proteins in melanocytes of normal skin vs. benign intradermal naevus and human metastatic melanoma biopsies. Pigment cell research / sponsored by the European Society for Pigment Cell Research and the International Pigment Cell Society. 2004;17(2):173-80. Epub 2004/03/16.

[124] Shattuck-Brandt RL, Richmond A. Enhanced degradation of I-kappaB alpha contributes to endogenous activation of NF-kappaB in Hs294T melanoma cells. Cancer research. 1997;57(14):3032-9. Epub 1997/07/15.

[125] Das R, Philip S, Mahabeleshwar GH, Bulbule A, Kundu GC. Osteopontin: it's role in regulation of cell motility and nuclear factor kappa B-mediated urokinase type plasminogen activator expression. IUBMB life. 2005;57(6):441-7. Epub 2005/07/14.

[126] Liu J, Suresh Kumar KG, Yu D, Molton SA, McMahon M, Herlyn M, et al. Oncogenic BRAF regulates beta-Trcp expression and NF-kappaB activity in human melanoma cells. Oncogene. 2007;26(13):1954-8. Epub 2006/09/27.

[127] Malumbres M, Pellicer A. RAS pathways to cell cycle control and cell transformation. Frontiers in bioscience : a journal and virtual library. 1998;3:d887-912. Epub 1998/08/11.

[128] Borner C, Schlagbauer Wadl H, Fellay I, Selzer E, Polterauer P, Jansen B. Mutated N-ras upregulates Bcl-2 in human melanoma in vitro and in SCID mice. Melanoma research. 1999;9(4):347-50. Epub 1999/09/30.

[129] Chin L, Merlino G, DePinho RA. Malignant melanoma: modern black plague and genetic black box. Genes & development. 1998;12(22):3467-81. Epub 1998/12/01.

[130] Davies H, Bignell GR, Cox C, Stephens P, Edkins S, Clegg S, et al. Mutations of the BRAF gene in human cancer. Nature. 2002;417(6892):949-54. Epub 2002/06/18.

[131] Erhardt P, Schremser EJ, Cooper GM. B-Raf inhibits programmed cell death downstream of cytochrome c release from mitochondria by activating the MEK/Erk pathway. Molecular and cellular biology. 1999;19(8):5308-15. Epub 1999/07/20.

[132] Wan PT, Garnett MJ, Roe SM, Lee S, Niculescu-Duvaz D, Good VM, et al. Mechanism of activation of the RAF-ERK signaling pathway by oncogenic mutations of B-RAF. Cell. 2004;116(6):855-67. Epub 2004/03/24.

[133] Smalley KS. Understanding melanoma signaling networks as the basis for molecular targeted therapy. The Journal of investigative dermatology. 2010;130(1):28-37. Epub 2009/07/03.

[134] Pollock PM, Harper UL, Hansen KS, Yudt LM, Stark M, Robbins CM, et al. High frequency of BRAF mutations in nevi. Nature genetics. 2003;33(1):19-20. Epub 2002/11/26.

[135] Michaloglou C, Vredeveld LC, Soengas MS, Denoyelle C, Kuilman T, van der Horst CM, et al. BRAFE600-associated senescence-like cell cycle arrest of human naevi. Nature. 2005;436(7051):720-4. Epub 2005/08/05.

[136] Lage H, Christmann M, Kern MA, Dietel M, Pick M, Kaina B, et al. Expression of DNA repair proteins hMSH2, hMSH6, hMLH1, O6-methylguanine-DNA methyltransferase and N-methylpurine-DNA glycosylase in melanoma cells with acquired drug resistance. International journal of cancer Journal international du cancer. 1999;80(5):744-50. Epub 1999/02/27.

[137] Ma S, Egyhazi S, Ringborg U, Hansson J. Immunohistochemical analysis of DNA mismatch repair protein and O6-methylguanine-DNA methyltransferase in melanoma metastases in relation to clinical response to DTIC-based chemotherapy. Oncology reports. 2002;9(5):1015-9. Epub 2002/08/09.

[138] Ma S, Egyhazi S, Martenhed G, Ringborg U, Hansson J. Analysis of O(6)-methylguanine-DNA methyltransferase in melanoma tumours in patients treated with dacarbazine-based chemotherapy. Melanoma research. 2002;12(4):335-42. Epub 2002/08/10.

[139] Li W, Melton DW. Cisplatin regulates the MAPK kinase pathway to induce increased expression of DNA repair gene ERCC1 and increase melanoma chemoresistance. Oncogene. 2012;31(19):2412-22. Epub 2011/10/15.

[140] Chen KG, Valencia JC, Gillet JP, Hearing VJ, Gottesman MM. Involvement of ABC transporters in melanogenesis and the development of multidrug resistance of melanoma. Pigment cell & melanoma research. 2009;22(6):740-9. Epub 2009/09/04.

[141] Depeille P, Cuq P, Mary S, Passagne I, Evrard A, Cupissol D, et al. Glutathione S-transferase M1 and multidrug resistance protein 1 act in synergy to protect melanoma cells from vincristine effects. Molecular pharmacology. 2004;65(4):897-905. Epub 2004/03/27.

[142] Ortega A, Benlloch M, Ferrer P, Segarra R, Asensi M, Obrador E, Estrela JM. GSH depletion in B16 melanoma cells: MRP 1-channeled drug extrusion, Bcl-2 antisense therapy and inhibition of {gamma}-glutamyltranspeptidase. AACR Meeting Abstracts 2004 2004: 122.

[143] Frank NY, Margaryan A, Huang Y, Schatton T, Waaga-Gasser AM, Gasser M, et al. ABCB5-mediated doxorubicin transport and chemoresistance in human malignant melanoma. Cancer research. 2005;65(10):4320-33. Epub 2005/05/19.

[144] Elliott AM, Al-Hajj MA. ABCB8 mediates doxorubicin resistance in melanoma cells by protecting the mitochondrial genome. Molecular cancer research : MCR. 2009;7(1): 79-87. Epub 2009/01/17.

[145] Frank NY, Pendse SS, Lapchak PH, Margaryan A, Shlain D, Doeing C, et al. Regulation of progenitor cell fusion by ABCB5 P-glycoprotein, a novel human ATP-binding cassette transporter. The Journal of biological chemistry. 2003;278(47):47156-65. Epub 2003/09/10.

[146] Chen KG, Szakacs G, Annereau JP, Rouzaud F, Liang XJ, Valencia JC, et al. Principal expression of two mRNA isoforms (ABCB 5alpha and ABCB 5beta) of the ATP-binding cassette transporter gene ABCB 5 in melanoma cells and melanocytes. Pigment cell research / sponsored by the European Society for Pigment Cell Research and the International Pigment Cell Society. 2005;18(2):102-12. Epub 2005/03/12.

[147] Huang Y, Anderle P, Bussey KJ, Barbacioru C, Shankavaram U, Dai Z, et al. Membrane transporters and channels: role of the transportome in cancer chemosensitivity and chemoresistance. Cancer research. 2004;64(12):4294-301. Epub 2004/06/19.

[148] Szakacs G, Annereau JP, Lababidi S, Shankavaram U, Arciello A, Bussey KJ, et al. Predicting drug sensitivity and resistance: profiling ABC transporter genes in cancer cells. Cancer cell. 2004;6(2):129-37. Epub 2004/08/25.

[149] Schatton T, Murphy GF, Frank NY, Yamaura K, Waaga-Gasser AM, Gasser M, et al. Identification of cells initiating human melanomas. Nature. 2008;451(7176):345-9. Epub 2008/01/19.

[150] Keshet GI, Goldstein I, Itzhaki O, Cesarkas K, Shenhav L, Yakirevitch A, et al. MDR1 expression identifies human melanoma stem cells. Biochemical and biophysical research communications. 2008;368(4):930-6. Epub 2008/02/19.

[151] Halliwell B. Oxidative stress and cancer: have we moved forward? The Biochemical journal. 2007;401(1):1-11. Epub 2006/12/08.

[152] Rasheed MH, Beevi SS, Geetha A. Enhanced lipid peroxidation and nitric oxide products with deranged antioxidant status in patients with head and neck squamous cell carcinoma. Oral Oncol. 2007;43(4):333-8. Epub 2006/07/22.

[153] Kumar B, Koul S, Khandrika L, Meacham RB, Koul HK. Oxidative stress is inherent in prostate cancer cells and is required for aggressive phenotype. Cancer research. 2008;68(6):1777-85. Epub 2008/03/15.

[154] Martin KR, Barrett JC. Reactive oxygen species as double-edged swords in cellular processes: low-dose cell signaling versus high-dose toxicity. Hum Exp Toxicol. 2002;21(2):71-5. Epub 2002/07/10.

[155] McCord JM. Superoxide radical: controversies, contradictions, and paradoxes. Proc Soc Exp Biol Med. 1995;209(2):112-7. Epub 1995/06/01.

[156] Lau A, Villeneuve NF, Sun Z, Wong PK, Zhang DD. Dual roles of Nrf2 in cancer. Pharmacological research : the official journal of the Italian Pharmacological Society. 2008;58(5-6):262-70. Epub 2008/10/08.

[157] Yanagawa T, Ishikawa T, Ishii T, Tabuchi K, Iwasa S, Bannai S, et al. Peroxiredoxin I expression in human thyroid tumors. Cancer letters. 1999;145(1-2):127-32. Epub 1999/10/26.

[158] Lee KW, Lee HJ. Biphasic effects of dietary antioxidants on oxidative stress-mediated carcinogenesis. Mech Ageing Dev. 2006;127(5):424-31. Epub 2006/03/08.

[159] Fruehauf JP, Meyskens FL, Jr. Reactive oxygen species: a breath of life or death? Clinical cancer research : an official journal of the American Association for Cancer Research. 2007;13(3):789-94. Epub 2007/02/10.

[160] Valko M, Rhodes CJ, Moncol J, Izakovic M, Mazur M. Free radicals, metals and antioxidants in oxidative stress-induced cancer. Chemico-biological interactions. 2006;160(1):1-40. Epub 2006/01/25.

[161] Campos AC, Molognoni F, Melo FH, Galdieri LC, Carneiro CR, D'Almeida V, et al. Oxidative stress modulates DNA methylation during melanocyte anchorage blockade associated with malignant transformation. Neoplasia. 2007;9(12):1111-21. Epub 2007/12/18.

[162] Donkena KV, Young CY, Tindall DJ. Oxidative stress and DNA methylation in prostate cancer. Obstet Gynecol Int. 2010;2010:302051. Epub 2010/07/31.

[163] Ziech D, Franco R, Pappa A, Malamou-Mitsi V, Georgakila S, Georgakilas AG, et al. The role of epigenetics in environmental and occupational carcinogenesis. Chemico-biological interactions. 2010;188(2):340-9. Epub 2010/07/06.

[164] Weitzman SA, Turk PW, Milkowski DH, Kozlowski K. Free radical adducts induce alterations in DNA cytosine methylation. Proceedings of the National Academy of Sciences of the United States of America. 1994;91(4):1261-4. Epub 1994/02/15.

[165] Turk PW, Laayoun A, Smith SS, Weitzman SA. DNA adduct 8-hydroxyl-2'-deoxyguanosine (8-hydroxyguanine) affects function of human DNA methyltransferase. Carcinogenesis. 1995;16(5):1253-5. Epub 1995/05/01.

[166] Turk PW, Weitzman SA. Free radical DNA adduct 8-OH-deoxyguanosine affects activity of Hpa II and Msp I restriction endonucleases. Free radical research. 1995;23(3): 255-8. Epub 1995/09/01.

[167] Christman JK, Sheikhnejad G, Marasco CJ, Sufrin JR. 5-Methyl-2'-deoxycytidine in single-stranded DNA can act in cis to signal de novo DNA methylation. Proceedings of the National Academy of Sciences of the United States of America. 1995;92(16): 7347-51. Epub 1995/08/01.

[168] Franco R, Schoneveld O, Georgakilas AG, Panayiotidis MI. Oxidative stress, DNA methylation and carcinogenesis. Cancer letters. 2008;266(1):6-11. Epub 2008/03/29.

[169] Sander CS, Hamm F, Elsner P, Thiele JJ. Oxidative stress in malignant melanoma and non-melanoma skin cancer. The British journal of dermatology. 2003;148(5):913-22. Epub 2003/06/06.

[170] Gidanian S, Mentelle M, Meyskens FL, Jr., Farmer PJ. Melanosomal damage in normal human melanocytes induced by UVB and metal uptake--a basis for the pro-oxidant state of melanoma. Photochemistry and photobiology. 2008;84(3):556-64. Epub 2008/03/12.

[171] Meyskens FL, Jr., McNulty SE, Buckmeier JA, Tohidian NB, Spillane TJ, Kahlon RS, et al. Aberrant redox regulation in human metastatic melanoma cells compared to normal melanocytes. Free radical biology & medicine. 2001;31(6):799-808. Epub 2001/09/15.

[172] Meyskens FL, Jr., Farmer P, Fruehauf JP. Redox regulation in human melanocytes and melanoma. Pigment cell research / sponsored by the European Society for Pigment Cell Research and the International Pigment Cell Society. 2001;14(3):148-54. Epub 2001/07/04.

[173] Meyskens FL, Jr., Berwick M. UV or not UV: metals are the answer. Cancer epidemiology, biomarkers & prevention : a publication of the American Association for Cancer Research, cosponsored by the American Society of Preventive Oncology. 2008;17(2):268-70. Epub 2008/02/13.

[174] Cooke MS, Evans MD, Dizdaroglu M, Lunec J. Oxidative DNA damage: mechanisms, mutation, and disease. FASEB journal : official publication of the Federation of American Societies for Experimental Biology. 2003;17(10):1195-214. Epub 2003/07/02.

[175] Pavel S, van Nieuwpoort F, van der Meulen H, Out C, Pizinger K, Cetkovska P, et al. Disturbed melanin synthesis and chronic oxidative stress in dysplastic naevi. Eur J Cancer. 2004;40(9):1423-30. Epub 2004/06/05.

[176] Smit NP, van Nieuwpoort FA, Marrot L, Out C, Poorthuis B, van Pelt H, et al. Increased melanogenesis is a risk factor for oxidative DNA damage--study on cultured melanocytes and atypical nevus cells. Photochemistry and photobiology. 2008;84(3): 550-5. Epub 2008/04/26.

[177] Leikam C, Hufnagel A, Schartl M, Meierjohann S. Oncogene activation in melanocytes links reactive oxygen to multinucleated phenotype and senescence. Oncogene. 2008;27(56):7070-82. Epub 2008/09/23.

[178] Gaudiano G, Koch TH. Redox chemistry of anthracycline antitumor drugs and use of captodative radicals as tools for its elucidation and control. Chemical research in toxicology. 1991;4(1):2-16. Epub 1991/01/01.

[179] Sengupta SK, Kelly C, Sehgal RK. "Reverse" and "symmetrical" analogues of actinomycin D: metabolic activation and in vitro and in vivo tumor growth inhibitory activities. Journal of medicinal chemistry. 1985;28(5):620-8. Epub 1985/05/01.

[180] Roller A, Weller M. Antioxidants specifically inhibit cisplatin cytotoxicity of human malignant glioma cells. Anticancer research. 1998;18(6A):4493-7. Epub 1999/01/19.

[181] Thrall BD, Raha GA, Springer DL, Meadows GG. Differential sensitivities of murine melanocytes and melanoma cells to buthionine sulfoximine and anticancer drugs. Pigment cell research / sponsored by the European Society for Pigment Cell Research and the International Pigment Cell Society. 1991;4(5-6):234-9. Epub 1991/12/01.

[182] Iacobini M, Menichelli A, Palumbo G, Multari G, Werner B, Del Principe D. Involvement of oxygen radicals in cytarabine-induced apoptosis in human polymorphonuclear cells. Biochemical pharmacology. 2001;61(8):1033-40. Epub 2001/04/05.

[183] Sakhi AK, Russnes KM, Thoresen M, Bastani NE, Karlsen A, Smeland S, et al. Pre-radiotherapy plasma carotenoids and markers of oxidative stress are associated with survival in head and neck squamous cell carcinoma patients: a prospective study. BMC Cancer. 2009;9:458. Epub 2009/12/23.

[184] Sabitha KE, Shyamaladevi CS. Oxidant and antioxidant activity changes in patients with oral cancer and treated with radiotherapy. Oral Oncol. 1999;35(3):273-7. Epub 2000/01/06.

[185] Kasapovic J, Pejic S, Stojiljkovic V, Todorovic A, Radosevic-Jelic L, Saicic ZS, et al. Antioxidant status and lipid peroxidation in the blood of breast cancer patients of different ages after chemotherapy with 5-fluorouracil, doxorubicin and cyclophosphamide. Clin Biochem. 2010;43(16-17):1287-93. Epub 2010/08/18.

[186] Gupta A, Bhatt ML, Misra MK. Assessment of free radical-mediated damage in head and neck squamous cell carcinoma patients and after treatment with radiotherapy. Indian J Biochem Biophys. 2010;47(2):96-9. Epub 2010/06/05.

[187] Kim SK, Yang JW, Kim MR, Roh SH, Kim HG, Lee KY, et al. Increased expression of Nrf2/ARE-dependent anti-oxidant proteins in tamoxifen-resistant breast cancer cells. Free radical biology & medicine. 2008;45(4):537-46. Epub 2008/06/10.

[188] Osburn WO, Kensler TW. Nrf2 signaling: an adaptive response pathway for protection against environmental toxic insults. Mutat Res. 2008;659(1-2):31-9. Epub 2008/01/01.

[189] Kim YJ, Ahn JY, Liang P, Ip C, Zhang Y, Park YM. Human prx1 gene is a target of Nrf2 and is up-regulated by hypoxia/reoxygenation: implication to tumor biology. Cancer research. 2007;67(2):546-54. Epub 2007/01/20.

[190] Maher JM, Dieter MZ, Aleksunes LM, Slitt AL, Guo G, Tanaka Y, et al. Oxidative and electrophilic stress induces multidrug resistance-associated protein transporters via the nuclear factor-E2-related factor-2 transcriptional pathway. Hepatology. 2007;46(5):1597-610. Epub 2007/08/03.

[191] Chan JY, Kwong M. Impaired expression of glutathione synthetic enzyme genes in mice with targeted deletion of the Nrf2 basic-leucine zipper protein. Biochimica et biophysica acta. 2000;1517(1):19-26. Epub 2000/12/19.

[192] Xu Z, Chen L, Leung L, Yen TS, Lee C, Chan JY. Liver-specific inactivation of the Nrf1 gene in adult mouse leads to nonalcoholic steatohepatitis and hepatic neoplasia. Proceedings of the National Academy of Sciences of the United States of America. 2005;102(11):4120-5. Epub 2005/03/02.

[193] Chen L, Kwong M, Lu R, Ginzinger D, Lee C, Leung L, et al. Nrf1 is critical for redox balance and survival of liver cells during development. Molecular and cellular biology. 2003;23(13):4673-86. Epub 2003/06/17.

[194] Ohtsuji M, Katsuoka F, Kobayashi A, Aburatani H, Hayes JD, Yamamoto M. Nrf1 and Nrf2 play distinct roles in activation of antioxidant response element-dependent genes. The Journal of biological chemistry. 2008;283(48):33554-62. Epub 2008/10/02.

[195] Khandrika L, Kumar B, Koul S, Maroni P, Koul HK. Oxidative stress in prostate cancer. Cancer letters. 2009;282(2):125-36. Epub 2009/02/03.

[196] Frohlich DA, McCabe MT, Arnold RS, Day ML. The role of Nrf2 in increased reactive oxygen species and DNA damage in prostate tumorigenesis. Oncogene. 2008;27(31): 4353-62. Epub 2008/04/01.

[197] Kaspar JW, Niture SK, Jaiswal AK. Nrf2:INrf2 (Keap1) signaling in oxidative stress. Free radical biology & medicine. 2009;47(9):1304-9. Epub 2009/08/12.

[198] Wang XJ, Sun Z, Villeneuve NF, Zhang S, Zhao F, Li Y, et al. Nrf2 enhances resistance of cancer cells to chemotherapeutic drugs, the dark side of Nrf2. Carcinogenesis. 2008;29(6):1235-43. Epub 2008/04/17.

[199] Padmanabhan B, Tong KI, Ohta T, Nakamura Y, Scharlock M, Ohtsuji M, et al. Structural basis for defects of Keap1 activity provoked by its point mutations in lung cancer. Molecular cell. 2006;21(5):689-700. Epub 2006/03/02.

[200] Singh A, Misra V, Thimmulappa RK, Lee H, Ames S, Hoque MO, et al. Dysfunctional KEAP1-NRF2 interaction in non-small-cell lung cancer. PLoS medicine. 2006;3(10):e420. Epub 2006/10/06.

[201] Ohta T, Iijima K, Miyamoto M, Nakahara I, Tanaka H, Ohtsuji M, et al. Loss of Keap1 function activates Nrf2 and provides advantages for lung cancer cell growth. Cancer research. 2008;68(5):1303-9. Epub 2008/03/05.

[202] Nioi P, Nguyen T. A mutation of Keap1 found in breast cancer impairs its ability to repress Nrf2 activity. Biochemical and biophysical research communications. 2007;362(4):816-21. Epub 2007/09/08.

[203] Shibata T, Kokubu A, Gotoh M, Ojima H, Ohta T, Yamamoto M, et al. Genetic alteration of Keap1 confers constitutive Nrf2 activation and resistance to chemotherapy in gallbladder cancer. Gastroenterology. 2008;135(4):1358-68, 68 e1-4. Epub 2008/08/12.

[204] Matundan HH, Dellinger RW, Jr. FLM. Nrf2 Mediates Chemoresistance in Melanoma. Free Radical Biology and Medicine. 1 November 2011.;51:S126.

[205] Takatori T, Ogura M, Tsuruo T. Purification and characterization of NF-R2 that regulates the expression of the human multidrug resistance (MDR1) gene. Jpn J Cancer Res. 1993;84(3):298-303. Epub 1993/03/01.

[206] Hayashi A, Suzuki H, Itoh K, Yamamoto M, Sugiyama Y. Transcription factor Nrf2 is required for the constitutive and inducible expression of multidrug resistance-associated protein 1 in mouse embryo fibroblasts. Biochemical and biophysical research communications. 2003;310(3):824-9. Epub 2003/10/11.

[207] You A, Nam CW, Wakabayashi N, Yamamoto M, Kensler TW, Kwak MK. Transcription factor Nrf2 maintains the basal expression of Mdm2: An implication of the regulation of p53 signaling by Nrf2. Archives of biochemistry and biophysics. 2011;507(2): 356-64. Epub 2011/01/08.

[208] Hayes JD, Ashford ML. Nrf2 orchestrates fuel partitioning for cell proliferation. Cell metabolism. 2012;16(2):139-41. Epub 2012/08/14.

[209] So HS, Kim HJ, Lee JH, Lee JH, Park SY, Park C, et al. Flunarizine induces Nrf2-mediated transcriptional activation of heme oxygenase-1 in protection of auditory cells from cisplatin. Cell death and differentiation. 2006;13(10):1763-75. Epub 2006/02/18.

[210] Beyer TA, Xu W, Teupser D, auf dem Keller U, Bugnon P, Hildt E, et al. Impaired liver regeneration in Nrf2 knockout mice: role of ROS-mediated insulin/IGF-1 resistance. The EMBO journal. 2008;27(1):212-23. Epub 2007/12/07.

[211] Mitsuishi Y, Taguchi K, Kawatani Y, Shibata T, Nukiwa T, Aburatani H, et al. Nrf2 redirects glucose and glutamine into anabolic pathways in metabolic reprogramming. Cancer cell. 2012;22(1):66-79. Epub 2012/07/14.

[212] Sun Z, Huang Z, Zhang DD. Phosphorylation of Nrf2 at multiple sites by MAP kinases has a limited contribution in modulating the Nrf2-dependent antioxidant response. PloS one. 2009;4(8):e6588. Epub 2009/08/12.

[213] Niture SK, Jaiswal AK. INrf2 (Keap1) targets Bcl-2 degradation and controls cellular apoptosis. Cell death and differentiation. 2011;18(3):439-51. Epub 2010/09/25.

[214] Niture SK, Jaiswal AK. Nrf2 protein up-regulates antiapoptotic protein Bcl-2 and prevents cellular apoptosis. The Journal of biological chemistry. 2012;287(13):9873-86. Epub 2012/01/26.

Chapter 17

Management of Acral Lentiginous Melanoma

Yoshitaka Kai and Sakuhei Fujiwara

Additional information is available at the end of the chapter

http://dx.doi.org/10.5772/54266

1. Introduction

Cutaneous malignant melanoma is the most common cause of mortality from skin cancers in Caucasian populations. The incidence rates of malignant melanoma show considerable variation worldwide. Annual incidence rates per 100,000 people vary between about 40 in Australia and New Zealand to about 20 in the United States [1,2]. In contrast, a significantly lower incidence rate has been reported in Asian populations with rates of 0.65 to 1/100,000 [3-5]. In addition, the most common sites of melanoma occurrence in Asians are the extremities at a rate of about 50% of all cases [6,7], compared to only 2-3% in Caucasian populations [8].

In 1976, RJ Reed first described the fourth variant of melanoma as "pigmented lesions on the extremities, particularly on palmoplantar regions, that are characterized by a lentiginous (radial) growth phase evolving over months or years to a dermal (vertical) invasive stage" [9]. He named this anatomical subgroup of melanoma as "plantar lentiginous melanoma (PLM) ", which had a characteristic lentiginous, radial component of melanocytic proliferation and mentioned for the first time that this subgroup was the most common in Blacks and the very poor prognosis group [10].

In 1986, malignant melanoma was classified into four subtypes by Clark et al. according to histological features; nodular melanoma (NM), superficial spreading melanoma (SSM), lentigo maligna melanoma (LMM) and acral lentiginous melanoma (ALM) [11]. In the United States, the incidence rates of SSM, NM, LMM and ALM are approximately 70%, 15%, 13% and 2-3% respectively [12,13]. Although, ALM is the most common expression of malignant melanoma in Asian and Black populations, the rate of ALM is 41% in Japan [14], 65% in Korea [15] and 62% in the American Blacks [16].

The prognosis of each subtype differs due to delayed diagnosis rather than an actual differences in the biological nature of tumour and the prognosis of ALM is generally poorer than other subtypes [17]. The lesion, especially on soles and nail beds, is likely to be overlooked by patients. Moreover, Metzger et al. found that ALM had a high likelihood of being clinically misdiagnosed as a benign melanocytic lesion, which leads to a delay in the initiation of treatment [18]. However, this report was made in the pre-dermoscopic era and now it has become much easier with dermoscopy to distinguish the early stage of ALM from a benign lesion.

Human extremities, especially palms and soles, are not exposed to ultraviolet light and there is no evidence of overexposure to UV light as a risk factor of ALM [19]. In contrast, UV light plays an important role in the pathogenesis of LMM.

In 2005, Bastian et al. proposed new classification of melanoma according to genetic alterations at different sites. They classified melanoma into four distinct groups, each of which has a different degree of exposure to UV light: chronic sun-damaged melanoma (CSD) which nearly corresponds to LMM, non-CSD melanoma which also corresponds to SSM, acral melanoma (AM) which also corresponds to ALM, and mucosal melanoma [20]. They found that 81% of non-CSD melanoma had mutations in BRAF or N-RAS and the other groups had no mutations in either gene. Otherwise, melanoma with wild-type BRAF or N-RAS frequently had an increase in the number of copies of the genes for cyclin-dependent kinase 4 (CDK4) and cyclin D1 (CCND1). Furthermore, a recent study showed that AM and mucosal melanoma had frequent mutation or amplification of the KIT gene [21]. Although these findings have led to molecular targeted therapy today, this new therapeutic approach has just begun and therefore we will only touch upon these new directions.

Today, there are some difficulties and controversies in the treatment of ALM caused by the anatomical and biological specificity of ALM. The standardized treatment of ALM is not easy to establish due to the unique characteristics. This chapter includes our experiences and a review of the literature focusing on the surgical treatment of ALM, and in particular, discusses the controversies surrounding the treatment of ALM.

Clinical presentation and dermoscopic findings of ALM

ALM occurs more frequently on lower extremities than on upper extremities. In our institute, 41 cases of all 61 ALM cases occurred on lower extremities. The soles of the feet are the most frequent sites of ALM, where 56% of ALM on lower extremities occurred. In contrast, most frequent sites on upper extremities are fingernails, where 45% of ALM on upper extremities appeared.

Clinically, ALMs begin with pale brown macules, enlarge slowly and form irregularly pigmented, asymmetric macular lesions with notching at the periphery over the years. After that, nodules appear on the pigmented lesion and form ulceration. In the past ALM was considered to occur from benign malanocytic lesions, however, de novo synthesis in major cases of ALM has been confirmed by dermoscopic findings (see below). Due to the very slow progress, it tends to be overlooked and even when the tumour becomes larger, it is easily underestimated.

Histologically, "(1) the radial growth phase consists of lentiginous dysplastic melanocytes, extending along the basal cell layer, with extension of single atypical melanocytes up into the thickened epidermis; (2) the vertical growth phase usually consists of a progressive central plaque-like thickening of malignant cells in the papillary dermis, with (3) extension of the spindle cells into the deeper levels, accompanied by prominent dysplasia; (4) there is epidermal hyperplasia with elongation of the rete ridges and acanthosis and central ulceration; and (5) host immune response is active, with areas of tumor regression" [22].

	Location	**Case Number (%)**
Lower extremities	Thigh	1 (1.6)
	Lower leg	6 (9.8)
	Dorsum of foot	1 (1.6)
	Sole	23 (37.7)
	Toe	8 (13.1)
	Toenail	2 (3.3)
	Total	41
Upper extremities	Upper arm	0 (0)
	Forearm	1 (1.6)
	Dorsum of Hand	1 (1.6)
	Palm	4 (6.6)
	Finger	4 (6.6)
	Fingernail	9 (14.8)
	Total	19
Unknown		1 (1.6)
Total		61 (100)

Table 1. Primary sites of cutaneous melanoma experienced in our institute from 2004 to 2011

Dermoscopic observations help the diagnosis in the early stage of ALM. In 66 cases of volar skin melanomas, irregular diffuse pigmentation (60%) with variable shades from tan to black without parallel disposition of pigment (figure 1a) and the parallel ridge pattern (53%) with pigmentation along the ridges (figure 1b) were the two most prevalent patterns [23]. According to Saida et al., the sensitivity and specificity of the parallel ridge pattern in diagnosing all melanoma on volar skins were 86% and 99% respectively and those of irregular diffuse pigmentation were 85% and 97% respectively. Only in diagnosing melanoma in situ on volar skin, the sensitivity of parallel ridge pattern (86%) was significantly higher than that of irregular diffuse pigmentation (69%) [24]. A parallel furrow pattern with pigmentation along the furrows (figure 1c) and a lattice-like pattern with longitudinal and transversal thicker lines surrounding the eccrine pores (figure 1d) are more common in melanocytic nevi. The sensitivity and specificity of a parallel furrow pattern or lattice-like pattern in diagnosing melanocytic nevi were 67% and 93% respectively [24].

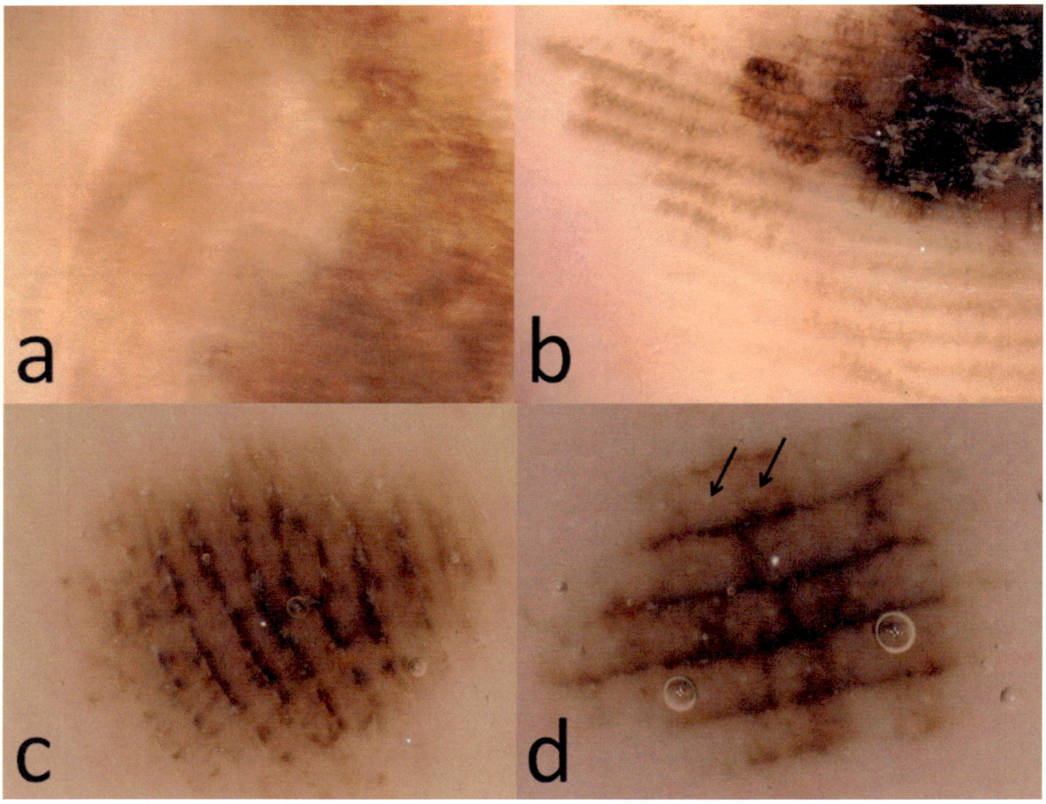

Figure 1. Dermoscopy of early stage ALM (a,b) and melanocytic nevi (c,d). (a) Irregular diffuse pigmentation, (b) parallel ridge pattern, (c) parallel furrow pattern, (d) lattice-like pattern with longitudinal and transversal thicker lines surrounding the eccrine pores (arrows).

Ulceration on nodules following pigmented macules reveals a polymorphous vascular pattern with a combination of milky-red areas (95%) which are larger areas of fuzzy or unfocused milky-red colour corresponding to an elevated part of the lesion, linear irregular vessels (49%), dotted vessels (43%) and hairpin vessels (41%) [25].

2. Subungual melanoma

The incidence of subungual melanoma also has a racial difference. It is more frequent in Asian and Blacks than in Caucasians. Its frequency has been reported to be approximately 2-4% in all cutaneous melanomas in Caucasians and 10% in Japanese [26]. Of the 108 subungual melanomas in Japan, the cases involving fingers and toes were 76% and 24% respectively. On both fingers and toes, the thumb and the great toe were the most common sites [26]. Among the subungual melanoma, the occurrence rate of ALM on the fingernail is higher than on toenails. According to the literature, of 64 cases of subungual melanoma, 55% cases occurred on the thumbnail, 27% on the nail of the great toe, 2-4% on the nail of the index, middle and ring finger, 1.6% on the nail of the second toe [27].

It is known that subungual melanoma has a very poor prognosis among all subtypes of cutaneous melanomas. The reason for this is because the majority of subungual melanomas are already been quite deep when diagnosed [28]. Delayed diagnosis of subungual melanoma is common because it is very difficult to distinguish the early stage of subungual melanoma from longitudinal melanonychia. According to Cohen et al., 38 of 43 patients (88%) had delayed diagnosis and the median delay time was 24 months (range 4 to 132) [29].

Subungual melanomas begin with fine pigmented striata which could not be clinically distinguished from benign longitudinal melanonychia at an early stage and grow wider with colour variegation and the presence of nail plate fissuring or splitting eventually forming a triangular shape which has a broader proximal lesion rather than a distal lesion, blurred lateral borders and Hutchinson's sign - indicating the peripheral pigmentation beyond the nail apparatus [30].

Baran et al. mentioned the clinical clues to the diagnosis of subungual melanoma in detail. Hutchinson's sign is the most important sign of subungual melanoma. Other clues are when longitudinal melanonychia (a) begins in a single digit of a person over six decades or more, (b) develops abruptly in a previous normal nail plate, (c) becomes suddenly darker or wider, (d) occurs in either the thumb, index finger or giant toe, (e) is accompanied by nail destruction or disappearance, (f) has colour variegation, (g) has a wide band and so on [31].

In addition to these clinical clues, dermoscopy provides useful information for the diagnosis of subungual melanoma. The prominent dermoscopic features of subungual melanoma are brown pigmentation of the background with longitudinal brown to black lines which are irregular in their colouration, spacing, thickness and parallelism [32]. This irregularity was significantly associated with melanoma when compared with all other benign diseases. The micro-Hutchinson's sign is the suspicious dermoscopic feature, which consists of the irregular lines in the cuticle area and can be observed only on dermoscopy [32,33].

Since the early stage of subungual melanoma has minimal histopathological change, it may be difficult to distinguish subungual melanoma from benign lesion with only histopathological findings. Thus, both clinical features, including present history and histopathological findings, are necessary for diagnosis.

We propose a diagnostic algorithm for the early stage of subungual melanoma (figure 2). When a case falls under any of the clinical features mentioned above (a-g), dermoscopic examination is recommended. If Hutchinson's sign and colour change in overall nail to dark black are present, excisional biopsy is recommended. When those characteristic appearances are absent, but a nail streak has irregularity, biopsy is also recommended. On the contrary, when nail streaks are monotonous pale brown, subungual melanoma is not suspicious. Even if a streak is dark brown or black, no irregularity of lines on dermoscopy allows careful follow-up without biopsies. If the streak increases in width or has colour variegation during a period of follow-up, the necessity of excision or biopsy should be discussed according to further dermoscopic examination.

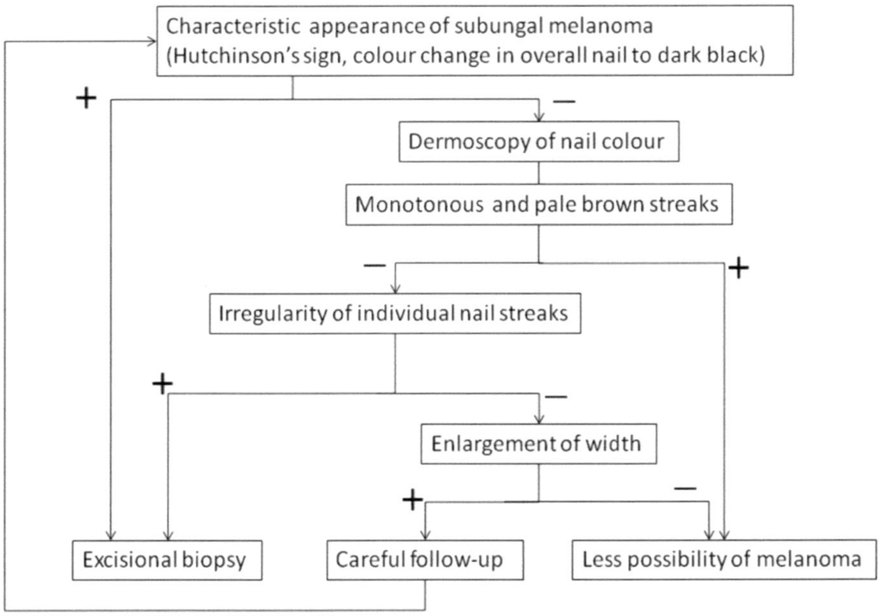

Figure 2. Diagnostic algorithm for early stage subungual melanoma.

Since nail biopsies cause cosmetic problems, biopsy methods should be selected as follows. If streaks are more likely to be melanoma, complete excisional biopsies are desirable. If it is less likely, punch biopsies around the origin of the longitudinal melanonychia (which is frequently located on the nail matrix) can be chosen. When excisional biopsies are performed, we should keep in mind that an insufficient margin at the proximal side of the nail may cause incision in between the lesional nail matrix without including the whole lesion. Ultrasound echography provides useful information on the location of the nail matrix [34], so that a sufficient margin can be ensured. Furthermore, it is desirable that extent of the excisional biopsy includes the periosteum of the distal phalanx. Since the distance between the nail matrix and bone is extremely close at the proximal side, excisional biopsies excluding periosteum may incise the nail matrix and leave some lesion on the body. Excisional biopsies including the periosteum causes very little disadvantage compared with those excluding the periosteum and afterwards good granulation tissue will be formed on the bone when the artificial dermis is used. If it is histopathologically diagnosed as subungual melanoma, a local wide excision is selected, excluding the case when a sufficient margin is ensured at the previous excisional biopsy.

Excisional biopsies in a good manner allow us to determine correct tumour thickness, which provides important information on the choice of SLNB, local wide excision and chemotherapy. However, biopsy specimens easily break down if the biopsy procedure for histological examination is not performed well, which may cause incorrect choices for treatment.

If nail destruction is present under diagnosis of subungual melanoma, amputation of the distal phalanx will be applied on the assumption that the lesion invades the periosteum or bone. However, not all cases of nail destruction are accompanied with invasion. Some cases of nail destruction may be melanomas in situ. Since the distance between nail bed and bone is wider at the distal side than at the proximal side, the possibility of avoiding amputation is higher when the nail destruction is modest and located at the distal side of the nail.

Moehrle et al. proposed 'functional' surgery for subungual melanoma, by which the amputation of the distal phalanx could be avoided and the more digital function could be preserved [35]. The tumour was surgically removed with measurable excision margins and a partial resection of the distal part of the distal phalanx was performed with a Luer instrument. After the resection, three-dimensional histology was performed as described in the literature [36]. Two of 31 patients had local recurrence after this operation. This method did not lead to shorter survival when compared to amputation, thus, it is worth considering.

3. Wide local excision

According to a review of the literature on the margins of radical excision for melanomas thinner than 2mm, the French Cooperative Group Trial [37] and the Scandinavian Melanoma Group Study [38] compared 2cm with 5cm margins and the World Health Organization (WHO) Melanoma Program Trial 10 [39] compared 1cm with 3cm margins. All three trials demonstrated no benefits for wider margins.

Although a 5mm margin for melanoma in situ is frequently recommended in some national guidelines, Kunishige et al. demonstrated that 86% of 1120 melanomas in situ were successfully excised with a 6mm margin and 98.9% with a 9mm margin. They concluded that a 6mm margin for melanomas in situ was inadequate and a 9mm margin was necessary [40].

A 1cm margin of excision has been proposed for melanomas less than 1mm thick and a wider margin for more than 1mm thick [41,42]. Although many national guidelines recommend that a 1 cm margin is appropriate for 1-2mm thick invasive melanoma, this is less clear because there has been very little data indicating that a 1cm margin for 1-2mm thick melanoma is safer than 2cm margin [43]. For more than 2mm thick melanomas, a 2cm margin is considered to be sufficient in almost all cases. Depth of excision has been recommended to be at least the level of muscle fascia and deeper excision under it has not been shown to improve outcome [43-45].

For melanomas on the extremities, especially on fingers, amputation impairs the function. Thus, even if finger amputation is necessary, it is desirable that the defect is smaller so that functional impairment can be minimal. Detailed histopathological examination of resected specimens may allow surgeons to excise a smaller part of the fingers. We show the pathological specimen as illustrated on Figure 3. Because the resected margins are usually intricately curved, the specimen is divided into several parts so that a marginal side of each part becomes planar and paraffin sections can be made so that the whole surface of the marginal side can be examined. This technique provides highly accurate detection of continuous lesions with a small possibility of missing skip lesions. If the margin is negative, additional excision is not necessary and that provides preservation of more digital functions.

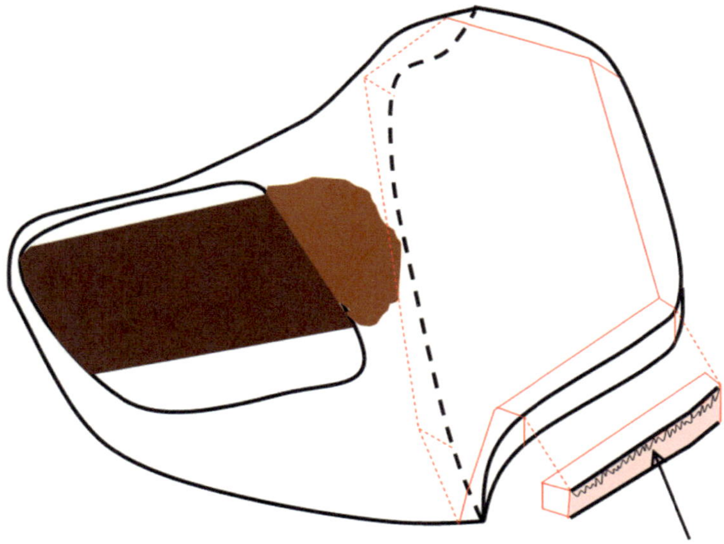

Figure 3. How to make pathological specimen of an amputated finger tip was illustrated. In order to examine the tumor cells at the marginal side accurately and continuously, curved rim of the excised margin was cut as linear as possible, and the outside of the margin is examined. (arrow)

4. Sentinel lymph node biopsy

Sentinel lymph node biopsy (SLNB) has become the standard procedure used to determine whether a tumour has metastasized to lymph nodes and more accurate staging of the melanoma. It is a less invasive technique than lymph node dissection allowing patients with node negative (N0) melanoma to avoid unnecessary lymph node dissection. In the case of SLN positive melanoma, additional surgery of lymph node dissection is necessary.

The false-negative rate in SLN mapping for melanoma has been reported to be very low with a rate of 0 to 2 % [46-49]. The multicenter selective lymphadenectomy trial-1 (MSLT-1) demonstrated immediate lymph node dissection following microscopic positive node at SLNB could bring about better prognosis than the lymph node dissection after clinical nodal observation [50].

For more correct mapping of SLNs, a combination of blue dye and radioisotope ^{99m}Tc labelled phytate is generally used. SLNs are identified by the presence of blue stained lymph vessels and lymph nodes, and the radioactivity measured by gamma probe. Furthermore, distinction between SLNs and secondary non-SLNs is achieved by using pre-operative dynamic cutaneous lymphoscintigraphy [51].

Although most melanomas drain to conventional regional nodes, unexpected drainage outside of these basins is observed in some cases. Pre-operative lymphscintigraphy and a hand-held gamma probe are required for detection of these interval SLNs. According to a single-institution study in Japan, SLNs were identified in 253 nodal basins from 117 patients and interval SLNs were found in six patients. They recognized 41 (17%) SLN metastases in 246 conventional nodal basins and one (14%) in seven interval SLNs [52].

5. Sentinel lymph node biopsy on upper extremities

Tumours on upper extremities almost always drain to the axillary region. The axillary region is divided into three parts based on the pectoralis minor. Level 1, 2 and 3 are located lateral, deep and medial to the pectoralis minor respectively. Outside this conventional region, SLNs are recognized in the cubital region and other areas. Figure 4 is the local sites of SLNs in our experience of 10 cases.

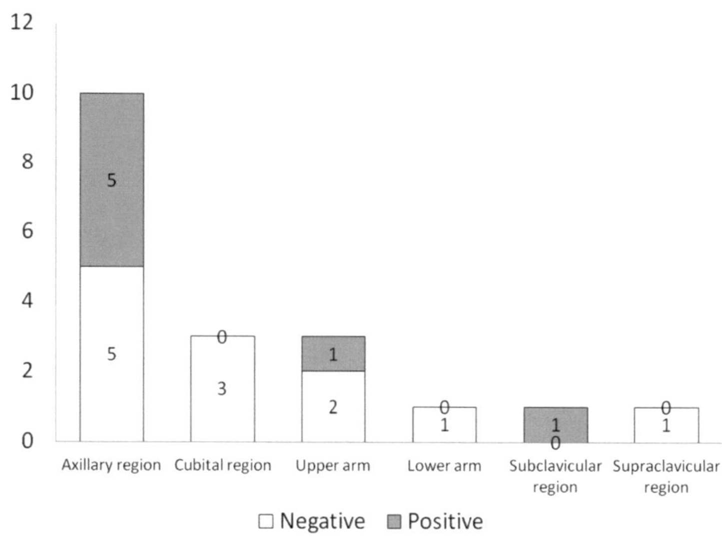

Figure 4. The sites of SLNs in primary melanomas on upper extremities.

SLNs were identified in all 10 cases (100%) for the axillary region, three cases (30%) for the cubital region, three cases (30%) for the upper arm, one case (10%) for the forearm, one case (10%) for the subclavicular region (level 3) and one case (10%) for the supraclavicular region. In all 10 cases, SLNs were present in anatomic level 1 of the axillary region. Although it has been considered that there is very little chance of finding SLNs in level 3, one case with SLN in level 3 was present in our data.

SLNs between the primary lesion and the axillary region are regarded as interval nodes on the upper extremities. Manganomi et al. reported that the interval SLN identification rate on upper extremities was 0.4% (two out of 480 cases) [53] and Kelly et al. reported 3.8% (16 out of 423 cases) [54]. Cubital region is the most common site of interval SLN on upper extremities. In our 3 cases of interval SLNs identified in cubital region, those were present on cubital fossa and on ulnar side of cubital region. We have experienced five cases of other interval region rather than cubital region.

Tumours on upper extremities rarely drain to the subclavicular region (level 3) rather than to level 1 or 2. Our case with SLNs on the subclavicular region had positive with non-positive SLNs in level 11 and no SLNs in level 2 (Figure 5).

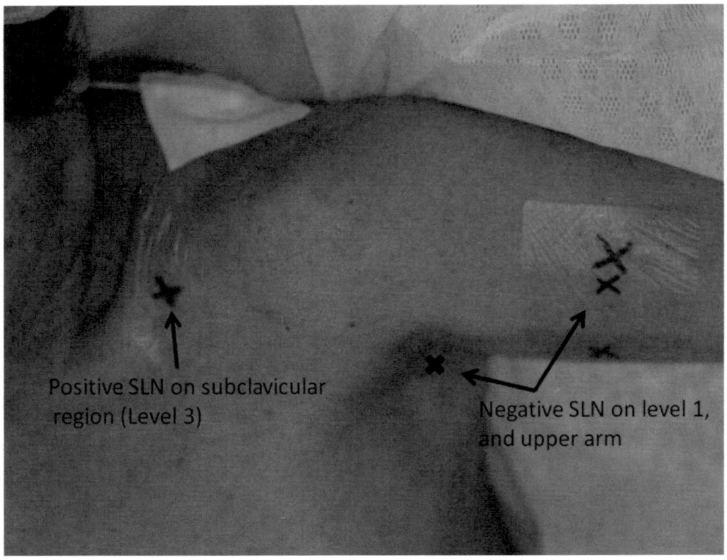

Figure 5. The case with positive SLN in level 3 and non-positive SLNs in level 1 and the upper arm. This metastatic pattern is extremely rare.

There may be cases where it is uncertain whether or not SLNB should be applied when tumour thickness is unknown. Some literature demonstrated that the patients with primary lesions on their extremities have a lower risk of misidentification of SLNs, even after wide local excision, than patients with axial primary lesions [55-59]. Tumors on central trunk may drain to both bilateral, or both axillary and inguinal regions. By contrast, tumours on extremities tend to drain more simply to the expected region. Although it is preferable that wide local excision and SLNB are performed at the same time, SLNB after wide local excision is less disruptive to lymphatic drainage in the case of primary lesions on the extremities than on axial sites.

6. Sentinel lymph node biopsy on lower extremities

In almost all cases, tumours on lower extremities drain to the inguinal region. Figure 6 demonstrates lymphatic drainage for 23 cases with tumours on lower extremities in our institute. Of all 23 cases, the lymph node identification rate was 23 cases (100%) for the inguinal region, five cases (21%) for the popliteal region and 10 cases (43%) for the pelvic region (nine cases for external iliac lymph nodes and one case for the obturator region). Three of the 23 cases with SLN on the inguinal region had positive nodes and there were no positive nodes on the popliteal and pelvic region.

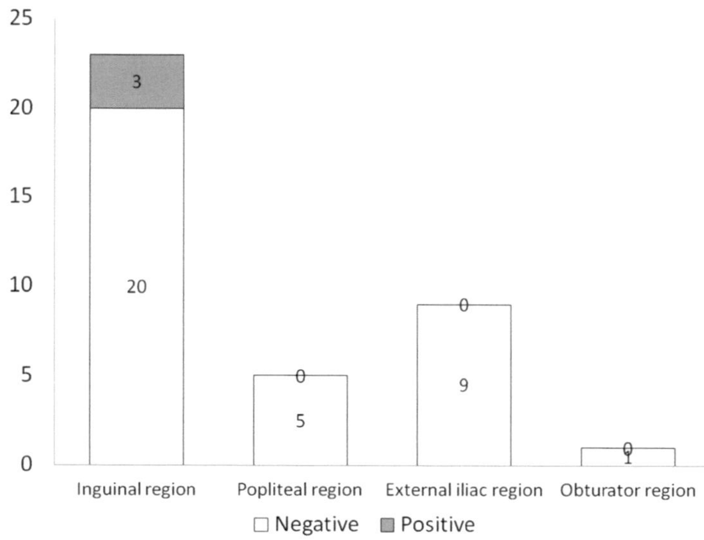

Figure 6. The sites of SLNs in primary melanomas on lower extremities.

One of the problems with SLNB of lower extremities is the presence of pelvic SLNs. Kaoutzanis et al. showed 11 of 82 cases with tumour on lower extremities had SLNs on the pelvic region and underwent SLNB [60]. They also showed that 19 of 82 cases (24%) had positive SLNs and all the positive SLNs were located in the inguinal region. No positive SLNs were present in the pelvic region as our cases.

Even in SLNB, removing the lymph nodes in the external iliac and obturator region is a relatively invasive technique. It is still controversial whether or not SLNs in the pelvic region should be harvested because SLNs in the pelvic region may be considered as secondary or third lymphatic basin, even when radioisotope is accumulated in pelvic lymph nodes.

Even now there is no consensus on the clinical definition of an SLN [61]. The SLN has been described as the hottest node, the blue node, first node visualized on lymphoscintigraphy and a node with radioactivity greater than twice or three times background radioactivity [61-63]. McMaster et al. recommended that all blue nodes and all nodes that measure 10% or higher of the 'ex vivo' radioactive count of hottest SLNs should be removed in order to decrease false-negative cases [64]. In our institute, SLN is defined as the node which showed higher than one tenth of the radioactivity of the hottest node. Because radioactivity depends on the distance from the surface of skin to the nodes, the measured radioactivity of the pelvic lymph nodes from the surface of skin is much less than superficial lymph nodes and tends to be underestimated [65]. Therefore, Bagaria et al. provided an answer that the background radioactivity of the regional nodal basin was measured before incision and all blue nodes and all hot nodes that have radioactivity greater than the background were harvested [61]. According to Soteldo et al., the rate of the cases that had metastasized lymph nodes in the pelvic region after SLNB that had indicated non-positive SLNs in the inguinal region was 2.4% [65]. This indicated that there might be cases with positive lymph nodes in the pelvic region with non-positive lymph nodes in the inguinal region. This rate should not be underestimated and gives a reason for removing SLNs in the pelvic region.

On the other hand, there have been no published results of positive pelvic lymph nodes with negative inguinal SLNs for melanoma located below the knee. Pelvic lymph nodes for melanoma located below the knee were considered as secondary lymphatic basin because they were not stained blue and the radioactivity of the pelvic lymph nodes was significantly less than that of the inguinal nodes removed from the same patients [66]. By contrast, the pelvic lymph nodes for melanoma located on the trunk and thigh are possibly SLNs. In the case of melanoma below the knee in which there is a risk or difficulty in removing the pelvic lymph nodes, for example the case of pelvic adhesion after surgery in the pelvis, SLNB could be clinically avoided in terms of the cost-benefit relationship.

There are two approaches to removing the pelvic lymph nodes. One is the technique with incision above the inguinal ligament and the other is the technique with median incision in the lower abdomen. Each technique has an advantage. With median incision, it is easier to approach a deep site in the pelvic region such as the obturator area or the external iliac region near to the common iliac region. By contrast, it is easier and less invasive to approach the external iliac region near to the inguinal ligament with an incision above the inguinal ligament.

7. Lymph node dissection

Lymph node dissection is the primary management for regional lymph node metastasis. It is applied in cases of clinical metastasis, positive SLNs after SLNB and histological lymphatic invasion for a resected or biopsied primary lesion. Surgical technique, extent of dissection, morbidity and complication vary widely in the published literature. Although lymph node dissection has been a standard treatment and the technique has not drastically changed for many years, even now there is much controversy surrounding lymph node dissection. Some of the controversies will be mentioned in the following section.

8. Axillary lymph node dissection

Since the tumours on upper extremities drain to the axillary region, axillary dissection is necessary and performed by way of cure or local control of the metastatic melanoma in the upper extremities. On the area of axillary dissection, it is controversial whether a level 3 dissection should be included. Namm et al. reported that the local recurrence rate of axillary dissection including level 1 and 2was 5 % (14 cases out of 270 cases) [67]. Guggenheim et al. also reported a rate of 4.5% after axillary dissection which mainly included level 1 and 2 [68]. On the other hand, according to Kretschmer et al., the local recurrence rate was 9.5% (six out of 63 cases) after dissection including level 1,2 and 3. There is no direct evidence that dissection including level 3 is superior to dissection without level 3 [69].

The complication rate of dissection for level 1and 2 is less severe than that of dissection for level 1,2 and 3. The rates of infection and seroma after the former operation were 8% and 2% respectively, whereas those for the latter operation were 20% and 18% [67,70].

There are very few reported cases in which positive SLNs in level 3 were harvested except for our case. In addition, the lymph node ratio (LNR: the ratio of involved lymph nodes to total retrieved nodes in lymph node dissection) provides prognostic information [71-73]. There is very little possibility that positive lymph nodes are harvested only in level 3 without positive SLNs in level 1 or 2. Although there is data not on upper extremities but on lower extremities, a larger number of cases involved lymph nodes in the inguinal region with a higher rate of pelvic lymph node metastases [74]. This indicates that the number of superficial involved lymph nodes is related to the possibility of metastasis in the deep region. It has been reported that the size of SLN metastases predicts other nodal disease and survival in malignant melanoma [75,76]. Due to these findings, axillary dissection including level 3 is not always necessary when there are one or two micrometastatic lymph nodes in level 1, but it is necessary when a case falls under any of the following conditions:

- There is a relatively large clinically involved lymph node in level 1 or 2.
- There are many metastatic lymph nodes in level 1 or 2.
- There is negative SLNs in level 3 with positive lymph nodes in level 1 or 2.
- There are positive SLNs in level 3.
- There are involved lymph nodes in level 3 evaluated with radiological examination such as computed tomography (CT).

9. Inguinal and pelvic lymph node dissection

There is also controversy surrounding inguinal and pelvic lymph node dissection. The most controversial question is whether routine dissection with the primary tumour on lower extremities includes only a superficial inguinal lymph node dissection (SLND) or includes additional iliac and obturator lymph node dissection (deep pelvic/inguinal lymph node dissection : DLND) [77]. Like the axillary dissection, decision on the area to be dissected is difficult from the viewpoint of local control, overall survival and complications.

Hughes et al. reported that in cases of palpable inguinal lymph node metastases, pelvic lymph node recurrence occurred in one of 72 patients who had DLND and seven of 60 patients who had SLND (p=0.01) [74]. In this study, patients with one positive superficial node and those with more than one positive superficial node were 17% and 51% of 72 patients with DLND respectively. The number of positive superficial lymph nodes and the presence of extracapsular spread were significant prognostic factors for overall survival [77].

In addition, the patients who had DLND with the presence of pelvic lymph node metastases had significantly poorer five year survival than the patients without the pelvic lymph node metastases. However, there was no difference in postoperative morbidity between SLND and DLND [74]. Van der Ploeg et al. also reported that survival and local control did not differ for patients with palpable inguinal metastases treated by DLND or SLND and pelvic lymph node metastases was a significant prognostic factor [78]. In their series of 169 patients with palpable nodes in the inguinal region, five year estimated overall survival rates were 33% for DLND and 29% for SLND.

However, there is no evidence on how the recurrence affects quality of life when DLND is not performed and how the recurrence occurs in the pelvic region for melanomas on lower extremities. It is likely that enlargement of a tumour in pelvic region causes lymphedema, congestion of lower extremities, ileus and so on. Although these symptoms may be due to DLND, also it is possible that DLND increases patients' quality of life during the remaining life time by decreasing the risk of recurrence in the pelvic region. However, there is no evidence indicating this.

Cloquet's node is an indicator of pelvic lymph node metastases. According to Shen et al.'s study, positive pelvic lymph nodes were identified in the DLND specimen from 20 of 30 (67%) patients with a positive Cloquet's node and negative pelvic lymph nodes were identified from 27 of 35 (77%) patients with a negative Cloquet's node ($p=0.0019$) [79].

Pre-operative computed tomography (CT) is also a good tool to use in predicting the metastasis. Out of 44 patients with negative pelvic lymph nodes evaluated with pre-operative CT, 40 patients had in fact histologically negative pelvic lymph nodes (negative predictive value = 90.9%). On the other hand, the positive predictive value of pre-operative CT for pelvic metastases, was 59% [78].

A recent study shows pre-operative lymphoscintigraphy can be used to guide the extent of inguinal lymph node dissection [66]. Chu et al. reported on 42 cases of DLND with positive inguinal SLNs. The frequency of synchronous pelvic disease was five of 42 (11.9%) [80]. All five cases with pelvic disease had primary melanomas on extremities. Upon review on the lymphoscintigraphic findings, pelvic drainage was present in four of five cases with pelvic disease (80%) and in 18 of the 32 cases (56%) without pelvic disease, though neither was statistically significant. This strategy is based on the idea that when lymphoscintigraphy shows secondary nodes to be located in the next drainage basin, this basin should be included as the dissecting area [66]. More data is necessary to prove that treatment based on the idea improves the mortality and local control.

For now, there is no guideline on choosing between SLND and DLND. However, many findings provide useful information and surgeons should actively select DLND when a case falls under any of the following conditions:

- There is a palpable inguinal metastasis.
- There is more than one superficial lymph node metastasis.
- CT indicates metastatic pelvic lymph nodes.
- There is a Cloquet's lymph node metastasis.
- Lymphoschintigraphy indicates SLNs in the pelvic region with a superficial lymph node metastasis.

10. Molecular targeted therapy

Recent discoveries in cell signalling have provided greater understanding of the biology that underlines melanoma and these advances are being exploited to provide targeted drugs and new therapeutic approaches [81]. In some cases of ALM and mucosal melanoma, the mutations of KIT, a transmenbrane receptor tyrosine kinase, are reported and these mutations lead to marked expression of KIT in tumour cells. These cases have marked a tendency to respond to imatinib mesylate which inhibits tyrosine kinase. Although case reports are accumulating [82,83], more data, including long-term control and prognostic data, will be necessary to confirm the effect of this agent.

11. Conclusion

Controversies remain regarding the surgical treatment of ALM as described above, thus, international guidelines are yet to be established.

It is not still known whether the thickness of the nail tumour is the same as that on other sites because the distance between the nail bed and bone is very narrow and a mild degree of invasion can reach the bone easily. Considering the poor prognosis of cases with subungual melanoma, the tumour thickness of the subungual melanoma needs to be evaluated. Because biopsies of the nail bed may cause cosmetic and occasionally functional problems, surgeons may hesitate to do biopsies and lose a vital chance of early diagnosis. Suspicious lesions should be actively biopsied with fully informed consent. When taking a wait-and-see approach, careful observation is necessary so as not to overlook any minor change of dermoscopic findings.

On the excision margins around the primary lesion, 2cm is regarded as sufficient for invasive melanomas. Although some guidelines suggest a 0.5 cm margin for melanomas in situ, some data indicated that resection with 0.5 cm margin caused significant high rates of local recurrence. As mentioned here according to the report, a 1cm surgical margin is a better answer for melanomas in situ, except for tumours on cosmetic or functional sites such as the face or fingers. When an excision margin is less than 1cm, more careful histological examination and follow-up are necessary.

Although SLNB is the standard technique for the management of malignant melanoma, the definition of SLN itself has not been established. This creates differences in the extent of SLNB between each institute. SLNs in patients with melanomas on upper extremities are very rarely located in level 3. There are very few cases with positive SLNs only in level 3 without positive SLNs in level 1or 2, thus, the lymph nodes in level 3 can be regarded as secondary nodes for melanomas on upper extremities in almost all cases. Surgeons should also pay additional attention to SLNs in other sites such as supraclavicular, the cubital region and interval nodes.

There is controversy around the management of lymph nodes in the pelvic region. According to the literature, there were patients without positive SLNs in the inguinal region, who had metastatic lymph nodes in the pelvic region during follow-up. Thus, at the moment, it is better not to regard all pelvic lymph nodes as secondary nodes and not to exclude all pelvic lymph nodes from SLNs. There are no reported cases with primary melanomas below the knee in which only positive pelvic lymph nodes are present without positive inguinal lymph nodes. Thus, surgeons should decide whether to harvest pelvic lymph nodes taking into consideration the sites of primary lesion, Brethlow thickness and the possibility of complication on a case by case basis.

Whether or not dissection in cases with primary lesions on upper extremities should include the extent of level 3 is controversial. When a case falls under any of the lists described above, the dissection including level 3 should be actively performed. However, not all cases with positive lymph nodes in level 1 or 2 need to undergo dissection including level 3.

Similarly, it is difficult to choose between SLND and DLND in the case of primary melanomas on lower extremities. The cases which are likely to have metastatic lymph nodes in the pelvic region were mentioned above. It is better that the indication of DLND is determined by referring to the list.

Author details

Yoshitaka Kai and Sakuhei Fujiwara*

*Address all correspondence to: fujiwara@oita-u.ac.jp

Department of Dermatology, Faculty of Medicine, Oita University, Oita, Japan

References

[1] Sneyd M, Cox B. The control of melanoma in New Zealand. New Zealand Medical Journal 2006;119 U2169.

[2] Parkin DM, Bray F, Ferlay J, Pisani P. Global cancer statistics, 2002. CA: A Cancer Journal for Clinicians 2005; 55(2) 74-108

[3] Ishihara K, Saida T, Otsuka F, Yamazaki N; Prognosis and Statistical Investigation Committee of the Japanese Skin Cancer Society. Statistical profiles of malignant melanoma and other skin cancers in Japan: 2007 update. International Journal of Clinical Oncology 2008; 13(1) 33-41.

[4] Makredes M, Hui SK, Kimball AB. Melanoma in Hong Kong between 1983 and 2002: a decreasing trend in incidence observed in a complex socio-political and economic setting. Melanoma Research 2010; 20(5) 427-430.

[5] Chang JW. Cutaneous melanoma: Taiwan experience and literature review. Chang Gung Medical Journal 2010; 33(6) 602-612.

[6] Luk NM, Ho CL, Choi CL, Wong KH, Yu KH, Yeung WK. Clinicopathological features and prognostic factors of cutaneous melanoma among Hong Kong Chinese. Clinical and Experimental Dermatology 2004;29(6) 600-604.

[7] Chen YJ, Wu CY, Chen JT, Shen JL, Chen CC, Wang HC. Clinicopathologic analysis of malignant melanoma in Taiwan. Journal of American Academy of Dermatology 1999;41(6) 945-949.

[8] Bradford PT, Goldstein AM, McMaster ML, Tucker MA. Acral lentiginous melanoma. Incidence and survival patterns in the United States 1986-2005. Archives of Dermatology 2009;145(4) 427-434.

[9] Reed, RJ. New Concepts in Surgical Pathology of the Skin. New York: John Wiley & Sons; 1976.

[10] Reed RJ, Ichinose H, Krementz ET. Plantar lentiginous melanoma: a distinctive variant of human cutaneous malignant melanoma. American Journal of Surgical Pathology 1977;1(2) 131-143.

[11] Clark, W. H., Jr., Elder, D. E. & Van Horn, M. The biologic forms of malignant melanoma. Human Pathology 1986; 17(5) 443-450.

[12] Surveillance, Epidemiology and End Results (SEER) Program. National Cancer Institute, DCCPS,Surveillance Research Program, Cancer Statistics Branch. 2008 SEER*Stat Database. (www.seer.cancer.gov).

[13] Markovic SN, Erickson LA, Rao RD, et al. Malignant Melanoma in the 21st Century, Part 1:Epidemiology, Risk Factors, Screening, Prevention, and Diagnosis. Mayo Clinic Proceedings 2007;82(3) 364-380.

[14] Ishihara, K., Saida, T., Otsuka, F. & Yamazaki, N. Statistical profiles of malignant melanoma and other skin cancers in Japan. International Journal of Clinical Oncology 2007; 13(1) 33-41.

[15] Mi Ryung Roh, Jihyun Kim, and Kee Yang Chung. Treatment and Outcomes of Melanoma in Acral Location in Korean Patients. Yonsei Medical Journal 2010;51(4) 562-568.

[16] Krementz ET, Sutherland CM, Carter RD, Ryan RF. Malignant melanoma in the American Black. Annals of Surgery 1976; 183(5) 533-542.

[17] Paek SC, Sober AJ, Tsao H, Mihm MC Jr, Johnson TM. Cutaneous melanoma. In: Wolff K, Goldsmith LA, Katz SI, Gilchrest BA, Paller AS, Leffell DJ.(ed.) Fitzpatrick's dermatology in general medicine. 7th ed. New York: McGraw-Hill; 2008. p1134-1157.

[18] Metzger S, Ellwanger U, Stroebel W, Schiebel U, Rassner G, Fierlbeck G. Extent and consequences of physician delay in the diagnosis of acral melanoma. Melanoma Research 1998;8(2) 181-186.

[19] Phan A, Touzet S, Dalle S, Ronger-Savlé S, Balme B, Thomas L. Acral lentiginous melanoma: a clinicoprognostic study of 126 cases. British Journal of Dermatology 2006; 155(3) 561-569.

[20] Curtin JA, Fridlyand J, Kageshita T, Patel HN, Busam KJ, Kutzner H, Cho KH, Aiba S, Bröcker EB, LeBoit PE, Pinkel D, Bastian BC. Distinct sets of genetic alterations in melanoma. New England Journal of Medicine 2005; 353(20) 2135-2147.

[21] Curtin JA, Busam K, Pinkel D, Bastian BC. Somatic activation of KIT in distinct subtypes of melanoma. Journal of Clinical Oncology 2006; 24(26) 4340-4346.

[22] Krementz ET, Feed RJ, Coleman WP 3rd, Sutherland CM, Carter RD, Campbell M. Acral lentiginous melanoma. A clinicopathologic entity.Annals of Surgery 1982; 195(5) 632-645.

[23] Phan A, Dalle S, Touzet S, Ronger-Savlé S, Balme B, Thomas L.British Journal of Dermatology 2010; 162(4) 765-771.

[24] Saida T, Miyazaki A, Oguchi S, Ishihara Y, Yamazaki Y, Murase S, Yoshikawa S, Tsuchida T, Kawabata Y, Tamaki K. Archives of Dermatology 2004; 140(10) 1233-1238.

[25] Moloney FJ, Menzies SW. Key points in the dermoscopic diagnosis of hypomelanotic melanoma and nodular melanoma. Journal of Dermatology 2011; 38(1) 10-15.

[26] Miura S, Jimbow K. Clinical characteristics of subungual melanomas in Japan: case report and a questionnaire survey of 108 cases. Journal of Dermatology 1985; 12(5) 393-402.

[27] Seui M, Takematsu H, Hosokawa M, Obata M, Tomita Y, Kato T, Takahashi M, Mihm MC Jr. Acral melanoma in Japan. Journal of Investigative Dermatology 1983; 80(1 Suppl):56s-60s

[28] Patterson RH, Helwig EB. Subungual malignant melanoma: a clinical-pathologic study. Cancer 1980; 46(9) 2074-2087.

[29] Cohen T, Busam KJ, Patel A, Brady MS. Subungual melanoma: management considerations. American Journal of Surgery 2008; 195(2) 244-248.

[30] Di Chiacchio N, Hirata SH, Enokihara MY, Michalany NS, Fabbrocini G, Tosti A. Dermatologists' accuracy in early diagnosis of melanoma of the nail matrix. Archives of Dermatology 2010; 146(4) 382-387.

[31] Baran R, Kechijian P. Longitudinal melanonychia (melanonychia striata): diagnosis and management. Journal of the American Academy of Dermatology 1989; 21(6) 1165-1175.

[32] Ronger S, Touzet S, Ligeron C, Balme B, Viallard AM, Barrut D, Colin C, Thomas L. Dermoscopic examination of nail pigmentation. Archives of Dermatology 2002; 138(10) 1327-1333.

[33] Koga H, Saida T, Uhara H. Key point in dermoscopic differentiation between early nail apparatus melanoma and benign longitudinal melanonychia. Journal of Dermatology 2011; 38(1) 45-52.

[34] Jemec GB, Serup J. Ultrasound structure of the human nail plate. Archives of Dermatology 1989; 125(5) 643-646.

[35] Moehrle M, Metzger S, Schippert W, Garbe C, Rassner G, Breuninger H. "Functional" surgery in subungual melanoma. Dermatologic Surgery 2003; 29(4) 366-374.

[36] Breuninger H, Schlagenhauff B, Stroebel W, Schaumburg-Lever G, Rassner G. Patterns of local horizontal spread of melanomas: consequences for surgery and histopathologic investigation. American Journal of Surgical Pathology 1999; 23(12) 1493-1498.

[37] Khayat D, Rixe O, Martin G, Soubrane C, Banzet M, Bazex JA, Lauret P, Vérola O, Auclerc G, Harper P, Banzet P; French Group of Research on Malignant Melanoma. Surgical margins in cutaneous melanoma (2 cm versus 5 cm for lesions measuring less than 2.1-mm thick). Cancer 2003; 97(8) 1941-1946.

[38] Cohn-Cedermark G, Rutqvist LE, Andersson R, Breivald M, Ingvar C, Johansson H, Jönsson PE, Krysander L, Lindholm C, Ringborg U. Long term results of a randomized study by the Swedish Melanoma Study Group on 2-cm versus 5-cm resection margins for patients with cutaneous melanoma with a tumor thickness of 0.8-2.0 mm. Cancer 2000; 89(7) 1495-1501.

[39] Veronesi U, Cascinelli N, Adamus J, Balch C, Bandiera D, Barchuk A, Bufalino R, Craig P, De Marsillac J, Durand JC, et al. Thin stage I primary cutaneous malignant melanoma. Comparison of excision with margins of 1 or 3 cm. New England Journal of Medicine 1988; 318(18) 1159-1162.

[40] Kunishige JH, Brodland DG, Zitelli JA. Surgical margins for melanoma in situ. Journal of the American Academy of Dermatology 2012; 66(3) 438-444.

[41] Karakousis CP. Surgical treatment of malignant melanoma. Surgical Clinics of North America 1996; 76(6) 1299-1312.

[42] Ng AK, Jones WO, Shaw JH. Analysis of local recurrence and optimizing excision margins for cutaneous melanoma. British Journal of Surgery 2001; 88(1) 137-142.

[43] Testori A, Rutkowski P, Marsden J, Bastholt L, Chiarion-Sileni V, Hauschild A, Eggermont AM. Surgery and radiotherapy in the treatment of cutaneous melanoma. Annals of Oncology 2009; Suppl 6:vi22-29.

[44] Kenady DE, Brown BW, McBride CM. Excision of underlying fascia with a primary malignant melanoma: effect on recurrence and survival rates. Surgery 1982; 92(4) 615-618.

[45] Holmström H. Surgical management of primary melanoma. Seminars in Surgical Oncology 1992; 8(6) 366-369.

[46] Morton DL, Wen DR, Wong JH, Economou JS, Cagle LA, Storm FK, Foshag LJ, Cochran AJ. Technical details of intraoperative lymphatic mapping for early stage melanoma. Archives of Surgery 1992; 127(4) 392-399.

[47] Ross MI, Reintgen D, Balch CM. Selective lymphadenectomy: emerging role for lymphatic mapping and sentinel node biopsy in the management of early stage melanoma. Seminars in Surgical Oncology 1993; 219-223.

[48] Reintgen D, Cruse CW, Wells K, Berman C, Fenske N, Glass F, Schroer K, Heller R, Ross M, Lyman G, et al. The orderly progression of melanoma nodal metastases. Annals of Surgery 1994; 220(6) 759-767.

[49] Thompson JF, McCarthy WH, Bosch CM, O'Brien CJ, Quinn MJ, Paramaesvaran S, Crotty K, McCarthy SW, Uren RF, Howman-Giles R. Sentinel lymph node status as an indicator of the presence of metastatic melanoma in regional lymph nodes.Melanoma Research 1995; 5(4) 255-260.

[50] Morton DL, Thompson JF, Cochran AJ, Mozzillo N, Elashoff R, Essner R, Nieweg OE, Roses DF, Hoekstra HJ, Karakousis CP, Reintgen DS, Coventry BJ, Glass EC, Wang HJ; MSLT Group. Sentinel-node biopsy or nodal observation in melanoma. New England Journal of Medicine 2006; 355(13) 1307-1317.

[51] Morton DL, Cochran AJ, Thompson JF, Elashoff R, Essner R, Glass EC, Mozzillo N, Nieweg OE, Roses DF, Hoekstra HJ, Karakousis CP, Reintgen DS, Coventry BJ, Wang HJ; Multicenter Selective Lymphadenectomy Trial Group. Sentinel node biopsy for early-stage melanoma: accuracy and morbidity in MSLT-I, an international multicenter trial. Annals of Surgery 2005; 242(3) 302-313.

[52] Matsumoto T, Shibata S, Yasue S, Sakakibara A, Yokota K, Sawada M, Kono M, Kato K, Shimoyama Y, Tomita Y. Interval sentinel lymph nodes in patients with cutaneous melanoma: a single-institution study in Japan. Journal of Dermatology 2010; 37(7) 629-634.

[53] Manganoni AM, Farfaglia R, Sereni E, Farisoglio C, Pizzocaro C, Marocolo D, Gavazzoni F, Pavoni L, Calzavara-Pinton P. Interval sentinel lymph nodes: an unusual lo-

calization in patients with cutaneous melanoma. Dermatology Research and Practice 2011; Epub 2011 May 4.

[54] McMasters KM, Chao C, Wong SL, Wrightson WR, Ross MI, Reintgen DS, Noyes RD, Cerrito PB, Edwards MJ; Sunbelt Melanoma Trial Group. Interval sentinel lymph nodes in melanoma. Archives of Surgery 2002; 137(5) 543-9.

[55] Gannon CJ, Rousseau DL Jr, Ross MI, Johnson MM, Lee JE, Mansfield PF, Cormier JN, Prieto VG, Gershenwald JE. Accuracy of lymphatic mapping and sentinel lymph node biopsy after previous wide local excision in patients with primary melanoma. Cancer 2006;107(11) 2647-2652.

[56] Leong SP, Thelmo MC, Kim RP, Gokhale R, Rhee JY, Achtem TA, Morita E, Allen RE Jr, Kashani-Sabet M, Sagebiel RW. Delayed harvesting of sentinel lymph nodes after previous wide local excision of extremity melanoma. Annals of Surgical Oncology 2003; 10(2) 196-200.

[57] Uren RF, Howman-Giles RB, Shaw HM, Thompson JF, McCarthy WH. Lymphoscintigraphy in high-risk melanoma of the trunk: predicting draining node groups, defining lymphatic channels and locating the sentinel node. Journal of Nuclear Medicine 1993; 34(9) 1435-1440.

[58] Sumner WE 3rd, Ross MI, Mansfield PF, Lee JE, Prieto VG, Schacherer CW, Gershenwald JE. Implications of lymphatic drainage to unusual sentinel lymph node sites in patients with primary cutaneous melanoma. Cancer 2002; 95(2) 354-360.

[59] Porter GA, Ross MI, Berman RS, Lee JE, Mansfield PF, Gershenwald JE. Significance of multiple nodal basin drainage in truncal melanoma patients undergoing sentinel lymph node biopsy. Annals of Surgical Oncology 2000; 7(4) 256-261.

[60] Kosmidis C, Efthimiadis C, Anthimidis G, Grigoriou M, Vasiliadou K, Ioannidou G, Makedou F, Baka S. Acral lentiginous melanoma: a case control study and guidelines update. Case Reports in Medicine 2011; Epub 2011 Apr 6.

[61] Bagaria SP, Faries MB, Morton DL. Sentinel node biopsy in melanoma: technical considerations of the procedure as performed at the John Wayne Cancer Institute. Journal of Surgical Oncology 2010; 101(8) 669-676.

[62] Nieweg OE, Tanis PJ, Kroon BB. The definition of a sentinel node. Annals of Surgical Oncology 2001; 8(6) 538-541.

[63] Morton DL, Bostick PJ. Will the true sentinel node please stand?. Annals of Surgical Oncology 1999; 6(1) 12-14.

[64] McMasters KM, Reintgen DS, Ross MI, Wong SL, Gershenwald JE, Krag DN, Noyes RD, Viar V, Cerrito PB, Edwards MJ. Sentinel lymph node biopsy for melanoma: how many radioactive nodes should be removed?. Annals of Surgical Oncology 2001; 8(3) 192-197.

[65] Soteldo J, Ratto EL, Gandini S, Trifirò G, Mazzarol G, Tosti G, Rastrelli M, Verrecchia F, Baldini F, Testori A. Pelvic sentinel lymph node biopsy in melanoma patients: is it worthwhile?. Melanoma Research 2010; 20(2) 133-137.

[66] Kaoutzanis C, Barabás A, Allan R, Hussain M, Powell B. When should pelvic sentinel lymph nodes be harvested in patients with malignant melanoma?. Journal of Plastic, Reconstructive & Aesthetic Surgery 2012; 65(1) 85-90.

[67] Namm JP, Chang AE, Cimmino VM, Rees RS, Johnson TM, Sabel MS. Is a level III dissection necessary for a positive sentinel lymph node in melanoma?. Journal of Surgical Oncology 2012; 105(3) 225-228.

[68] Guggenheim MM, Hug U, Jung FJ, Rousson V, Aust MC, Calcagni M, Künzi W, Giovanoli P. Morbidity and recurrence after completion lymph node dissection following sentinel lymph node biopsy in cutaneous malignant melanoma. Annals of Surgery 2008; 247(4) 687-693.

[69] Kretschmer L, Preusser KP. Standardized axillary lymphadenectomy improves local control but not survival in patients with palpable lymph node metastases of cutaneous malignant melanoma. Langenbeck's Archives of surgery 2001; 386(6) 418-425.

[70] Kretschmer L, Thoms KM, Peeters S, Haenssle H, Bertsch HP, Emmert S. Postoperative morbidity of lymph node excision for cutaneous melanoma-sentinel lymphonodectomy versus complete regional lymph node dissection. Melanoma Research 2008; 18(1) 16-21.

[71] Xing Y, Badgwell BD, Ross MI, Gershenwald JE, Lee JE, Mansfield PF, Lucci A, Cormier JN. Lymph node ratio predicts disease-specific survival in melanoma patients. Cancer 2009; 115(11) 2505-2513.

[72] Spillane AJ, Cheung BL, Winstanley J, Thompson JF. Lymph node ratio provides prognostic information in addition to american joint committee on cancer N stage in patients with melanoma, even if quality of surgery is standardized. Annals of Surgery 2011; 253(1) 109-115.

[73] Spillane AJ, Winstanley J, Thompson JF. Lymph node ratio in melanoma: A marker of variation in surgical quality?. Cancer 2009; 115(11) 2384-2387.

[74] Hughes TM, A'Hern RP, Thomas JM. Prognosis and surgical management of patients with palpable inguinal lymph node metastases from melanoma. British Journal of Surgery 2000; 87(7) 892-901.

[75] Pearlman NW, McCarter MD, Frank M, Hurtubis C, Merkow RP, Franklin WA, Gonzalez R, Lewis K, Roaten JB, Robinson WA. Size of sentinel node metastases predicts other nodal disease and survival in malignant melanoma. Americal Journal of Surgery 2006; 192(6) 878-881.

[76] Carlson GW, Murray DR, Lyles RH, Staley CA, Hestley A, Cohen C. The amount of metastatic melanoma in a sentinel lymph node: does it have prognostic significance?. Annals of Surgical Oncology 2003; 10(5) 575-581.

[77] Mack LA, McKinnon JG. Controversies in the management of metastatic melanoma to regional lymphatic basins. Journal of Surgical Oncology 2004; 86(4) 189-199.

[78] van der Ploeg AP, van Akkooi AC, Schmitz PI, van Geel AN, de Wilt JH, Eggermont AM, Verhoef C. Therapeutic surgical management of palpable melanoma groin metastases: superficial or combined superficial and deep groin lymph node dissection. Annals of Surgical Oncology 2011; 18(12) 3300-3308.

[79] Shen P, Conforti AM, Essner R, Cochran AJ, Turner RR, Morton DL. Is the node of Cloquet the sentinel node for the iliac/obturator node group?. Cancer Journal 2000; 6(2) 93-97.

[80] Chu CK, Delman KA, Carlson GW, Hestley AC, Murray DR. Inguinopelvic lymphadenectomy following positive inguinal sentinel lymph node biopsy in melanoma: true frequency of synchronous pelvic metastases. Annals of Surgical Oncology 2011; 18(12) 3309-3315.

[81] Gray-Schopfer V, Wellbrock C, Marais R. Melanoma biology and new targeted therapy. Nature 2007; 445(7130) 851-857.

[82] [82]Yamaguchi M, Harada K, Ando N, Kawamura T, Shibagaki N, Shimada S. Marked response to imatinib mesylate in metastatic acral lentiginous melanoma on the thumb. Clinical and Experimental Dermatology 2011; 36(2) 174-177.

[83] Itoh M, Goto A, Wakasugi H, Yoshida Y, Matsunaga Y, Fujii K, Suzuki K, Yonezawa K, Abe T, Arimura Y, Shinomura Y. Anorectal melanoma with a KIT-activating mutation, which is a target for tyrosine kinase inhibitor. International Journal of Clinical Oncology 2011; 16(4) 428-434.

Chapter 18

Sentinel Lymph Node Biopsy for Melanoma and Surgical Approach to Lymph Node Metastasis

Yasuhiro Nakamura and Fujio Otsuka

Additional information is available at the end of the chapter

http://dx.doi.org/10.5772/53625

1. Introduction

The surgical approach to cutaneous melanoma patients with clinically uninvolved regional lymph nodes has been controversial. Although most patients with melanoma have no clinically palpable nodal disease at the time of presentation, some patients whose primary tumor increases in thickness, has ulceration, and shows a high mitotic rate histologically harbor clinically undetectable regional lymph node metastasis[1].

While some authors have advocated wide excision of the primary tumor with elective lymph node dissection (ELND), others had recommended excision of the primary site alone and therapeutic lymph node dissection (TLND) only when clinical nodal disease is present. ELND is based on the concept that metastasis arises by passage of the tumor from the primary to the regional lymph nodes and distant sites, in which case early LND will prevent this metastatic progression. In contrast, TLND, which is a "watch and wait" approach, suggests that regional lymph node metastases are markers for disease progression and that hematogenous distant metastases could occur without lymph node metastasis. Four randomized prospective studies comparing ELND with TLND were reported[2-5]. The earlier 2 studies conducted in the 1970s demonstrated no overall survival advantage for ELND[2, 3]. Accordingly, ELND was once contested and largely abandoned. Thereafter, the latter 2 studies conducted in the 1990s suggested the tendency, albeit statistically insignificant, that patients with early regional metastases may benefit from ELND[4, 5]. However, in most melanoma patients with no clinical nodal disease, microscopic nodal disease is absent at presentation. These patients cannot benefit from ELND; if ELND were to be performed, they would suffer from the cost, time, and morbidity of an unnecessary operation.

With respect to this controversy surrounding ELND, the technique of lymphatic mapping and sentinel lymph node biopsy (SLNB) was introduced as a minimally invasive method for detection of microscopic regional lymph node metastases in the early 1990s[6]. Lymphatic mapping is based on the concept that the lymphatic drainage from the skin to the regional lymph node basins runs in an orderly, stepwise fashion. These lymphatic drainage patterns would be the same as the dissemination of melanoma through the lymphatic system and therefore predict the routes of metastatic spread of melanoma cells to the regional lymph nodes (Fig. 1). Morton et al. first reported the details of the SLN technique using intradermal blue dye injection around the primary site and reported that the SLN identification rate was 82% among 237 patients[6], which was considered a high identification rate at that time. In the early 1990s, several authors evaluated this concept by performing synchronous ELND at the time of SLNB[7-9]. A "false-negative" SLN was defined as microscopic metastasis in a non-SLN despite the SLN showing no metastasis. These studies indicated that 5.8% of patients had a false-negative SLN. In addition, Gershenwald et al. reported that only 4.1% (10/243) of patients with a histologically negative SLN developed a nodal recurrence in the previously mapped basin during a follow-up period of over 3 years[10]. This low false-negative rate supported the SLN concept described above.

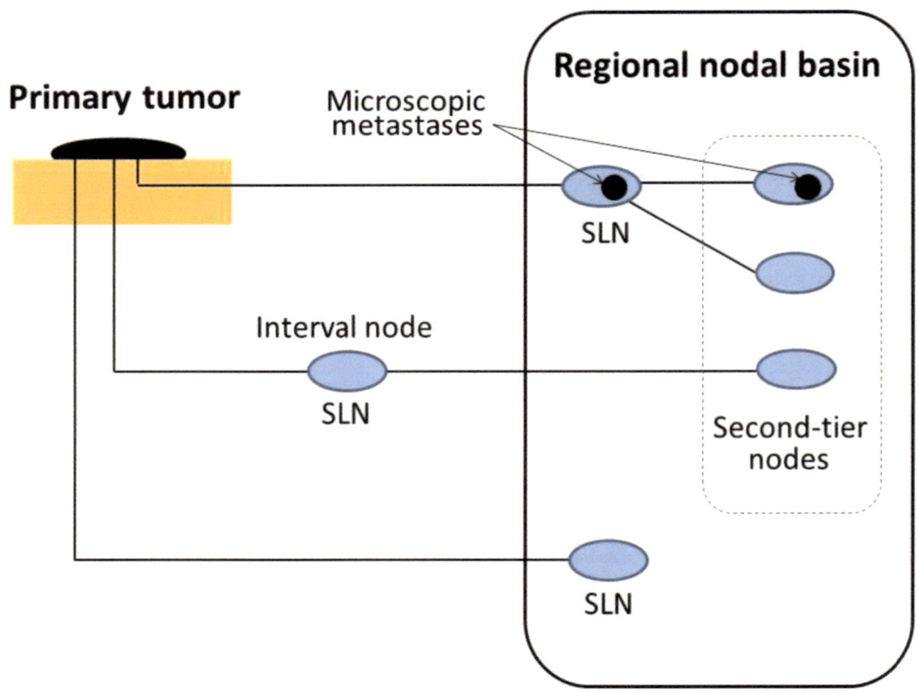

Figure 1. Lymphatic drainage from a primary tumor to sentinel lymph nodes. A sentinel node is sometimes located between the primary tumor and the regional nodal basins, in which case it is called an interval (unusual, in-transit, ectopic) node. If the SLN has microscopic nodal metastasis, some of the second-tier nodes may also have metastasis.

2. Technical advances in SLNB

Although the initial SLN identification rate using blue dye injections alone was approximately 82%[6], the advent of lymphoscintigraphy and the intraoperative hand-held gamma probe drastically improved the SLN identification rate. Studies comparing blue dye injection alone with combined techniques using blue dye, lymphoscintigraphy, and an intraoperative hand-held gamma probe showed a significant increase in SLN identification of up to 99% with the combined techniques[11, 12], which has come to be recognized as the standard technique of SLNB (Fig. 2). This combined technique also enables the surgeon to identify the interval (unusual, in-transit, ectopic) nodes located outside the named regional nodal basins (Fig. 3)[13-17]. The rate of interval SLN identification is reported to be approximately 5% to 10%, and the rate of microscopic metastasis in the interval nodes is approximately the same as that in the SLN in the regional nodal basins[14].

However, SLNB in the head and neck has particular problems because the lymphatic drainage in the head and neck is much more complex than those in the axillary and inguinal regions. Furthermore, the cervical and parotid lymph nodes are smaller and located in sites that are not easily accessible, for example in the parotid gland, through which the facial nerve passes [18, 19]. In addition, it is sometimes difficult to detect the lymphatic drainage and SLN with lymphoscintigraphy because the SLN is often close to the highly radioactive site where the tracer was injected, the so-called shine-through phenomenon[18, 19]. In addition, in some cases the naked eye cannot confirm that an SLN has been dyed blue even after injection of the blue dye because of the short staining period for blue dye in cervical SLNs resulting from the rapid and complex cervical lymphatic flow[19]. In our experience too, over half of the SLNs did not show any blue staining. Furthermore, some authors reported a high false-negative rate of up to 44%, which leads to increased morbidity[20-22]. This high rate may be caused by partially obstructed lymphatic vessels that do not allow for smooth flow of nanocolloids with a size of 6 to 12 nm[23]. Although several authors have reported a high identification rate in SLNB for head and neck melanoma[24-26], the identification rate of SLNs for the standard technique in the cervical region is generally less than that in the inguinal or axillary regions. In the MSLT-I trial reported by Morton et al., the SLN identification rate in the cervical region (84.5%) was clearly lower than that in the inguinal (99.3%) or axillary regions (96.6%)[18].

Several studies on the SLNB technique using indocyanine green (ICG) injection in skin cancer patients have demonstrated high SLN detection and identification rates, although these studies involved mainly axillary and inguinal SLNBs and only a small number of cervical SLNBs[23, 27-29]. ICG is a diagnostic reagent used in various examinations such as examination for cardiac output or hepatic function and retinal angiography. It has a size of only 2.1 nm, binds with albumin, and generates a peak wavelength of 840 nm near-infrared fluorescence when excited with 765-nm light[30]. Using a near-infrared camera intraoperatively, it is possible to observe the ICG as a subcutaneous lymphatic flow as well as SLNs in the fluorescence images after intradermal injection of ICG around the primary tumor. (Fig. 4) In our experience, the mean and median numbers of SLNs per basin were higher in the ICG group than in the standard-technique group. The small size of ICG allows a smooth flow along the lymphatic vessels. It may lead to detection of SLNs not detectable by lymphoscintigraphy (Fig. 4C, D) owing to poor flow of the radioactive tracer and may reduce the false-negative rate. Indeed, Stoffels et al. reported that 2 of 11 additional SLNs that were only identified by the ICG technique showed microscopic metastasis[23].

In addition, the recently introduced hybrid single-photon emission computed tomography with computed tomography (SPECT/CT) can visualize the exact anatomic location of the SLN and second-tier nodes, which would be of great help in identifying the SLN, especially those in the head and neck region[31, 32], as well as the interval nodes.

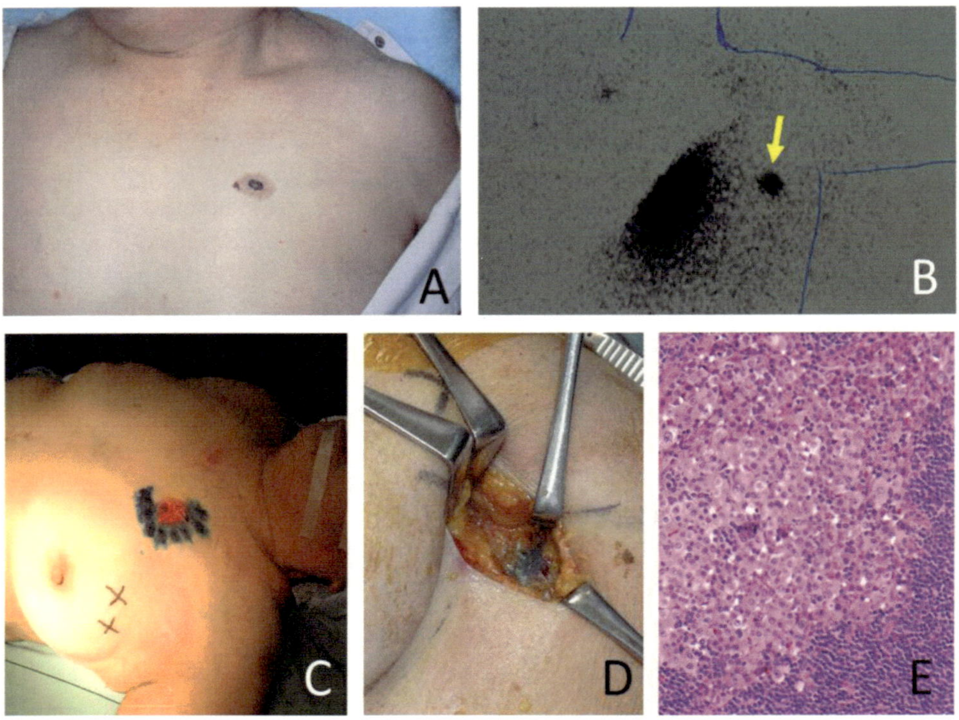

Figure 2. The technique of lymphatic mapping and sentinel lymph node biopsy (SLNB). (A) Primary melanoma on the left chest. (B) Lymphoscintigraphy shows accumulation of 99Tc-tin colloid which was intradermally injected around the primary tumor in the left axilla (arrow). (C) Intradermal injection of 2% isosulfan blue injection around the primary site. (D) The exploration of the location of SLN using a hand-held gamma-probe and identification of a blue-stained SLN. (E) Histopathologic detection of microscopic nodal metastasis.

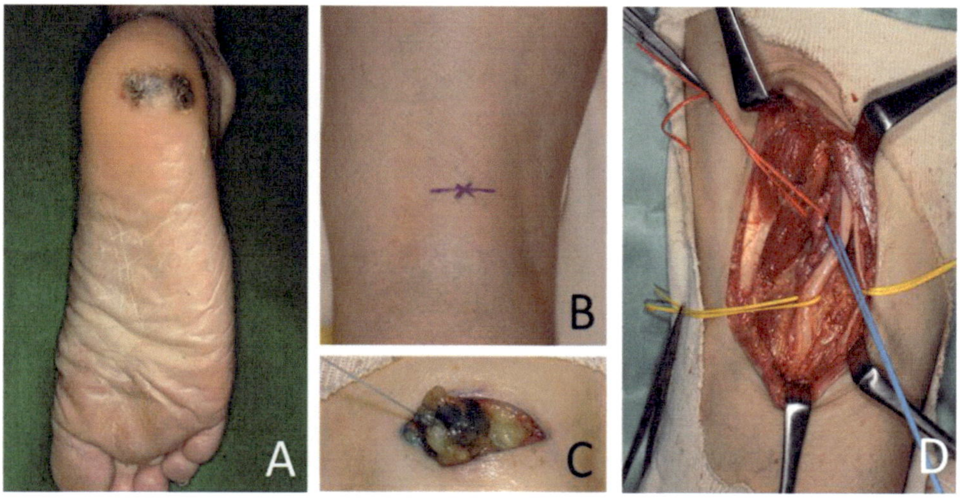

Figure 3. Detection of interval SLN. (A) Primary melanoma on the right heel. (B) Lymphoscintigraphy revealed accumulation in the right popliteal fossa. (C) Radioactive and blue-stained popliteal node, which had microscopic metastasis. (D) Popliteal lymph node dissection was performed.

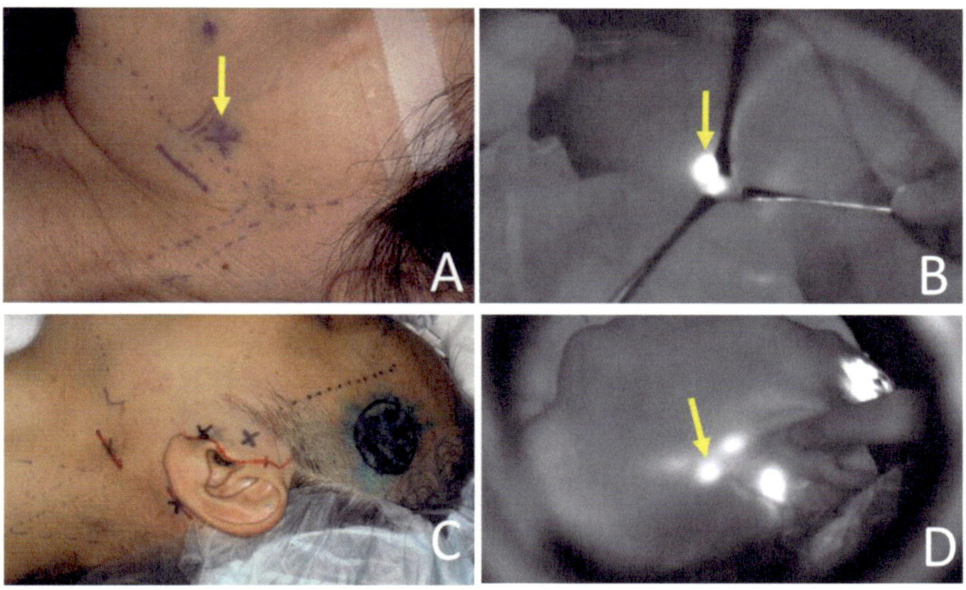

Figure 4. SLNB using ICG. (A) SLNB for melanoma of the nose. The X mark on the left mandible indicates accumulation of radioisotope (arrow). (B) A fluorescent submandibular SLN is visible through the incision using the near-infrared camera (arrow). (C) SLNB for melanoma of the left temporal region. The X marks indicate accumulation of radioisotope. (D) An additional fluorescent SLN (arrow), which was not detected by lymphoscintigraphy, is observed through the overlying skin.

3. Does SLNB-guided early lymph node dissection improve survival rate?

Whether patients who undergo complete lymph node dissection (CLND) after confirmation of a positive SLN have a better prognosis than patients who undergo TLND after occurrence of clinical nodal disease is controversial. The results of retrospective studies that compared survival after CLND for a positive SLN with survival after TLND for clinical nodal disease remain controversial. Several retrospective studies, including a multicentric study and a matched control study, demonstrated a significant survival benefit for patients who underwent CLND for a positive SLN[33, 34]. In addition, a survival benefit was also demonstrated for patients whose primary tumor thickness was between 1 mm and 4 mm and who underwent CLND for a positive SLN[35]. In contrast, other retrospective studies demonstrated no significant difference in overall survival between patients who underwent CLND for a positive SLN and those who underwent TLND for clinical nodal disease[36, 37].

The third interim analysis of the Multicenter Selective Lymphadenectomy Trial 1 (MLST-1), the only randomized control trial with available results, failed to demonstrate a 5-year survival advantage for the SLNB group when compared with the observation group and only a disease-free survival benefit for the SLNB group[38]. In a subgroup analysis, patients who underwent CLND for a positive SLN showed an improvement in 5-year survival of about 20% when compared with patients who underwent TLND after nodal observation and subsequently occurring clinical nodal disease (72.3% vs 52.4%; P=.004). The nodal recurrence was lower in patients who had a negative SLN (4.0%) than in those who had a positive SLN but were observed without early CLND (15.6%). From these results, the authors concluded that microscopic metastasis would develop within the lymph nodes and that early LND may lead to accurate staging and survival improvement.

However, whether SLNB and/or CLND would be a therapeutic procedure remains unclear, and several authors have questioned this conclusion from the results of the MLST-1. First, they claim that it was inappropriate to conclude that early CLND would improve survival because this result was based on a postrandomization subgroup analysis[39]. Second, they question whether all microscopic metastases will develop into clinical nodal disease. That is, some microscopic metastases may show indolent behavior and not develop into clinical nodal disease for a long time. In that case, comparison of the nodal recurrence rate between the 2 arms described above is an inappropriate analysis[37]. As a result, all that is currently clear is that SLNB can provide staging information that predicts prognosis and may impact clinical management.

4. Complete lymph node dissection

4.1. The role of complete lymph node dissection

The therapeutic value of CLND and appropriate selection of patients for CLND remain questionable. The role of CLND in patients with positive SLNs is also a clinically important question because only 10% to 25% of patients with positive SLNs will have additional microscopic metastasis in non-SLNs[40-42], which means that approximately 80% of patients with positive SLNs may be spared CLND. Several authors categorized the SLN as several variables and tried to find a reliable indicator of non-SLN status[43, 44]. However, it remains unclear what size of microscopic metastasis of the SLN or which histopathologic location of metastasis in the SLN, such as subcapsular, parenchymal, multifocal, and extensive, would be a reliable indicator of non-SLN status[44].

The choice of the extent of CLND is ultimately decided by the individual surgeon. Few specific recommendations are available in the published guidelines, with the common description being "a thorough dissection" and reports of low levels of evidence supporting the appropriate surgical extent of CLND of the cervical, axillary, and inguinal regions[45-47].

5. Neck dissection

5.1. Extent of dissection and regional recurrence rate

The purpose of neck dissection is to control regional disease; it has little impact on overall survival. However, the extent of neck dissection is still controversial and various extents of neck dissection have been advocated by several authors. Radical neck dissection (RND) including removal of level I-V (Fig. 5A) and nonlymphatic tissue such as the sternocleidomastoid muscle, the internal jugular vein, and the spinal accessary nerve has been the gold standard for neck dissection for melanoma[48]. Despite extensive areas of dissection, O'Brien et al. reported that regional control with RND was unsatisfactory, with regional recurrence of 28% in patients with all nodal disease and of 34% in patients with clinical nodal disease[48].

Generally, RND is associated with significant morbidity. Therefore, some authors have considered modified RND (MRND) or functional neck dissection including preservation of any or all of the sternocleidomastoid muscle, the internal jugular vein, and the spinal accessory nerve[49, 50]. In studies of patients with clinical nodal disease, several authors demonstrated that regional recurrence rates were 14-32% after RND, 0% after MRND, and 23% to 29% after selective neck dissection (SND), which is not statistically significant among the groups[51-53]. Byers also reported a 16% recurrence rate after MRND[54]. From these studies, MRND has been advocated even in the setting of clinical nodal disease.

In addition, as an even more selective approach, the lymphatic drainage patterns of head and neck melanoma have been described by O'Brien et al. based on a consecutive series of over 270 neck dissections and parotidectomies (Fig. 5B)[52]. As described above, although several authors reported relatively high regional recurrence rates of 23% to 29% after SND, these studies include clinical N2-N3 (multiple involved nodes) disease, which will have a higher risk of recurrence than N1 disease[51, 52]. In a study of 37 consecutive patients with clinically N1 neck disease reported by White et al., 6 patients underwent RND, 24, MRND, and 7, SND. None of the 3 groups had any cases of local recurrence during a mean follow-up of 46 months[55], indicating that SND may be an alternative to RND or MRND for the clinically N1 neck in melanoma[55].

Furthermore, the appropriate extent of dissection is also unclear in patients with positive SLNs. Pu et al. reported 23 consecutive patients with positive SLNs who underwent MRND or superficial parotidectomy. Of those patients, 21 (91.3%) had no additional positive non-SLNs and only 2 (8.7 %) had 1 additional positive non-SLN[56]. No patient developed a regional local recurrence during a mean follow-up period of 23.7 months. The low prevalence of additional positive non-SLNs in MRND specimens suggests that when microscopic SLN metastasis exists, nodal disease is confined to the SLN alone in most patients [56] and SND may be selected.

As for parotid gland nodes, patients with clinically palpable parotid nodes have a 28% to 58% risk of microscopic metastasis in the cervical nodes[57-59]. Although neck dissection should be included when clinical parotid disease is present, the need to treat the parotid nodes when clinical nodal disease of the neck is present is controversial. In such cases, many surgeons selectively perform superficial parotidectomy combined with a neck dissection based on O'Brien's lymphatic map (Fig. 5B) or the protocol of the individual institute[60].

However, the lymphatic drainage in the head and neck is generally complex and 8% to 43% of patients have unexpected drainage patterns in the occipital, postauricular, and contralateral nodes (Fig. 5A).[26, 61-64] Therefore, SND should be tailored to the individual patient according to the location of the SLN and second-tier nodes.

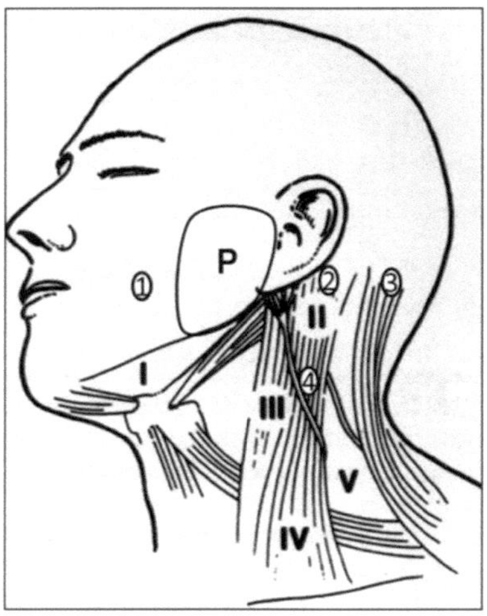

P: Parotid node
1: Buccal node
2: Postauricular node
3: Occipital node
4: Superficial cervical node

A

Primary site of melanoma	Predicted lymphatic drainage
Anterior scalp	I-III or IV, P
Coronal scalp	I-V, P
Posterior scalp	I-V, 3
Preauricular	I-III or IV, P
Ear	II-V, 3
Upper face	I-III or IV, P
Nose	I-III or IV, P
Lower face	I-III or IV, P
Anterior upper neck	I-III or IV, P
Anterior lower neck	II-V
Coronal upper neck	I-V, P
Coronal lower neck	III-V
Posterior upper neck	II-V, 3
Posterior lower neck	III-V

B

Figure 5. A)Lymphatic anatomy of the head and neck showing the 5 major lymph node levels and superficial nodes (B) Predicted lymphatic drainage and extent of neck dissection recommended by O'Brien et al.

5.2. Complication rate and technical variables

Significant complications associated with radical neck dissection may include injury to the facial and spinal accessory nerves, chylous fistula, and skin flap necrosis[65]. Although it is generally accepted that the rate of morbidity is reduced by MRND and further reduced by SND, detailed complication rates in the treatment of melanoma have not been reported. According to the literature, neck dissection and parotidectomy is usually safe when appropriately planned preoperatively and when performed by well-experienced surgeons.

Technical variables mainly include skin incisions. Commonly used incisions are single Y, T, or double Y-type incisions, which provide optimal exposure of the entire neck. However, the edge of the flap sometimes has a poor blood supply and breakdown can result in the exposure of the major vessels. The three-point suture line gives a high incidence of postoperative scar contracture[66, 67]. The Mcfee incision was designed to eliminate the three-point exposure line, giving a good cosmetic result. However, the exposure is difficult, particularly in a short fat neck, and excessive traction of the skin flaps can result in damaging of the skin edges[67]. Large, single incisions such as the curtain flap, apron flap, U-flap, and Hockey stick incision offer a good blood supply and most of the scar lies within the relaxed skin tension lines of the neck[68]. Each incision should be selected appropriately according to the extent of the neck dissection.

6. Axillary lymph node dissection

6.1. Extent of dissection and regional recurrence

Axillary LND for patients with melanoma is performed for local control and staging[69]; the therapeutic value is still unclear. The axillary nodes are divided into level I, II, and III nodes. Level I nodes are lateral to the lateral edge of the pectoralis minor muscle. Level II nodes are between the medial and lateral edges of the pectoralis minor muscle. Level III nodes are medial to the medial edge of the pectorarlis minor muscle, in the apex of the axilla. The generally recommended extent of dissection is from level I to III nodes because of the various drainage patterns in the second-tier nodes as well as the potentially increased risk of recurrence with a lesser dissection[70, 71]. Several authors recommended a more extensive dissection including the supraaxillary fat pad because approximately 14% of patients will have metastatic nodes in this area[69, 72]. In contrast, several authors have questioned whether a level III dissection is necessary in all melanoma patients with a positive SLN and advocated that level III dissection should be included only when suspicious nodes are present in this level [73-75]. Namm et al. also advocated that level I and II dissection should be performed for positive-SLN patients because of the low regional recurrence rate and low postoperative morbidity and concluded that level III dissection is not necessary for regional control in patients with microscopic metastasis[76].

As for the regional recurrence rate, unfortunately, most studies grouped together all of the dissected levels. Several authors reported a 10% to 19% regional recurrence rate during about a 30-month median follow-up[77-79]; however, in all 3 of those studies, the extent of dissection was not documented. Veenstra et al. reported a 4% regional recurrence rate and documented which levels were included when axillary LND was performed; however, they did not tease out the axillary recurrence rate specifically[80]. In the case of level I and II dissection for patients with a positive SLN, a low recurrence rate of 4% during a median follow-up of approximately 39-month was reported[76].

6.2. Complication rate and technical variables

Wrightson et al. reported a 19.9% complication rate among 262 patients undergoing axillary LND, most of which was thought to be level I-III dissection, for a positive SLN[81]. Several authors reported a complication rate of 14% to 21% for wound infection and of 19% to 36% for lymphocele when performing level I–III dissections[82, 83]. In contrast, Numm et al. reported that postoperative complications occurred in 11% of patients, with infectious complications in 8% when performing level I and II dissection. However, comparative studies of level I-II dissection with and level I-III dissection have not been published. Although the definition of lymphedema varies among studies, a long-term lymphedema rate was reported to be 1% to 12%[72, 75, 81].

Evidence of an optimal surgical technique for axillary LND has not been shown. As technical modifications, 2 incisions are mainly used. One is a transverse incision from the lateral edge of the pectoralis major muscle to the border of the latissimus dorsi muscle, and the other is an extended incision following the contour of the pectoralis major into the axillary apex and then down the medial arm[72, 84]. However, these incision variables would not affect the complication rate. Lawton et al. advocated preservation of the pectoralis major, the interpectoral, and the latissimus dorsi fascia during axillary LND to try to reduce lymphedema[84]. Over 110 elective and therapeutic fascia-preserving axillary LNDs developed a 5% incidence of long-term lymphedema, which is the same as or slightly lower than the incidence rates reported by the studies [72, 75, 81] described above. Optimal surgical exposure for level III dissection sometimes requires transection of the pectoralis minor muscle, and several authors suggested routine en bloc dissection of the pectoralis minor for TLND[16, 72, 75]. The long thoracic and thoracodorsal nerves are routinely preserved, although the intercostobrachial nerves are often sacrificed in TLND[73, 75]. As a result, no modifications clearly improve the complication rate, and only the extent of dissection impacts the complication rate.

7. Ilioinguinnal lymph node dissection

7.1. Extent of dissection and regional recurrence rate

The dissection areas subject to most controversy are inguinal LND alone or ilioinguinal LND (inguinal LND + iliac/obturator (pelvic) LND). When iliac or obturator node involvement is suspected clinically or radiologically, additional pelvic LND is generally recommended[74, 85-87]. For patients with clinically palpable nodal disease in the inguinal region alone, additional pelvic LND has not been widely accepted because of the lack of overall survival advantage[88, 89]. However, some authors advocated ilioinguinal LND because the rate of pelvic lymph node involvement in patients with palpable inguinal disease is 27% to 52%[87-92]. In a study of predictive factors for pelvic nodal status, Strobbe et al. reported that the Cloquet node has a limited sensitivity of 65% to predict involvement of the pelvic nodes and that the negative predictive value is 78%. In patients with clinical inguinal nodal disease, a tumor-positive Cloquet node had a 69% risk (positive predictive value) of additional positive nodes[91]. They also showed that the number of positive nodes in the inguinal region is not a reliable predictive factor for the pelvic nodal status, with a sensitivity of 41% and a negative predictive value of 78%[91].

Furthermore, the extent of dissection is more controversial in positive inguinal SLN patients. Van der Ploeg et al. reported that there is no lymphatic drainage to the inferior lateral zone, which is just lateral to the femoral artery and inferior to the level of saphenofemoral junction in the inguinal area, in patients with a positive SLN and advocated that this area need not be included in LND for such patients[93]. Pelvic nodes also seem unlikely to be involved when an inguinal SLN shows only microscopic metastasis[94, 95]. Several authors reported that 9% to 17 % of patients with a positive inguinal SLN also have positive pelvic nodes when ilioinguinal LND is performed[96-98]. In addition, a study evaluating lymphatic flow using lymphoscintigraphy and/or SPECT/CT demonstrated that over 50% of patients with a positive SLN showed second-tier nodal drainage to the pelvic nodes[93]. This study suggests that a selective pelvic LND based on the location of the second-tier nodes may be appropriate in positive SLN patients[93, 99].

As for the regional recurrence rate, published recurrence rates after inguinal or ilioinguinal LND for patients with clinical nodal disease is 0% to 33.6% (inguinal LND: 11.7%-13%; ilioinguinal LND: 0%-17.9%)[74, 85-89]. Sterne et al. reported that patients with palpable nodal disease who underwent inguinal LND alone had a regional recurrence rate of 12.5% (2 of 16 patients), whereas for those who underwent ilioinguinal LND, it was 0% (0 of 25 patients) [85]. Pearlman et al. reported a modification of inguinal LND that does not violate the femoral sheath. However, a 16% rate of regional recurrence was reported[100].

7.2. Complication rate and technical variables

In the field of urology, classical inguinal LND has traditionally been associated with an 80% to 100% risk of surgical morbidity[101]. In the treatment of melanoma, several authors reported that 20% to 77% of patients who underwent inguinal LND had postoperative morbidity such as skin necrosis and wound dehiscence (7%-55%), wound infection (5%-15%), lymphocele/seroma (2%-46%), and lymphedema (5%-64%).[102] Although concerns have been raised about the potential for increased morbidity in patients undergoing an additional pelvic LND[87, 103], the addition of pelvic LND to inguinal LND did not significantly increase the risk for postoperative wound complication[87, 101, 104, 105]. However, lymphedema was more common after inguinal LND alone in some studies, although 1 study specifically evaluating the incidence of lymphedema found no difference between the 2 procedures[87, 106, 107]. The lack of consensus about the complications of additional pelvic LND may suggest that when clinically indicated, concern about increased morbidity should not be a reason to avoid ilioinguinal LND, although patients may suffer from the operating time and cost.

The commonly described technical variables of ilioinguinal LND include different type of skin incision, thick skin flap, preservation of the large saphenous vein, transposition of the sartorius muscle over the femoral vessels, continuity dissection with division of the inguinal ligament, and trimming of the skin edges at the time of closure[108].

Several skin incisions are used: a Lazy-S incision from just medial to the anterior superior iliac spine to the inferior margin of the femoral triangle, paired oblique incisions (Fig. 6A), or an oblique/transverse incision above the inguinal crease with a longitudinal incision below and a skin bridge between[73, 84, 100]. Lazy-S incision provides optimal exposure and less subcutaneous lymphatic disruption[108]. In contrast, paired oblique incisions or an oblique/transverse incision can avoid an incision in the inguinal crease to reduce skin necrosis and wound dehiscence[84]. Recently, however, Spillane et al. reported minimal-access 3- to 6-cm-long paired incisions above and below the inguinal ligament, which showed no significant difference in wound and lymphedema complications[109]. A thick skin flap elevated at the level of the Scarpa fascia may improve skin necrosis and wound dehiscence rates; however, a 26% to 34% rate of skin necrosis and wound infection was reported[84, 100]. The preservation of the saphenous vein and the sartorius transposition flap for vessel coverage were designed to improve lymphedema rates, with no incidence of lymphedema[100]. When performing ilioinguinal LND, technical variables include a continuity dissection by dividing the inguinal ligament or an abdominal wall incision above and parallel to the inguinal ligament (Fig. 6B) to expose the retroperitoneal space[73, 84, 86]. Although advantages of inguinal ligament division include optimal exposure and possible continuity dissection, the main disadvantage is possible long-term abdominal wall weakness that may lead to abdominal incisional hernia. As another modification, Lawton et al. advocated fascia-preserving ilioinguinal LND, which is similar to the modified axillary dissection described above in the section on axillary LND, and the long-term lymphedema rate was 14%. Video-assisted endoscopic inguinal LND is currently investigated as a minimally invasive and less morbid approach but is not widely used[110, 111].

Despite such modifications, a comparative study reported by Sabel et al. demonstrated no significant difference in wound and lymphedema complications between modified inguinal LND (incision avoiding the inguinal crease, saphenous vein preservation, or sartorius transposition) and conventional inguinal LND[107]. However, although insignificant, saphenous vein preservation decreased the lymphedema rate from 30% to 13% and the wound complication rate from 20% to 7%. An incision avoiding the inguinal crease also decreased the wound complication rate from 21% to 9%, which is also statistically insignificant. Thus, these modifications seem to offer promise in decreasing morbidity.

http://dx.doi.org/10.5772/53625

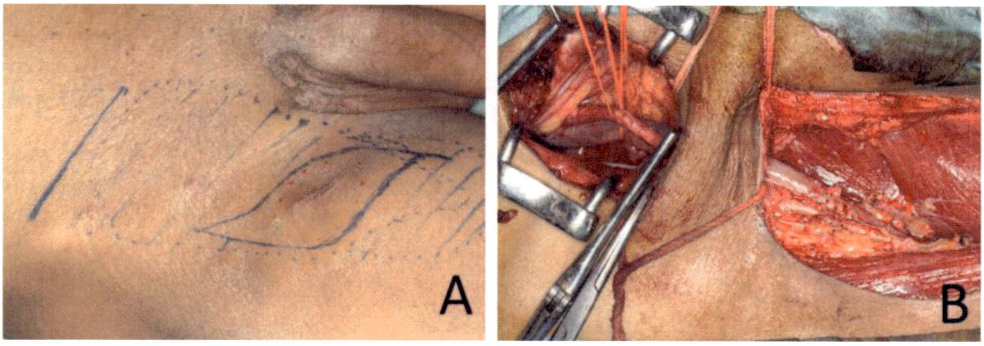

Figure 6. Ilioinguinal LND using paired incisions. (A) Incision lines. The incision below the inguinal crease is fusiform to include the skin overlying the metastatic node. (B) Operating field after dissection. The abdominal wall was incised parallel to the inguinal ligament, which was preserved under the bipedicle flap.

As another procedure in an attempt to decrease lymphocele, Nakamura et al. reported a simple method using intraoperative injection of isosulfan blue during inguinal LND without modifications to identify leakage from an injured lymphatic vessels for the prevention of lymphocele (Fig. 7)[112]. There was no incidence of lymphocele in the isosulfan blue injection group and the lymphatic drainage output from the inguinal region was clearly less, leading to early removal of the suction catheter.

Despite many technical variables, it is difficult to evaluate each technique because of the different study designs, variable definitions of complications, and different patient populations. Multicenter, randomized prospective trials with a standardized definition of complications are required in the future.

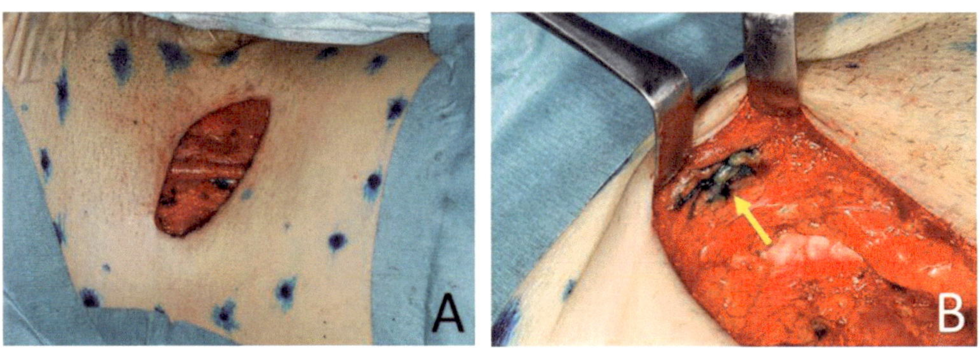

Figure 7. Intraoperative injection of blue dye during inguinal LND for detection of injured lymphatic vessels. (A) Intracutaneous injection of isosulfan blue around the right inguinal region just after inguinal LND. (B) Blue-staining lymphatic leak (arrow) in the surgical field, which was ligated.

8. Adjuvant radiation therapy

Regional recurrence occurs in 20% to 50% of patients after TLND. High-risk factors associated with regional recurrence include a cervical lymph node basin, large lymph nodes, multiple positive lymph nodes, and extracapsular extension[113]. Patients with such risk factors are appropriate candidates for adjuvant radiation therapy, and several nonrandomized studies have demonstrated that adjuvant radiation therapy after CLND for patients with regional nodal disease can reduce the risk of regional recurrence to between 5% and 20% [114-118]. In a prospective phase II study by the Trans Tasman Radiation Oncology Group (TROG Study 96.06) of adjuvant radiation therapy after CLND for patients with regional nodal disease, the regional control rate was 91%[118].

Although adjuvant radiation therapy can be effective in achieving regional control after TLND, it increases chronic lymphedema, particularly in the inguinal region, which is the major morbidity associated with TLND[119].

9. Conclusions

The surgical approach to regional lymph node metastasis of cutaneous melanoma is challenging. SLNB allows accurate staging of nodal status and prediction of prognosis. A positive SLN should be treated with CLND for regional control. However, the impact on SLNB on overall survival remains unclear, and the appropriate surgical extent of CLND in the cervical, axillary, and inguinal regions is also debated. More research is required to provide evidence-based guidelines for surgeons about the extent of LND and to investigate the factors that may lead to a more patient-tailored approach.

Acknowledgements

We thank Ms F. Miyamasu, associate professor of the Medical English Communications Center, University of Tsukuba, for expert English revision.

This work was partly supported by the National Cancer Center Research and Development Fund (23-A-22), and the Japanese Association of Dermatologic Surgery.

Author details

Yasuhiro Nakamura* and Fujio Otsuka

*Address all correspondence to: ynakamurta3@yahoo.co.jp

Department of Dermatology, Faculty of Medicine, University of Tsukuba, Tsukuba, Japan

References

[1] Balch CM, Soong SJ, Gershenwald JE et al. Prognostic factors analysis of 17,600 melanoma patients: validation of the American Joint Committee on Cancer melanoma staging system. J Clin Oncol 2001; 19: 3622-34.

[2] Sim FH, Taylor WF, Pritchard DJ, Soule EH. Lymphadenectomy in the management of stage I malignant melanoma: a prospective randomized study. Mayo Clin Proc 1986; 61: 697-705.

[3] Veronesi U, Adamus J, Bandiera DC et al. Inefficacy of immediate node dissection in stage 1 melanoma of the limbs. N Engl J Med 1977; 297: 627-30.

[4] Cascinelli N, Morabito A, Santinami M, MacKie RM, Belli F. Immediate or delayed dissection of regional nodes in patients with melanoma of the trunk: a randomised trial. WHO Melanoma Programme. Lancet 1998; 351: 793-6.

[5] Balch CM, Soong S, Ross MI et al. Long-term results of a multi-institutional randomized trial comparing prognostic factors and surgical results for intermediate thickness melanomas (1.0 to 4.0 mm). Intergroup Melanoma Surgical Trial. Ann Surg Oncol 2000; 7: 87-97.

[6] Morton DL, Wen DR, Wong JH et al. Technical details of intraoperative lymphatic mapping for early stage melanoma. Arch Surg 1992; 127: 392-9.

[7] Ross MI, Reintgen D, Balch CM. Selective lymphadenectomy: emerging role for lymphatic mapping and sentinel node biopsy in the management of early stage melanoma. Semin Surg Oncol 1993; 9: 219-23.

[8] Reintgen D, Cruse CW, Wells K et al. The orderly progression of melanoma nodal metastases. Ann Surg 1994; 220: 759-67.

[9] Thompson JF, McCarthy WH, Bosch CM et al. Sentinel lymph node status as an indicator of the presence of metastatic melanoma in regional lymph nodes. Melanoma Res 1995; 5: 255-60.

[10] Gershenwald JE, Colome MI, Lee JE et al. Patterns of recurrence following a negative sentinel lymph node biopsy in 243 patients with stage I or II melanoma. J Clin Oncol 1998; 16: 2253-60.

[11] Kapteijn BA, Nieweg OE, Liem I et al. Localizing the sentinel node in cutaneous melanoma: gamma probe detection versus blue dye. Ann Surg Oncol 1997; 4: 156-60.

[12] Gershenwald JE, Tseng CH, Thompson W et al. Improved sentinel lymph node localization in patients with primary melanoma with the use of radiolabeled colloid. Surgery 1998; 124: 203-10.

[13] Uren RF, Howman-Giles R, Thompson JF et al. Lymphoscintigraphy to identify sentinel lymph nodes in patients with melanoma. Melanoma Res 1994; 4: 395-9.

[14] Sumner WE, 3rd, Ross MI, Mansfield PF et al. Implications of lymphatic drainage to unusual sentinel lymph node sites in patients with primary cutaneous melanoma. Cancer 2002; 95: 354-60.

[15] Thompson JF, Uren RF, Shaw HM et al. Location of sentinel lymph nodes in patients with cutaneous melanoma: new insights into lymphatic anatomy. J Am Coll Surg 1999; 189: 195-204.

[16] Uren RF, Howman-Giles R, Thompson JF et al. Interval nodes: the forgotten sentinel nodes in patients with melanoma. Arch Surg 2000; 135: 1168-72.

[17] Uren RF, Thompson JF, Howman-Giles R. Sentinel nodes. Interval nodes, lymphatic lakes, and accurate sentinel node identification. Clin Nucl Med 2000; 25: 234-6.

[18] Morton DL, Cochran AJ, Thompson JF et al. Sentinel node biopsy for early-stage melanoma: accuracy and morbidity in MSLT-I, an international multicenter trial. Ann Surg 2005; 242: 302-11; discussion 11-3.

[19] Hayashi T, Furukawa H, Oyama A et al. Sentinel lymph node biopsy using real-time fluorescence navigation with indocyanine green in cutaneous head and neck/lip mucosa melanomas. Head Neck 2012; 34: 758-61.

[20] Thomas JM. Sentinel lymph node biopsy in malignant melanoma. BMJ 2008; 336: 902-3.

[21] Veenstra HJ, Wouters MW, Kroon BB, Olmos RA, Nieweg OE. Less false-negative sentinel node procedures in melanoma patients with experience and proper collaboration. J Surg Oncol 2011; 104: 454-7.

[22] Thomas JM. Caution with sentinel node biopsy in cutaneous melanoma. Br J Surg 2006; 93: 129-30.

[23] Stoffels I, von der Stuck H, Boy C et al. Indocyanine green fluorescence-guided sentinel lymph node biopsy in dermato-oncology. J Dtsch Dermatol Ges 2012; 10: 51-7.

[24] Wagner JD, Park HM, Coleman JJ, 3rd, Love C, Hayes JT. Cervical sentinel lymph node biopsy for melanomas of the head and neck and upper thorax. Arch Otolaryngol Head Neck Surg 2000; 126: 313-21.

[25] Chao C, Wong SL, Edwards MJ et al. Sentinel lymph node biopsy for head and neck melanomas. Ann Surg Oncol 2003; 10: 21-6.

[26] Fincher TR, O'Brien JC, McCarty TM et al. Patterns of drainage and recurrence following sentinel lymph node biopsy for cutaneous melanoma of the head and neck. Arch Otolaryngol Head Neck Surg 2004; 130: 844-8.

[27] Namikawa K, Yamazaki N. Sentinel lymph node biopsy guided by indocyanine green fluorescence for cutaneous melanoma. Eur J Dermatol 2011; 21: 184-90.

http://dx.doi.org/10.5772/53625

[28] Fujisawa Y, Nakamura Y, Kawachi Y, Otsuka F. A custom-made, low-cost intraoperative fluorescence navigation system with indocyanine green for sentinel lymph node biopsy in skin cancer. Dermatology 2011; 222: 261-8.

[29] Polom K, Murawa D, Rho YS, Spychala A, Murawa P. Skin melanoma sentinel lymph node biopsy using real-time fluorescence navigation with indocyanine green and indocyanine green with human serum albumin. Br J Dermatol 2012; 166: 682-3.

[30] Benson RC, Kues HA. Fluorescence properties of indocyanine green as related to angiography. Phys Med Biol 1978; 23: 159-63.

[31] Uren RF. SPECT/CT Lymphoscintigraphy to locate the sentinel lymph node in patients with melanoma. Ann Surg Oncol 2009; 16: 1459-60.

[32] Vermeeren L, van der Ploeg IM, Olmos RA et al. SPECT/CT for preoperative sentinel node localization. J Surg Oncol 2010; 101: 184-90.

[33] Morton DL, Hoon DS, Cochran AJ et al. Lymphatic mapping and sentinel lymphadenectomy for early-stage melanoma: therapeutic utility and implications of nodal microanatomy and molecular staging for improving the accuracy of detection of nodal micrometastases. Ann Surg 2003; 238: 538-49; discussion 49-50.

[34] Kretschmer L, Hilgers R, Mohrle M et al. Patients with lymphatic metastasis of cutaneous malignant melanoma benefit from sentinel lymphonodectomy and early excision of their nodal disease. Eur J Cancer 2004; 40: 212-8.

[35] Nowecki ZI, Rutkowski P, Michej W. The survival benefit to patients with positive sentinel node melanoma after completion lymph node dissection may be limited to the subgroup with a primary lesion Breslow thickness greater than 1.0 and less than or equal to 4 mm (pT2-pT3). Ann Surg Oncol 2008; 15: 2223-34.

[36] Pasquali S, Mocellin S. The anticancer face of interferon alpha (IFN-alpha): from biology to clinical results, with a focus on melanoma. Curr Med Chem 2010; 17: 3327-36.

[37] van Akkooi AC, Bouwhuis MG, de Wilt JH, Kliffen M, Schmitz PI, Eggermont AM. Multivariable analysis comparing outcome after sentinel node biopsy or therapeutic lymph node dissection in patients with melanoma. Br J Surg 2007; 94: 1293-9.

[38] Morton DL, Thompson JF, Cochran AJ et al. Sentinel-node biopsy or nodal observation in melanoma. N Engl J Med 2006; 355: 1307-17.

[39] Ross MI, Gershenwald JE. How should we view the results of the Multicenter Selective Lymphadenectomy Trial-1 (MSLT-1)? Ann Surg Oncol 2008; 15: 670-3.

[40] Govindarajan A, Ghazarian DM, McCready DR, Leong WL. Histological features of melanoma sentinel lymph node metastases associated with status of the completion lymphadenectomy and rate of subsequent relapse. Ann Surg Oncol 2007; 14: 906-12.

[41] Gershenwald JE, Andtbacka RH, Prieto VG et al. Microscopic tumor burden in sentinel lymph nodes predicts synchronous nonsentinel lymph node involvement in patients with melanoma. J Clin Oncol 2008; 26: 4296-303.

[42] Vuylsteke RJ, Borgstein PJ, van Leeuwen PA et al. Sentinel lymph node tumor load: an independent predictor of additional lymph node involvement and survival in melanoma. Ann Surg Oncol 2005; 12: 440-8.

[43] Francischetto T, Spector N, Neto Rezende JF et al. Influence of sentinel lymph node tumor burden on survival in melanoma. Ann Surg Oncol 2010; 17: 1152-8.

[44] van der Ploeg AP, van Akkooi AC, Schmitz PI, Koljenovic S, Verhoef C, Eggermont AM. EORTC Melanoma Group sentinel node protocol identifies high rate of submicrometastases according to Rotterdam Criteria. Eur J Cancer 2010; 46: 2414-21.

[45] Marsden JR, Newton-Bishop JA, Burrows L et al. Revised U.K. guidelines for the management of cutaneous melanoma 2010. Br J Dermatol 2010; 163: 238-56.

[46] Garbe C, Peris K, Hauschild A et al. Diagnosis and treatment of melanoma: European consensus-based interdisciplinary guideline. Eur J Cancer 2010; 46: 270-83.

[47] Gershenwald JE, Ross MI. Sentinel-lymph-node biopsy for cutaneous melanoma. N Engl J Med 2011; 364: 1738-45.

[48] O'Brien CJ, Gianoutsos MP, Morgan MJ. Neck dissection for cutaneous malignant melanoma. World J Surg 1992; 16: 222-6.

[49] Calearo CV, Teatini G. Functional neck dissection. Anatomical grounds, surgical technique, clinical observations. Ann Otol Rhinol Laryngol 1983; 92: 215-22.

[50] O'Brien CJ, Coates AS, Petersen-Schaefer K et al. Experience with 998 cutaneous melanomas of the head and neck over 30 years. Am J Surg 1991; 162: 310-4.

[51] Turkula LD, Woods JE. Limited or selective nodal dissection for malignant melanoma of the head and neck. Am J Surg 1984; 148: 446-8.

[52] O'Brien CJ, Petersen-Schaefer K, Ruark D, Coates AS, Menzie SJ, Harrison RI. Radical, modified, and selective neck dissection for cutaneous malignant melanoma. Head Neck 1995; 17: 232-41.

[53] Jonk A, Strobbe LJ, Kroon BB et al. Cervical lymph-node metastasis from cutaneous melanoma of the head and neck: a search for prognostic factors. Eur J Surg Oncol 1998; 24: 298-302.

[54] Byers RM. The role of modified neck dissection in the treatment of cutaneous melanoma of the head and neck. Arch Surg 1986; 121: 1338-41.

[55] White N, Yap LH, Srivastava S. Lymphadenectomy for melanoma in the clinically N1 neck: radical, modified radical, or selective? J Craniofac Surg 2009; 20: 385-8.

[56] Pu LL, Wells KE, Cruse CW, Shons AR, Reintgen DS. Prevalence of additional positive lymph nodes in complete lymphadenectomy specimens after positive sentinel lymphadenectomy findings for early-stage melanoma of the head and neck. Plast Reconstr Surg 2003; 112: 43-9.

[57] O'Brien CJ, McNeil EB, McMahon JD, Pathak I, Lauer CS. Incidence of cervical node involvement in metastatic cutaneous malignancy involving the parotid gland. Head Neck 2001; 23: 744-8.

[58] Caldwell CB, Spiro RH. The role of parotidectomy in the treatment of cutaneous head and neck melanoma. Am J Surg 1988; 156: 318-22.

[59] Barr LC, Skene AI, Fish S, Thomas JM. Superficial parotidectomy in the treatment of cutaneous melanoma of the head and neck. Br J Surg 1994; 81: 64-5.

[60] Klop WM, Veenstra HJ, Vermeeren L, Nieweg OE, Balm AJ, Lohuis PJ. Assessment of lymphatic drainage patterns and implications for the extent of neck dissection in head and neck melanoma patients. J Surg Oncol 2011; 103: 756-60.

[61] O'Brien CJ, Uren RF, Thompson JF et al. Prediction of potential metastatic sites in cutaneous head and neck melanoma using lymphoscintigraphy. Am J Surg 1995; 170: 461-6.

[62] Pathak I, O'Brien CJ, Petersen-Schaeffer K et al. Do nodal metastases from cutaneous melanoma of the head and neck follow a clinically predictable pattern? Head Neck 2001; 23: 785-90.

[63] Lin D, Franc BL, Kashani-Sabet M, Singer MI. Lymphatic drainage patterns of head and neck cutaneous melanoma observed on lymphoscintigraphy and sentinel lymph node biopsy. Head Neck 2006; 28: 249-55.

[64] Reynolds HM, Smith NP, Uren RF, Thompson JF, Dunbar PR. Three-dimensional visualization of skin lymphatic drainage patterns of the head and neck. Head Neck 2009; 31: 1316-25.

[65] Leong SP. Role of selective sentinel lymph node dissection in head and neck melanoma. J Surg Oncol 2011; 104: 361-8.

[66] Attie JN. A single transverse incision for radical neck dissection. Surgery 1957; 41: 498-502.

[67] Macfee WF. Transverse incisions for neck dissection. Ann Surg 1960; 151: 279-84.

[68] Dancey AL, Srivastava S. Experience with the modified hockey stick incision for block dissection of neck. J Plast Reconstr Aesthet Surg 2006; 59: 1276-9.

[69] Balch CM. Axillary lymph node dissection: differences in goals and techniques when treating melanoma and breast cancer. Surgery 1990; 108: 118-9.

[70] Garbe C, Hauschild A, Volkenandt M et al. Evidence-based and interdisciplinary consensus-based German guidelines: systemic medical treatment of melanoma in the adjuvant and palliative setting. Melanoma Res 2008; 18: 152-60.

[71] Essner R. Surgical treatment of malignant melanoma. Surg Clin North Am 2003; 83: 109-56.

[72] Karakousis CP, Hena MA, Emrich LJ, Driscoll DL. Axillary node dissection in malignant melanoma: results and complications. Surgery 1990; 108: 10-7.

[73] Karakousis CP. Therapeutic node dissections in malignant melanoma. Ann Surg Oncol 1998; 5: 473-82.

[74] Meyer T, Merkel S, Gohl J, Hohenberger W. Lymph node dissection for clinically evident lymph node metastases of malignant melanoma. Eur J Surg Oncol 2002; 28: 424-30.

[75] Serpell JW, Carne PW, Bailey M. Radical lymph node dissection for melanoma. ANZ J Surg 2003; 73: 294-9.

[76] Namm JP, Chang AE, Cimmino VM, Rees RS, Johnson TM, Sabel MS. Is a level III dissection necessary for a positive sentinel lymph node in melanoma? J Surg Oncol 2012; 105: 225-8.

[77] Gershenwald JE, Berman RS, Porter G, Mansfield PF, Lee JE, Ross MI. Regional nodal basin control is not compromised by previous sentinel lymph node biopsy in patients with melanoma. Ann Surg Oncol 2000; 7: 226-31.

[78] Clary BM, Brady MS, Lewis JJ, Coit DG. Sentinel lymph node biopsy in the management of patients with primary cutaneous melanoma: review of a large single-institutional experience with an emphasis on recurrence. Ann Surg 2001; 233: 250-8.

[79] Leiter U, Buettner PG, Bohnenberger K et al. Sentinel lymph node dissection in primary melanoma reduces subsequent regional lymph node metastasis as well as distant metastasis after nodal involvement. Ann Surg Oncol 2010; 17: 129-37.

[80] Veenstra HJ, van der Ploeg IM, Wouters MW, Kroon BB, Nieweg OE. Reevaluation of the locoregional recurrence rate in melanoma patients with a positive sentinel node compared to patients with palpable nodal involvement. Ann Surg Oncol 2010; 17: 521-6.

[81] Wrightson WR, Wong SL, Edwards MJ et al. Complications associated with sentinel lymph node biopsy for melanoma. Ann Surg Oncol 2003; 10: 676-80.

[82] Kretschmer L, Thoms KM, Peeters S, Haenssle H, Bertsch HP, Emmert S. Postoperative morbidity of lymph node excision for cutaneous melanoma-sentinel lymphonodectomy versus complete regional lymph node dissection. Melanoma Res 2008; 18: 16-21.

[83] de Vries M, Vonkeman WG, van Ginkel RJ, Hoekstra HJ. Morbidity after axillary sentinel lymph node biopsy in patients with cutaneous melanoma. Eur J Surg Oncol 2005; 31: 778-83.

[84] Lawton G, Rasque H, Ariyan S. Preservation of muscle fascia to decrease lymphedema after complete axillary and ilioinguinofemoral lymphadenectomy for melanoma. J Am Coll Surg 2002; 195: 339-51.

[85] Sterne GD, Murray DS, Grimley RP. Ilioinguinal block dissection for malignant melanoma. Br J Surg 1995; 82: 1057-9.

[86] Strobbe LJ, Jonk A, Hart AA, Nieweg OE, Kroon BB. Positive iliac and obturator nodes in melanoma: survival and prognostic factors. Ann Surg Oncol 1999; 6: 255-62.

[87] Hughes TM, A'Hern RP, Thomas JM. Prognosis and surgical management of patients with palpable inguinal lymph node metastases from melanoma. Br J Surg 2000; 87: 892-901.

[88] Mann GB, Coit DG. Does the extent of operation influence the prognosis in patients with melanoma metastatic to inguinal nodes? Ann Surg Oncol 1999; 6: 263-71.

[89] Kretschmer L, Neumann C, Preusser KP, Marsch WC. Superficial inguinal and radical ilioinguinal lymph node dissection in patients with palpable melanoma metastases to the groin--an analysis of survival and local recurrence. Acta Oncol 2001; 40: 72-8.

[90] Shen P, Conforti AM, Essner R, Cochran AJ, Turner RR, Morton DL. Is the node of Cloquet the sentinel node for the iliac/obturator node group? Cancer J 2000; 6: 93-7.

[91] Strobbe LJ, Jonk A, Hart AA et al. The value of Cloquet's node in predicting melanoma nodal metastases in the pelvic lymph node basin. Ann Surg Oncol 2001; 8: 209-14.

[92] Allan CP, Hayes AJ, Thomas JM. Ilioinguinal lymph node dissection for palpable metastatic melanoma to the groin. ANZ J Surg 2008; 78: 982-6.

[93] van der Ploeg IM, Kroon BB, Valdes Olmos RA, Nieweg OE. Evaluation of lymphatic drainage patterns to the groin and implications for the extent of groin dissection in melanoma patients. Ann Surg Oncol 2009; 16: 2994-9.

[94] Jansen L, Nieweg OE, Peterse JL, Hoefnagel CA, Olmos RA, Kroon BB. Reliability of sentinel lymph node biopsy for staging melanoma. Br J Surg 2000; 87: 484-9.

[95] Estourgie SH, Nieweg OE, Valdes Olmos RA, Hoefnagel CA, Kroon BB. Review and evaluation of sentinel node procedures in 250 melanoma patients with a median follow-up of 6 years. Ann Surg Oncol 2003; 10: 681-8.

[96] Santinami M, Carbone A, Crippa F et al. Radical dissection after positive groin sentinel biopsy in melanoma patients: rate of further positive nodes. Melanoma Res 2009; 19: 112-8.

[97] Spillane AJ, Haydu L, McMillan W, Stretch JR, Thompson JF. Quality assurance parameters and predictors of outcome for ilioinguinal and inguinal dissection in a contemporary melanoma patient population. Ann Surg Oncol 2011; 18: 2521-8.

[98] Chu CK, Delman KA, Carlson GW, Hestley AC, Murray DR. Inguinopelvic lymphadenectomy following positive inguinal sentinel lymph node biopsy in melanoma: true frequency of synchronous pelvic metastases. Ann Surg Oncol 2011; 18: 3309-15.

[99] van der Ploeg IM, Valdes Olmos RA, Kroon BB, Nieweg OE. Tumor-positive sentinel node biopsy of the groin in clinically node-negative melanoma patients: superficial or superficial and deep lymph node dissection? Ann Surg Oncol 2008; 15: 1485-91.

[100] Pearlman NW, Robinson WA, Dreiling LK, McIntyre RC, Jr., Gonzales R. Modified ilioinguinal node dissection for metastatic melanoma. Am J Surg 1995; 170: 647-9; discussion 9-50.

[101] Spiess PE, Hernandez MS, Pettaway CA. Contemporary inguinal lymph node dissection: minimizing complications. World J Urol 2009; 27: 205-12.

[102] Chang SB, Askew RL, Xing Y et al. Prospective assessment of postoperative complications and associated costs following inguinal lymph node dissection (ILND) in melanoma patients. Ann Surg Oncol 2010; 17: 2764-72.

[103] Hughes TM, Thomas JM. Combined inguinal and pelvic lymph node dissection for stage III melanoma. Br J Surg 1999; 86: 1493-8.

[104] Ravi R. Morbidity following groin dissection for penile carcinoma. Br J Urol 1993; 72: 941-5.

[105] Karakousis CP, Driscoll DL. Groin dissection in malignant melanoma. Br J Surg 1994; 81: 1771-4.

[106] Beitsch P, Balch C. Operative morbidity and risk factor assessment in melanoma patients undergoing inguinal lymph node dissection. Am J Surg 1992; 164: 462-5; discussion 5-6.

[107] Sabel MS, Griffith KA, Arora A et al. Inguinal node dissection for melanoma in the era of sentinel lymph node biopsy. Surgery 2007; 141: 728-35.

[108] Karakousis CP. Therapeutic node dissections in malignant melanoma. Semin Surg Oncol 1998; 14: 291-301.

[109] Spillane AJ, Tucker M, Pasquali S. A pilot study reporting outcomes for melanoma patients of a minimal access ilio-inguinal dissection technique based on two incisions. Ann Surg Oncol 2011; 18: 970-6.

[110] Delman KA, Kooby DA, Rizzo M, Ogan K, Master V. Initial experience with videoscopic inguinal lymphadenectomy. Ann Surg Oncol 2011; 18: 977-82.

[111] Ising IM, Bembenek A, Gutzmer R, Kockerling F, Moesta KT. Enhanced postoperative lymphatic staging of malignant melanoma by endoscopically assisted iliacoinguinal dissection. Langenbecks Arch Surg 2012; 397: 429-36.

[112] Nakamura Y, Fujisawa Y, Maruyama H, Furuta J, Kawachi Y, Otsuka F. Intraoperative mapping with isosulfan blue of lymphatic leakage during inguinal lymph node dissection (ILND) for skin cancer for the prevention of postoperative lymphocele. J Surg Oncol 2011; 104: 657-60.

http://dx.doi.org/10.5772/53625

[113] Lee RJ, Gibbs JF, Proulx GM, Kollmorgen DR, Jia C, Kraybill WG. Nodal basin recurrence following lymph node dissection for melanoma: implications for adjuvant radiotherapy. Int J Radiat Oncol Biol Phys 2000; 46: 467-74.

[114] Ballo MT, Strom EA, Zagars GK et al. Adjuvant irradiation for axillary metastases from malignant melanoma. Int J Radiat Oncol Biol Phys 2002; 52: 964-72.

[115] Ballo MT, Bonnen MD, Garden AS et al. Adjuvant irradiation for cervical lymph node metastases from melanoma. Cancer 2003; 97: 1789-96.

[116] Ballo MT, Zagars GK, Gershenwald JE et al. A critical assessment of adjuvant radiotherapy for inguinal lymph node metastases from melanoma. Ann Surg Oncol 2004; 11: 1079-84.

[117] Ballo MT, Ross MI, Cormier JN et al. Combined-modality therapy for patients with regional nodal metastases from melanoma. Int J Radiat Oncol Biol Phys 2006; 64: 106-13.

[118] Burmeister BH, Mark Smithers B, Burmeister E et al. A prospective phase II study of adjuvant postoperative radiation therapy following nodal surgery in malignant melanoma-Trans Tasman Radiation Oncology Group (TROG) Study 96.06. Radiother Oncol 2006; 81: 136-42.

[119] Agrawal S, Kane JM, 3rd, Guadagnolo BA, Kraybill WG, Ballo MT. The benefits of adjuvant radiation therapy after therapeutic lymphadenectomy for clinically advanced, high-risk, lymph node-metastatic melanoma. Cancer 2009; 115: 5836-44.

Chapter 19

Cutaneous Melanoma – Surgical Treatment

Mario Santinami, Roberto Patuzzo,
Roberta Ruggeri, Gianpiero Castelli,
Andrea Maurichi, Giulia Baffa and Carlotta Tinti

Additional information is available at the end of the chapter

http://dx.doi.org/10.5772/54105

1. Introduction

1.1. Excision margins for primary tumor

Although surgical excision of the primary melanoma is internationally accepted as the treatment of choice, several questions concerning the follow-up schedule are still debated controversially. Incision biopsies should be avoided, except in selected cases (wide lesions or critical anatomic locations). Excision biopsy is preferred to give the dermatopathologist an optimal specimen and to allow evaluation of the excision margins for residual tumor. Since the beginning of the last century, the recommendation has been to excise a primary melanoma with safety margins. In 1907 Handley [1] analyzed the pattern of satellite metastases in melanoma and recommended excision of the primary tumor with a margin of 1 inch (2.54 cm) from the edge of the tumor. In the 1970s and 1980s, safety margins of 5 cm, independent of tumor thickness, were the surgical standard.[2] The World Health Organization Melanoma Group performed the first surgical trial to compare lower safety margins of 1 and 3 cm in primary melanomas with less than 2 mm of tumor thickness.[3] The group found no differences in survival and only slightly increased local recurrence rates in the patients with narrower excision margins. These results led to the recommendation of 1-cm margins in patients with primary melanomas with less than 1 mm tumor thickness. Later comparisons of 5- and 2-cm safety margins in thick primary melanomas revealed no significant advantages for the 5-cm margins.[4] A recent trial, however, comparing 1- and 3-cm safety margins in thick primary melanoma with 2 mm and more tumor thickness showed an increased rate of local recurrence in those with the small safety margins and a simultaneous trend towards decreased survival rates. These findings indicate that the safety margin cannot be reduced to zero in melanoma.[5] Different national guidelines now give uniform recommendations for the excision of primary melanoma.[6-9]

2. Sentinel lymph node biopsy and lymph node dissection

Metastasis to regional nodes is the most important prognostic factor in patients with early-stage melanoma and has been shown to occur in approximately 20% of patients with intermediate-thickness tumors.[10,11] As such, it is critically important to identify those patients for whom the expected benefits of resecting regional lymph nodes outweigh the risks of surgical morbidity. The technique of lymphatic mapping and sentinel lymph node (SLN) biopsy for melanoma has emerged during the last 2 decades as a minimally invasive approach to evaluate regional lymph node basins in patients with intermediate- and high-risk primary cutaneous melanoma. Goals of SLN biopsy include accurate nodal staging, identification of patients with clinically occult, microscopic lymph node disease who may benefit from further treatment, regional nodal control, and a possible survival benefit.[12,13] Moreover, this approach may also identify a subset of patients for whom further treatment is not indicated, sparing them from unnecessary surgical procedures or systemic therapies.[12,13] In this review, we examine the evolution of SLN biopsy as a technique, the preoperative assessment and operative strategy, the pathologic evaluation of the SLN, the current practice guidelines, the prognostic significance of SLN biopsy findings, and the potential complications of the procedure and address some of the current areas of controversies in the field. Sentinel lymph node (SLN) biopsy is commonly used in melanoma and has been endorsed by the American Joint Committee on Cancer (AJCC) as a valuable staging procedure for patients with melanoma who are at risk of clinically occult nodal metastases. This highly accurate and low-morbidity staging procedure should be used to guide treatment decisions (ie, completion lymph node dissection [CLND] and adjuvant therapy) as well as entry into clinical trials.[14] To develop and formalize guideline recommendations for the use of SLN biopsy in oncology practice, the American Society of Clinical Oncology (ASCO) and Society of Surgical Oncology (SSO) convened a joint Expert Panel in order to better define what are the indications for SLN biopsy as well as what is the role of CLND. SLN biopsy is recommended for patients with intermediate-thickness cutaneous melanomas (Breslow thickness, 1 to 4 mm) of any anatomic site. Routine use of SLN biopsy in this population provides accurate staging. Although there are few studies focusing specifically on patients with thick melanomas (T4; Breslow thickness, > 4 mm), use of SLN biopsy in this population may be recommended for staging purposes and to facilitate regional disease control. There is insufficient evidence to support routine SLN biopsy for patients with thin melanomas (T1; Breslow thickness, < 1 mm), although it may be considered in selected patients with high-risk features when the benefits of pathologic staging may outweigh the potential risks of the procedure. Such risk factors may include ulceration or mitotic rate $\geq 1/mm^2$, especially in the subgroup of patients with melanomas 0.75 to 0.99 mm in Breslow thickness. After a positive SLN biopsy, 97.5% of patients underwent CLND, and 20.1% were found to have additional positive lymph nodes. Overall, the recurrence rate in the same nodal basin after a positive

SLN biopsy was 7.5%, despite CLND in nearly all patients.[15] Overall, the SLN biopsy procedure is well tolerated and associated with low complication rates.[16] Although clinical variables such as older age have been variably reported as lower risk factors,[17-19] there are no specific variables that can reliably identify patients with intermediate-thickness melanomas at low risk for metastases. The definition of intermediate-thickness melanoma varied by study. Nevertheless, it is clinically consistent with contemporary staging systems to define intermediate-thickness melanomas as those measuring 1 to 4 mm.[20] Clinical judgment must be used when considering SLN biopsy in patients with comorbid medical conditions. The individual risks and benefits of the procedure should be weighed against the operative and anesthetic risks as well as potential competing causes of mortality. Complications after SLN biopsy are uncommon. The overall complication rate reported in the Multicenter Selective Lymphadenectomy Trial I (MSLT I) was 10.1% after SLN biopsy compared with 32.7% after CLND.[21] The most common complications after SLN removal documented in MSLT I included seroma (5.5%), infection (4.6%), and wound separation (1.2%). The Sunbelt Melanoma Trial similarly showed a low overall rate of complications from SLN biopsy (4.6%) compared with CLND (23.2%).[16,17] Most complications were noted to be short-term issues that resolved over time with wound care and selective use of antibiotics. Accurate identification of patients with node-negative (stage I or II) or node-positive (stage III) disease improves staging and may facilitate regional disease control and decision making for treatment with adjuvant therapy.[14,22] With substantive changes in the melanoma staging guidelines in 2002, the AJCC staging system effectively linked disease stage and prognosis.[23,24] At that time, the number of nodal metastases and whether nodal disease was occult or clinically apparent (ie, how the N category was defined with regard to burden of disease) were noted to be the most significant independent predictors of survival in patients with stage III melanomas. With later iterations of the last AJCC staging system,[10] additional refinements were made in the N category based on the prognostic value of distinguishing micrometastases (as would be diagnosed after SLN biopsy) from macrometastases.[25,26] A melanoma macrometastasis is detected by clinical examination (not by size criteria) and confirmed pathologically, whereas a melanoma micrometastasis is a clinically occult nodal metastasis that is detected by a pathologist on microscopic examination of lymph nodes, with or without immunohistochemistry, and is not limited by any minimum or maximum size threshold. Recognizing the value of examining SLNs to detect low volumes of metastatic disease (aggregates of only a few cells), the current staging system[10,27] incorporates the use of immunohistochemistry and eliminates any minimum size threshold for defining nodal metastases. Molecular diagnostics, such as reverse transcriptase-polymerase chain reaction, have unproven prognostic significance, and these results are not used to define positive nodes. As a result, more refined definitions of the N category are now used for classification. Distinct differences in classifications have validated prognostic significance. For example, 5-year survival ranges from 70% for patients with one SLN positive with micrometastatic disease to 39% for patients with > four involved nodes or with nodes that are extensively involved (eg, matted nodes).[1] Although SLN biopsy has been widely accepted for the pathologic staging of patients with intermediate-thickness melanomas, somewhat more controversy exists regarding the value of this procedure for patients with thick primary tumors

(T4; Breslow thickness, > 4 mm). Conventional wisdom asserts that patients with thick melanomas have a high risk of systemic disease at the time of diagnosis and that no survival benefit can be derived from removal of regional lymph nodes. However, among patients without distant disease, it can be argued that those with thick melanomas have indications for SLN biopsy similar to those of patients with intermediate-thickness melanomas and derive the same benefits from SLN biopsy as a pathologic staging procedure. One of the main advantages of SLN biopsy in patients with thick melanomas is better regional disease control, which is especially important in a population with > 30% chance of lymph node involvement.[25,28] Evidence from multiple retrospective studies has demonstrated that SLN biopsy provides important staging and prognostic information for patients with thick melanomas. Seven of eight published studies-each evaluating SLN biopsy in > 100 patients with T4 melanomas-have shown that SLN biopsy is a significant predictor of overall survival.[11,25,26,28-33] The one study that did not show a significant difference in overall survival demonstrated a significant difference in disease-free survival.[29] A majority (70%) of melanomas diagnosed are thin melanomas (T1; Breslow thickness, < 1 mm).[34] In general, the routine use of SLN biopsy in patients with thin melanomas has not been advocated, because the overall risk of nodal involvement is estimated to be only approximately 5.1%,[35] although there are reports of positive SLNs in up to 20% of patients in subsets with thin melanomas (especially those that are 0.75 to 0.99 mm in thickness with ulceration and/or mitotic rate $\geq 1/mm^2$).[27] An individualized approach to SLN biopsy for patients with thin melanomas has been advocated in many treatment centers based on risk factors that have been shown to be associated with SLN metastasis. Further investigation is also needed to better identify the subgroups of patients with thin melanomas with a greater risk of nodal metastasis. CLND is recommended for all patients with a positive SLN biopsy. CLND achieves regional disease control, although whether CLND after a positive SLN biopsy improves survival is the subject of the ongoing Multicenter Selective Lymphadenectomy Trial II (MSLT II). Currently, CLND is the standard recommendation for patients with tumor-positive SLNs. The goals of CLND are to improve survival rates, maximize regional disease control, and minimize operative morbidity. Whether CLND improves survival is the subject of the ongoing prospective randomized MSLT II study.[36] The main objective of MSLT II is to determine if there is a therapeutic benefit to removing any non-SLNs in patients who have already had their tumor-positive SLN removed. In MSLT I, patients with demonstrated nodal metastases had a survival advantage with early intervention compared with those who had a delayed lymphadenectomy when they presented with clinically evident nodal metastases.[5] Hence, although two goals of CLND are regional disease control and cure, there is currently insufficient evidence to determine whether omission of CLND is safe. In the two large prospective randomized trials (ie, the Sunbelt Melanoma Trial and MSLT I), the rate of positive non-SLNs among patients who underwent CLND for a tumor-positive SLN was 16%.[17,37] In a retrospective multi-institutional study by Wong et al,[38] which included 134 highly selected patients with positive SLNs who did not undergo CLND, regional nodal metastasis was a component of first recurrence in 15% of these patients. Therefore, it is reasonable to conclude from these data that the risk of developing regional nodal metastasis as a first site of recurrence, if no CLND is performed, is at least 15% to 20%.[39,40] In MSLT I, the rate of regional nodal recurrence after CLND was 4.2%[5]; in the Sunbelt Melanoma Trial, it was 4.9% (unpublished data). These rates are much lower than the 15% rate of regional nodal recurrence as a site of first metastasis and the 41% overall regional nodal recurrence rate when CLND was not performed, reported in the study by Wong et al.[37] Until final results of MSLT II are available, we will not be able to determine, with higher-level evidence, the impact of CLND on regional disease control. Until that time, the best available evidence suggests that CLND is effective at achieving regional disease control in the majority of patients with positive SLNs. MSLT I showed no benefit of CLND with regard to overall survival, likely because only a minority of patients (16%) had tumor-positive SLNs, and the majority of the patients in the study would not have been helped by removal of regional lymph nodes.[37] However, the 5-year survival rate for patients with tumor-positive SLNs who underwent CLND was 72.3% compared with 52.4% for patients who did not undergo SLN biopsy and developed palpable nodal disease (hazard ratio, 0.51; 95% CI, 0.32 to 0.81; P =.004). CLND should be performed until there is convincing evidence that it does not improve regional disease control or survival. CLND is associated with risks of long-term morbidity, especially lymphedema. However, morbidity with CLND may be considerably worse when it is delayed until there is clinically evident disease. The observed increases in morbidity for patients who have undergone therapeutic lymphadenectomy for palpable disease and the increased morbidity associated with radiation therapy support the continued use of CLND for patients with a positive SLN biopsy rather than delayed CLND for palpable disease. There is a need for future clinical trials to address many unresolved research questions related to the use of SLN biopsy in patients with melanoma. These include: determining precise criteria for selecting which patients should undergo SLN biopsy, determining whether early identification of metastases in the SLN truly improves survival or merely represents lead-time bias, identifying which criteria for individualized risks best inform appropriate risk stratification for patients at high risk for relapse and those for whom CLND and/or adjuvant therapy are suitable, and establishing the role of prognostic markers from the primary melanoma and SLN to help assign appropriate risk stratification. Results from MSLT II, in which patients were randomly assigned to CLND or observation, will help determine whether there is any benefit to CLND after a positive sentinel node in patients with melanoma. Answers to these questions will assist clinicians and patients with making decisions and ultimately help to identify patients who may avoid expensive and intrusive procedures in staging and follow-up.

3. Treatment of *in transit* metastases

In 5–8% of cases, melanoma patients will develop in-transit metastasis (IT-mets). Standard regional treatment options include surgical resection, isolated limb perfusion (ILP), isolated limb infusion (ILI) and Electrochemotherapy. As regional recurrence often precedes systemic disease, amputative surgery is in general no longer practiced, although old series of radical surgery have demonstrated that some patients with IT-mets confined to the limb can be cured.[42,43] Simple surgical resection may suffice for incidental and low numbers of IT-mets. In cases of rapid recurrences and multiple IT-mets, other techniques must provide an attractive treatment option that can improve local control markedly and thereby quality of life. ILP, developed by Creech et al., achieves a 20-fold higher concentration of chemotherapeutic drugs when compared with systemic therapy.[44,45] Melphalan-based ILP (M-ILP) has been the standard treatment and has been reported to achieve overall complete response (CR) rates in the range of about 50%.[46]In general large IT-mets showed a poor response and inhomogeneous uptake comparable with locally advanced soft tissue sarcomas (STS). The introduction of tumor necrosis factor-α (TNF) changed this situation dramatically. Large tumors now reacted very well to ILP.[47] This led to a successful multicenter trial in Europe and the approval of TNF-based ILP (TM-ILP) for unresectable extremity soft tissue sarcomas (STS).[48] Similar encouraging results were reported for the use of TNF in ILP for melanoma patients.[49] Preclinical and clinical studies suggested that a reduction of the dose of TNF to 1 mg for the arm and 2 mg for the leg might be as effective as the higher doses.[50-53]Isolated limb infusion (ILI) is a minimally invasive technique for delivering high-dose regional chemotherapy in locally advanced melanoma. It was first described by Thompson et al. in 1994 from the Sydney Melanoma Unit as a simplified alternative to ILP [54,55]. Percutaneous arterial and venous catheters are placed in the affected extremity by interventional radiologists and a tourniquet is placed proximal to the catheter tips to allow isolation of the limb from the systemic circulation. High-dose chemotherapy (e.g. melphalan and actinomycin-D) is infused into a hyperthermic, hypoxic limb via the arterial catheter and blood is withdrawn from the venous catheter to be re-infused into the arterial side. Therefore, it is a quicker, safer, and cheaper procedure with reported response rates comparable to ILP.[56,57] Although the primary indication for this technique is melanoma, it has been successfully applied to other tumors such as soft-tissue sarcomas,[58] Merkel cell tumor,[59] and cutaneous T-cell lymphoma.[60]

Electrochemotherapy (ECT) represents an effective therapeutic option for skin tumors that has received experimental and clinical support in recent years.[61-71] The European standard operating procedures for ECT emphasize the technical aspects of the procedure and have established this treatment in clinical practice.[72,73] In recent years, the effectiveness of ECT treatment has been confirmed in several small series of patients with melanoma.[71] At present, ECT is employed routinely with encouraging results not only for superficial tumor control but also to preserve quality of life.[70]Patients with regional or distant skin or subcutaneous metastases, with or without visceral disease, could undergo this technique. Eligibility criteria were the following: melanoma stage IIIC–IV (American Joint Committee on Cancer, 6th edition)[74] lesions no deeper than 3 cm suitable for electrode insertion; no anticancer treatments 4 weeks before and 8 weeks after ECT; age more than 18 years; and an Eastern Cooperative Oncology Group performance status equal to or less than 2. Exclusion criteria included: allergy to Bleomycin; pulmonary, cardiac or liver impairment; epilepsy; life expectancy less than 3 months; active infection; brain metastases; and cardiac pacemaker in patients with chest wall metastases. Bleomycin is administered intravenously (15 000 units/m^2 in a bolus administered over 60 s) and was followed, within 8 min after intravenous injection, by the application of brief electric pulses to each tumor nodule. Electric currents were delivered by means of a 2–3-cm long needle electrode according to lesion size.

The electrodes were connected to a pulse generator (Cliniporator™; Igea, Modena, Italy). This generator produces high voltages (up to 1000 V), but delivered as a compressed train of eight pulses at a frequency of 5000 Hz and 100 μs duration, and therefore well tolerated by the patient. The software controls and stores the applied voltage and the actual current delivered to each tumor. ECT could be repeated every 8–12 weeks according to local response, the appearance of new lesions and the patient's tolerance of the treatment.

4. Surgical approach for distant metastases

Conventional teaching maintains that resection is not indicated in patients with distant metastases, except for palliation. This dogma stems from the concept that patients with multiple metastases usually also have occult micrometastases and circulating tumor cells. However the results of surgical treatment of stage IV melanoma patients have improved considerably over the past two decades. Recent studies [75] provide further evidence of the beneficial role of surgery for distant metastases of melanoma. Our findings indicate a survival advantage for a surgical approach, even in patients with high-risk visceral metastases or multiple metastases that may require multiple operations for complete resection. At least 55 % of stage IV patients may be eligible to undergo surgery as part of their treatment plan and the surgeon should play an integral role in evaluation and treatment planning for all patients with stage IV recurrence of melanoma. One potential therapeutic advantage of resection is that it may delay disease progression by interrupting the metastatic cascade associated with hematogenous seeding of cells to other sites.[76]In addition, it immediately reduces tumor burden and thereby decreases tumor-induced immune suppression.[77] Finally, metastasectomy may enhance the patient's endogenous immune defences or response to adjuvant immunotherapy and thus maintain a complete clinical remission. Surgery for distant metastases has been improved by development of more advanced imaging techniques that can detect lesions as small as 5–10 mm.[78] These techniques can differentiate patients with multiple versus limited metastases, allowing surgeons to better judge the extent of disease and plan the operative procedure necessary for complete resection. In addition, modern advances in anaesthesia, surgical techniques and supportive care have reduced operative mortality from multiple metastasectomy with a corresponding reduction in morbidity and finally, shorter postsurgical hospitalizations have decreased the total costs of cancer surgery. Surgical therapy for stage IV disease remains controversial. The development of metastases is a complex process and the rationale for surgical resection of metastatic melanoma is multifactorial. First, reduction of tumor burden through surgical resection limits disease progression by interrupting the metastatic cascade associated with haematogenous seeding of cells to other sites. Unlike chemotherapy, surgery can easily eradicate tumor masses 2 cm or larger. Second, surgery may reverse tumor-induced immunosuppression, restoring immune function and inhibiting metastatic progression. Third, most patients tolerate surgical resection to a much greater extent than they can tolerate adverse effects of systemic therapy and recurrences after initial metastasectomy can also be treated through a secondary resection of metastases. Last, metastasectomy does not preclude systemic therapy;

however, if metastasectomy is delayed, increasing tumor burden may make disease unresectable. In addition the advent of newer and better systemic therapies makes the role of surgical resection more relevant today than ever before. Timing of surgery versus systemic treatment is another important end point. The development of new and effective drugs in the systemic treatment of stage IV melanoma patients have been reported recently, with the BRAF inhibitor Vemurafinib and the monoclonal antibody Ipilimumab; other targeted drugs are being developed, and some are currently being tested in the clinical setting. Thus a therapeutic strategy combining new drugs with aggressive surgery in selected cases of melanoma metastatic disease could be designed in the following years.

Author details

Mario Santinami[1], Roberto Patuzzo[1], Roberta Ruggeri[1], Gianpiero Castelli[1], Andrea Maurichi[1], Giulia Baffa[1] and Carlotta Tinti[1]

1 Melanoma Sarcoma Unit Fondazione Istituto Tumori Milano, Italy

Dermatology Unit Ospedale Umberto I Siracusa, Italy

References

[1] W.S. Handley. The pathology of melanotic growths in relation to their operative treatment. Lancet, i: 927-996,1907

[2] R. Kaufmann. Surgical management of primary melanoma. Clin Exp Dermatol 25: 476–481, 2000

[3] U. Veronesi, N. Cascinelli, J. Adamus et al.Thin stage I primary cutaneous malignant melanoma. Comparison of excision with margins of 1 or 3 cm. N Engl J Med 318:1159–1162,1988.

[4] U. Ringborg, R. Andersson, J. Eldh et al. Resection margins of 2 versus 5 cm for cutaneous malignant melanoma with a tumor thickness of 0.8 to 2.0 mm: randomized study by the Swedish Melanoma Study Group. Cancer 77:1809–1814,1996.

[5] J.M. Thomas, J. Newton-Bishop, R. A'Hern et al.Excision margins in high-risk malignant melanoma N Engl J Med 350:757–766, 2004.

[6] R. Dummer, R. Panizzon, P.H. Bloch, et al.Updated Swiss guidelines for the treatment and follow-up of cutaneous melanoma.Dermatology 210: 39–44, 2005.

[7] R. Dummer, A. Hauschild, L. Jost. Cutaneous malignant melanoma: ESMO clinical recommendations for diagnosis, treatment and follow-up. Ann Oncol 19 (Suppl 2): ii86–ii88, 2008.

http://dx.doi.org/10.5772/54105

[8] C. Garbe, A. Hauschild, M. Volkenandt et al.Evidence and interdisciplinary consensus-based German guidelines: surgical treatment and radiotherapy of melanoma. Melanoma Res, 18: 61–67, 2008.

[9] R. Essner, J.H. Lee, L.A. Wanek, et al.Contemporary surgical treatment of advanced-stage melanoma. Arch Surg 139: 961–966, 2004.

[10] Balch CM, Gershenwald JE, Soong SJ, et al. Final version of 2009 AJCC melanoma staging and classification. J Clin Oncol 27:6199-6206, 2009.

[11] Balch CM, Gershenwald JE, Soong SJ. Multivariate analysis of prognostic factors among 2,313 patients with stage III melanoma: Comparison of nodal micrometastases versus macrometastases. J Clin Oncol 28:2452–2459, 2010.

[12] Gershenwald JE, Ross MI. Sentinel-lymph-node biopsy for cutaneous melanoma. N Engl J Med 364: 1738–1745, 2011.

[13] Ross MI, Thompson JF, Gershenwald JE. Sentinel lymph node biopsy for melanoma: critical assessment at its twentieth anniversary. Surg Oncol Clin North Am 20: 57–78, 2011.

[14] Balch CM, Morton DL, Gershenwald JE, et al.Sentinel node biopsy and standard of care for melanoma. J Am Acad Dermatol 60:872–875, 2009.

[15] Valsecchi ME, Silbermins D, de Rosa N, et al. Lymphatic mapping and sentinel lymph node biopsy in patients with melanoma: A meta-analysis. J Clin Oncol 29:1479–1487,2011.

[16] Wrightson WR, Wong SL, Edwards MJ, et al. Complications associated with sentinel lymph node biopsy for melanoma. Ann Surg Oncol 10:676–680,2003.

[17] McMasters KM, Noyes RD, Reintgen DS, et al. Lessons learned from the Sunbelt Melanoma Trial. J Surg Oncol 86:212–223, 2004.

[18] Sondak VK, Taylor JM, Sabel MS, et al. Mitotic rate and younger age are predictors of sentinel lymph node positivity: Lessons learned from the generation of a probabilistic model. Ann Surg Oncol 11:247–258,2004.

[19] Sabel MS, Rice JD, Griffith KA, et al.Validation of statistical predictive models meant to select melanoma patients for sentinel lymph node biopsy. Ann Surg Oncol 19:287–293, 2012.

[20] Edge SB, Byrd DR, Compton CC, et al. AJCC Cancer Staging Manual, Springer, New York, NY,ed 7, 2010.

[21] Morton DL, Cochran AJ, Thompson JF, et al.Sentinel node biopsy for early-stage melanoma: Accuracy and morbidity in MSLT-I, an international multicenter trial. Ann Surg 242:302–311, discussion 311-313, 2005.

[22] Eggermont AM, Suciu S, Santinami M, et al. Adjuvant therapy with pegylated interferon alfa-2b versus observation alone in resected stage III melanoma: Final results of EORTC 18991, a randomised phase III trial. Lancet 372:117–126, 2008.

[23] Balch CM, Buzaid AC, Soong SJ, et al.Final version of the American Joint Committee on Cancer staging system for cutaneous melanoma. J Clin Oncol 19:3635–3648, 2001.

[24] Balch CM, Soong SJ, Gershenwald JE, et al. Prognostic factors analysis of 17,600 melanoma patients: Validation of the American Joint Committee on Cancer melanoma staging system. J Clin Oncol 19:3622–3634, 2001.

[25] Gershenwald JE, Mansfield PF, Lee JE, et al.Role for lymphatic mapping and sentinel lymph node biopsy in patients with thick (≥ 4 mm) primary melanoma. Ann Surg Oncol 7:160–165, 2000.

[26] Ferrone CR, Panageas KS, Busam K, et al.Multivariate prognostic model for patients with thick cutaneous melanoma: Importance of sentinel lymph node status. Ann Surg Oncol 9:637–645, 2002.

[27] Balch CM, Gershenwald JE, Soong SJ, et al. Update on the melanoma staging system: The importance of sentinel node staging and primary tumor mitotic rate. J Surg Oncol 104:379–385, 2011.

[28] Gajdos C, Griffith KA, Wong SL, et al.Is there a benefit to sentinel lymph node biopsy in patients with T4 melanoma? Cancer 115:5752–5760,2009.

[29] Essner R, Chung MH, Bleicher R, et al.Prognostic implications of thick (≥ 4 mm) melanoma in the era of intraoperative lymphatic mapping and sentinel lymphadenectomy. Ann Surg Oncol 9:754–761,2002.

[30] Carlson GW, Murray DR, Hestley A, et al.Sentinel lymph node mapping for thick (≥ 4 mm) melanoma: Should we be doing it? Ann Surg Oncol 10:408–415,2003.

[31] Thompson JF, Shaw HM.The prognosis of patients with thick primary melanomas: Is regional lymph node status relevant, and does removing positive regional nodes influence outcome? Ann Surg Oncol 9:719–722,2002.

[32] Gutzmer R, Satzger I, Thoms KM, et al.Sentinel lymph node status is the most important prognostic factor for thick (≥ 4 mm) melanomas. J Dtsch Dermatol Ges 6:198–203,2008.

[33] Scoggins CR, Bowen AL, Martin RC 2nd, et al.Prognostic information from sentinel lymph node biopsy in patients with thick melanoma. Arch Surg 145:622–627,2010.

[34] Criscione VD, Weinstock MA. Melanoma thickness trends in the United States 1988-2006. J Invest Dermatol 130:793–797,2010.

[35] Andtbacka RH, Gershenwald JE. Role of sentinel lymph node biopsy in patients with thin melanoma. J Natl Compr Canc Netw 7:308–317,2009.

[36] Amersi F, Morton DL.The role of sentinel lymph node biopsy in the management of melanoma. Adv Surg 41:241–256,2007.

[37] Morton DL, Thompson JF, Cochran AJ, et al.Sentinel-node biopsy or nodal observation in melanoma. N Engl J Med 355:1307–1317,2006

[38] Wong SL, Morton DL, Thompson JF, et al. Melanoma patients with positive sentinel nodes who did not undergo completion lymphadenectomy: A multi-institutional study. Ann Surg Oncol 13:809–816, 2006

[39] Kingham TP, Panageas KS, Ariyan CE, et al. Outcome of patients with a positive sentinel lymph node who do not undergo completion lymphadenectomy. Ann Surg Oncol 17:514–520, 2010

[40] Calabro A, Singletary SE, Balch CM. Patterns of relapse in 1,001 consecutive patients with melanoma nodal metastases. Arch Surg 124:1051–1055, 1989.

[41] Wong SL, Brady MS, Busam KJ, et al.Results of sentinel lymph node biopsy in patients with thin melanoma. Ann Surg Oncol 13:302–309,2006.

[42] Jaques DP, Coit DGet al. Major amputation for advanced malignant melanoma. Surg Gynecol Obstet 169:1–6,1989.

[43] Karakousis CP, Choe KJ, Holyoke ED. Biologic behavior and treatment of intransit metastasis of melanoma. Surg Gynecol Obstet 150:29–32,1980.

[44] Creech O, Jr., Krementz ET, Ryan RF, et al. Chemotherapy of cancer: regional perfusion utilizing an extracorporeal circuit. Ann Surg 148:616–32,1958.

[45] Benckhuijsen C, Kroon BB, van Geel AN, et al. Regional perfusion treatment with melphalan for melanoma in a limb: an evaluation of drug kinetics. Eur J Surg Oncol 14:157–63, 1988.

[46] Vrouenraets BC, Nieweg OE, Kroon BB. Thirty-five years of isolated limb perfusion for melanoma: indications and results. Br J Surg 83:1319–28,1996.

[47] Eggermont AM, Schraffordt Koops H, Lienard D, et al. Isolated limb perfusion with high-dose tumor necrosis factor-alpha in combination with interferon-gamma and melphalan for nonresectable extremity soft tissue sarcomas: a multicenter trial. J Clin Oncol 14:2653–65,1996

[48] Eggermont AM, Schraffordt Koops H, Klausner JM, et al. Isolated limb perfusion with tumor necrosis factor and melphalan for limb salvage in 186 patients with locally advanced soft tissue extremity sarcomas. The cumulative multicenter European experience. Ann Surg 224:756–64; discussion 764–5,1996

[49] Lejeune FJ, Lienard D, Leyvraz S, et al. Regional therapy of melanoma. Eur J Cancer 29A: 606–12, 1993.

[50] de Wilt JH, Manusama ER, van Tiel ST, et al. Prerequisites for effective isolated limb perfusion using tumour necrosis factor alpha and melphalan in rats. Br J Cancer 80:161–6, 1999

[51] Bonvalot S, Laplanche A, Lejeune F, et al. Limb salvage with isolated perfusion for soft tissue sarcoma: could less TNF-alpha be better? Ann Oncol 16:1061–8, 2005.

[52] Hill S, Fawcett WJ, Sheldon J, et al. Low-dose tumour necrosis factor alpha and melphalan in hyperthermic isolated limb perfusion. Br J Surg 80:995–7, 1993

[53] Rossi CR, Foletto M, Mocellin S, et al. Hyperthermic isolated limb perfusion with low-dose tumor necrosis factor-alpha and melphalan for bulky in-transit melanoma metastases. Ann Surg Oncol 11:173–7, 2004.

[54] J.F. Thompson, R.C. Waugh, C.W. Schacherer et al. Isolated limb infusion with melphalan for recurrent limb melanoma: a simple alternative to isolated limb perfusion. Reg Cancer Treat 7:188–192, 1994.

[55] J.F. Thompson, P.C. Kam, R.C. Waugh et al.Isolated limb infusion with cytotoxic agents: a simple alternative to isolated limb perfusion. Semin Surg Oncol 14: 238–247,1998.

[56] P. Lindnér, A. Doubrovsky, P.C.A. Kam et al.Prognostic factors after isolated limb infusion with cytotoxic agents for melanoma.Ann Surg Oncol, 9: 127–136, 2002.

[57] H.M. Kroon, M. Moncrieff, P.C.A. Kam et al.Outcomes following isolated limb infusion for melanoma. A 14-year experience.Ann Surg Oncol, 15: 3003–3013, 2008.

[58] M.S. Brady, K. Brown, A. Patel et al.A phase II trial of isolated limb infusion with melphalan and dactinomycin for regional melanoma and soft tissue sarcoma of the extremity.Ann Surg Oncol, 13: 1123–1129, 2006.

[59] A.S. Gupta, S. Heinzmann, E.A. Levine. Successful treatment of in transit metastases in Merkel's cell carcinoma with isolated hyperthermic limb perfusion. South Med J, 91: 289–292, 1998.

[60] E. Elhassadi, E. Egan, G. O'Sullivan et al. Isolated limb infusion with cytotoxic agent for treatment of localized refractory cutaneous T-cell lymphoma. Clin Lab Haematol, 4: 279–281, 2006.

[61] Belehradek M, Domenge C, Luboinski B, et al. Electrochemotherapy, a new antitumor treatment: first clinical phase I–II trial report. Cancer 72: 3694–3700, 1993.

[62] Mir LM, Orlowski S. Mechanisms of electrochemotherapy. Adv Drug Del Rev 35: 107–118,1999.

[63] Mir LM, Glass LF, Sersa G, et al. Effective treatment of cutaneous and subcutaneous malignant tumours by electrochemotherapy. Br J Cancer 77: 2336–2342,1998.

[64] Rols MP, Bachaud JM, Giraud P, et al. Electrochemotherapy of cutaneous metastases in malignant melanoma. Melanoma Res 10: 468–474,2000.

[65] Byrne MC, Thompson JF, Johnston H, et al. Treatment of metastatic melanoma using electroporation therapy with bleomycin (electrochemotherapy). Melanoma Res 15: 45–51,2005.

[66] Gaudy C, Richard MA, Folchetti G, et al. Randomized controlled study of electrochemotherapy in the local treatment of skin metastases of melanoma. J Cutan Med Surg 10: 115–121,2006.

[67] Larkin JO, Collins CG, Aarons S, et al. Electrochemotherapy: aspects of preclinical development and early clinical experience. Ann Surg 245: 469–479,2007.

[68] Serša G, Štabuc B, Čemažar M, et al. Electrochemotherapy with cisplatin: the systemic antitumour effectiveness of cisplatin can be potentiated locally by the application of electric pulses in the treatment of malignant melanoma skin metastases. Melanoma Res 10: 381–385,2000.

[69] Domenge C, Orlowski S, Luboinski B, et al. Antitumour electrochemotherapy: new advances in the clinical protocol. Cancer 77: 956–963,1996.

[70] Campana LG, Mocellin S, Basso M, et al. Bleomycin-based electrochemotherapy: clinical outcome from a single institution's experience with 52 patients. Ann Surg Oncol 6: 191–199,2009.

[71] Kis E, Oláh J, Ócsai H, et al. Electrochemotherapy of cutaneous metastases of melanoma—a case series study and systematic review of the evidence. Dermatol Surg 37: 816–824,2011.

[72] Marty M, Serša G, Garbay JR, et al. Electrochemotherapy—an easy, highly effective and safe treatment of cutaneous and subcutaneous metastases: results of ESOPE study. EJC Suppl 4: 3–13,2006.

[73] Mir LM, Gehl J, Sersa G, et al. Standard operating procedures of the electrochemotherapy: instructions for the use of bleomycin or cisplatin administered either systemically or locally and electric pulses delivered by the Cliniporator by means of invasive or non-invasive electrodes. EJC Suppl 4: 14–25, 2006.

[74] Balch CM, Buzaid AC, Soong SJ, et al. Final version of the American Joint Committee on Cancer staging system for cutaneous melanoma. J Clin Oncol 19: 3635–3648, 2001.

[75] Howard JH, Thompson JF, Mozzillo N, et al. Metastasectomy for Distant Metastatic Melanoma: Analysis of Data from the First Multicenter Selective Lymphadenectomy Trial (MSLT-I). Ann Surg Oncol 19:2547-55, 2012.

[76] Roth JA, Silverstein MJ, Morton DL. Metastatic potential of metastases. Surgery 79:669–73, 1976.

[77] Morton DL, Holmes EC, Golub SH. Immunologic aspects of lung cancer. Chest 71:640–3, 1977.

[78] Gulec SA, Faries MB, Lee CC, et al. The role of fluorine-18 deoxyglucose positron emission tomography in the management of patients with metastatic melanoma: impact on surgical decision making. Clin Nucl Med 28:961–5, 2003.

Chapter 20

Therapeutic Agents for Advanced Melanoma

Zhao Wang, Wei Li and Duane D. Miller

Additional information is available at the end of the chapter

http://dx.doi.org/10.5772/53632

1. Introduction

Melanoma is an extremely complicated disease, with many gene mutations and alternations in signaling pathways. Because effective treatment for melanoma is lacking, the prognosis for metastatic melanoma patients remains very poor. Over the past 30 years, significant efforts have been made to search for better agents or strategies to fight this deadly disease. Numerous clinical trials at different stages have been carried out. Although most of them have failed, some did show very promising results. New treatment strategies have resulted in paradigm shift in our approach to melanoma therapy. These shining examples may markedly change our philosophy about melanoma treatment.

The year 2011 marked a fruitful year for melanoma research. The FDA approved three drugs for advanced melanoma treatment: ipilimumab (an anti-cytotoxic T lymphocyte antigen-4 monoclonal antibody), vemurafenib (a selective BRAF inhibitor), and pegylated interferon-α2b for adjuvant setting usage [1]. However, there are still significant limitations for melanoma treatment. Ipilimumab only prolonged the survival time for metastatic melanoma patient from an average of 6.5 months to an average of 10 months. This treatment also has been associated with strong immunological adverse effects; severe to fatal autoimmune reactions were seen in 12.9% of patients treated with ipilimumab in a clinical trial that enrolled 676 melanoma patients [2]. Vemurafenib is not effective for melanoma patients with wide type BRAF, and confirmation of BRAFV600E mutation-positive melanoma using an FDA-approved test is required before treatment with vemurafenib. This treatment also only prolonged the median survival time for advanced melanoma patients 2~3 months [1]. More importantly, despite the high initial response rate for patients with BRAFV600E mutation to vemurafenib, virtually all the patients developed primary or acquired resistance to this drug in the end [3]. With the rapidly rising incidents of this disease and the high resistance to current therapeutic agents, developing more effective drugs for melanoma is very important.

In this chapter, we will review available therapeutic agents for advanced melanoma as well as agents that are still under clinical development. We will focus on their mechanism of action, development history, and therapeutic effects. In learning from our efforts in the past, we must continue to challenge the current paradigms of treatment as we forge new paths to more effective treatment options. This will likely involve a multimodal approach to therapy utilizing all of the available tools in our arsenal.

2. Chemotherapy agents

According to the current 7th edition American Joint Committee of Cancer (AJCC) staging system, melanoma can be pathologically classified in the following stages: 0, IA, IB, IIA, IIB, IIC, IIIA, IIIB, IIIC, and IV. Stage 0 is in situ melanoma. Stage I and II are growth phase of localized cutaneous melanoma with increasing thickness. Stage III has regional involvement of lymph node. Stage IV means distant metastasis. Normally stage III and IV melanoma are called metastatic melanoma. Localized melanoma is curable with complete surgical excision in most patients. But currently treatment for metastatic melanoma is still very challenging. Only two chemotherapy drugs in current use have been approved by the Food and Drug Administration (FDA) for metastatic melanoma: dacarbazine (DTIC) and vemurafenib. Other agents that have been tried on melanoma patients are also discussed below.

2.1. Dacarbazine (DTIC)

DTIC is the first FDA approved chemotherapy drug for metastatic melanoma. This drug gained FDA approval in May 1975 as DTIC-Dome for the treatment of metastatic melanoma. It was initially marketed by Bayer. The therapeutic effect of DTIC is believed to be produced through alkylation of DNA. While its anticancer mechanism of action is still not fully understood, DTIC is believed to be first metabolically bioactivated through a series of reactions involving CYP450. Initial demethylation to MTIC [3-methyl-(triazen-1-yl)imidazole-4-carboxamide] is followed by formation of diazomethane, the active moiety of DTIC and a potent methylating agent [4].

DTIC has produced response rates of from 15% to 25% in single-institution trials. But the overall response rate has fallen over the years from 15% to 7% and less than 5% of responses are complete in phase 3 trials. The median response durations to DTIC are 5 to 6 months. Long-term follow-up of patients treated with DTIC alone shows that only <2% can be anticipated to survive for more than 6 years. In recent phase 3 trials that used strict response assessment criteria, the response rates with single-agent DTIC did not exceed 12% [5].

Over the past 30 years after its approval by the FDA, DTIC remains the only currently used cytotoxic drug for the treatment of metastatic melanoma. Despite its low single-agent activity, DTIC has remained the mainstay of many combination chemotherapy regimens and evaluations of resistance-reversing agents. After more than 20 years of research, DTIC is still the standard against which most new chemotherapy agents are compared [6].

As for the dose, it has been demonstrated that 850~1000 mg/m^2 single dose of DTIC is tolerated. This single dose administration appears to deliver clinical improvements similar to those observed with multiple doses that provide the same total dose per cycle. This should be the reference standard for randomized trials comparing new therapies with DTIC [7].

2.2. Temozolomide

Temozolomide (TMZ) is an orally active alkylating agent. It's a prodrug of MTIC and congener of DTIC. It has been available in the US since August 1999 and in other countries since the early 2000s. The therapeutic benefit of temozolomide depends on its ability to alkylate/methylate DNA, which most often occurs at the N-7 or O-6 positions of guanine residues. This methylation damages the DNA and triggers the death of tumor cells. However, some tumor cells are able to repair this type of DNA damage, and therefore diminish the therapeutic efficacy of temozolomide, by expressing an enzyme called O-6-methylguanine-DNA methyltransferase (MGMT) or O-6-alkylguanine-DNA alkyltransferase [8].

The single agent activity of TMZ in metastatic melanoma has been established in several phase 1 and 2 studies [9]. In a randomized trial of 305 patients with advanced melanoma, TMZ showed efficacy at least equivalent to that of DTIC in terms of objective response rate, time to progression, and overall disease-free survival [10]. TMZ was tolerated very well and showed an advantage in terms of improvement in the quality of life. More patients showed improvement or maintenance of physical functioning at Week 12. That trial excluded patients who had brain metastases. Because the trial design was intended to demonstrate the superiority of TMZ over DTIC, rather than equivalence, the FDA did not accept the results of that trial as grounds for approving a melanoma indication for TMZ. But in clinical practice, patients with metastatic melanoma often are treated off-label with TMZ.

TMZ has demonstrated efficacy in the treatment of variety of solid tumors, especially in brain malignancies, which is a manifestation of its far greater ability to penetrate the central nervous system (CNS). Taking into account the high rate of CNS recurrence as a site of failure after cytotoxic chemotherapy, TMZ may represent a viable alternative to DTIC, which is ineffective against melanoma CNS metastases.

2.3. Sorafenib

Sorafenib (BAY43-9006, developed by Bayer Pharmaceuticals, West Haven CT, trade name Nexavar) is an orally administered tyrosine kinase inhibitor. It is a potent inhibitor of the BRAF kinase that is frequently mutated in melanoma, as well as an inhibitor of the Vascular Endothelial Growth Factor (VEGF) receptor and other kinases. It targets the adenosine triphosphate-binding site of the BRAF kinase and inhibits both wild-type and mutant BRAF *in vitro*. Sorafenib was approved by the FDA in December 2005 for use in the treatment of advanced renal cancer. Preclinical studies demonstrated a significant retardation in the growth of human melanoma tumor xenografts with Sorafenib. In a phase 1 study, the maximum tolerated dose of Sorafenib as a single agent was established at 400 mg twice daily, and the most common toxicities were gastrointestinal (mainly diarrhea), dermatologic (skin rash, hand-foot syndrome), and fatigue [11].

But in further phase 2 clinical trials, Sorafenib had shown relatively little activity in metastatic melanoma when using alone. In a phase 2 trial that was conducted in 20 patients with refractory metastatic melanoma, Sorafenib showed modest activity with 1 partial response and 3 patients who achieved stable disease [12]. In another phase 2, randomized, discontinuation trial, no objective responses were achieved, and 19% of patients achieved stable disease [13].

Sorafenib combined with other chemotherapy drugs were also tested clinically. In a phase 1 and 2 study that combined carboplatin and paclitaxel with escalating doses of Sorafenib in 35 patients, a promising response rate of 31% was observed, and another 54% of patients experienced stable disease that lasted longer than 3 months. That study recently was updated to include 105 patients, and the current response rate is 27% [14]. On this basis, 2 phase 3 trials have been launched to assess the efficacy of carboplatin and paclitaxel plus Sorafenib versus placebo in chemotherapy-naive patients and in previously treated patients. In December 2006, Bayer reported the combinations failed to show significant improvement of progression-free survival in melanoma patients [15].

2.4. Vemurafenib

Vemurafenib established a successful model for extracellular chemotherapeutic targeted therapy based on deep understanding cancer biology. It's a paradigm of structured-based drug development. It was first discovered in 2002 that the protein kinase BRAF is mutated in about 70% of malignant melanomas and a significant number of colorectal, ovarian and papillary thyroid cancers, implicating mutated BRAF as a critical promoter of malignancy. Then scientists determined the structure of the BRAF catalytic domain and identified a class of BRAF inhibitors that bind to the active conformation of the protein. Further lead series were developed and crystal structures of complexes combined with molecular modeling studies have resulted in potent selective inhibitors. Vemurafenib is the first one that went into clinical trials and gained FDA approval in August 2011.

Vemurafenib (PLX4032/RG7204) is developed by Plexxikon (now part of the Daiichi Sankyo group and Hoffmann–La Roche) for the treatment of late-stage melanoma. Vemurafenib can induce programmed cell death in melanoma cell lines. It interrupts the BRAF/MEK step on the BRAF/MEK/ERK pathway – if the BRAF has the common V600E mutation [16].

Vemurafenib has very impressive single-agent clinical activity, with unprecedented response rates of about 80% and a clear impact on progression-free survival longer than 6 months. An international randomized open-label trial in patients with previously untreated metastatic or unresectable melanoma with the $BRAF^{V600E}$ mutation led to the FDA approval of Vemurafenib for melanoma. This clinical trial enrolled 675 patients. 337 patients were randomly assigned to vemurafenib with 960 mg orally twice daily. 338 patients were randomly assigned to dacarbazine with 1000 mg/m^2 intravenously every three weeks. Treatment end-points are disease progression, unacceptable toxicity, and/or consent withdrawal.

Vemurafenib's efficacy was measured by overall survival (OS), investigator-assessed progression-free survival (PFS) and confirmed investigator-assessed best overall response rate. Overall survival was significantly improved in patients receiving vemurafenib compared with those receiving dacarbazine. The median survival of patients receiving vemurafenib had not been reached and was 7.9 months for those receiving dacarbazine. Progression-free survival (PFS) was also significantly improved in patients receiving vemurafenib. The median PFS was 5.3 months for patients receiving vemurafenib and 1.6 months for patients receiving dacarbazine. 48.4% for patients who received vemurafenib showed complete or partial response while only 5.5% patients who received dacarbazine showed complete or partial response [17].

Arthralgia, rash, photosensitivity, fatigue, alopecia, pruritis, and skin papilloma were observed in at least 30% of patients treated with vemurafenib. Cutaneous squamous cell carcinomas were detected in approximately 24% of patients. Other adverse reactions reported in patients treated with vemurafenib included hypersensitivity, Stevens-Johnson syndrome, toxic epidermal necrolysis, uveitis, QT prolongation, and liver enzyme laboratory abnormalities [18].

2.5. Other single chemotherapy agents

Cisplatin and carboplatin have shown modest activity as single agents in patients with metastatic melanoma. Cisplatin as single-agent therapy induced a 15% response rate with a short median duration of 3 months [19]. A response rate of 19% has been reported in 26 chemotherapy-naive patients with metastatic melanoma who received carboplatin. In those patients, there were 5 partial responses, and thrombocytopenia was the dose-limiting toxicity [20]. *In vitro* studies suggested that oxaliplatin may be more active than cisplatin or carboplatin. But a small phase 2 trial in 10 patients who had received and failed prior chemotherapy produced no objective responses [21].

The nitrosoureas (carmustine, lomustine, and semustine) induce objective responses in 13~18% patients. They can cross the blood-brain barrier. But at conventional doses, little or no activity was observed against melanoma brain metastases [22]. Another drawback of the nitrosureas is they induce prolonged myelosuppression. Despite these, they have been included frequently in multi-agent chemotherapy combinations, presumably for their ability to penetrate into the CNS and lack of viable alternatives for metastatic melanoma.

The vinca alkaloids (vindesine and vinblastine) have produced responses in approximately 14% of patients [23]. The taxanes have produced responses in 16~17% patients [24]. All of these response rate data were obtained from phase 2 trials. None of those drugs have been evaluated as single agents in phase 3 trials. Based on the experience with DTIC, it is likely that the phase 3 trial objective response rates would be less than the rates reported from phase 2 trials. All of these drugs are rarely used currently as single-agent therapy in metastatic melanoma, but they frequently have been incorporated into combination chemotherapy and biochemotherapy regimens.

2.6. Chemotherapy drug combinations

Theoretically drug combination should be based on laboratory or clinical evidence of synergistic effect. But since single-agent chemotherapy regimens only provided modest activity against metastatic melanoma and lack of viable alternatives, many combination regimens have been evaluated in clinical trials. Initially two-agent combinations were tested in which DTIC was combined with a nitrosourea, vinca alkaloid, or platinum compound. In most of these trials, only 10~20% response rates were observed. There was little evidence to suggest superiority of these combinations compared with DTIC treatment alone [25-27].

In order to improve response rates, more aggressive multi-drug combinations using 3 or 4 different drugs were also tested clinically. Two most widely studied combinations are cisplatin, vinblastine, and DTIC (CVD) and the Dartmouth regimen. The latter is a 4-drug combination consisting of cisplatin, DTIC, carmustine, and tamoxifen (also called CDBT). Both combinations showed improved response rates that ranged from 30% to 50% in single-institution phase 2 studies [28, 29]. But in further randomized phase 3 trials which involved more patients, they all showed much lower efficiency: In a randomized trial comparing CVD with single-agent DTIC that involved approximately 150 patients, the CVD arm produced a 19% response rate compared with 14% for the DTIC arm, and there was no differences in either response duration or survival. In another randomized phase 3 trial, the CDBT combination was compared with single-agent DTIC. That cooperative group trial involved 240 patients, and the response rate was 10% for the DTIC regimen compared with 19% for the CDBT regimen (P=0.09). The median survival was 7 months, with no significant difference between the 2 treatment arms [6].

The main reason for such discrepancies between the results from single-institution studies and those from large, multicenter, cooperative trials probably is selection bias. Differences in performance status, percentages of patients with visceral involvement, and number of metastatic sites easily could account for some of the observed differences. In fact, all of those factors are known to have an impact on both response rate and survival [30].

Overall, controlled trials have produced no compelling evidence to support the value of combination chemotherapy, with or without tamoxifen, in patients with metastatic melanoma. Toxicity was substantially greater for the combination regimen, with bone marrow suppression, nausea, emesis, and fatigue significantly more frequent with CDBT than with DTIC [6]. So it is difficult to justify the use of either CVD or CDBT instead of single-agent DTIC or TMZ for the treatment of most patients with metastatic melanoma.

3. Immunotherapy agents

3.1. Interleukin-s (IL-2)

In 1998, the FDA approved intermittent high-dose bolus IL-2 based on its ability to mediate durable complete response in metastatic melanoma patients [31]. IL-2 is a type of cytokine immune system signaling molecule, which is a leukocytotrophic hormone that is instrumental in the body's natural response to microbial infection and in discriminating between foreign (non-self) and self. It's a glycosylated 15,500 dalton single protein molecule. IL-2 mediates its effects by binding to IL-2 receptors, which are expressed by lymphocytes, the cells that are responsible for immunity. It is one of the only two FDA approved agents for the treatment of metastatic melanoma. Although the overall response rate is only about 15% and less than 5% of patients achieve complete remission with IL-2, its performance on melanoma is better than DTIC.

One of the major immunologic effects of IL-2 upon the immune system is to expand the total number of T-lymphocytes (CD4+ and CD8+) and to prevent lymphocyte apoptosis. Another key role of IL-2 is to provide the appropriate cytokine milieu necessary to overcome tumor-induced immune tolerance. But the exact molecular and genetic mechanisms involved in this complex interaction between the tumor and the host immune response is still largely unknown [32].

There is currently a wide spectrum of dosing schedules and regimens for IL-2 therapy, with the current standard used by most oncologists being 600,000 to 720,000 IU/kg/dose, given at 8 h intervals. Although the optimal dosing schedule resulting in the best clinical response is currently unknown, previous data would suggest that the higher dose regimens as well as the number of total doses received correlates best with clinical response. Thus, several groups have begun to look at alternative dosing strategies to achieve an increased drug tolerance and tolerability profile, such as the continuous infusion of IL-2 (18 mIU/m^2/day) over an extended period of 72 h [33]. But the multiorgan toxicity of many IL-2 regimens limits its use. In addition, the tumor-killing cytotoxic T cells and natural killer cells, which are the presumed target cells for IL-2, are frequently inefficient in the tumor environment, partly due to suppressive and apoptosis-inducing signals from tumor-infiltrating mononuclear phagocytes [34].

3.2. Interferon α

Interferons (IFNs) are proteins made and released by the cells of most vertebrates in response to the presence of pathogens or tumor cells. They allow communication between cells to trigger the protective defenses of the immune system that eradicate pathogens or tumors. IFNs belong to the large class of glycoproteins known as cytokines. They are named after their ability to "interfere" with viral replication within host cells. IFNs have other functions: they activate immune cells, such as natural killer cells and macrophages; they increase recognition of infection or tumor cells by up-regulating antigen presentation to T lymphocytes; and they increase the ability of uninfected host cells to resist new infection by virus.

Based on the type of receptors through which they signal, human interferons have been classified into three major types. The type I interferons present in human are IFN-α, IFN-β and IFN-ω [35]. High-dose IFN therapy using IFN-α was the first form of medical therapy to be approved by the FDA for use in high-risk melanoma in the adjuvant setting. Adjuvant normally means using IFN- α weeks after the surgical excision of the melanoma tumor. Common treatment scheme is IFN-α2b at 20 million units (MU)/m^2/day intravenous injection 5 days a week for 4 weeks, then 10 MU/m^2/day subcutaneous injection 3 days a week for the next 48 weeks for a full year's. But IFN-α2b can also be used one month before definitive surgical lymphadenectomy. This is called 'neoadjuvant' treatment [36].

The first randomized comparison of high-dose IFN versus observation found the median relapse-free survival was 1.72 years in the high-dose IFN arm versus 0.98 year in the observation arm (P=0.0023) and the median overall survival was 3.82 versus 2.78 years (P=0.0237) respectively [37]. But in a later pooled analysis of more patients in more clinical trials, the relapse-free survival benefit was maintained but no overall survival benefit was seen [38].

The exact mechanism of IFN IFN-α's anti-tumor efficacy is still unknown. But it was found that the STAT1/STAT3 expression ratios rose in association with IFN treatment. The clinical effects of IFN-α2b in human melanoma are also found to be inversely related to STAT3 expression (41). Induction of apoptosis has been shown to be important *in vitro,* if not *in vivo.* IFN-α can induce apoptosis in transformed cell lines as well as primary tumor cells [39].

High-dose IFN is the standard of care for high-risk melanoma patients in the adjuvant setting. However, it is associated with significant toxicity. The incidence and severity of these adverse events is clearly dose-related. Consequently, there has been a great deal of interest in intermediate- and low-dose regimens administered through subcutaneous injection. However, none of the trials using intermediate or low dosing so far have been able to demonstrate any reliable benefit in terms of relapse-free survival or overall survival [40].

3.3. Pegylated interferon-α2b

Pegylated interferon-α2b gained its approval from the FDA in March 2011 in the adjuvant setting for melanoma patients with lymph-node-positive disease (stage III) after lymph-node dissection. The approval was based on a randomized controlled phase-III trial in 1256 stage-III melanoma patients. This trial compared treatment with pegylated interferon- α2b for up to 5 years with observation. The results revealed a significant and sustained impact on relapse free survival (RFS) in the intention-to-treat (ITT) population. This trial also showed that interferon-α2b treatment didn't significantly improve distant metastasis-free survival (DMFS) or overall survival (OS) [41]. Pegylated interferon-α2b also showed much better effect in patients with sentinel-node-positive disease (stage III-N1: microscopic involvement only) compared with patients with palpable nodal disease (stage III-N2). It also significantly improved DMFS in sentinel-node-positive patients in contrast to a marginal effect in patients with palpable nodes. The authors identified tumor stage as a predictive factor in trials. One very important finding from clinical trials was that ulceration of the primary melanoma indicated a distinct biology that was clearly IFN sensitive in contrast to the non-ulcerated type of melanoma.

3.4. Anti-CTLA4 antibodies: Ipilimumab and tremelimumab

Cytotoxic T-Lymphocyte Antigen 4 (CTLA4) also known as CD152 (Cluster of differentiation 152) is a member of the immunoglobulin super family, which is expressed on the surface of Helper T cells and transmits an inhibitory signal to T cells that eventually shuts off the activated state. The rationale for involving this in treatment of metastatic melanoma is to block the negative signal sending by CTLA4 by using anti-CTLA4 antibodies, thus reduce the sensitivity of activated T cells to negative regulatory signals and enhance the immune response of the host to tumor cells.

As of October 2007 there are two fully human monoclonal anti-CTLA4 antibodies in advanced clinical trials, one from Medarex, Inc. (Princeton, NJ) and Bristol-Myers Squibb (New York), called ipilimumab (MDX-010), and one from Pfizer (New York), called tremelimumab (formerly ticilimumab, CP-675,206) [42]. These antibodies were produced using different types of mice with engineered immune systems, and are thus fully human, with long half-lives of 2– 4 weeks.

Ipilimumab (MDX-010) is an IgG1 monoclonal antibody. Preclinical and early clinical studies of patients with metastatic melanoma show that ipilimumab promotes antitumor activity as monotherapy and in combination with treatments such as chemotherapy, vaccines, or cytokines. The initial success with these antibodies has encouraged the rapid development of new agonistic and antagonistic antibodies that alter immune regulation, such as anti-PD-1, anti-4-1BB, anti-CD40, and anti-OX-40. On December 10, 2007, Bristol-Myers Squibb and Medarex released the results of three studies on ipilimumab [42]. The three studies tested 487 patients with metastatic melanoma. Short-term tumor progression prior to delayed regression has been observed in ipilimumab-treated patients, and objective responses may be of prolonged duration. In some patients clinical improvement manifests as stable disease, which may also extend for months or years. One of the three studies failed to meet its primary goal of shrinking tumors in at least 10% of the study's 155 patients. Overall the medication produced weaker-than-anticipated efficacy on melanoma patients.

In the meantime, the side effect profile was high in the ipilimumab treated group, with the generation of autoimmune-like effects, such as diarrhea, dermatitis and effects upon the thyroid and pituitary glands. Several patients also experienced vitiligo, indicative of anti-melanocyte autoimmunity. However, the majority of the side effects were noted to be transient (except the vitiligo), improving or disappearing after the completion of therapy. Early clinical data suggest a correlation between these side effects and response to ipilimumab treatment and most likely reflect the drug mechanism of action and corresponding effects on the immune system [42].

In 2011, the first-line pivotal trial data for ipilimumab was released. The median survival of patients treated with ipilimumab at a dose of 10 mg/kg in combination with dacarbazine was 11.2 months. Patients treated with dacarbazine alone showed a median survival of 9.1 months. The improvement in the median survival was 2.1 months. The estimated survival rates in the two groups of, respectively, 47.3% and 36.3% at 1 year, 28.5% and 17.9% at 2 years, and 20.8% and 12.2% at 3 years. These results are not better than those observed with the 3 mg/kg dose in second-line treatment. One possible reason is that a significant and unexpectedly high rate of hepatitis in the dacarbazine + ipilimumab arm did take a significant percentage of patients off treatment before the third or especially the fourth dose of ipilimumab could be administered, thus limiting both the number of administrations of dacarbazine as well as of ipilimumab in the combination arm. Other immune-related adverse events were not increased compared to those with the 3 mg/kg dose experience. The overall interpretation therefore is that dacarbazine did not help, but may rather have mitigated the results in the dacarbazine plus ipilimumab arm. Based on all the data available, the large cumulative phase-II experience, and the two phase-III trials, the FDA approved treatment of melanoma with ipilimumab alone at the 3mg/kg dose [43].

Tremelimumab is an IgG2 monoclonal antibody produced by Pfizer. It blocks the binding of the antigen-presenting cell ligands B7.1 and B7.2 to CTLA-4, resulting in inhibition of B7-CTLA-4-mediated down-regulation of T-cell activation. Subsequently, B7.1 or B7.2 may interact with another T-cell surface receptor protein, CD28, resulting in a B7-CD28-mediated T-cell activation unopposed by B7-CTLA-4-mediated inhibition. Tremelimumab is thought to stimulate patients' immune systems to attack their tumors. It has been shown to induce durable tumor responses in patients with metastatic melanoma in phase 1 and phase 2 clinical studies [44].

On April 2, 2008, Pfizer announced that it has discontinued a phase 3 clinical trial for patients with metastatic melanoma after the review of interim data showed that the trial would not demonstrate superiority to standard chemotherapy [45]. Studies for other tumors are planned as of October 2009, namely for prostate cancer and bladder cancer.

3.5. Anti-integrin antibody: Etaracizumab

Etaracizumab (also known as etaratuzumab, MEDI-522, trade name Abegrin) is an IgG1 humanized monoclonal antibody directed against the $\alpha V\beta 3$ integrin. $\alpha V\beta 3$ is essential for endothelial cell proliferation, maturation, and survival. When it is blocked, proliferating endothelial cells undergo apoptosis and regress. In addition, $\alpha V\beta 3$ is highly expressed in melanomas and is associated with tumor growth and invasion. In preclinical studies using $\alpha V\beta 3$ antagonists, inhibition of melanoma tumor growth independent of its antiangiogenic effects was reported [46]. Etaracizumab has been investigated in 3 phase 1, dose-escalation studies in patients with refractory melanoma. In the phase 2 trial, 57 patients received etaracizumab alone, and 55 patients received etaracizumab plus DTIC. Etaracizumab with or without DTIC generally was well tolerated and was active in patients with metastatic melanoma. The median survival was 12.6 months for the group that received etaracizumab with DTIC and 9.4 months for the group that received etaracizumab without DTIC [47]. These results encouraged people to further test this antibody in more clinical trials.

Early 2010, a study by the Etaracizumab Melanoma Study Group was reported. In this study, 112 patients were randomized to receive etaracizumab alone or etaracizumab plus DTIC. None of the patients in the etaracizumab alone study arm and 12.7% of patients in the etaracizumab plus DTIC study arm achieved an objective response. Stable disease occurred in 45.6% of patients in the etaracizumab alone study arm and 40.0% of patients in the etaracizumab plus DTIC study arm. Despite a modest increase in survival, 12.6 months in the etaracizumab alone arm, versus 9.4 months in the etaracizumab plus DTIC arm, the researchers concluded that the survival results in both treatment arms of this study were considered unlikely to result in clinically meaningful improvement over DTIC alone [48]. At the present time, clinical development of etaracizumab has been interrupted.

3.6. Vaccines based on tumor cells: Canvaxin, melacine, and MVax

The basic idea is to use tumor cell-based vaccine to stimulate and activate the host immune system to recognize, contain and eliminate cancer cells. This effect may be based on the following two pathways: direct migration of the tumor cells to the draining lymph node basin after injection, or uptake of apoptotic or necrotic tumor cells by host dendritic cells located within the skin [49].

The most extensively studied tumor cell-based vaccine is a polyvalent, antigen-rich whole cell vaccine called Canvaxin (CancerVax Corp., Carlsbad, CA). It is comprised of three melanoma cell lines that contain over 20 immunogenic melanoma tumor antigens, given intradermally every two weeks for 3 to 5 doses, followed by monthly injections for the remainder of the first year. However, several small, single-institution phase 1 and 2 clinical trials of Canvaxin have not yielded a striking clinical benefit in most patients when administered with BCG as an immunoadjuvant [50]. But the rare complete responder to Canvaxin therapy has prompted the initiation of two multicenter phase 3 randomized trials of Canvaxin therapy in 1998. In these trials, patients who have undergone complete resection of regional (stage III) or distant (stage IV) metastatic melanoma receive postoperative adjuvant immunotherapy with Canvaxin plus Bacillus of Calmette and Guerin (BCG) or BCG alone. In April 2005, CancerVax announced the discontinuation of their phase 3 clinical trial of Canvaxin in patients with Stage IV melanoma based upon the clinical funding that it was unlikely that the trial would provide significant evidence of a survival benefit for Canvaxin-treated patients versus those receiving placebo. On October 3, 2005, CancerVax announced the discontinuation of another phase 3 clinical trial of Canvaxin in patients with Stage III melanoma base on a similar reason [51].

The second tumor cell-based vaccine that has been well studied since 1988 is Melacine. It is an allogeneic melanoma cell lysate combined with an immunologic adjuvant which is composed of a mixture of detoxified endotoxin, cell wall cytoskeleton and monophosphoryl lipid A. Early phase 1 and 2 clinical trials in 1987 and 1988 revealed some promising results, with one complete and three partial responses seen in 25 patients treated with Melacine. These results prompted the completion of seven open-label phase 2 trials involving 139 patients with stage III/IV melanoma and a multicenter phase 3 clinical trial of Melacine versus the Dartmouth regimen. The objective response rates for all of the above studies have been between 5 and 10%. Based largely upon these former results and the clinical results of other phase 3 trials, a phase 3 observation controlled trial of Melacine in melanoma patients was conducted. But the results revealed no evidence of a benefit from Melacine in patients with melanoma [52].

One very promising autologous cell vaccine is MVax which is now in active phase 3 clinical trial sponsored by AVAX Technologies, Inc. This vaccine is derived from autologous tumor cells that have been irradiated and then modified with the hapten dinitrophenyl (DNP) [53]. In February 2004 the Journal of Clinical Oncology published an article by Dr. David Berd on the treatment of 214 Stage IIIb and IIIc melanoma patients that showed a five-year survival rate of 44%. Comparison to published results of similar patients treated with surgery alone showed five-year survival figures of 22%. In stage IV patients MVax has demonstrated significant response rates as a monotherapy and in published reports MVax plus adjuvant IL-2 have reported response rate of 35% (13% Complete Response, 22% Partial Response). This compares to published response rates in low dose IL-2 of 3% [54].

In October 2006, AVAX obtained a Special Protocol Assessment (SPA) agreement with the FDA for its phase 3 protocol. The SPA allows for the start of the phase 3 registration clinical trial for MVax for the treatment of patients with metastatic melanoma. In addition, the SPA addressed AVAX's ability to use a surrogate endpoint as a basis for accelerated approval. Based on this SPA, a phase 3 trial for stage IV melanoma was started on May 2007. AVAX plans to enroll up to 387 patients who will be assigned in a double-blind fashion at a 2:1 ratio to MVax or placebo vaccine. The MVax arm will consist of an initial dose of MVax followed by cyclophosphamide and then six weekly doses of MVax administered with BCG. Following vaccine administration patients will receive a specific schedule of low dose IL-2. Patients assigned to the control group will receive a treatment identical to the MVax group, except that a placebo vaccine will replace MVax. The primary endpoints of the study are best overall anti-tumor response rate and the percentage of patients surviving at least 2 years. Secondary endpoints of the study will include overall survival time, response duration, percentage complete and partial responses, progression free survival and treatment related adverse events [55].

3.7. Vaccines based on peptides: MDX-1379, astuprotimut-R, and others

The identification of tumor antigens that are present on the surface of melanoma cells is the basis for developing cancer vaccines that utilize peptide based immunotherapy. There are several melanoma differentiation antigens known involved in the synthesis of melanin and recognized by melanoma-reactive T cells, for example, gp100, MART-1/Melan-A, tyrosinase, TRP-1 and TRP-2, NY-ESO-1and the melanoma-associated antigen (MAGE) *etc.* One big advantage of peptide based-vaccination is that it has few toxic side effects or adverse reactions. Data suggests that most tumor cell lines established from fine needle aspiration biopsies of patients with metastatic melanoma exhibit a relatively homogeneous co-expression of MART-1 and tyrosinase, with a much more heterogeneous expression of other tumor antigens, such as gp100, NY-ESO 1 and the MAGE antigens [56].

Rosenberg and his colleagues developed a with a peptide based-vaccine using modified immunodominant peptide of the gp100 antigen, g209-2M. They used this agent vaccinated stage IV melanoma patients subcutaneously every three weeks. Following two immunizations, 10 of 11 (91%) of patients showed a consistently high level of immunization against the native g209~217 peptide, but not against the control peptide g280~288. This study also demonstrated that the majority of patients immunized with the g209-2M peptide in incomplete Freund's adjuvant (IFA) consistently developed high levels of circulating immune precursors reactive against the native g209~217 peptide. Clinically, one of nine patients who received the g209~217 peptide in IFA experienced an objective cancer regression that lasted 4 months. Three of the eleven patients exhibited mixed responses with complete or partial regression of several lesions. However, all patients eventually developed progressive disease [57].

MDX-1379 vaccine consists of two gp100 melanoma peptides. These peptides are part of a protein normally found on melanocytes, or pigmented skin cells, and on melanoma cells. These melanoma peptides are recognized by cytotoxic T cells in melanoma patients that are positive for HLA-A2, a human immune system compatibility antigen that is expressed in approximately half of the melanoma population. Phase II data show limited evidence of MDX-1379's clinical activity although there is strong proof-of-concept for therapeutic vaccines based on gp100 in melanoma. Medarex is currently conducting a phase 3 clinical trial with ipilimumab and MDX-1379 combination therapy in stage III and IV melanoma at multiple sites within the United States. Preliminary data showed MDX-1379 plus ipilimumab induced a modest percentage of durable response in stage IV melanoma. But autoimmune events could make the risk/benefit ratio for MDX-1379 plus ipilimumab unfavorable [58].

Astuprotimut-R (also called recombinant MAGE-A3 antigen-specific cancer immunotherapeutic GSK1203486A) is a cancer vaccine consisting of a recombinant form of human melanoma antigen A3 (MAGE-A3) combined with a proprietary adjuvant with potential immunostimulatory and antineoplastic activities. Upon administration, astuprotimut-R may stimulate a cytotoxic T-lymphocyte response against tumor cells expressing the MAGE-A3 antigen, resulting in tumor cell death. MAGE-A3, a tumor-associated antigen (TAA) originally discovered in melanoma cells, is expressed by various tumor types including melanoma, non-small cell lung cancer, head and neck cancer, bladder cancer, with no expression in normal cells. MAGE-A3 protein has been in-licensed by GlaxoSmithKline (GSK) from the Ludwig Institute for Cancer Research. The proprietary immunostimulating adjuvant in this agent is composed of a specific combination of immunostimulating compounds selected to increase the anti-tumor immune response to MAGE-A3. Using this vaccine as intramuscular administration together with GSK's two proprietary adjuvant systems, AS15 or AS02B, they have developed a treatment regimen for cancer patients called Antigen-Specific Cancer Immunotherapeutic (ASCI).

In 2008, GSK reported a randomized, open-label phase 2 study designed to evaluate Astuprotimut-R. A total of 72 patients with measurable metastatic MAGE-A3-positive cutaneous melanoma (unresectable or in transit stage III or stage IV M1a) were randomized to receive immunization with MAGE-A3 protein combined with either AS15 or AS02B as first-line metastatic treatment. Patients were to receive a maximum of 24 immunizations over four years. Clinical activity is assessed by the Response Evaluation Criteria In Solid Tumors (RECIST) criteria, the international standards for evaluation of solid tumors. Complete response (CR) and partial response (PR) *i.e.*, disappearance or significant reduction of tumor, were reported in 4 patients in the AS15 group (3 CR and 1 PR) with two of these ongoing for more than two years; in the AS02B arm, 1 patient showed a partial response which lasted for 6 months. The safety profile was similar in both groups with the majority of reported adverse events being mild or moderate local or systemic reactions [59]. Currently this agent still is under phase 2 clinical development for progressive metastatic cutaneous melanoma.

Because melanoma tumors are heterogeneous in their antigenic profile, it is very difficult to make vaccines that can elicit cytotoxic T-cell responses universally in all the host immune systems. Rosenberg's group analyzed 28 different peptide-based vaccines utilized in stage

IV melanoma patients. A total of 381 patients were treated with 370 patients showing no response, 9 patients showing a partial response and 2 patients with a complete response, for an overall objective response rate of only 2.9%. This suggested the lack of effectiveness with this single peptide based vaccination approach [60].

Next logical step is to make vaccines with multiple peptides to overcome tumor cell antigenic heterogeneity. A recent randomized phase 2 trial was performed in 26 patients with metastatic melanoma, vaccinating with four melanoma peptides. Although a high level of specific T-cell responses were noted (in 42% of the peripheral blood, 80% of sentinel lymph nodes), only three patients had a clinical response [61].

Here is the biggest issue in this area, actually many peptide based-vaccinations have resulted in a significant increase in the number of lymphocyte precursors reactive against a variety of tumor differentiation antigens by immunization with native or modified peptides. However, such immunological responses to peptide-based therapy have not translated into meaningful clinical responses for the vast majority of patients. To date, there is no study that has clearly shown a direct correlation between an immunologic response to therapy (immune cell activation) and a clinical response (regression of established tumor).

3.8. Vaccines based on dendritic cells

In the normal human epidermis and dermis, dendritic cells (DC) are present as relatively immature antigen presenting cells, exhibiting relatively low levels of class II major histocompatibility complex (MHC) molecules and co-stimulatory molecules. But these immature DC are quite capable of capturing various soluble protein antigens, such as apoptotic and necrotic tumor cells and then cross-presenting such tumor-associated antigens to cytotoxic CD8+ T cells. When relatively immature DC in the skin is triggered to enter afferent lymphatic channels, this migrating pathway also initiates a phenotypic conversion that has profound immunological consequences [30]. When the DC arrives in the lymph node, it is characterized by an abundant levels of class II MHC antigens, as well as high surface levels of costimulatory molecules, such as CD40, CD54, CD80, CD83, and CD86. The matured DC is then capable of forming stable MHC class II-peptide complexes available to activate antigen specific CD4+ T cells [62].

To make the dendritic cell-based vaccine, the monocyte-derived, autologous DC can be pulsed *in vitro* with either whole irradiated, autologous tumor cells or tumor cell lysate. Once the tumor cells are "fed" to the DC *in vitro*, the apoptotic or necrotic cells are then processed and tumor-specific peptide antigens are then transported to the surface in both an MHC class I- and II-restricted fashion. Both immature and mature DC can be administered to patients as vaccine safely with few adverse side effects. The administration of DC via various routes of vaccination (intradermal, intranodal and intravenous) is also feasible. The first published clinical trial of DC vaccination was in 1995 and has since been followed by 98 additional clinical trials describing more than 1,000 DC-based vaccines performed in 15 different countries. Twenty-eight trials focused on patients with various advanced stages of melanoma. The safety profile was again noted to be quite remarkable, however, despite the

http://dx.doi.org/10.5772/53632

treatment of over 1,000 patients with DC-based vaccines, the record of effectiveness have been disappointing [63].

One very successful DC-based trial for patients with advanced, metastatic melanoma was reported by Nestle *et al.* He used plastic adherent monocytes matured with a xenogeneic-based 10% fetal calf serum, subsequently pulsed with either tumor cell lysate or multiple HLA-matched peptides injected intranodally. This trial involved 16 patients who were immunized on an outpatient basis. Overall, 5 of 16 patients experienced an objective response, 2 complete and 3 partial responses. The side effects were noted to be minimal in all cases, with the development of vitiligo in a few patients. One dramatic feature of this treatment was the durability of the clinical responses, with the 2 complete responders remaining free of disease for over 15 months [64].

One phase 3 clinical trial about using DC-based vaccine to treat metastatic melanoma was report by Schadendorf and colleagues recently [65]. The trial was a prospective, randomized trial that analyzed the therapeutic effects of an autologous peptide-pulsed DC-based vaccine in patients with stage IV melanoma compared to standard chemotherapy with DTIC alone. The results revealed that the overall response in the vaccine group was 3.8% compared to 5.5% in the DTIC group, with no statistically significant differences noted in response, toxicity, overall and progression-free survival between the two groups. The median time to progression was 2.8 months versus 3.2 months respectively and the median survival was 11 months for the DTIC arm but only 9 months for the vaccine arm [65].

Although disappointed by many trials, several new avenues of DC-based immunotherapy are actively being pursued and in various stages of development, focusing on different ways to enhance the therapeutic efficacy of DC in combination with various immunoadjuvants and other anticancer agents.

3.9. Individual therapy based on activated T-cells

One very promising approach to treat metastatic melanoma is to use fully activated anti-tumor T-cells as warhead. This regimen involves the adoptive autologous transfer of highly selective tumor-reactive T-cells directed against over-expressed self-derived differentiation antigens after lymphodepleting chemotherapy. Rosenberg group reported in 2004 a clinical trial using this method. Cancer regression in patients with refractory metastatic melanoma with large, vascularized tumors was noted in a remarkable 18 of 35 patients (51% response rate), including four patients with a complete regression of all metastatic disease. Such results may stem from the ability to infuse a large number of fully activated tumor infiltrating lymphocytes with anti-tumor activity into a host that is depleted of regulatory T-cells [66].

4. Gene therapy agents

The recent developments in the field of gene transfer have advanced the use of gene therapy as a novel strategy against a variety of human malignancies. Because of its unique set of characteristics, melanoma represents a suitable target for gene therapy. Several strategies have been used by gene therapy to treat melanoma. First is to target melanoma cells to introduce "suicide" genes. Second is to transfer tumor suppressor genes. Third is to inactivate aberrant oncogene expression. Fourth is to introduce genes encoding immunologically relevant molecules. Last is to target the host's immune cells to redirect immune responses against melanoma. Clinical trials have shown the feasibility and safety of gene therapy against malignant melanoma. Although no major successes have been reported, the positive results observed in some patients support the potential for gene therapy in the management of this disease. To make gene therapy as an effective modality of treatment for malignant melanoma, better vector technology as well as increased understanding of the "bystander effect" triggered by gene transfer approaches are needed [67].

The gene therapy in our discussion is to introduce oligonucleotide or DNA sequence into host body thus to stimulate immune response to tumor cells. So it is also called DNA vaccination. This approach has been shown to induce long-lasting immunity against infectious agents and protection from tumor outgrowth in several animal models [68]. Likewise, intramuscular injections of DNA (composed of naked DNA expression plasmids) into humans have also resulted in the development of an immunologic response [69]. It is hypothesized that one mechanism of tumor antigen expression may involve the DNA introducing the appropriate genes into dendritic cells for subsequent processing and presentation to the host immune system. One of the obvious advantages of DNA vaccinations is that they can be administered to patients regardless of HLA-phenotype and without identifying immunogenic epitopes.

4.1. Anti-BCL2 antisense oligonucleotide genasense

Genasense (Oblimersan sodium developed by Genta Inc. which is a biopharmaceutical company based in Berkeley Heights, New Jersey) is a phosphorothioate antisense oligonucleotide directed against the first six codons of the Bcl-2 messenger RNA. Binding of the drug to the mRNA recruits RNAse H, resulting in cleavage of the mRNA. As a result, further translation is halted and intracellular protein concentrations of Bcl-2 decrease with time. Melanoma cell lines having Bcl-2 overexpression have been shown to enhance activity of metastasis-related proteinases, *in vitro* cell invasion, and *in vivo* tumor growth [70]. Many *in vitro* studies have demonstrated increased sensitivity of melanoma cells to chemotherapy when combined with antisense Bcl-2 therapy [71]. Genasense is the first oncology drug of its kind to directly target the biochemical pathway (known as apoptosis) whereby cancer cells are ultimately killed by chemotherapy. Genasense is believed to inhibit the production of Bcl-2, a protein that is believed to be a fundamental cause of resistance to anticancer therapy. By inhibiting Bcl-2, Genasense may greatly improve the activity of anticancer therapy.

Encouraged by previous data, numerous clinical trials were started to evaluate the addition of oblimersan to chemotherapy in various solid tumors, including melanoma. Updated analysis from a randomized phase 3 trial, comparing DTIC combined with oblimersan, with DTIC alone in 771 patients with Stage IV or unresectable Stage III melanoma who had not previously received chemotherapy has shown a response rate of 12.4% in the former compared with 6.8% in the latter group (P=0.007) [72]. Median progression-free survival for the oblimersan group was 2.4 months as compared with 1.6 months for the DTIC group, with a relative risk reduction of 27% (P=0.0003). The median survival was increased from 7.8 months in the DTIC arm to 9 months in the oblimersan arm with a P value of 0.077, which became significant when the patients with normal baseline LDH were analyzed. In terms of toxicity, no new or unexpected adverse events were observed in this study, which had not been seen with DTIC alone.

However, in May 2004, a new drug application (NDA) based on 6-months of minimum follow-up data from this trial failed to receive an affirmative vote for approval by an advisory committee to the FDA. Genta subsequently withdrew that application, and the Company has not yet made a decision regarding re-filing the U.S. application [73].

4.2. DNA Plasmid-lipid complex allovectin-7

Allovectin-7 is a bicistronic plasmid formulated with a cationic lipid system containing the DNA sequences encoding HLA-B7 and beta-2 microglobulin, which together form a MHC1 antigen. Injection of Allovectin-7 directly into tumors is designed to stimulate an immune response against both local and distant metastatic tumors. Allovectin-7 is a novel gene therapy approach for cancer with a unique mechanism of action that is fundamentally different from currently approved treatments. The following three mechanisms were believed to play roles in this agent's efficacy. Mechanism one, in HLA-B7 negative patients, a vigorous allogeneic immune response may be initiated against the foreign MHC class I antigen. Mechanism two, in all patients, ß2 microglobulin may reconstitute normal class I antigen presentation and/or increase tumor antigen presentation to the immune system. Mechanism three, in some patients, an innate pro-inflammatory response may occur that induces tumor responses following intralesional injection of the DNA/lipid complex. The final outcome of all these mechanisms is to initially cause recognition of the tumor at the local site to allow a then sensitized immune response to recognize un-injected tumors at distant metastatic sites [74].

In 2001, Dr. Richards and his colleagues began a high-dose, 2 mg, phase 2 trial evaluating the Allovectin-7 immunotherapeutic alone for patients with stage III or stage IV melanoma, who have few other treatment options. The high-dose phase 2 trial completed enrollment in 2003. The data showed that the trial had a total of 15 responders among the 127 patients receiving the high dose (11.8%), with four of the patients having complete responses and 11 having partial responses. The Kaplan-Meier estimated median duration of response was 13.8 months. The Kaplan-Meier median survival was 18 months. The safety profile was excellent with no reported Grade 3 or Grade 4 adverse events associated with Allovectin-7 [75].

Allovectin-7 has been granted orphan drug designation for the treatment of invasive and metastatic melanoma by the FDA's Office of Orphan Products Development. Orphan drug designation provides U.S. marketing exclusivity for seven years if marketing approval is received from the FDA

Vical is conducting the AIMM (Allovectin-7 Immunotherapeutic for Metastatic Melanoma) trial, a phase 3 pivotal trial of Allovectin-7 as first-line therapy in approximately 375 patients with Stage III or IV recurrent metastatic melanoma in accordance with a SPA agreement completed with the FDA. The trial is being conducted at approximately 60 clinical sites worldwide. They designed the trial to include patients most likely to benefit from our treatment, and specifically excluded patients with brain or liver metastases, patients previously treated with chemotherapy, and patients with elevated lactate dehydrogenase (LDH) levels.

In January 2010 Vical announced that the company has completed enrollment of the planned 375 subjects in its multinational phase 3 trial of Allovectin-7 in patients with metastatic melanoma. Allovectin-7®'s safety profile is excellent with no drug-related serious adverse events reported to date in the phase 3 trial [74].

4.3. Herpes simplex virus based oncoVEX

OncoVEX (GM-CSF) is an enhanced potency, immuneenhanced oncolytic herpes simplex virus type 1 (HSV-1). It is deleted for infected-cell protein gene 34.5 (ICP34.5), providing tumor selective replication, and ICP47 gene which otherwise blocks antigen presentation. In addition, ICP47 deletion increases unique short region protein 11 (US11) gene expression thereby enhancing virus growth and replication in tumor cells. The coding sequence for human granulocyte-macrophage colony-stimulating factor (GM-CSF) is inserted, replacing ICP34.5, to enhance the immune response to tumor antigens released following virus replication.

OncoVEX is developed by BioVex (Woburn, MA). It is a first-in-class oncolytic, or cancer destroying virus, that works by replicating and spreading within solid tumors (leaving healthy cells unaffected), thereby causing cancer cell death and stimulating the immune system to destroy un-injected metastatic deposits. Both modes of action have been clearly validated in the clinic, where multiple patients with metastatic disease progressing at enrollment have been declared disease free.

BioVex recently concluded a 50-patient phase 2 trial for OncoVEX (GM-CSF) as a standalone therapy in patients with Stage IIIc and Stage IV melanoma. The trial was designed to measure overall objective response, which is defined as a complete response, where disease is completely eliminated, or partial response, where there is a >50% reduction in disease burden. 74% of patients who entered the study were progressing after having failed prior therapy. 13 objective systemic responses (26% objective response rate) were achieved including eight CRs, seven of which remain free of disease. 12 responses have so far continued for more than 6 months (ranging from 6 to more than 29 months). Responses were observed in patients with all stages of disease, including the complete resolution of un-injected visceral deposits. Adverse effects were primarily limited to transient flu-like symptoms [76].

In April 2009, BioVex Inc. announced that its OPTiM (OncoVEX Pivotal Trial in Melanoma) phase 3 study with OncoVEX (GM-CSF) in previously treated patients with Stage III and Stage IV melanoma had initiated. The study has commenced recruiting patients in the U.S. and with sites in the United Kingdom, Germany and Australia. The OPTiM trial is a multinational, open label, randomized study designed to assess the efficacy and safety of treatment with OncoVEX (GM-CSF) as compared to subcutaneously administered GM-CSF in patients with unresectable stage III (b-c) and stage IV (M1a-c) disease. Patients will have received at least one prior therapy for active disease which includes any type of therapy including investigational drugs. A total of 360 patients will be enrolled (240 to the OncoVEX (GM-CSF) arm and 120 to the control arm). The study design was agreed with the FDA under the special protocol assessment process [77].

5. Possible reasons for extremely high resistance of metastatic melanoma

Despite an epic number of clinical trials to test a wide variety of anticancer strategies, the average survival rate for patients with metastatic melanoma remains unimproved during the past 30 years (41). Though constant clinical trials effort, although some approaches showed promising intermediate results, still no agent has been granted FDA approval for the treatment of metastatic melanoma. There are several reasons that may account for the extremely high resistance of metastatic melanoma to current treatment modalities.

5.1. Reasons for chemotherapy resistance

Melanoma cells are quite resistant to most chemotherapy reagents. This is associated with the specific feature of melanoma cells. In nature, these cells have low levels of spontaneous apoptosis *in vivo* compared with other tumor cell types, and they are relatively resistant to drug-induced apoptosis *in vitro* [78]. The natural role of melanocytes is to protect inner organs from UV light, a potent DNA damaging agent. Therefore, it is not surprising that melanoma cells may have special DNA damage repair systems and enhanced survival properties [79]. Moreover, recent studies showed that, during melanoma progression, it acquired complex genetic alterations that led to hyperactivation of efflux pumps, detoxification enzymes, and a multifactorial alteration of survival and apoptotic pathways. All these have been proposed to mediate the multi-drug resistant phenotype of melanoma [80].

5.2. Barriers for successful immunotherapy

The major barrier is immunosuppressive effects activated by tumors. Tumor cell can escape immune rejection and induce immunosuppression through the following five major paths. Firstly, tumor cells may lose or down-regulate either the melanoma associated antigens or MHC molecules. Secondly, tumor cells may produce a plethora of immunosuppressive factors such as interleukin-10, VEGF and transforming growth factor. These factors create an inherently unfavorable microenvironment that limits the host immune response, in addition to tolerating the T-cell response to established tumor. Third possible reason is intrinsic inefficiency of DC whereby the appropriate co-stimulatory molecules are not being presented on the cell surface. Fourth possible reason is tumor-related alterations in T-cell signaling and a skewing of the immune response from a Th1 (immunoactivating) to a Th2 response (immunotolerant). Lastly, the concept of tumor cell escape and immune tolerance is an exceedingly complex process. We need to further understand these mechanisms before we can have successful immunotherapy to melanoma [32].

Specifically for cancer vaccines, there are some further barriers. First is the characterization of vaccines potency and toxicity. This is especially important in the transition from phase 2 to phase 3 trials. To select a meaningful and validated end point for trials is a big challenge most of the time. Second barrier is selection of the maximum tolerated dose of cancer vaccine, particularly compared with traditional anticancer agents. Cancer vaccines are typically not very toxic. So the optimum dose often has to be based on the immune response of patients. But if the patients have previously been heavily treated with other anticancer agents, this can lead to a compromised immune system that makes it difficult to detect an evoked immune response. The third barrier is appropriate trial design and statistical data process. This is also a key part and can substantially affect final trial outcome [53].

6. Future directions

With the rapidly rising incidence and the high resistance to current therapeutic agents, developing more effective drugs for metastatic melanoma is urgently needed. But before we can thoroughly understand all the major molecular pathological changes associated with melanoma malignancy, it is very difficult to reach a cure for it.

Melanoma is an extremely complicated disease, with many gene mutation and signaling pathway changes. Elevated signaling pathway in melanoma including mitogen-activated protein kinase (MAPK) pathway, phosphatidylinositol 3 kinase (PI3K)-AKT pathway, Wnt-Frizzled-β-catenin pathway, JAK/Stat pathway and α-MSH-MC1R or microphthalmia-associated transcription factor (MITF) pathway. The first two are crucial pathway accounting for melanoma malignance. Gene mutation that are involved in melanoma include the following oncogenes: BRAF, N-ras, akt3; tumor suppressors: CDKN2A, PTEN, p53, APAF-1, p16, p15, p19; others: Cyclin D1, MITF etc [81].

The binding of growth factors to their respective receptors leads to activation of RAS proteins. Ras will then activate Raf. Raf activate mitogen-activated protein kinase (MEK), which then act on extracellular-related kinase (ERK). Phosporylated ERK kinases (ERK-P) translocate to the nucleus and activate transcription factors, which promote cell cycle progression and proliferation. The PI3K-AKT pathway mediates cell survival signaling via growth factors. Phosphatase and tensin homolog (PTEN) inhibits growth factor signaling by inactivating phosphatidylinositol triphosphate (PIP3) generated by PI3K. Activated PI3K converts the plasma membrane lipid phosphatidylinositol 4,5-bisphosphonate to PIP3, which acts as a second messenger leading to the phosphorylation AKT and subsequent up-regulation of cell cycle, growth, and survival proteins. AKT can also up-regulate mTOR (mammalian target of rapamycin), S6K, and NFκb leading to cell growth and inhibition of apoptosis.

Knowing the huge complexity of melanoma, it's easy to understand why so many random trials of single agents or combinational treatment have failed. So targeted therapy in a systemic way based on the understanding about melanoma molecular pathology seems to be a reasonable way to fight this disease.

Individualized T-cell-based therapy is a very promising approach. Combined with other suitable tumor killing agents, it could improve the patient survival rate and time. Unfortunately, the selective tumor-reactive T-cells isolated from a patient can only be used for this same patient. Thus the cost associated with this treatment method is very high. Such an expensive treatment may not be available to all the patients in the near future.

In learning from our efforts in the past, we must continue to challenge the current paradigms of treatment as we forge new paths to more effective treatment options. This will likely involve a multimodal approach to therapy utilizing all of the available tools in our arsenal. Several agents given in unique combinations may then synergize with standard chemotherapeutic regimens resulting in prolonged clinical responses and long term survival. Take Sorafenib as an example, its failure maybe largely due to the fact that it only blocks the RAF-MEK-ERK signaling pathway. Melanoma cells can still survive by compensatory upregulation in other survival pathways such as the PI3K-AKT pathway. Melanoma can also develop drug resistance with time by over-expressing MDR genes. Ideally, if we can use drugs to synergistically block all the major survival pathways in melanoma cells and then educate our immune system to fight the tumor cells, we will have a much better chance to conquer this deadly disease.

Author details

Zhao Wang, Wei Li* and Duane D. Miller

*Address all correspondence to: wli@uthsc.edu

Department of Pharmaceutical Sciences, University of Tennessee Health Science Center, Memphis, USA

References

[1] Eggermont, A.M. and C. Robert, *New drugs in melanoma: It's a whole new world.* Eur J Cancer, 2011. 47(47): p. 2150-2157.

[2] Kahler, K.C. and A. Hauschild, *Treatment and side effect management of CTLA-4 antibody therapy in metastatic melanoma.* J Dtsch Dermatol Ges, 2011. 9(4): p. 277-86.

[3] Roukos, D.H., *PLX4032 and melanoma: resistance, expectations and uncertainty.* Expert Rev Anticancer Ther, 2011. 11(3): p. 325-8.

[4] Williams, D.A. and T.L. Lemke, *Foye's Principles of Medicinal Chemistry*. Fifth Edition ed2002, Philadelphia, PA: Lippincott Williams & Wilkins.

[5] Falkson, C.I., et al., *Phase III trial of dacarbazine versus dacarbazine with interferon alpha-2b versus dacarbazine with tamoxifen versus dacarbazine with interferon alpha-2b and tamoxifen in patients with metastatic malignant melanoma: an Eastern Cooperative Oncology Group study.* J Clin Oncol, 1998. 16(5): p. 1743-51.

[6] Chapman, P.B., et al., *Phase III multicenter randomized trial of the Dartmouth regimen versus dacarbazine in patients with metastatic melanoma.* J Clin Oncol, 1999. 17(9): p. 2745-51.

[7] Eggermont, A.M. and J.M. Kirkwood, *Re-evaluating the role of dacarbazine in metastatic melanoma: what have we learned in 30 years?* Eur J Cancer, 2004. 40(12): p. 1825-36.

[8] Jacinto, F.V. and M. Esteller, *MGMT hypermethylation: a prognostic foe, a predictive friend.* DNA Repair (Amst), 2007. 6(8): p. 1155-60.

[9] Newlands, E.S., et al., *Phase I trial of temozolomide (CCRG 81045: M&B 39831: NSC 362856).* Br J Cancer, 1992. 65(2): p. 287-91.

[10] Middleton, M.R., et al., *Randomized phase III study of temozolomide versus dacarbazine in the treatment of patients with advanced metastatic malignant melanoma.* J Clin Oncol, 2000. 18(1): p. 158-66.

[11] Strumberg, D., et al., *Phase I clinical and pharmacokinetic study of the Novel Raf kinase and vascular endothelial growth factor receptor inhibitor BAY 43-9006 in patients with advanced refractory solid tumors.* J Clin Oncol, 2005. 23(5): p. 965-72.

[12] Ahmad T, M.R., Pyle L, James M, Schwartz B, Gore M, Eisen T., *BAY 43-9006 in patients with advanced melanoma: The Royal Marsden experience.* Journal of Clinical Oncology 2004 ASCO Annual Meeting Proceedings., 2004. 22(14s).

[13] Eisen, T., et al., *Sorafenib in advanced melanoma: a Phase II randomised discontinuation trial analysis.* Br J Cancer, 2006. 95(5): p. 581-6.

[14] Flaherty KT, B.M., Schucter L, et al, *Phase I/II trial of BAY 43-9006, carboplatin (C) and paclitaxel (P) demonstrates preliminary antitumor activity in the expansion cohort of patients with metastatic melanoma.* Journal of Clinical Oncology 2004 ASCO Annual Meeting Proceedings., 2004. 22(14s): p. 7507.

[15] Herlyn, M., *recent development in melanoma research (review on literature).* 2007.

[16] Sala, E., et al., *BRAF silencing by short hairpin RNA or chemical blockade by PLX4032 leads to different responses in melanoma and thyroid carcinoma cells.* Mol Cancer Res, 2008. 6(5): p. 751-9.

[17] Chapman, P.B., et al., *Improved survival with vemurafenib in melanoma with BRAF V600E mutation.* N Engl J Med, 2011. 364(26): p. 2507-16.

[18] Young, K., A. Minchom, and J. Larkin, *BRIM-1, -2 and -3 trials: improved survival with vemurafenib in metastatic melanoma patients with a BRAF(V600E) mutation.* Future Oncol, 2012. 8(5): p. 499-507.

[19] Atkins, M.B., *The treatment of metastatic melanoma with chemotherapy and biologics.* Curr Opin Oncol, 1997. 9(2): p. 205-13.

[20] Evans, L.M., E.S. Casper, and R. Rosenbluth, *Phase II trial of carboplatin in advanced malignant melanoma.* Cancer Treat Rep, 1987. 71(2): p. 171-2.

[21] Gogas, H.J., J.M. Kirkwood, and V.K. Sondak, *Chemotherapy for metastatic melanoma: time for a change?* Cancer, 2007. 109(3): p. 455-64.

[22] Boaziz, C., et al., *[Brain metastases of malignant melanomas].* Bull Cancer, 1991. 78(4): p. 347-53.

[23] Quagliana, J.M., et al., *Vindesine in patients with metastatic malignant melanoma: a Southwest Oncology Group study.* J Clin Oncol, 1984. 2(4): p. 316-9.

[24] Bedikian, A.Y., et al., *Phase II trial of docetaxel in patients with advanced cutaneous malignant melanoma previously untreated with chemotherapy.* J Clin Oncol, 1995. 13(12): p. 2895-9.

[25] Avril, M.F., et al., *Combination chemotherapy of dacarbazine and fotemustine in disseminated malignant melanoma. Experience of the French Study Group.* Cancer Chemother Pharmacol, 1990. 27(2): p. 81-4.

[26] Fletcher, W.S., et al., *Evaluation of cis-platinum and DTIC combination chemotherapy in disseminated melanoma. A Southwest Oncology Group Study.* Am J Clin Oncol, 1988. 11(5): p. 589-93.

[27] Vorobiof, D.A., R. Sarli, and G. Falkson, *Combination chemotherapy with dacarbazine and vindesine in the treatment of metastatic malignant melanoma.* Cancer Treat Rep, 1986. 70(7): p. 927-8.

[28] Legha, S.S., et al., *A prospective evaluation of a triple-drug regimen containing cisplatin, vinblastine, and dacarbazine (CVD) for metastatic melanoma.* Cancer, 1989. 64(10): p. 2024-9.

[29] Del Prete, S.A., et al., *Combination chemotherapy with cisplatin, carmustine, dacarbazine, and tamoxifen in metastatic melanoma.* Cancer Treat Rep, 1984. 68(11): p. 1403-5.

[30] Flaherty, L.E., et al., *Comparison of patient characteristics and outcome between a single-institution phase II trial and a cooperative-group phase II trial with identical eligibility in metastatic melanoma.* Am J Clin Oncol, 1997. 20(6): p. 600-4.

[31] Smith, F.O., et al., *Treatment of metastatic melanoma using interleukin-2 alone or in conjunction with vaccines.* Clin Cancer Res, 2008. 14(17): p. 5610-8.

[32] Riker, A.I., et al., *Immunotherapy of melanoma: a critical review of current concepts and future strategies.* Expert Opin Biol Ther, 2007. 7(3): p. 345-58.

[33] Quan, W., Jr., et al., *Repeated cycles with 72-hour continuous infusion interleukin-2 in kidney cancer and melanoma.* Cancer Biother Radiopharm, 2004. 19(3): p. 350-4.

[34] Kiessling, R., et al., *Tumor-induced immune dysfunction.* Cancer Immunol Immunother, 1999. 48(7): p. 353-62.

[35] Liu, Y.J., *IPC: professional type 1 interferon-producing cells and plasmacytoid dendritic cell precursors.* Annu Rev Immunol, 2005. 23: p. 275-306.

[36] Moschos, S.J., et al., *Neoadjuvant treatment of regional stage IIIB melanoma with high-dose interferon alfa-2b induces objective tumor regression in association with modulation of tumor infiltrating host cellular immune responses.* J Clin Oncol, 2006. 24(19): p. 3164-71.

[37] Kirkwood, J.M., et al., *Interferon alfa-2b adjuvant therapy of high-risk resected cutaneous melanoma: the Eastern Cooperative Oncology Group Trial EST 1684.* J Clin Oncol, 1996. 14(1): p. 7-17.

[38] Kirkwood, J.M., et al., *High-dose interferon alfa-2b does not diminish antibody response to GM2 vaccination in patients with resected melanoma: results of the Multicenter Eastern Cooperative Oncology Group Phase II Trial E2696.* J Clin Oncol, 2001. 19(5): p. 1430-6.

[39] Sangfelt, O., et al., *Induction of apoptosis and inhibition of cell growth are independent responses to interferon-alpha in hematopoietic cell lines.* Cell Growth Differ, 1997. 8(3): p. 343-52.

[40] Kirkwood, J.M., et al., *Mechanisms and management of toxicities associated with high-dose interferon alfa-2b therapy.* J Clin Oncol, 2002. 20(17): p. 3703-18.

[41] Eggermont, A.M., et al., *Adjuvant therapy with pegylated interferon alfa-2b versus observation alone in resected stage III melanoma: final results of EORTC 18991, a randomised phase III trial.* Lancet, 2008. 372(9633): p. 117-26.

[42] Weber, J., *Review: anti-CTLA-4 antibody ipilimumab: case studies of clinical response and immune-related adverse events.* Oncologist, 2007. 12(7): p. 864-72.

[43] Robert, C., et al., *Ipilimumab plus dacarbazine for previously untreated metastatic melanoma.* N Engl J Med, 2011. 364(26): p. 2517-26.

[44] Reuben, J.M., et al., *Biologic and immunomodulatory events after CTLA-4 blockade with ticilimumab in patients with advanced malignant melanoma.* Cancer, 2006. 106(11): p. 2437-44.

[45] Johnston, R.L., et al., *Cytotoxic T-lymphocyte-associated antigen 4 antibody-induced colitis and its management with infliximab.* Dig Dis Sci, 2009. 54(11): p. 2538-40.

[46] Mitjans, F., et al., *In vivo therapy of malignant melanoma by means of antagonists of alphav integrins.* Int J Cancer, 2000. 87(5): p. 716-23.

[47] Hersey, P., et al., *A phase II, randomized, open-label study evaluating the antitumor activity of MEDI-522, a humanized monoclonal antibody directed against the human metastatic melanoma (MM),* in *Proc Am Soc Clin Oncol*2005. p. 711s..

[48] Hersey, P., et al., *A randomized phase 2 study of etaracizumab, a monoclonal antibody against integrin alpha(v)beta(3), +/- dacarbazine in patients with stage IV metastatic melanoma.* Cancer.

[49] Ward, S., et al., *Immunotherapeutic potential of whole tumour cells.* Cancer Immunol Immunother, 2002. 51(7): p. 351-7.

[50] Hsueh, E.C. and D.L. Morton, *Antigen-based immunotherapy of melanoma: Canvaxin therapeutic polyvalent cancer vaccine.* Semin Cancer Biol, 2003. 13(6): p. 401-7.

[51] *CancerVax Announces Results of Phase 3 Clinical Trials of Canvaxin(TM) in Patients With Stage III and Stage IV Melanoma.* Market Wire, 2006.

[52] Sondak, V.K., et al., *Adjuvant immunotherapy of resected, intermediate-thickness, node-negative melanoma with an allogeneic tumor vaccine: overall results of a randomized trial of the Southwest Oncology Group.* J Clin Oncol, 2002. 20(8): p. 2058-66.

[53] *Rethinking therapeutic cancer vaccines.* Nat Rev Drug Discov, 2009. 8(9): p. 685-6.

[54] Berd, D., et al., *Immunopharmacologic analysis of an autologous, hapten-modified human melanoma vaccine.* J Clin Oncol, 2004. 22(3): p. 403-15.

[55] Avax Technologies, I., *Harnessing the patient's immune system for the treatment of cancer.* Avax fact sheet, 2007.

[56] Riker, A.I., et al., *Development and characterization of melanoma cell lines established by fine-needle aspiration biopsy: advances in the monitoring of patients with metastatic melanoma.* Cancer Detect Prev, 1999. 23(5): p. 387-96.

[57] Rosenberg, S.A., et al., *Immunologic and therapeutic evaluation of a synthetic peptide vaccine for the treatment of patients with metastatic melanoma.* Nat Med, 1998. 4(3): p. 321-7.

[58] Report, D., *Pipeline Insight: Therapeutic Cancer Vaccines - Prospect of first approval set to reinvigorate interest from major companies.* PipelineReview, 2009.

[59] Kruit W, S.S., Dreno B, et al, *Immunization with recombinant MAGE-A3 protein combined with adjuvant systems AS15 or AS02B in patients with unresectable and progressive metastatic cutaneous melanoma: a randomized open-label phase II study of the EORTC Melanoma Group.* J Clin Oncol, 2008. 26: p. abstr 9065.

[60] Rosenberg, S.A., J.C. Yang, and N.P. Restifo, *Cancer immunotherapy: moving beyond current vaccines.* Nat Med, 2004. 10(9): p. 909-15.

[61] Slingluff, C.L., Jr., et al., *Clinical and immunologic results of a randomized phase II trial of vaccination using four melanoma peptides either administered in granulocyte-macrophage colony-stimulating factor in adjuvant or pulsed on dendritic cells.* J Clin Oncol, 2003. 21(21): p. 4016-26.

[62] Albert, M.L., B. Sauter, and N. Bhardwaj, *Dendritic cells acquire antigen from apoptotic cells and induce class I-restricted CTLs.* Nature, 1998. 392(6671): p. 86-9.

[63] Ridgway, D., *The first 1000 dendritic cell vaccinees.* Cancer Invest, 2003. 21(6): p. 873-86.

[64] Nestle, F.O., et al., *Vaccination of melanoma patients with peptide- or tumor lysate-pulsed dendritic cells.* Nat Med, 1998. 4(3): p. 328-32.

[65] Schadendorf D, N.F., Broecker EB, Enk A, Grabbe S, Ugurel S, Edler L, Schuler G, De-COG-DC Study Group., *Dacarbacine (DTIC) versus vaccination with autologous peptide-pulsed dendritic cells (DC) as first-line treatment of patients with metastatic melanoma: Results of a prospective-randomized phase III study.* Journal of Clinical Oncology, ASCO Annual Meeting Proceedings, 2004. 22(14s): p. 7508.

[66] Rosenberg, S.A. and M.E. Dudley, *Cancer regression in patients with metastatic melanoma after the transfer of autologous antitumor lymphocytes.* Proc Natl Acad Sci U S A, 2004. 101 Suppl 2: p. 14639-45.

[67] Sotomayor, M.G., et al., *Advances in gene therapy for malignant melanoma.* Cancer Control, 2002. 9(1): p. 39-48.

[68] Piechocki, M.P., S.A. Pilon, and W.Z. Wei, *Complementary antitumor immunity induced by plasmid DNA encoding secreted and cytoplasmic human ErbB-2.* J Immunol, 2001. 167(6): p. 3367-74.

[69] Ulmer, J.B., et al., *Heterologous protection against influenza by injection of DNA encoding a viral protein.* Science, 1993. 259(5102): p. 1745-9.

[70] Trisciuoglio, D., et al., *Bcl-2 overexpression in melanoma cells increases tumor progression-associated properties and in vivo tumor growth.* J Cell Physiol, 2005. 205(3): p. 414-21.

[71] Jansen, B., et al., *Chemosensitisation of malignant melanoma by BCL2 antisense therapy.* Lancet, 2000. 356(9243): p. 1728-33.

[72] Millward MJ, B.A., Conry RM, Gore ME, Pehamberger HE, Sterry W, Pavlick AC, De Conti RC, and I.L. Gordon D, *Randomized multinational phase 3 trial of dacarbazine (DTIC) with or without Bcl-2 antisense (oblimersen sodium) in patients (pts) with advanced malignant melanoma (MM): Analysis of long-term survival.* Journal of Clinical Oncology, (Post-Meeting Edition), 2004. 22(14S (July 15 Supplement)).

[73] Genta, A.a., *FDA Advisory Committee Reviews Genasense(reg) For Use in Advanced Melanoma.* Medical News Today, 2004.

[74] Vical, *Vical Completes Enrollment in Allovectin-7(r) Phase 3 Trial for Metastatic Melanoma.* Globe Newswire, 2010.

[75] J. M. Richards, A.B., R. Gonzalez, M. B. Atkins, E. Whitman, J. Lutzky, M. A. Morse, T. Amatruda, E. Galanis, J. Thompson Vical Clinical Research Operations Team *High-dose Allovectin-7 in patients with advanced metastatic melanoma: final phase 2 data and design of phase 3 registration trial* Journal of Clinical Oncology 2005 ASCO Annual Meeting Proceedings., 2005. 23(16s): p. 7543.

[76] Nemunaitis., N.N.S.H.K.T.A.M.N.T.R.G.D.R.G.J.G.E.W.K.H.R.C.J., *Updated Results of a Phase II Clinical Trial with a Second Generation, Enhanced Potency, Immune-enhanced,*

Oncolytic Herpesvirus in Unresectable Metastatic Melanoma. American Society of Clinical Oncology, 2009. annual meeting: p. poster.

[77] biovex, *BioVex Commences OncoVEX (GM-CSF) Phase 3 Trial In Metastatic Melanoma.* Medical News Today, 2009.

[78] Gray-Schopfer, V., C. Wellbrock, and R. Marais, *Melanoma biology and new targeted therapy.* Nature, 2007. 445(7130): p. 851-7.

[79] Dothager, R.S., et al., *Synthesis and identification of small molecules that potently induce apoptosis in melanoma cells through G1 cell cycle arrest.* J Am Chem Soc, 2005. 127(24): p. 8686-96.

[80] Fernandez, Y., et al., *Differential regulation of noxa in normal melanocytes and melanoma cells by proteasome inhibition: therapeutic implications.* Cancer Res, 2005. 65(14): p. 6294-304.

[81] Smalley, K.S. and M. Herlyn, *Targeting intracellular signaling pathways as a novel strategy in melanoma therapeutics.* Ann N Y Acad Sci, 2005. 1059: p. 16-25.

Chapter 21

Update in Ocular Melanoma

Victoria de los Ángeles Bustuoabad,
Lucia Speroni and Arturo Irarrázabal

Additional information is available at the end of the chapter

http://dx.doi.org/10.5772/53633

1. Introduction

1.1. Ocular anatomy

In order to understand the pathophysiology of this condition we will describe the *uvea* anatomy.

The Iris is a contractile diaphragm that controls the degree of retinal illumination, it has a central aperture, the pupil, located slightly nasally. It consists of the following layers from anterior to posterior:

1. Stroma: a thin avascular layer with fibroblasts and melanocytes. It is heavily pigmented in persons with brown eyes less pigmented in green and hazel irises and least in blue. Posteriorly, the stroma contains the sphincter pupillae muscle (parasympathetic, miosis).

2. Pigment epithelium: consists of 2 layers of cells: -anterior layer, which intermingles with the dilator pupillae muscle (sympathetic, mydriasis) -posterior layer, which is continuous with the pigment epithelium of the ciliary body and RPE of the retina, all having the same embryologic origin.

The cilliary body is one of the three parts of the uvea and extends for 6 mm from the end of the retina (ora serrata) till the scleral spur. Its epithelial portion (adjacent to vitreous) consists of a posterior portion (pars plana) and an anterior portion (pars plicata). The latter has 60-70 folds called the ciliary processes which secrete the aqueous humor into the posterior chamber. Its uveal portion contains the ciliary muscle which has 3 parts, all under parasympathetic innervation: longitudinal (outermost), radial and circular.

The choroid is a dark brown vascular sheet, 0.25mm thick, lying between the sclera and the retina. The outer vascular bed has large vessels (layer of Haller) and the inner bed consists of an extensive network of fenestrated vessels, the choriocapillaris which is the major blood supply to the outer layers of the retina and to the whole macula The inner layers, up to the middle of the Pigmented Epithelium are supplied by the central retinal artery.

1.2. Difference between ocular melanoma and cutaneous melanoma

Ocular and cutaneous melanomas show several differences despite they both derive from melanocytes. Both malignancies show a high tendency to metastasize though they display different preferential sites. Skin melanomas spread to distant skin sites, lung, liver, central nervous system and bone. However uveal melanoma, the most frequently diagnosed of the ocular melanomas, gives rise to metastases almost exclusively in the liver which is affected in 90% of the cases.

Interestingly, both malignancies display similar chromosomal aberrations as well as a similar gene expression profile [1]. The similarity in this aspect, despite the difference in tumor behaviour, serves as a proof of the role of the microenvironment in tumor development.

With respect to the early diagnosis, in the skin melanoma the suspected diagnosis and the subsequent clinical follow-up are based on the ABCDE rule.On the other hand, in the diagnosis of ocular melanoma the most relevant information comes from the ophthalmoscopy and the ultrasonography. Finally, consulting times for patients and prognosis are different for both types of melanoma.

2. Objectives

In this chapter we will focus in the clinical management of ocular melanoma from the diagnosis to the treatment.

3. Immunopathology

The eye is an immunologically privileged site; from an evolutionary point of view this condition helps to control or eliminate pathogens while generating the least inflammatory damage to the ocular tissues. However, the counterpart of this phenomenon is that it favors the escape of the tumor cells from the controls of the immune system, facilitating the growth of the uveal melanoma and its metastatic dissemination. Experiments in mice it have shown that cytotoxic cell activity in the ocular tissue might be modulated by two mechanisms:

1. By direct interference of the specific effector function of CD8 + lymphocytes.

2. Indirectly affected by stimulation of macrophages [2].

The inhibition of macrophage action was expressed by an insufficient production of nitric oxide in the ocular tissue, which is known to modulate the tumoricidal activity of cytotoxic T lymphocytes [3]. It has also been shown that tumor rejection in mice by the CD8 + CTL is mediated by TNF-α [4].

The study of the mechanisms that facilitate the growth of an immunogenic tumor in the anterior chamber, demonstrated an influx of CD8 + CTL infiltrating the tumor. This phenomenon was preceded by intratumoral accumulation of CD11 + myeloid cells B, which exert a powerful immunosuppressive activity on the CTL, facilitating tumor escape from the immune system. Regulatory T cells, myeloid suppressor cells and stroma cells could also reduce the delayed type hypersensitivity reaction to induce apoptosis of CD8 + and NK cells [5]

4. Demographic and epidemiological data

The *racial* background of the patient is an important factor. Whites have been shown to be eight times more likely to develop choroidal melanoma than African-Americans. This trend is also observed in skin melanoma, whites are six times. More likely to develop this malignancy than African-Americans [6-7]. The individuals with light iris are at increased risk of developing uveal melanoma. This is a finding that implicates *sunlight exposure* as an important environmental risk factor. The protective effect of melanin may be particularly important in the iris as it is the only part of the uveal tract positioned in front of the lens, which serves as an effective ultraviolet filter.

The median *age* at diagnosis is about 55-65 years and the incidence decreases after 70 years of age. With regards to incidence depending on *sex*, there is a slight predominance of males [8].

In a study involving 4500 patients with uveal melanoma, only 0.6% of the cases had a family history of this disease [9]. Thus *heredity* does not seem to be a significant determinant of uveal melanoma. With respect to *occupational and chemical exposures*, the only specific occupational exposure that has been linked to uveal melanoma is welding. Ocular melanomas have been induced in laboratory animals after administration of *radium, methylcholanthrene, N-2fluorenylacetamide, ethionine and nickel subsulfide.*

5. Diagnosis of ocular melanoma

Accuracy in the early diagnosis of ocular melanoma is crucial to improve the prognosis. Currently the diagnosis of ocular melanoma is based on both the clinical experience of the specialists and on the use of modern diagnostic techniques.

The rate of misdiagnosis for eyes enucleated for choroidal melanoma was 20 % until the 1970's but it has decreased to 1% since then. [10-16]

5.1. Clinical

The most common symptoms include *visual loss, photopsias and visual field defects*. None of these symptoms are specific of choroidal melanoma. Pain is very atypical in ocular melanoma, except in those cases that present massive extraocular extension, inflammation or neovascular glaucoma.

Indirect Ophthalmoscopy through a well-dilated pupil is the most important examination in the diagnosis of choroidal melanoma. The classic image is a pigmented, dome-shaped or collar button-shaped tumor in a minority of cases and an associated exudative retinal detachment, orange tumor pigmentation (Lipofuscin) and sentinel vessels (prominent epiescleral vessels especially in those involving ciliary body). Scleral transillumination has been advocated by Reese. [17]

The lesions most commonly mistaken for choroidal melanoma are choroidal nevus (49%), periphereal exudative hemorrhagic chorioretinopathy (8%), congenital hypertrophy of the retinal pigment epithelium (6%), hemorrhagic detachment of the retina or pigment epithelium (5%), circumscribed choroidal hemangioma (8%) and age related macular degeneration (4%) [18]

5.2. Complementary studies

Ultrasonography: The most important ancillary test in the evaluation of a patient with intraocular mass lesions is the combination of both A-mode and B-mode ultrasonography (see Box 1). For tumors larger than 3 mm in thickness, a combination of both scans in skilled hands can diagnose choroidal melanomas with greater than 95% accuracy [19].

A-mode:

1. medium to low internal echoes with smooth attenuation.

2. vascular pulsations within the tumor

B-mode: 3 classic futures

1. Low to medium reflectivity within the melanoma.

2. Choroidal excavation.

3. Shadowing in the orbit.

Box 1. Ultrasonography

Fluorescein angiography: Early hyperfluorescence with late leakage and multifocal punctate hyperfluorescence. This study is of major importance in order to distinguish lesions that simulate choroidal melanoma.

http://dx.doi.org/10.5772/53633

Other studies like Optical Coherence Tomography and Indocyanine Green angiography may be useful in the diagnosis of this pathology. Magnetic resonance imaging, nuclear magnetic resonance spectography, color Doppler ultrasonography, electrophysiologic testing and inmmunologic testing do not offer reliable results. [20-26]

6. Current medical management of patients with Ocular Melanoma

a. Cytogenetic: Personalized Targeted Therapy

Currently much effort is directed toward understanding uveal melanoma genetics and genomics [27], hoping that this knowledge will contribute to the development of effective molecular therapies

Inhibitors of B.Raf and MEK kinases hold promise for treatment of cutaneous melanomas harboring BRAF mutations. BRAF are rare in ocular melanomas, but somatic mutations in the G protein alfa subunits G alfa q and G alfa 11 (encoded by *Gnaq* and *Gna11*, respectively) occur, in a mutually exclusive pattern, in 80% of uveal melanomas. The impact of the B-Raf inhibitor PLX4720 and the MEK inhibitor AZD6244, the AKT inhibitor MK2206 and the PKC inhibitors bisindolylmaleimide I (GF109203X) has been assessed [28].

A randomized phase II study compared MEK inhibition (AZD6244) to temozomide in advanced uveal melanoma. MEK inhibition seems to be a rationale therapeutic strategy in uveal melanoma, using Gnaq/11 as a potential predictor of sensitivity [29].

b. Surgery: Resection/Enucleation

Enucleation is indicated when the tumor size exceeds 16 mm of base and 10 mm of height, is diffuse and with bad prognosis; however it is very important to emphasize that there is no scientific evidence of increased survival after enucleation. Also, enucleation does not prevent metastases.

A novel minimally invasive surgical technique for resection of selected cases of small iris tumours has been described. This technique avoids the potential morbidity associated with a large corneoescleral incision allowing for rapid visual recovery [30].

Radiotherapy, *Brachytherapy* (BT: I125, 103 Pd, 131 Cs, Ru) and Proton Beam Radiotherapy (PBRT)

The most commonly employed form of radiotherapy has been the application of an epiescleral radioactive plaque and the most frequently employed isotopes include *60 Co (Cobalt), 106 Ru (Ruthenium), 192 Ir (Iridium) and 125 I (Iodine)* [31-32].

It is extremely important to highlight the conservative treatment of melanoma, proposed by *Irarrazabal A. et al* using brachytherapy. This procedure has shown positive results in preserving the eye, without increase in mortality. Moreover useful vision was retained in more than half of the treated patients [33].

In a study comparing patients treated with *Ruthenium* brachytherapy with patients undergoing simultaneous thermotherapy or BT alone, combined treatment provided higher local control, eye globes preservation, better recurrence-free survival rates, lower rates of metastases and prolonged survival than treatment with BT alone.

I125 episcleral brachytherapy in uveal melanoma is effective in tumor control, allowing preservation of the eye and useful visual function for the majority of patients [34].

It has been suggested that length of remaining life after diagnosis of uveal melanoma is similar following enucleation (removal of the eye) to local eye-conserving radiotherapy. The multidisciplinary COMS Group emphasized that there were no differences in survival outcomes and a small difference in quality-of-life outcomes between patients in the brachytherapy arm and those in the enucleation arm [35].

Radiation treatment was found to reduce the tumor in 94% of the cases. Mean tumor thickness decreased from 3.7 to 2.5 and 2.1 after 3 and 5 years respectively. Recurrence occured in 6% of the treated patients. Although this therapy is associated with complications like radiation optic neuropathy in 81% and vitreous bleeding in 30% of cases, it is a promising treatment given that enucleation was necessary in only 3% of patients and metastasis developed in 15% during follow up. Even though the visual acuity decreases considerably after optic disc irradiation with proton beam therapy, the rates of tumor control and eye retention are favourable.

The second most frequent method of radiotherapy is the use of heavy ions such as *Proton Beam Radiotherapy* [36]. In a comparison of the efficacy of PBRT and Ruthenium-106 notched plaque radiotherapy with or without TTT for the treatment of juxtapapillary choroidal melanoma, it was found that the tumors were successfully treated using either proton beam or notched plaque combined with adjuvant TTT [37].However, vision is often sacrificed. On the other hand, Notched plaque alone is not as efficient in reducing the tumor but results in improved visual outcome [37].

Proton beam irradiation of uveal melanoma has great advantages over brachytherapy because of the homogenous dose delivered to the tumor and the possibility of sparing normal tissue close to the tumor. Complications such as retinal detachment, maculopathy, papillopathy, cataract, glaucoma, vitreous hemorrhage and dryness are described. The severest complication that usually leads to secondary enucleation is neovascular glaucoma and it is encountered after irradiation of large to extra-large tumors. It is hypothesized that the residual tumor scar may produce proinflammatory cytokines and Vascular endothelial growth factor- VEGF (toxic tumor syndrome) leading to intraocular inflammation and neovascular glaucoma. Additional treatments after proton beam such as transpupillary thermotherapy, endoresection of the tumor scar or intravitreal injections of anti-VEGF may reduce the rate of these complications [38].

c. Monoclonal Antibodies

Current systemic treatments for metastatic uveal melanoma have not improved overall survival. The fully human anti-cytotoxic T-lymphocyte antigen-4 (CTLA-4) monoclonal anti-

http://dx.doi.org/10.5772/53633

body, *ipilimumab*, improved overall survival of patients with advanced cutaneous melanoma in a phase 3 trial. However, uveal melanoma patients were excluded from this study. A sub-analysis, performed by the ipilimumab-ocular melanoma expanded access program (I-OMEAP) study group, aimed at assessing the activity and safety of ipilimumab in patients with uveal melanoma in a setting similar to daily clinical practice. The results indicated that uveal melanoma is a potential target for ipilimumab treatment and that it should be further investigated in clinical trials [39].

The *R24 monoclonal antibody,* that recognizes the disialoganglioside GD3 expressed on the surface of malignant melanoma cells, could mediate destruction of these cells. A combination of R24 with a low dose of IL-2 was found to promote destruction of cultured melanoma cells and it can be safely administered to patients with metastatic melanoma [40].

d. Transpupillary Thermotherapy (TTT):

Choroidal melanomas should be diagnosed and treated at the very early stage as the initial spread of metastases is thought to occur during the proliferative stage of tumor development.

TTT is recomended for the management of posterior choroidal nevi suspected for malignant transformation or small choroidal melanomas that are less than 2-5 mm in thickness [41]. TTT might be the treatment of choice for selected, very small melanomas. However, studies with long follow-up and large number of patients are needed to evaluate its effectiveness.

Choroidal melanomas treated with TTT as stand-alone procedure need a close monitoring since these tumors developed a significant rate of local recurrences and ocular side-effects in the long run.

e. Antiangiogenic drugs (Bevacizumab)

Anti-angiogenic therapy is based on the assumption that a tumor cannot grow beyond the limits of diffusion (about 1-2 mm) of oxygen and nutrients from capillaries, unless angiogenesis takes place. VEGF plays a key role in angiogenesis, regulating vasopermeability and the proliferation and migration of endothelial cells. VEGF levels are significantly elevated in uveal melanoma patients with metastatic disease compared to patients without metastases. Anti-angiogenic therapy, such as bevacizumab, is currently used for the treatment of metastases of several malignancies. [43].

Bevacizumab may be used as an adjuvant agent when used following plaque brachytherapy in the treatment of choroidal melanoma. The combination of this treatments was assessed in an interventional case series of 100 patients treated from 2006-2008 for choroidal melanoma and the results were satisfactory. Melanoma specific mortality was 0% at 9 months after treatment. Mean visual acuity for combined treatment at 6 months was 20/30 [42]

The *bevacizumab - radiotherapy combination* could be a promising clinical approach for the management of human uveal melanoma, since it may allow the use of lower doses of radiotherapy without compromising the antitumor effect [44].

f. Chemotherapy

There is no current evidence that chemotherapy has a significant role in the primary management of uveal melanoma. Such treatment may prolong survival for a few months but it is unlikely that it will be curative.

Uveal melanoma metastases develop in 6.5-35% of patients, most commonly to the liver. Metastatic uveal melanoma survival is poor, with 5-7 months of median survival. A retrospective study including 58 patients with uveal melanoma metastases showed that the median overall survival (OS) for all the patients was 10.83 months. Patients who had undergone chemotherapy presented 10.83 months of median OS whereas the patients who did not undergo this treatment had an OS of 8.033 months. Patients with metastatic uveal melanoma should be included in clinical trials evaluating other options with newer agents [45].

g. Others (Adjuvant therapy with interferon, Imatinilo Mesylate, Paclitaxeldocosahexaenoico Acid, Factionated Radiosurgery Cyberknife, aflibercept, vaccine).

7. Medical prognosis: Mortality (Hepatic metastasis), loss of the eye, loss of vision

These three variables will affect directly the patient survival:

Variable	Importance for prognosis
A Size (Base more than 16 mm and altura more than 10 mm).	+
B Cell Type (Epithelloid Cells)	++
C Genetic Type (GEP: Gene Expression Profile)	+++

Prognosis: GEP (Gene Expression Profile) In a prospective evaluation involving 514 uveal melanoma patients [46], the gene expression profile prognostic assay helped in classifying the primary tumor into two prognostic subgroups:

Class I (60% of the cases)

Low metastatic risk :

IA (87%) almost without metastasis (0.8% of the patients).

IB (13%) few metastasis (10.8%) + disomy cr3 few metastasis.

Class II (40% of the cases)

High metastatic risk: metastasis (29.8%) + monosomy or pseudodisomy cr3 metastasis is not sure, + Trisomy cr6: 80 % of patients will show metastasis 4 years after diagnosis.

http://dx.doi.org/10.5772/53633

This classification might be helpful for the prognosis in three aspects: in the screening targeted to metastasis, in the earlier diagnosis of the metastasis and for an earlier preventing treatment of the metastasis in high risk cases. In this regard, it is important to highlight that there is no scientific evidence about increased survival due to metastasis treatment [47].

8. Uveal melanoma TNM staging and survival: Implications in patient management and prognosis

Damato, B; Eleuteri, A [48] support the idea that Kaplan-Meier survival curves based only in tumour size and extend do not provide a true indication of prognosis. This is because the survival prognosis in uveal melanoma correlates not only with clinical stage but also with histologic grade, genetic type and competing causes of death. They propose an online predictor tool using the following data:

8.1. Parameters

Age

Sex

Large ultrasound diameter

Cilliary body involvement

Extraocular extension

Years since treatment

Epithelloid Cells

Closed PAS+ ve loops

Mitotic rate/40

Monosomy 3

Regional Lymph nodes

Distant metastasis

First scan (years)

Threshold for next scan (number)

8.2. TNM Stage

C.

Survival

Controls

Subjects

Difference

Relative

9. Conclusion

The uveal melanoma, which arises from melanocytes residing in the stroma, is the most common primary intraocular tumour in adults. More than 90% involve the choroid, the remainder being confined to the ciliary body and iris.

The most common symptoms in uveal melanoma include visual loss, photopsias and visual field defects but none of these symptoms are specific of this malignancy. Diagnosis is based on slit-lamp biomicroscopy and/or ophthalmoscopy, with ultrasonography, autofluorescence photography. Although each day we count with more variety and helpful complementary studies, suspicious lesions should be closely monitored. Uveal melanomas are diverse in their clinical features and behaviour. Despite ocular treatment almost 50% of patients with primary uveal melanoma will develop distance metastasis [50]. The metastatic disease occurs almost exclusively in patients whose tumour show chromosome 3 loss and/or class 2 gene expression profile. When the tumour shows such lethal genetic changes, the survival time depends on the anatomical stage and the histological grade of the malignancy.

Prognostication has improved as a result of progress in multivariate analysis including all the major risk factors.

Screening for metastases is more sensitive as a consequence of the advances in liver scanning with magnetic resonance imaging and other methods. More patients with metastases are living longer, benefiting from therapies such as: partial hepatectomy; radiofrequency ablation; ipilumumab immunotherapy; selective internal radiotherapy; intra-hepatic chemotherapy, possibly with isolated liver perfusion; and systemic chemotherapy [48].

Conservation of the eye with useful vision has improved thanks to the advances in brachytherapy, proton beam radiotherapy, transpupillary thermotherapy. The current trend is to try to preserve the affected eye by all means, as there is no scientific evidence that shows that removing the affected eye will improve survival.. This is a great difference in the treatment of ocular vs cutaneous melanoma. The specialists must take into consideration the need to protect the eye with melanoma and preserve as much vision as possible as the other eye may be affected by another pathology in the future with the consequent loss of vision.

On the basis of the currently available information it appears that patients treated with radiotherapy have a survival rate at least as good, if not better than those treated with enucleation [36].

Several drugs, such as bortezomib, celecoxib, dacarbazine, anti-angiogenic agents (such as bevacizumab, sorafenib and sunitinib), temsirolimus, mitogen-activated protein kinase kinase (MEK) inhibitors, ipilimumab and AEB071 are candidate drugs, and studies are underway to determine the therapeutic effects of these drugs in uveal melanoma [51].

Currently, the aim is to improve the detection of uveal melanoma so as to maximize the opportunities for conserving the eye and vision, as well as preventing metastatic spread. Patient management has been enhanced by the formation of multidisciplinary teams in specialized ocular oncology centers all over the world.

Acknowledgements

This publication was supported by grants from Raymos S.A.C.I. laboratory.

Author details

Victoria de los Ángeles Bustuoabad[1], Lucia Speroni[2] and Arturo Irarrázabal[3]

1 German Hospital, Buenos Aires, Argentina

2 Department of Anatomy and Cellular Biology, Tufts University, Boston, USA

3 Consultores Oftalmológicos Institute, Montevideo, Buenos Aires, Argentina

References

[1] Van den Bosch T, Kilic E, Paridaens D, de Klein A. Genetics of uveal melanoma and cutaneous melanoma: two of a kind? Dermatol Res Pract. 2010;2010:360136.

[2] Vicetti Miguel RD, Cherpes TL, Watson LJ, Mc Kenna KC: CTL induction of tumoricidal nitric oxide production by intratumoral macrophages is critical for tumor elimination. J Immunol 2010, 185:6706-18.

[3] Dace DS, Chen PW, Niederkorn JY: CD8+ Tcells circumvent privilege in the eye and mediate intraocular tumor rejection by aTNF-alfa dependent mechanism. J Immunol, 2007, 178:6115-22

[4] McKenna KC, Kapp JA: Accumulation of immunosuppressive CD11B+ myeloid cells correlates with the failure to prevent tumor grouth in the anterior chamber of the eye. J Immunol, 2006, 177:1599-608.

[5] Poggi A, Zocchi MR: Mechanisms of tumor escape: role of tumor microenviroment inducing apoptosis of cytolytic effector cells. Arch. Immunol The Exp (Warsz) 2006, 54:323-33.

[6] Margo CE, Mc Lean IW: Malignant melanoma of the choroid and ciliary body in black patiens. Arch Ophthalmol 1984; 102:77-79.

[7] Graham BJ, Duane TD: Meetings, conferences, symposia: report of ocular melanoma task force. Am J Ophthalmol 1981; 90:728-733.

[8] Gragoudas ES: First 1000 patients with uveal melanoma treated by proton beam irradiation. Presented at the second International Meeting in the Diagnosis and Treatment of Intraocular Tumors in Nyon, Switzerland, November, 1987.

[9] Singh AD, Shields CL, De Potter P, Shields JA, Trock B, Cater J, Pastore D. Familial uveal melanoma. Clinical observations on 56 patients. Arch Ophthalmol.1996 Apr; 114(4):392-9.

[10] Ferry AP: Lesions mistaken for malignant melanoma of the posterior uvea: a clinicopathologic analysis of 100 cases with ophthalmoscopically vivible lesions. Arch, Ophthalmol 1964; 72:463-469.

[11] Shields JA, Zimmerman LE: Lesions simulating malignant melanoma of the posterior uvea. Arch Ophthalmol 1973; 89:466-471.

[12] Zimmerman LE: Bedell Lecture. Problems in the diagnosis of malignant melanoma of the choroid and ciliary body. Am J Phthalmol 1973; 75:917-929.

[13] Chang M, Zimmerman LE. Mc Lean IW: The persisting pseudomelanoma problem. Arch Ophthalmol 1984, 102:726-727.

[14] Shields JA, Augsburger JJ, Brown GC, Stephens RF: The Differential diagnosis of posterior uveal melanoma. Ophthalmology 1980; 87:518-522.

[15] Shields JA, Mashayekhi A, Ra S, Shields CL: Pseudomelanomas of the posterior uveal tract. Retina 2005; 25:767-771.

[16] Char DH, Stone RD, Irvine AR, et al: Diagnostic modalities in choroidal melanoma. Am J Ophthalmol 1980; 89:223-230.

[17] Reese AB: Tumors of the eye 3rd edn. Hagerstown, MD: Harper & Row; 1976:174-262.

[18] Shields JA, Mashayekhi A, Ra S, Shields CL: Pseudomelanomas of the posterior uveal tract. Retina 2005; 25:767-771

[19] Char DH, Stone RD, Irvine AR, et al: Diagnostic modalities in choroidal melanoma. Am J Ophthalmol 1980; 89:223-230.

[20] Char DH: Inhibition of leukocyte migration with melanoma-associated antigens in choroidal tumors. Invest Ophthalmol Vis Sci 1977; 16:176-179.

[21] Brownstein S, Phillips TM, Lewis MG: Specificity of tumor-associated antibodies in serum of patients with uveal melanoma. Can J Ophthalmol 1978; 13:190-193.

[22] Felberg NT, Donoso LA, Federman JL: Tumor-associated antibodies in the serum of patients with ocular melanoma. Ophthalmology 1980; 87:529-533.

[23] Felberg NT, Pro-Landazuri JM, Shields JA, Federman JL: Tumor-associated antibodies in the serum of patients with ocular melanoma. Arch Ophthalmol 1979; 97:256-259.

[24] Donoso LA, Felberg NT, Edelberg K, et al: Metastasic uveal melanoma: an ocular melanoma-associated antigen in the serum of patients with metastatic deasease.

[25] Meyer F, Naron d, Zonix S: The role of carcinoembryonic antigen in surveillance of patients with choroidal melanoma: a prospectibe study. Ann Ophthalmol 1987; 19:24-25.

[26] Bomanji J, Hungerford JL, Granowska M, Britton Ke: Radioimmunoscintigraphy of ocular melanoma with 99m Tc labeled cutaneous melanoma antibody fragments. Br J Ophthalmol 1987; 71:651-658.

[27] Leyvraz S, Keilholz U: Ocular Melanoma: whats new? Curr Opin Oncol. 2012 Mar; 24(2):162-9.

[28] Vasiliki Poulaki, Sue Anne Chew, Bin He, Nicholas Mitsiades. Personalized Targeted Therapy harboring GNAq and GNA 11 Mutations. Inhibition of genes (Mek, B-Raf, Akt, PkC). Uveal Melanoma. XVth Biannual Meeting ISOO International Society of Ocular Oncology, 2011, Nov 14-17.

[29] Carvajal R, Wolchok JD, Chapman PB, Dickson M, Bluth M, Ambrosini G, Marr B, Heinemann M, Fusco A, Nalysnyk, Martin N, Doyle A, Bastian B, Abramson D, Schwartz G: Rationale, study design and accrual status of a randomized phase II study of AZD6244, a MEK inhibitor, vs temozomide in advanced uveal melanoma. XVth Biannual Meeting ISOO International Society of Ocular Oncology, 2011, Nov 14-17.

[30] Singh A: Resection of iris tumours: Internal approach. XVth Biannual Meeting ISOO International Society of Ocular Oncology, 2011, Nov 14-17.

[31] Shields JA, Augsburger JJ, Brady LW, Day JL: Cobalt plaque therapy of posterior uveal melanomas. Ophthalmology 99:1201-1207, 1982.

[32] Shields JA: Diagnosis and Management of Intraocular Tumours. St. Louis, the CV Mosby Co, 1983.

[33] Irarrázabal A, Cazon P: Results of melanoma brachytherapy in Argentina. XVth Biannual Meeting ISOO (International Society of Ocular Oncology), 2011, Nov 14-17.

[34] García-Álvarez C, Saornil MA, López-Lara F, Almaraz A, Muñoz MF, Frutos-Baraja J, Muiños Y: Episcleral brachytherapy for uveal melanoma: analysis of 136 cases. Clin Transl Oncol. 2012 May;14(5):350-5.

[35] Hawkins BS: Collaborative ocular melanoma study randomized trial of I-125 brachytherapy. Clin Trials. 2011 Oct;8(5):661-73.

[36] Gragoudas ES, Goiten M, Verhey L, Munzenreider J, Suit HD, Kohler A: Proton Beam irradiation, an alternative to Enucleation for intraocular melanoma. Ophthalmology 87:571-581, 1980.

[37] Tsimpida M, Hungerford J, Cohen V: Treatment of juxtapapillary choroidal melanoma. XVth Biannual Meeting ISOO International Society of Ocular Oncology, 2011, Nov 14-17.

[38] Damato B: Progress in the management of patients with uveal melanoma. Eye (Lond). 2012 Jun 29. The 2012 Ashton Lecture. [Epub ahead of print]

[39] Danielli R, Ridolfi R, Chiarion-Sileni V, Queirolo P, Testori A, Plummer R, Boitano M, Calabró L, Rossi CD, Giacomo AM, Ferrucci Pf, Ridolfi L, Altomonte M, Miracco C, Balestrazzi A, Maio M: Ipilimumab in pretreated patients with metastatic uveal melanoma.: safety and clinical efficacy. Cancer Immunol Immunother, 2012 Jan; 61(!): 41-8. Epub 2011 Aug 11.

[40] Soiffer RJ, Chapman PB, Murray C, Williams L, Unger P, Collins H, Houghton AN, Ritz J: Administration of R24 monoclonal antibody and low-dose interleukin 2 for malignant melanoma. Clin Cancer Res, 1997 Jan; 3(1):17-24.

[41] Mordechai R, Moroz I, Moisseiev J, Vishnevskia-Dai V: Our experience with transpupillary thermo therapy for suspected or small choroidal melanomas. XVth Biannual Meeting ISOO International Society of Ocular Oncology, 2011, Nov 14-17.

[42] Houston SK, Murray T, Markoe A, Pina Y, Decataur C: Intravitreal bevacizumab as an adjuvant agent when used immediately after treatment with plaque brachytherapy. XVth Biannual Meeting ISOO International Society of Ocular Oncology, 2011, Nov 14-17.

[43] el Filali M, van der Velden PA, Luyten GP, Jager MJ: Anti-angiogenic therapy in uveal melanoma. Dev Ophthalmol. 2012;49:117-36. Epub 2011 Oct 21.

[44] Sudaka A, Susini A, Lo Nigro C, Fischel JL, Toussan N, Formento P, Tonissi F, Lattanzio L, Russi E, Etienne-Grimaldi MC, Merlano M, Milano G: Combination of bevacizumab and irradiation on uveal melanoma: an in vitro and in vivo preclinical study. Invest New Drugs. 2012 Jun 20. [Epub ahead of print]

[45] Pons F, Plana M, Caminal JM, Pera J, Fernandes I, Perez J, Garcia-Del-Muro X, Marcoval J, Penin R, Fabra A, Piulats JM: Metastatic uveal melanoma: is there a role for conventional chemotherapy? - A single center study based on 58 patients. Melanoma Res. 2011 Jun;21(3):217-22.

[46] Harbour JW, Onken M, Worley L, Augsburger J, Correa Z, Devron HC, Nudleman E, Aaberg TJr, Altaweel MM, Bardenstein D, Finger P, Gallie B, Harocopos GJ, Hovland PG, McGowan H, Milman T, Mruthyunjaya P, Simpson ER, Smith M, Wilson D, Wirostko WJ: Prospective evaluation of a gene expression profile prognostic assay for uveal melanoma in 514 patients. XVth Biannual Meeting ISOO International Society of Ocular Oncology, 2011, Nov 14-17.

[47] Augsburger JJ, Correa ZM, Shaikh AH: Quality of evidence about effectiveness of treatments for metastatic uveal melanoma, Trans Am Ophthalmol Soc, 2008; 106:128-35; discussion 135-7.

[48] Damato B, Eleuteri A, Taktak AF, Coupland SE: Estimating prognosis for survival after treatment of choroidal melanoma. Prog Rtin Eye Res, 2011 Sep; 30(5):285-95. Epub 2011 May 30.

[49] Eye (Lond). 2012 Jun 29. doi: 10.1038/eye.2012.126. [Epub ahead of print]

[50] Spagnolo F, Caltabiano G, Queirolo P: Uveal Melanoma. Cancer Treat Rev 2012 Aug; 38(5):549-53. Epub 2012 Jan 24.

[51] Velho TR, Kapiteijn E, Jager MJ: New therapeutic agents in uveal melanoma. Anticancer Res. 2012 Jul;32(7):2591-8.

Section 3

Melanoma Related Features

Chapter 22

The Menace of Melanoma: A Photodynamic Approach to Adjunctive Cancer Therapy

L.M. Davids and B. Kleemann

Additional information is available at the end of the chapter

http://dx.doi.org/10.5772/53676

1. Introduction

Metastatic malignant melanoma (MMM) remains one of the most dreaded skin cancers worldwide. Numerous factors contribute to its resistance to hosts of treatment regimes and despite significant scientific advances over the last decade in the field of chemotherapeutics and melanocytic targets, there still remains the need for improved therapeutic modalities. Photodynamic therapy (PDT), a minimally invasive therapeutic modality has been shown to be effective in a number of oncologic and non-oncologic conditions. Using second-generation stable, lipophillic photosensitizers with optimised activation wavelengths, PDT may be a promising tool for adjuvant therapy and even pre-treatment in combating melanoma. Potential targets for PDT in melanoma eradication include cell proliferation inhibition, activation of cell death and reduction in pro-survival autophagy, a decrease in the cellular melanocytic antioxidant system and a disruption in the endogenous multi-drug resistant (MDR) cellular machinery. This chapter highlights the current knowledge with respect to these characteristics and suggests that PDT be considered as a good candidate for adjuvant treatment in post-resected malignant metastatic melanoma. Furthermore, it suggests that primary consideration must be given to organelle-specific destruction in melanoma specifically targeting the melanosomes – the one organelle that is specific to cells of the melanocytic lineage that houses the toxic compound, melanin. We believe that using this combined knowledge may eventually lead to an effective therapeutic tool to combat this highly intractable disease.

1.1. Melanoma clinical statistics

Melanoma accounts for 4% of all dermatologic cancers but remains responsible for 80% of deaths from skin cancer with the average patient diagnosed with disseminated metastases surviving for an average of 5 years (Cancer facts and figures, 2003, Atlanta, American Cancer Society, 2003]. According to the World Health Organization (WHO) melanoma skin cancer has been increasing over the past decades with a global estimation of 132 000 melanoma-related skin cancers reported to occur each year. Over the past 50 years, melanoma incidence has risen by 3–8% per year in most people of European background, with the greatest increases in elderly men [1]. In Europe, the current estimates at 15-20 per 100 000 people predominating in the 20-35 year old age group in Caucasians [2]. South Africa, next to Australia, has one of the highest incidences of malignant melanoma in the world. Reliable statistics for South Africa are lacking, however currently an estimate figure for the South African Cape region is 69 new cases per year per population of 100 000 Caucasians (Australia is 65 per 100 000). This means that 1 in 1429 people will develop malignant melanoma. The age-standardised incidence of melanoma was 27.2 per 100 000 for males and 22.2 per 100 000 for females from 1990-1999 but this increased to 36.9 for males and 33.5 per 100 000 for females (2000-2003) (CANSA association of South Africa www.melanoma.co.za/D_doccnr_MFS.asp) (Table 1).

	Age-standardised incidence(10^5 /yr)	Lifetime risk (incidence)	Incidence trend over 10 years	Mortality trend over 10 years	Most common cancer (ranking)
Australia (2001)					
Men	41.4 (world)	1 in 25	22% increase	2% increase	4th
Women	31.1 (world)	1 in 35	12% increase	0% increase	3rd
South Africa (2000)					
Men	36.9 (world)	1 in 29	33% increase	1.5% increase	4th
Women	33.5 (world)	1 in 40	27% increase	1% increase	3rd
USA (2001)					
Men	21.4 (world)	1 in 53	31% increase	0% increase	5th
Women	13.8 (world)	1 in 78	25% increase	1% decrease	7th
UK (2000)					
Men	9.7 (world)	1 in 147	59% increase	20% increase	12th
Women	11.2 (world)	1 in 117	41% incraese	3% increase	7th

Table 1. Melanoma statistics in 2 southern and northern hemisphere countries

Despite extensive research and clinical trials, the prognosis and survival of metastatic melanoma remains dismal. Early detection of localized melanoma may be cured through surgery however there is no therapy for metastatic melanoma or melanoma with metastatic potential. In addition, recurrence rates of resected melanoma remain high. Because melanoma is inherently resistant to traditional forms of chemotherapy and radiotherapy [3], various strategies have been developed for treatments which include immunotherapy eg. interleukin-2 (IL-2) [4], radiotherapy [5] biochemotherapy [6-9] and gene therapy [4,10]. A limited number of these therapies have progressed to human clinical trials but their outcomes remain negligible. One promising therapy is high-dose interferon (IFN) alpha-2b therapy which has just recently been approved as the only adjuvant therapy for melanoma approved by the US Food and Drug Administration [11]. The other is the use of BRAF kinase inhibitors such as vemurafenib [12]. Despite convincing evidence of improved disease-free survival associated with this therapy, the overall survival remains negligible or very small [13-15]. In addition, a number of melanoma-specific and melanoma-associated tumor antigens such as gp100, MART-1 and MAGE3 have been cloned [16] and the hope is that these potential antigens may be developed to stimulate tumor-specific T cells to eliminate melanoma cells [17]. Despite these advances, there remains the need for the development of novel and effective approaches to treat melanoma and this review explores the possibility of using photodynamic therapy (PDT) as an adjuvant therapy alone or in combination with current therapeutics to combat melanoma.

1.2. Melanoma origins

Melanoma represents the malignant phenotype of a skin melanocyte. Melanoma occurs most frequently after intermittent exposure to UV radiation and in people with chronic sunburns. Epidemiologic data suggest that chronic or low-grade exposures to UV induce protection against DNA damage, whereas acute, intense UV exposure leads to DNA damage and concomitant genetic alterations in the melanocyte genome [18]. It develops as a result of accumulated abnormalities in genetic pathways within the melanocyte which give way to increased cell proliferation and prevent normal pathways of apoptosis in response to DNA damage. Furthermore, this damage results in the selection for genetic mutations that allow all aspects of the malignant phenotype, including stimulation of blood vessel growth, evasion of the immune response, tumour invasion, and metastasis [19]. Although the mechanisms of differential cancer cell killing are poorly understood [20], selection of cells that are resistant to apoptotic mechanisms might contribute to the resistance of melanoma cells to the cytotoxic effects of chemotherapy, radiotherapy, and immunotherapy, especially through the expression of apoptosis inhibitors such as B-cell lymphoma derived protein 2 (Bcl-2) and BclxL [21].

Melanocytes progress through a series of steps toward malignant transformation by the acquisition of various phenotypic features. The particular histological features characterising each step of progression are the visible manifestations of underlying genetic changes [22].

Originating from a benign nevus, melanocytes undergo aberrant growth within the lesion subsequently displaying irregular borders, a change in colour and often an associated allergic response. At this stage the lesion is considered dysplastic. At a molecular level, these changes are associated with abnormal activation of the mitogen-activated protein kinase (MAPK) signalling pathway resulting in somatic mutations in the N-RAS and BRAF genes which are associated with about 15 and 50% of melanomas, respectively [23,24]. There is complementarity between the presence of *NRAS* and *BRAF* mutations in any individual melanoma since each has the same effect of causing unrestrained cell proliferation.

In addition, mutations in both the cyclin-dependent kinase inhibitor 2A (CDKN2A) and the phosphatase and tensin homologue (PTEN) gene increases the probability of dysplastic naevi becoming malignant [25]. This genetic locus is frequently targeted for disruption in melanomas [26]. When defective, p16 is unable to inactivate CDK4 and CDK6, which phosphorylate Rb, releasing the transcription factor E2F and leading to cell cycle progression [27].The molecule that is usually central to protection against DNA damage, p53, is rarely mutated early in melanoma, which is possibly one of several adaptations to permit survival of cells responsible for generating sun-protective pigment, melanin [28]. Interestingly, by-products of melanin biosynthesis can themselves cause oxidative stress and contribute to malignant change.

Further progression of melanoma is associated with decreased differentiation and clonal proliferation leading to the radial growth phase (RGP). Clinically, RGP presents as patches or plaques which can measure up to 2.5cm. Superficial spreading melanoma lesions are slightly raised and show striking variations of red, blue, white, brown, and black coloration. In RGP, melanoma mitoses are frequently seen in the epidermis but rarely in the dermis. After complete surgical excision of the tumor, RGP melanomas are usually associated with longterm metastasis-free survival [29-33]. RGP cells can progress to vertical growth phase (VGP) cells which breach the basement membrane and invade the dermis as nodules or nests of cells. Vertical growth phase (VGP) melanomas usually present as gray-black, blue-black, or even amelanotic nodules. In late or developed VGP, melanomas form expansile nodules in the dermis with cytology different from melanoma cells in the overlying epidermis. Mitotic figures are variably present, and tumor aggregates may extend into the reticular dermis or even subcutaneous fat. Dermal tumoral nests are larger in VGP than in RGP. Moreover, these cells are considered to have metastatic potential. Interestingly, not all melanomas pass through each of these individual phases – RGP and VGP can both develop directly from melanocytes or naevi and both can progress directly to metastatic malignant melanoma [34]. Moreover, the transition from RGP to VGP in cutaneous melanoma isassociated with the loss of c-KIT expression and the gain of the melanoma cell adhesion molecule (MCAM/MUC18) [35].

Increased proliferation and survival, chemoresistance, the ability to resist apoptosis, the induction of autophagy and the presence of the pigment melanin have all been listed as reasons contributing to the high mortality rates associated with cutaneous melanoma. Each of these topics will be dealt with in the context of targeting them with PDT.

1.3. Photodynamic Therapy (PDT) as a cancer treatment

PDT is a minimally invasive therapeutic modality which has been shown to be effective in several types of cancer including non-melanoma skin cancer (NMSC) and other skin tumors such as lymphoma as well as non-oncological conditions such as psoriasis vulgaris, acne vulgaris and human papilloma virus-induced skin disease [36,37]. The basis of PDT is the systemic or topical application and preferential uptake of a photosensitizer (PS). The PS is then activated at a specific wavelength of light and in the presence of oxygen, produces reactive oxygen species (ROS). The accumulative presence of these cytotoxic photoproducts start a cascade of molecular and biochemical events resulting in cell death via apoptotic or necrotic mechanisms [38,39].

The main advantage of PDT over conventional cancer treatments are i) it has a very low systemic cumulative toxicity allowing repeated dosing, ii) its ability to destroy tumors selectively (this seems to be related to the lipophillic nature of photosensitizers). Due to this selectivity, damage to normal surrounding cells is minimal. Finally, iii) PDT can be applied alone or in combination as an adjuvant therapeutic modality with chemotherapy, surgery, radiotherapy and immunotherapy [40,41]. These properties have led to PDT receiving increased support from preclinical research [42,43]. PDT requires three elements to be efficacious - a good PS, a coherent light source and the presence of molecular oxygen. A large amount of data with regard to these three elements over the last few years have resulted in the development of more naturally-derived, efficacious, second-generation photosensitizers.

1.3.1. Photosensitizers and melanoma-PDT

Photosensitizers are critical to the successful eradication of malignant cells and numerous first and second-generation photosensitizers have been tested both clinically (in vivo) and in vitro over the past years (for a detailed summary of melanoma-PDT research see Table 2). The structure of many PS is based on the tetrapyrrol ring eg. protoporphyrin IX, Photofrin and chlorines related to it eg. phthalocyanines. Newer, more stable second-generation PS include natural hydroxyquinone chromophores such as hypericins and porphycenes [44-47]. It is now accepted that a good PS for PDT is – i) chemically pure with good stability, ii) preferentially accumulated and retained by target tissue, iii) minimal toxicity in the absence of light with maximal efficacy upon activation, iv) high quantum yield of $^1O_2$ with an associated high molecular extinction coefficient [40]. Due to these properties, a number of synthetic or natural compounds have thus far been studied for a variety of cancers however these have been limited to porphycenes (structural isomers of porphyrins) such as aminolevulinic acid (ALA, trade name, Levulan®) and methylaminolevulinic acid (MAL, trade name, Metvix®) for the treatment of squamous cell (SCC) and basal cell carcinomas (BCC) as well as actinic keratoses [48-50] (Table 2).

Type of study	Tumour/Cell line	Photosensitizer	Ref
in vitro	B16-F10 melanoma cells	magnetoliposomes (MLs) loaded with zinc phthalocyanine (ZnPc) complexed with cucurbituril (CB) (CB:ZnPc-MLs)	[51]
in vivo	mice carrying B16-F10 melanoma xenografts	butadiyne-linked conjugated porphyrin dimer (Oxdime)	[52]
in vivo	subcutaneous amelanotic melanoma transplanted in C57/BL6 mice	pheophorbide a (Pba) and monomethoxy-polyethylene glycol-Pba	[53]
in vitro	A375, UCT Mel-1 human melanoma cells	hypericin and kojic acid (depigmenting agent)	[54]
in vitro/ in vivo	B16F10 mouse melanoma cells and lung melanomas in C57BL/6 mice	aminolevulic acid, gaussia luciferase, and its' substrate coelenterazine; murine neural stem cells (NSCs) and rat umbilical cord matrix-derived stem cells (RUCMSCs) with a plasmid expressing gaussia luciferase	[55]
in vitro	C32 human melanoma cells	Ficus carica L. cultivar Dottato extracts	[56]
in vitro	Melanoma, keratinocyte and fibroblast cells	aluminum tetrasulfophthalocyanines	[57]
in vivo	B16-F1 and Cloudman S9 melanoma-bearing mice	chlorin e(6) and modular nanotransporters targeted to α-melanocyte-stimulating hormone (αMSH) and epidermal growth factor (EGF) receptor	[58]
in vivo	malignant melanoma mouse model	methylene blue	[59]
in vitro	A549 and S91 melanoma cells	halogenated sulfonamide bacteriochlorins	[60]
in vitro	A375 melanoma cells	carotenoids (neoxanthin, fucoxanthin and siphonaxanthin)	[61]
in vitro	melanoma cells	2 cationic octanuclear metalla-cubes dual photosensitizers and chemotherapeutics	[62]
in vitro	A375 melanoma cells	Cachrys pungens Jan extracts from Italy	[63]
in vitro	B16F10 murine melanoma	indocyanine green (ICG) and hyperthermia	[64]
in vitro	B78-H1 murine melanoma cells	pheophorbide a	[65]
in vitro	S91 Cloudman melanoma cells and DBA mice	synthetic chlorin derivative ($TCPCSO_3H$)	[66]
in vitro/ in vivo	Melanoma cells and xenograft melanoma model	cis-Dichlorobis [3,4,7,8-tetramethyl-1,10-phenanthroline) rhodium(III) chloride (OCTBP)	[67]
in vitro	M21 human melanoma cells	Hedyotis corymbosa extracts	[68]
in vitro	A375, UCT Mel-1 human melanoma cells	hypericin and phenylthiourea (depigmenting agent)	[69]
in vitro	melanoma, keratinocyte and fibroblast cells	zinc tetrasulfophthalocyanines (ZnTSPc)	[70]

Type of study	Tumour/Cell line	Photosensitizer	Ref
in vitro	melanoma cells	PDT and Lycopene, β-carotene, vitamin C, N-acetylcysteine, trolox, N-tert-butyl-α-phenylnitrone and HO-1 activity inhibitor zinc protoporphyrine IX (ZnPPIX)	[71]
in vivo	mice bearing mouse melanomas	verteporfin	[72]
in vitro/ in vivo	S91 mouse melanoma cells and DBA mice	5,10,15,20-tetrakis[2-chloro-5-sulfophenyl)bacteriochlorin (TCPBSO3H)	[66]
in vitro	WM451LU melanoma cells	photosensitizers and heme oxygenase I (HO-I) and poly(ADP-ribose) polymerase (PARP) inhibitors	[73]
in vitro	A375 melanoma cells	5-aminolevulinic acid [5-ALA) and novel metallophthalocyanine (MPc)	[74]
in vivo	transplanted B16 melanoma	novel derivatives of chlorin e[6]	[75]
in vitro/ in vivo	melanoma bearing mice	C(60)-(Glc)1 (D-glucose residue pendant fullerene) and C(60)-(6Glc)1 (a maltohexaose residue pendant fullerene)	[76]
in vitro	SK-MEL-188 (human melanoma) cells	chlorin and bacteriochlorin derivatives of 5,10,15,20-tetrakis[2-chloro-5-sulfophenyl)porphyrin	[77]
in vitro	B16 melanoma cells	IPL and IPL plus 5-ALA	[78]
in vitro	melanoma cells	bacteriochlorins and photofrin	[79]
in vitro	C57 mice bearing a sub-cutaneously transplanted melanoma	Zn(II)-phthalocyanine disulphide (C11Pc)	[80]
in vitro	WM 1552C human melanoma cells	liposomes (LP) and nanocapsules (NC) containing Chloroaluminum phthalocyanine (ClAlPc)	[81]
in vitro	A375 melanoma cells	5,15-Diarylporphyrins (1-5) and Photofrin	[82]
in vivo	B16 melanoma tumours on mice	2 doses of photosensitizer	[83]
in vitro	B16 mouse melanoma cells	chlordiazepoxide (CDZ)	[84]
in vitro/ in vivo	B78H1 amelanotic mouse melanoma cells and C57BL/6 mice bearing a subcutaneously transplanted B78H1 amelanotic melanoma.	octabutoxy-naphthalocyanines	[85]
in vitro	G361 human melanoma cells	zinc-5,10,15,20-tetrakis(4-sulphonatophenyl) porphyrine (ZnTPPS(4)), chloraluminium phtalocyanine disulfonate (ClAlPcS(2)) and 5-aminolevulinic acid (ALA)	[86]
in vitro	A375 human melanoma cells B16F10 mouse melanoma cells	Pc4 encapsulated in silica nanoparticles	[87]

Type of study	Tumour/Cell line	Photosensitizer	Ref
in vitro	Sk-Mel-28 human skin melanoma cells	indocyanine green	[88]
in vitro	UCT Mel-1 and A375 human melanoma cells	hypericin	[89]
in vitro	G361 human melanoma cells	chloroaluminum phthalocyanine (ClAlPc) and ultrasound	[90]
in vitro	A375 human melanoma cells	5-aminolevulinic acid (ALA)	[91]
in vitro/ in vivo	B16F1 mouse melanoma cells and C57BL6 mice bearing a subcutaneously injected B16F1 melanoma.	methylene blue	[92]
in vitro/ in vivo	B16F1 mouse melanoma cells and C57BL6 mice bearing a subcutaneously injected B16F1 melanoma.	carboranyl-containing chlorin (TPFC)	[93]
in vitro/ in vivo	human malignant melanoma cells (MMCs)	porfimer sodium	[94]
in vivo	B57BL/6 mice bearing a B16BL6 melanoma	porfimer sodium and antibodies neutralizing decay-accelerating factor (DAF), complement-receptor-1-related protein y (Crry), and protectin	[95]
in vitro	G361 human melanoma cells	porphyrines (TPPS4, ZnTPPS4 and PdTPPS4	[96]
in vitro/ in vivo	B-16 mouse melanoma cells and subcutaneous B-16 melanoma-bearing C57BL/6 mice	5,10,15,20-tetraphenylporphin-loaded PEG-PE micelles	[97]
in vitro	UCT Mel-1 and UCT Mel-3 human melanoma cells	hypericin	[98]
in vitro	Me300 human melanoma cells	Five 5,10,15,20-tetra[4-pyridyl)porphyrin (TPP) areneruthenium(II) derivatives and a p-cymeneosmium and two pentamethylcyclopentadienyliridium and -rhodium analogues	[99]
in vitro	B16F10 melanotic melanomas transplanted to nude mice	methyl 5-aminolevulinate (MAL) and depigmentation with violet light	[100]
in vitro	S-91 mouse melanoma cells	titanium dioxide modified with platinum(IV) chloride complexes ($TiO_2/PtCl_4$)	[101]
in vitro	G361 human melanoma cells	zinc-5,10,15,20-tetrakis(4-sulphonatophenyl) porphyrine (ZnTPPS4) and atomic force microscopy	[102]
in vitro	WM451Lu metastatic human melanoma cells	5-aminolevulinic acid (ALA)	[103]
in vitro	B16F1 mouse melanoma cells	meso-tetra[4-nido-carboranylphenyl)porphyrin (H2TCP)	[104]

Type of study	Tumour/Cell line	Photosensitizer	Ref
in vitro	B16F10 mouse melanoma cells	solketal-substituted phthalocyanine (Si(sol)2Pc in mPEG-b-p(HPMAm-Lac2) micelles	[105]
in vitro	B19 mouse and G361 human melanoma cells	phthalocyanine ClAlPcS(2)	[106]
in vitro	S91 mouse and SKMEL 188 human melanoma cells	5,10,15,20-tetrakis[2-chloro-3-sulfophenyl)porphyrin (TCPPSO(3)H),	[107]
in vivo	choroidal melanomas in 46 New Zealand albino rabbit eyes	hematoporphyrin monomethyl ether	[108]
in vitro	G361 human melanoma cells	3 porphyrin sensitizers (TPPS(4), ZnTPPS[4] and PdTPPS(4))	[109]
in vitro	YUSAC2/T34A-C4 human melanoma cell line	porfimer sodium	[110]
in vivo	subcutaneous B16BL6 melanoma-bearing C57BL/6 mice	BPD, ce6, Photofrin, and mTHPC and gamma-inulin	[111]
in vitro	A375 human melanoma cells	acridine orange	[112]
in vitro	Cloudman S91/I3 mouse melanoma cells	photofrin II (PfII- porfirmer sodium), verteporfin, and merocyanine 540 (MC540)	[113]
in vivo	A-Mel-3 melanomas implanted in the dorsal skin fold chamber of Syrian Golden hamsters	5-aminolaevulinic acid (ALA)	[114]
in vivo	B-16 melanoma-bearing C57BL/6 mice	ATX-S10 No (II) and intratumoral injection of naïve dendritic cells (IT-DC)	[115]
in vitro/ in vivo	B16F1 mouse melanoma cells and C57BL6 mice bearing a subcutaneously injected B16F1 melanoma.	Zn(ii)-phthalocyanine derivative bearing four 10B-enriched o-carboranyl units [10B-ZnB4Pc)	[116]
in vitro	human Beidegröm Melanoma (BM) cell line	porfirmer sodium (photofrin II)	[117]
in vitro	G361 human melanoma cells	ZnTPPS(4) sensitizer bound to cyclodextrin hpbetaCD	[118].
in vitro	B78H1 mouse melanoma cells	Ni(II)-octabutoxy-naphthalocyanine (NiNc)	[119]
in vitro	G361 human melanoma cells	ZnTPPS(4) sensitizer bound to cyclodextrin hpbetaCD	[120]
in vitro	M2R mouse melanoma cells	O-[Pd-bacteriochlorophyllide]-serine methyl ester (Pd-Bchl-Ser)	[121]
in vitro	B78H1 melanoma cells	liposome-delivered Ni(II)-octabutoxy-naphthalocyanine	[119]
in vitro	human choroidal melanoma (CM) cells	tetrahydroporphyrin tetratosylat (THPTS)	[122]

Type of study	Tumour/Cell line	Photosensitizer	Ref
in vivo	M2R mouse melanoma xenografts	WST11	[123]
in vitro	B16 mouse melanoma cells	5-aminolevulinic acid [5-ALA) ester derivatives	[124]
in vivo	B-16 melanoma-bearing C57BL/6 mice	metal-free sulfonated phthalocyanine (H(2)PcS(2.4))	[125]
in vitro	A375 human melanoma cells	alpha-methylene-gamma-butyrolactone-psoralen heterodimer 2	[126]
in vitro	B16 mouse melanoma cells	5-aminolevulinic acid (ALA)	[127]
in vivo	C57BL6 mice bearing a subcutaneously injected B16F10 melanoma	silkworm excreta (SPbalpha) porfirmer sodium	[128]
in vitro	M3Dau human melanoma cells	silicon-phthalocyanines (SiPc) and chloro-aluminium Pc (ClAlPc),	[129]
in vitro	Me45 human melanoma cells	meso-tetra-4-N-methylpyridyl-porphyrin iodide and 5,10-di-[4-acetamidophenyl)-15,20-di-[4-N-methylpyridyl) porphyrin	[130]
in vitro	G361 human melanoma cells	meso-tetrakis[4-sulphonatophenyl)porphine (TPPS4) and zinc metallocomplex (ZnTPPS4)	[131]
in vitro	G361 human melanoma cells	ATX-S10(Na)	[132]
in vivo	syrian Golden hamsters fitted with dorsal skinfold chambers containing A-Mel-3 melanoma cells	5-aminolaevulinic acid (ALA)	[133]
in vitro	B16 mouse melanoma cells	5-aminolaevulinic acid (ALA)	[134]
in vivo	UB900518 human melanoma cells transplanted on nude (*nu/nu*) CD-1 mice	Liposomal meso-tetrakis-phenylporphyrin (TPP)	[135]
in vivo	pigmented choroidal melanoma 44 New Zealand albino rabbit eyes	liposomal preparation of benzoporphyrin derivative (BPD), verteporfin	[136]
in vitro	S91 mouse and SKMEL 188 human melanoma cells	indocyanine green (ICG)	[137]
in vitro	B16A45 (B16) mouse melanoma cells	delta-aminolevulinic acid (ALA) and meta(tetrahydroxyphenyl)chlorin or m-THPC	[138]
in vitro	B16 mouse melanoma cells	m-THPC and four apoptosis inhibitors: BAPTA-AM, Forskolin, DSF, and Z.VAD.fmk	[47]
in vitro	Bro, SKMel-23, SKMel-28	5-aminolevulinic acid (ALA)	[139]
In vitro	SKMEL 188 human melanoma cells	tritolylporphyrin dimer (T-D).	[140]
in vivo	Syrian Golden hamsters fitted with dorsal skinfold chambers containing A-Mel-3 melanoma cells	5-aminolaevulinic acid (ALA)	[141]
in vivo	Nude CD1 mice bearing malignant M2R melanoma xenografts	bacteriochlorophyll-serine (Bchl-Ser),	[142]

Type of study	Tumour/Cell line	Photosensitizer	Ref
in vitro	SK-23 mouse melanoma and SK-Mel 28 human melanoma	methylene blue	[143]
in vitro	B78H1 melanoma cells	liposome-incorporated Ni(II)-octabutoxy-naphthalocyanine (NiNc),	[144]
in vitro	B78H1 melanoma cells	Cu(II)-hematoporphyrin (CuHp)	[145]
in vivo	Syrian Golden hamsters fitted with dorsal skinfold chambers containing A-Mel-3 melanoma cells	5-aminolaevulinic acid (ALA)	[146]
in vitro	M6 human melanoma cells	dichlorosilicon phthalocyanine (Cl2SiPc) and bis(tri-n-hexylsiloxy) silicon phthalocyanine (HexSiPc)	[147]
in vivo	C57/BL6 mice bearing a subcutaneously transplanted B1 melanoma	benzoporphyrin derivative monoacid ring A (verteporfin, BPD-MA)	[148]
in vitro	SkMel-23 melanoma cells	5-aminolaevulinic acid (ALA)	[149]
in vivo	C57/BL6 mice bearing a subcutaneously transplanted B16 melanoma	Si(i.v.)-naphthalocyanine (isoBO-SiNc)	[150]
in vivo	C57/BL6 mice bearing a subcutaneously transplanted B16 melanoma	aluminum phthalocyanine (AlpcS4	[151]
in vivo	C57/BL6 mice bearing a subcutaneously transplanted B16F10 melanoma	lutetium texaphyrin (PCI-0123),	[152]
in vivo	Syrian Golden hamsters fitted with dorsal skinfold chambers containing A-Mel-3 melanoma cells	9-acetoxy-2,7,12,17-tetrakis-(beta-methoxyethyl)-porphycene (ATMPn)	[153].
in vivo	C57/BL6 mice bearing a subcutaneously transplanted B16 melanoma	Si(IV)-methoxyethylene-glycol-naphthalocyanine	[154]
in vivo	Syrian Golden hamsters fitted with dorsal skinfold chambers containing A-Mel-3 melanoma cells	5-aminolaevulinic acid (ALA)	[155]
in vivo	10 choroidal melanomas in rabbits	liposomal preparation of benzoporphyrin derivative	[156]
in vivo	M2R mouse melanoma tumors implanted in CD1 nude mice	bacteriochlorophyll-serine (Bchl-Ser),	[157]
in vitro	uveal melanoma cells	hematoporphyrin esters (HPE)	[158]
in vivo	Syrian Golden hamsters fitted with dorsal skinfold chambers containing A-Mel-3 melanoma cells	5-aminolaevulinic acid (ALA)	[159]
in vivo	C57/BL6 mice bearing a subcutaneously transplanted B16 melanoma	Zn(II)-2,3 naphthalocyanine (ZnNc)	[160]

Type of study	Tumour/Cell line	Photosensitizer	Ref
in vivo	32 choroidal tumours in New Zealand albino rabbit eyes.	benzoporphyrin derivative	[161]
in vitro	G361,M18 and M6 human melanoma cells	hypericin	[162]
in vitro	melanoma cell lines	hypericin	[163]

Table 2. Comprehensive update of in vivo and in vitro photodynamic therapy studies from 1996-present.

For melanoma treatment, where PDT will be more effective as a post-operative adjunctive treatment, very few reports highlight its effectiveness even though laboratory studies using melanoma cells show promise. Clinically, PDT has shown promise in the treatment of both ocular amelanotic melanomas [164] and skin metastases [165] however, more extensive clinical studies need to be conducted before PDT is accepted as the adjunctive therapy of choice [166] (Table 3).

Type of study	Tumour	Pigmentary phenotype	Photosensitizer	Outcome of study	Ref
clinical	choroidal melanoma	unpigmented	verteporfin	Dramatic tumor regression over 2 months to a completely flat scar [1.3 mm thickness), and remained stable at 50 months of follow-up.	[167]
clinical	3 choroidal melanomas	pigmented	PDT and intravitreal bevacizumab	The tumors treated with PDT and bevacizumab showed a marked reduction in tumor vascularity. The tumors receiving PDT as a primary treatment were followed by progressive tumor growth that led to enucleation years after.	[168]
clinical	9 posteriorly located choroidal melanomas	unpigmented	verteporfin	Eight tumors demonstrated apparent complete regression over 1 month to 14 months with no recurrence during follow-up of between 34 months and 81 months. One case developed 2 separate local recurrences at 21 months and 34 months.	[169]
clinical	11 late stage melanomas (cutaneous metastases)	ND	indocyanine green and imiquimod (immune modifier)	Complete response was observed in 6 patients. All lesions in the treatment area of the patients responded to photo-immunotherapy, 8 of which achieved complete local response (CLR). CLR was observed in the non-treatment site (regional) lesions in four patients. Five patients were still alive at the time of last follow-up.	[170]

Type of study	Tumour	Pigmentary phenotype	Photosensitizer	Outcome of study	Ref
clinical	1 duodenal metastatic melanoma	ND	porfirmer sodium	Successful treatment.	[171]
clinical	6 brain metastasis of malignant melanoma	ND	porfirmer sodium	All 6 patients [100%) remained free of brain disease till death, 50% died of malignant melanoma elsewhere and 50% died of unrelated causes.	[172]
clinical	melanoma in situ	unigmented	methyl aminolevulinate (MAL)	Recurrence at the original tumour site 4 months after PDT.	[173]
clinical	choroidal melanoma	unpigmented	benzoporphyrin derivative (BPD)	The tumor fully disappeared 1 month after the treatment, the visual acuity improved from 4/16 to 4/4. The disease did not recur during 24-month follow-up.	[174]
clinical	2 late-stage melanoma. Patient 1 had the primary tumour and local metastases on the left arm and metastatic tumours in the lungs. Patient 2 had a head and neck melanoma with multiple local metastases, which had failed repeated attempts at surgical resection and high-dose radiation therapy.	pigmented	indocyanine green (ICG) + imiquimod (toll-like receptor agonist)	Patient 1 free of all clinically detectable tumours (including the lung metastases) "/>20 months after the first treatment cycle. Patient 2 has been free of any clinical evidence of the tumour for over 6 months.	[175]
clinical	4 uveal melanoma, PDT on actual tumour site	mildly to heavily pigmented	benzoporphyrin derivative (BPD)	Vascular occlusion and thrombosis in mildly pigmented melanoma but no response in pigmented ones.	[176]
clinical	25 small and medium choroidal melanomas	ND	indocyanine green and transpupillary thermotherapy	After a mean of 2.4 treatments (range, 1 to 5 treatments), all of the tumors but one showed a significant volume reduction without clinical evidence of recurrences. Complications included retinal vascular occlusions, edema and superficial scarring of the macula, and rhegmatogenous retinal detachment.	[177]

Type of study	Tumour	Pigmentary phenotype	Photosensitizer	Outcome of study	Ref
clinical	14 skin metastasis from malignant melanoma, despite multiple courses of chemotherapy	pigmented	chlorin e_6	Complete regression after the first PDT treatment in eight cases and complete regression after multiple treatments in six cases. 11 of 14 patients died due to the progression of the melanoma, the median survival time after surgery was 883 days.	[165]
clinical	38 choroidal melanomas	ND	indocyanine green (ICG)	Changes in microcirculation 6 months after PDT, as well as significant decrease of tumors thickness in ultrasonography (mean 38%), were detected in all cases. Complete regression of intrinsic vessels was demonstrated by ICGA in 26 cases, and partial regression of pathological vascularization was found in 12 patients.	[178]
clinical	4 choroidal melanomas	ND	benzoporphyrin derivative (BPD)	One tumor decreased in size and remained stable for 18 months. One tumor had no growth for 11 months. Two melanomas continued to grow, necessitating enucleation.	[179]
clinical	3 uveal melanoma, PDT on unaffected areas before enucleation	ND	benzoporphyrin derivative (BPD)	Vascular thrombosis. No damage to the photoreceptors.	[180]
clinical	36 uveal melanomas	various	hematoporphyrin derivative	76 % of tumours were not growing at the end of the first year, 62 % after the second year and 38% after the fifth year. No eyes were lost as a result of PDT. The degree of tumour pigmentation and patient age at therapy significantly influence the tumour response to PDT.	[181]

Table 3. Clinical reports and outcomes of photodynamic effectiveness of photodynamic therapy protocols including the melanoma pigmentary phenotype.

1.3.2. Hypericin, a second generation photosensitizer for PDT

Hypericin, a second generation PS isolated from the plant *Hypericum perforatum,* is a phenanthroperylenequinone with two broad peaks of absorption – 300-400nm (ultraviolet) and 500-600nm (white light) (Figure 1). This may be considered as a disadvantage as a number of current second-generation photosensitizers have absorption peaks beyond 630nm allowing for increased penetration into tissues [182]. However, white light, used to activate hypericin, does penetrate deep into the dermis of the skin. Moreover, activation with ultraviolet light could be a distinct advantage for the use of hypericin in daylight-mediated PDT. This type of PDT is more convenient for patients and clinicians and causes less pain. It poses a particularly interesting avenue to explore for hospitals in developing countries where space is limited and budgets are inadequate. Daylight-mediated PDT is an effective treatment for thin actinic keratosis, as shown in three randomized controlled clinical studies (reviewed in Wiegell et al., 2011) [183]. The potential of hypericin in clinical practice has been highlighted by reports on its use to treat squamous and basal cell carcinomas [184-187], pancreatic tumors [188], bladder carcinomas [189-193], nasophyrangeal tumors [194,195] and recently melanomas [196].

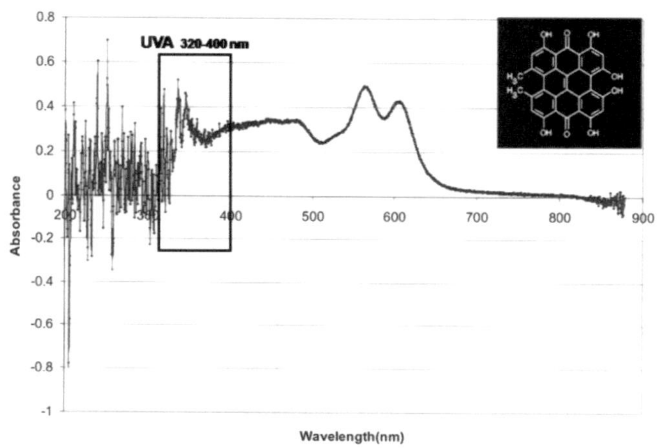

Figure 1. Absorbance spectrum of hypericin. Box, the wavelength of light used in our studies [98,197] representing one of the two activation peaks. Inset, chemical structure of hypericin.

1.3.3. *Melanoma cell death and biological mechanisms induced by hypericin-PDT*

Despite these promising studies, very few reports have highlighted hypericin's role in targeting melanoma. For the most part, cytotoxicity testing of new photosensitizers are tested on cell lines in vitro using assays such as the 3-[4,5-Dimethylthiazol-2-yl)-2,5-diphenyltetrazolium bromide (MTT), which is a colorimetric assays for measuring the activity of enzymes that reduce MTT to formazan dyes, giving a purple color [198,199]. Other tests for cytotoxicity include dead cell protease tests. Despite being used as the "gold standard" for cytotoxicity testing, it must be borne in mind that these assays are based on cellular metabolic activity and could result in a false positive result were the treatment to produce a cytostatic effect in cells. Moreover, as these are colorimetric-based tests, the photosensitizer used itself may interfere with the wavelength at which these tests are read.

One of the first few reports testing 1 to 20mg/ml hypericin efficacy on squamous carcinoma, sarcoma and melanoma cell lines found that a combination of activating laser light sources resulted in a reduction in cell viability of 90% [163]. Following this, Hadjur et al. (1996) exposed human pigmented and unpigmented melanoma cell lines to hypericin and showed minimal cytotoxicity on uptake but upon activation with white light, increased cell death in all three cell lines. Their findings thus suggest that amelanotic melanomas may be more susceptible to hypericin-PDT than pigmented melanomas. Their possible reasons for this related to the presence of melanin and antioxidant status of melanomas [162].

Work from our laboratory has shown a pigmentation dependant susceptibility of melanoma cells to hypericin-PDT, with pigmented cells being less susceptible than unpigmented cells [54,98,200,201]. Upon depigmentation with tyrosinase inhibitors, kojic acid and phenylthiourea, pigmented melanoma cells become more susceptible to hypericin-PDT [54,69]. Moreover, 72 hours after hypericin-PDT the cell viability of the depigmented melanoma cells remained significantly less than the control cells. Over the same time period the cells not treated with kojic acid approached a cell viability similar to the control.

Melanin is a potent antioxidant which could be a reason for the increased resistance of pigmented melanoma cells to PDT due to the scavenging of ROS produced by this therapy. Indeed we have shown that after depigmenting melanoma cells with kojic acid more ROS is produced upon treatment with hypericin-PDT compared to pigmented melanoma cells which were not depigmented [54]. We did not find a difference between the caspase 3, 7 activity after hypericin-PDT for both the depigmented and pigmented melanoma cells, which was lower than control. This suggests that pigmented melanoma cells might induce a caspase-independent mode of cell death such as the activation of apoptosis-inducing factor (AIF). Moreover, these cells might also undergo necrosis, necroptosis or autophagy in response to hypericin-PDT. We have further shown induction of autophagy at 4hours after hypericin-PDT in both pigmented and unpigmented melanoma cells [197]. Interestingly, pigmented melanoma cells (UCT Mel-1) show higher levels of externalisation of Annexin V, an early apoptotic event, compared to mildy and unpigmented melanoma cells [501mel and A375, respectively) after hypericin-PDT (Figure 2). However, the cell death response of pigmented and unpigmented melanoma cells is very complex and does seem to be cell type dependant. A possible explanation for this may be that the cell lines used in our studies are from different genetic origins and they thus might differ in various biochemical characteristics, including their antioxidant systems. The subcellular localisation of the photosensitizer is another factor determining the cell death mode initiated by PDT. Upon activation by light, photosensitizers produce ROS which are short-lived species acting directly in their vicinity of production. Localisation to different cellular compartments thus induces different modes of cell death.

Note: Since the discovery of programmed cell death in the 1960's the cell death field has evolved immensely. Researchers have shifted from morphological classifications to using more biochemical criteria. The increase in cell death studies necessitated a systemic classification of cell death modalities, which led to the formation of the Nomenclature Committee on Cell Death (NCCD). The main mission of this committee is 'to provide a forum in which names describing distinct modalities of cell death are critically evaluated and recommendations on their definition and use are formulated, hoping that a non-rigid, yet uniform nomenclature will facilitate the communication among scientists and ultimately accelerate the pace of discovery' [202-204].

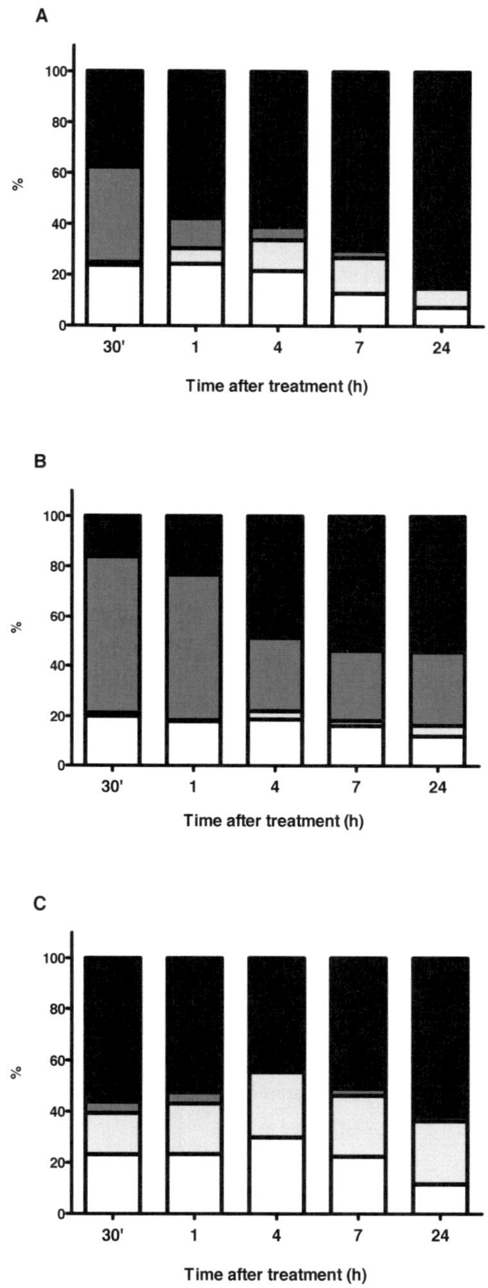

Figure 2. Graphs representing fluorescent activated cell sorting (FACS) analyses of melanoma cells at 30min, 1, 4, 7 and 24h after hypericin-PDT treatment (3μM hypericin with 1 J/cm^2 UVA). A: unpigmented A375, B: mildly pigmented 501mel and C: pigmented UCT Mel-1. Cells were stained for early apoptosis (FITC Annexin V, BD Biosciences) and necrosis (LIVE/DEAD Fixable Violet stain, Invitrogen). Different modes of cell death are represented as proportional percentages normalised to the control, black: late apoptotic/ necrotic, dark grey: necrotic, light grey: apoptotic, white: live; n=3.

1.4. PDT targets to treat melanoma

1.4.1. Cell proliferation and survival

It is now well established that one of the chief characteristics of cancer cells is their ability to overcome cellular control of proliferation [205]. In melanocytes, proliferation is caused by a combination of several mitogenic growth factors such as stem cell factor (SCF), epidermal growth factor (EGF), fibroblast growth factor (FGF) and hepatocyte growth factor (HGF) which cause a sustained extracellular receptor kinase (ERK) activity [206]. In melanoma, the RAS/Raf/MEK/ERK pathway is a key regulating pathway in proliferation with ERK being hyperactivated in up to 90% of human melanomas [207]. BRAF and PTEN mutations (see above) are co-incident in about 20% of cases [208]. The most common mutation in BRAF is a glutamic acid for valine substitution at position 600 (^{V600E}BRAF) [209]. This mutation leads to constitutive ERK signalling resulting in hyperproliferation and cell survival [210]. This pathway, through the EGF receptor as an extracellular ligand, has been a worthwhile target for PDT in that sustained activation of the ERK pathway protected cells from photofrin-based PDT as well as a reduction in the Raf protein levels in treated cells [211].

Nuclear factor kappa beta (NF-κβ) signalling leads to transcriptional regulation of a number of genes involved in responses ranging from proliferation, metastasis, and survival to inflammation. It therefore is an important target in PDT to stop aberrant cell proliferation. PDT-induced oxidative stress through increased ROS production has been shown to activate (NF-κβ) [212] and inactivate its inhibitor (Iκβ). Moreover, Ryter and Gomer showed increased NF-κβ binding in response to PDT stress in mouse cancer cells leading to a reduction in proliferation [213].

1.4.2. Inhibition of apoptosis

Apoptosis, a controlled mode of cell death, is characterised by cell shrinkage, chromatin condensation, DNA fragmentation, membrane blebbing and activation of caspases [214]. It is now well established that activation of the caspase cascade occurs through death receptor activation (extrinsic pathway) or through mitochondrial outer membrane permeabilization (intrinsic pathway). Both of these pathways have been shown to be activated through PDT. Several biochemical studies have established that PDT with different photosensitizers, including hypericin, utilise the mitochondrial-mediated pathway of caspase activation [215,216] although PDT has recently been shown to also engage caspase-independent pathways [217]. It is further known that several anti-cancer agents induce apoptosis and may share common pathways leading to cell killing with Fas/APO-1/CD95 [218,219]. Ali et al. (2002) elegantly showed that hypericin-PDT induces human nasopharyngeal cancer cells to undergo apoptosis through the Fas/FasL system. Moreover, they showed that the upregulation of Fas/FasL results in the release of cytochrome c into the cytoplasm with subsequent caspase induction – results that suggest that although apoptosis is considered a product of either an extrinsic or intrinsic mechanism; the overall response to PDT may be a combination of mechanisms [220].

Cancer cells are known to resist cell death by upregulation of anti-apoptotic proteins, mutations in pro-apoptotic proteins, inhibition of cell senescence or through protective mechanisms such as autophagy. PDT that is targeted for cancer therapy aims to invoke cell cytoxicity through attacking these characteristics – topics of a number of recent reviews [36,221-223].

Intriguingly, the emergence of a defined 'immunogenic apoptosis' seems to be a new 'subset' of apoptosis and autophagic cell death which has been shown to have the ability to release/expose damage-associated membrane proteins (DAMPs) [224-227]. Therapeutically, the immunogenicity of apoptosis is preferable for application rather than necrosis (or for that matter autophagic cell death) since necrosis can lead to harmful immunological reactions [228] (on the other hand, the extent of immunological impact of autophagic cell death is as yet uncharacterized, thereby making it an uncertain modality to use in the context of 'immunochemotherapy') [229]. The cell killing effectiveness is however dependent on parameters such as the PS used, the light dose and most importantly, the subcellular localization of the PS. It is crucial for photosensitizers to effectively enter the cell and accumulate in specific intracellular organelles in order to be efficient in their killing ability. Clearly, the final destination of the PS and its immediate vicinity will lead to different modes of cell death and consequently different efficiencies. Recent reports have highlighted that hypericin not only localises to different subcellular organelles but that this localization is exposure and dose-dependent in addition to being tumour cell-specific [230-234]. As a start however, the lipophillic nature of hypericin dictates its association with cellular membranes [235]. The fact that hypericin has been shown to associate with serum proteins (LDL and HDL lipoproteins [236] ensues that it enters cells quickly and is preferentially taken up by cancer cells in the 3-dimensional milieu as recent reports showed that these cells have high levels of LDL surface receptors [237]. This is further supported by a recent report showing that cholesterol serves as a key determinant for the uptake of hypericin into cellular membranes [238].

Noteworthy however is that even though high levels of hydrophobicity ensues, high levels of intracellular accumulation of the photosensitizer, changes in the physical structure of the PS due to aggregation and other modifications, may lead to reduced PDT efficiency [239]. Overall, the consensus emerging is that hypericin localises to three intracellular organelles namely, the endoplasmic reticulum (ER)-Golgi network [230,231,240,241], mitochondria (Mt) [242-245] and lysosomes [237,246] where through synergistic action, apoptosis is induced. More recent work by the Agostinis group show that hypericin-based PDT would produce photo-oxidative ER (p-ox ER stress) stress while 5-ALA (localizes in the mitochondria)-based PDT would produce photo-oxidative mitochondrial stress [36,247]. They also observed that Hyp-PDT induces 'pre-apoptotic' active exo-ATP secretion and late stage passive release of DAMPs like HSP70, HSP90 and CRT [223]. Overall they suggest that the potential of Hyp-PDT in causing exposure/secretion of 'critical' DAMPs add to the apoptotic cell death modality in a rather 'small club' of anti-cancerous therapeutic agents/modalities capable of exposing immunogenic signals like ecto-CRT [227,248].

1.4.3. Induction of autophagy

A recent finding is the induction of the cytoprotective programme of autophagy in melanomas in response to PDT-induced oxidative stress [89]. In addition, recent reports showed that cancer cells may respond to chemotherapeutics or other forms of oxidative stress such as PDT, through the induction of autophagy initially but continued stress leads to an overwhelming of the endogenous antioxidant enzymes along with a shift from autophagy to a possible senescent phenotype in an attempt to prolong cellular survival. Consequently however, the cell enters an apoptotic or necrotic mode of cell death [249-251]. Autophagy, defined as a cellular response to nutrient deprivation with consequent organelle breakdown, could converge with PDT at a number of cellular locations. Although more work relating to this aspect in melanomas is needed, reports on other cancer cells have shown that autophagy can be induced if the lysosomal system, needed for the clearance of ROS-damaged organelles, is affected by PDT [252]. Another cellular location is the mitochondria, where the PDT-induced loss of anti-apoptotic protein Bcl-2, may lead to an initation of autophagy [253].

1.4.4. Chemoresistance due to increased antioxidants

Cancer cells are considered to be under continuous oxidative stress which has been suggested to aid in tumor progression [254]. In support, several studies have shown tumor cell lines producing higher levels of ROS compared to their normal counterparts [255,256]. Due to this increased level of ROS and hence constitutive increased level of oxidative stress, it is not surprising that cancer cells have an extensive and advanced intracellular antioxidant network – a characteristic which further increases their chemoresistant property. Interestingly, the antioxidant status of melanomas differs from that of other skin cancers such as basal and squamous cell carcinomas in that their antioxidant activity levels (i.e. catalase, glutathione peroxidise, superoxide dismutase) are much higher [257]. In contrast, melanocytes, their normal untransformed phenotype, have lower levels of antioxidant activities and associated lower levels of resistance to oxidative stress [258]. It is therefore reasonable to postulate whether breaking this tolerance to oxidative stress may increase therapeutic efficacy in targeting melanoma. A number of studies have therefore suggested that treating melanoma by inhibiting cellular antioxidants may be efficacious [259-261]. One example of this was the addition of the superoxide dismutase (SOD) activity inhibitor, 2-methoxyestradiol (2-ME_2), to a mouse transplant model which induced growth arrest of melanoma cells after injection [262]. Paradoxically, several studies have suggested that antioxidants can enhance the action of cancer chemotherapeutics drugs in their in vitro models through inhibition of a variety of factors which contribute to the malignant phenotype [263,264]. A recent study however, using six different combinations of antioxidants and chemotherapeutic drugs in combination, failed to identify a single combination in which an antioxidant reduced the survival of malignant breast carcinoma cells [265]. To our knowledge the use of PDT as an inhibitor of antioxidants has not been tested in cancer cells.

1.4.5. Melanin and melanosomes as pro-survival agents

All the potential intracellular organelle targets for PDT mentioned above are consistent with most cancer cells. However, the one aspect that sets melanoma apart from other cancers is the presence of its cell-specific organelle called the melanosome and its associated product, melanin pigment. It is thus not inconceivable to believe that the intractability of this skin disease may in some way be related to this organelle and its function [266,267]. It follows logically then, that treatment regimes need to consider the melanosome as another potential target organelle in the fight against melanoma [268].

Melanosomes are membrane-bound organelles in melanocytic cells which house the pathway that results in the formation of the polymeric pigment, melanin [269,270]. The enzymes which participate in this pathway are translated in the cytoplasm and chaperoned to the melanosomes. Tyrosinase (TYR), the rate-limiting enzyme of the pathway, and its related proteins tyrosinase-related proteins 1 and 2 (TYRP-1 and TYRP-2) act in concert to first convert tyrosine to 3,4-dihydroxy-phenylalanine (DOPA) via tyrosine hydroxylase activity and then convert DOPA to DOPAquinone via dopa oxidase activity. Both of these activities occur via separate tyrosinase catalytic sites. During melanin synthesis toxic intermediates such as 5, 6-dihydroxyindole and 5,6-dihydroxyindole-2-carboxylic acid are produced. Structurally, the melanosomes are designed to compartmentalise these cytotoxic melanin intermediates from spilling into the cytoplasm [271]. Melanosomal biogenesis progresses through four distinct stages of maturation where the first two stages contain no melanin and the later stages constitute intermediates required to generate a matrix favourable for the formation of melanin [269,272]. The Pmel17/gp100/Silv/ME20 protein, a product of the Silver locus in melanocytic cells [273], is capable of polymerizing into fibrillar arrays that form the backbone of melanosomes. As a major component of the fibrillar matrix of early stage melanosomes, Pmel-17 serves as the best marker to follow intracellular trafficking steps that regulate melanosomal formation [274].

Moreover, as Pmel-17 facilitates melanin deposition and plays a pivotal role in melanosome biogenesis, it remains a strategic target when trying to combat melanoma through the fact that melanosomes are involved in scavenging endogenous cytotoxic metabolites and storing their waste products - a function that has been suggested to be a key in creating multi-drug resistance [267]. With the premise that melanosomes may be acting as cytotoxic drug "sinks" through the sequestration of chemotherapeutic drugs [267], it would be considered an effective therapy for a PS to enter the melanosomal membrane and damage the wall of the melanosome thus allowing the leakage of toxic melanin intermediates resulting in cell death. The drawback is that melanosomes, which are classified into stages along their biogenesis [269,270] only produce the toxic intermediates during their final maturing stages III and IV [268-270,275-277]. Most pigmented melanomas do however present with a majority of these end-stage melanosomes in their cytoplasm making the melanosomal membrane an attractive target for PDT. On the basis of this information, one may imagine that pigmented melanomas are therefore more susceptible to PDT-induced cell death. In contrast, our work has shown that pigmented melanomas are much less susceptible to hypericin-PDT than unpigmented/amelanotic melanomas despite hypericin readily entering the melanosomes [89].

We hypothesize that the reason for this is due to the presence of the pigment melanin. In support of this, pigmented human xenograft melanotic melanoma in mice, was shown to be far less responsive to PDT than amelanotic melanoma [278].

Melanin has been shown to act as both an oxidant and antioxidant [266,279] and in parallel studies, its presence in melanomas have been linked to chemoresistance. In support, further studies have shown that a lack of pigment in melanomas decreases their resistance to cell death. Our ongoing investigation into susceptibility to PDT-induced cell death in depigmented melanomas supports this hypothesis [54,69].

1.4.6. Cancer stem cells as future PDT targets

The cancer stem cell hypothesis purports the idea that a subset of cancer cells is capable of maintaining and driving disease progression [280,281]. With the identification of cancer stem cell populations in colon, breast and brain tumors [282-285], it is believed that these cells are integrally related to tumor formation, resistance to chemotherapy and escape from remission [286]. While the qualifications for melanoma stem cells have generally been defined as tumorigenicity in xenograft spheroid formation and self-renewal in non-adherent cultures, the markers used to identify these cells from the general tumor population remain debatable. A brief summary of these markers and their potential as targets for novel PDT-based therapy, follow.

ATP-binding cassette (ABC) transporters are a vast family of transmembrane proteins that have been studied for their ability to actively transport cytotoxic substances out of cells [287]. Intriguingly, some of these transporters have been demonstrated to be highly expressed in highly tumorigenic subpopulations of melanoma suggesting that they may be markers of melanoma stem cells [286]. One of these includes the ABCB5 transporter. Known for increased expression during melanoma progression in human tumor samples, ABCB5+ cells were able to resist treatment with doxorubicin [288]. While ABCB5+ cells were not able to renew in culture (a "stemness trait"), a subpopulation of cells that were indeed able to renew expressed the ABC transporter, Multi-drug Resistant-1 (MDR1) [289]. In vitro, MDR1+ cells exhibited less pigmentation than MDR1- cells, possessed the ability to continuously self-renew in soft agar and expressed the pluripotency and self-renewal regulators, human telomerase reverse transcriptase (hTERT) – all characteristics pointing towards "stemness". Interestingly, while MDR+ cells did exhibit cancer stem-cell like properties in vitro, they also co-expressed ABCB5 and ABCC2 mRNAs suggesting that a number of ABC transporters may be expressed in sub-populations [289]. To further add to the complication of delineating melanoma stem cell markers as potential targets for PDT is the fact that a number of recent markers are co-expressed with ABC transporters. These include CD133/prominin-1/AC133, which is co-expressed with ABCB5 and ABCG2 [288,290] and Nestin ([286].

Accumulating evidence suggests that another transporter, ABCG2, has physiological relevance in terms of photosensitivity and hence, PDT [291,292]. It has been shown that clinical photosensitizers and chemotherapeutic drugs have been transported out of cells by ABCG2 whereas this effect was abrogated by co-administration of its inhibitor, imatinib mesylate [293]. It is fascinating to speculate that a PDT protocol using a new, more stable photosensitizer such as hypericin may, through optimized concentrations, inhibit the action of the

ABCG2 transporter and thus create an intracellular pool of ROS resulting in efficacious cell death. This is definitely an avenue for exploration.

Overall, the ability to halt melanoma cancer progression through targeting melanoma stem cells could be extremely advantageous. However, with such a large number of potential markers and their interaction with PDT unknown, it may be a better option to focus on ABC transporters and investigate their susceptibility to second generation PS-based PDT as a means to an end for melanoma progression.

2. Conclusion and future directions

There is no doubt that our understanding of the molecular and cellular basis of melanoma has grown substantially over the past decade. However, due to its multifunctional nature, the nee d for better, improved therapies to combat or target melanoma remain essential. In addition, better understanding of the heterogenous nature of this diverse disease will likely lead to re-evaluation of the basic concepts underlying melanoma therapeutics development and clinical trial design. Till then however, novel adjuvant treatment modalities such as PDT using photostable, second-generation photosensitizers such as hypericin remain an option and need to be investigated further. Moreover, optimization of this type of therapy with regard to subcellular localization and its effect on cell death mechanisms within melanoma cells is needed. Targeting the integrity of melanocytes-specific organelles such as the melanosomes and producing an over-riding increase in ROS with consequent cytotoxicity remains a good therapeutic option but needs a systematic, scientific approach. Intriguingly, as more avenues of therapeutic targets such as melanoma stem cells and ABC transporters become illuminated, the ability to invoke cell death modalities in combination with PDT become more evident. Finally, it is clear that all these factors need to be considered in synergy if progress is to be made toward combating the menace that is metastatic melanoma.

Acknowledgements

This work was supported by the University of Cape Town Research Committee, the National Research Foundation of South Africa (LMD) and Postgraduate funding (BK) from the NRF and DAAD.

Author details

L.M. Davids and B. Kleemann

Redox Laboratory, Department of Human Biology; Faculty of Health Sciences; University of Cape Town Medical School; Cape Town, South Africa

References

[1] Armstrong B. Epidemiology of cutaneous melanoma and current trends. In: Thompson J, Morton D, Kroon B, editors. Textbook of Melanoma London, UK: Martin Dunitz; 2004. p. 65-80.

[2] Bataille V. Early detection of melanoma improves survival. Practitioner 2009 Oct; 253(1722):29-32, 3.

[3] Zbytek B, Carlson JA, Granese J, Ross J, Mihm MC, Slominski A. Current concepts of metastasis in melanoma. Expert Rev Dermatol 2008 Oct;3(5):569-585.

[4] Carlson JA, Ross JS, Slominski A, Linette G, Mysliborski J, Hill J, et al. Molecular diagnostics in melanoma. J Am Acad Dermatol 2005 May;52(5):743-75; quiz 775-8.

[5] Moncrieff MD, Martin R, O'Brien CJ, Shannon KF, Clark JR, Gao K, et al. Adjuvant postoperative radiotherapy to the cervical lymph nodes in cutaneous melanoma: is there any benefit for high-risk patients? Ann Surg Oncol 2008 Nov;15(11):3022-3027.

[6] Yamamura H, Ugawa S, Ueda T, Morita A, Shimada S. TRPM8 activation suppresses cellular viability in human melanoma. Am J Physiol Cell Physiol 2008 Aug; 295(2):C296-301.

[7] Chudnovsky Y, Khavari PA, Adams AE. Melanoma genetics and the development of rational therapeutics. J Clin Invest 2005 Apr;115(4):813-824.

[8] Slominski A, Tobin DJ, Shibahara S, Wortsman J. Melanin pigmentation in mammalian skin and its hormonal regulation. Physiol Rev 2004 Oct;84(4):1155-1228.

[9] Slominski A, Wortsman J, Carlson AJ, Matsuoka LY, Balch CM, Mihm MC. Malignant melanoma. Arch Pathol Lab Med 2001 Oct;125(10):1295-1306.

[10] Thompson JF, Scolyer RA, Kefford RF. Cutaneous melanoma. Lancet 2005 Feb 19-25;365(9460):687-701.

[11] McMasters KM, Edwards MJ, Ross MI, Reintgen DS, Martin RC,2nd, Urist MM, et al. Ulceration as a predictive marker for response to adjuvant interferon therapy in melanoma. Ann Surg 2010 Sep;252(3):460-5; discussion 465-6.

[12] Chapman PB, Hauschild A, Robert C, Haanen JB, Ascierto P, Larkin J, et al. Improved survival with vemurafenib in melanoma with BRAF V600E mutation. N Engl J Med 2011 Jun 30;364(26):2507-2516.

[13] Wheatley K, Ives N, Hancock B, Gore M, Eggermont A, Suciu S. Does adjuvant interferon-alpha for high-risk melanoma provide a worthwhile benefit? A meta-analysis of the randomised trials. Cancer Treat Rev 2003 Aug;29(4):241-252.

[14] Mocellin S, Pasquali S, Rossi CR, Nitti D. Interferon alpha adjuvant therapy in patients with high-risk melanoma: a systematic review and meta-analysis. J Natl Cancer Inst 2010 Apr 7;102(7):493-501.

[15] Janku F, Kurzrock R. Adjuvant interferon in high-risk melanoma: end of the era? J Clin Oncol 2010 Jan 10;28(2):e15-6; author reply e17-8.

[16] Boon T. Tumor antigens recognized by cytolytic T lymphocytes: present perspectives for specific immunotherapy. Int J Cancer 1993 May 8;54(2):177-180.

[17] Vogel TU, Visan L, Ljutic B, Gajewska B, Caterini J, Salha D, et al. Preclinical qualification of a new multi-antigen candidate vaccine for metastatic melanoma. J Immunother 2010 Oct;33(8):743-758.

[18] Gilchrest BA, Eller MS, Geller AC, Yaar M. The pathogenesis of melanoma induced by ultraviolet radiation. N Engl J Med 1999 Apr 29;340(17):1341-1348.

[19] Satyamoorthy K, Herlyn M. Cellular and molecular biology of human melanoma. Cancer Biol Ther 2002 Jan-Feb;1(1):14-17.

[20] Vogelstein B, Kinzler KW. Cancer genes and the pathways they control. Nat Med 2004 Aug;10(8):789-799.

[21] Soengas MS, Lowe SW. Apoptosis and melanoma chemoresistance. Oncogene 2003 May 19;22(20):3138-3151.

[22] Clark WH,Jr, Elder DE, Guerry D,4th, Epstein MN, Greene MH, Van Horn M. A study of tumor progression: the precursor lesions of superficial spreading and nodular melanoma. Hum Pathol 1984 Dec;15(12):1147-1165.

[23] Brunet A, Roux D, Lenormand P, Dowd S, Keyse S, Pouyssegur J. Nuclear translocation of p42/p44 mitogen-activated protein kinase is required for growth factor-induced gene expression and cell cycle entry. EMBO J 1999 Feb 1;18(3):664-674.

[24] Lin AW, Barradas M, Stone JC, van Aelst L, Serrano M, Lowe SW. Premature senescence involving p53 and p16 is activated in response to constitutive MEK/MAPK mitogenic signaling. Genes Dev 1998 Oct 1;12(19):3008-3019.

[25] Miller AJ, Mihm MC,Jr. Melanoma. N Engl J Med 2006 Jul 6;355(1):51-65.

[26] Kefford R, Bishop JN, Tucker M, Bressac-de Paillerets B, Bianchi-Scarra G, Bergman W, et al. Genetic testing for melanoma. Lancet Oncol 2002 Nov;3(11):653-654.

[27] Serrano M. The tumor suppressor protein p16INK4a. Exp Cell Res 1997 Nov 25;237(1):7-13.

[28] Gilchrest BA, Eller MS. DNA photodamage stimulates melanogenesis and other photoprotective responses. J Investig Dermatol Symp Proc 1999 Sep;4(1):35-40.

[29] Johnson TM, Dolan OM, Hamilton TA, Lu MC, Swanson NA, Lowe L. Clinical and histologic trends of melanoma. J Am Acad Dermatol 1998 May;38(5 Pt 1):681-686.

[30] Rossi CR, Foletto M, Vecchiato A, Alessio S, Menin N, Lise M. Management of cutaneous melanoma M0: state of the art and trends. Eur J Cancer 1997 Dec;33(14): 2302-2312.

[31] Slominski A, Ross J, Mihm MC. Cutaneous melanoma: pathology, relevant prognostic indicators and progression. Br Med Bull 1995 Jul;51(3):548-569.

[32] Clark WH,Jr, Elder DE, Guerry D,4th, Braitman LE, Trock BJ, Schultz D, et al. Model predicting survival in stage I melanoma based on tumor progression. J Natl Cancer Inst 1989 Dec 20;81(24):1893-1904.

[33] Guerry D,4th, Synnestvedt M, Elder DE, Schultz D. Lessons from tumor progression: the invasive radial growth phase of melanoma is common, incapable of metastasis, and indolent. J Invest Dermatol 1993 Mar;100(3):342S-345S.

[34] Gray-Schopfer V, Wellbrock C, Marais R. Melanoma biology and new targeted therapy. Nature 2007 Feb 22;445(7130):851-857.

[35] Jean D, Gershenwald JE, Huang S, Luca M, Hudson MJ, Tainsky MA, et al. Loss of AP-2 results in up-regulation of MCAM/MUC18 and an increase in tumor growth and metastasis of human melanoma cells. J Biol Chem 1998 Jun 26;273(26): 16501-16508.

[36] Buytaert E, Dewaele M, Agostinis P. Molecular effectors of multiple cell death pathways initiated by photodynamic therapy. Biochim Biophys Acta 2007 Sep;1776(1): 86-107.

[37] Babilas P, Schreml S, Landthaler M, Szeimies RM. Photodynamic therapy in dermatology: state-of-the-art. Photodermatol Photoimmunol Photomed 2010 Jun;26(3): 118-132.

[38] Dougherty TJ, Gomer CJ, Henderson BW, Jori G, Kessel D, Korbelik M, et al. Photodynamic therapy. J Natl Cancer Inst 1998 Jun 17;90(12):889-905.

[39] Henderson BW, Dougherty TJ. How does photodynamic therapy work? Photochem Photobiol 1992 Jan;55(1):145-157.

[40] Juarranz A, Jaen P, Sanz-Rodriguez F, Cuevas J, Gonzalez S. Photodynamic therapy of cancer. Basic principles and applications. Clin Transl Oncol 2008 Mar;10(3): 148-154.

[41] Ortel B, Shea CR, Calzavara-Pinton P. Molecular mechanisms of photodynamic therapy. Front Biosci 2009 Jan 1;14:4157-4172.

[42] Gomer CJ, Ferrario A, Luna M, Rucker N, Wong S. Photodynamic therapy: combined modality approaches targeting the tumor microenvironment. Lasers Surg Med 2006 Jun;38(5):516-521.

[43] Verma S, Watt GM, Mai Z, Hasan T. Strategies for enhanced photodynamic therapy effects. Photochem Photobiol 2007 Sep-Oct;83(5):996-1005.

[44] Detty MR, Gibson SL, Wagner SJ. Current clinical and preclinical photosensitizers for use in photodynamic therapy. J Med Chem 2004 Jul 29;47(16):3897-3915.

[45] Stockert JC, Canete M, Juarranz A, Villanueva A, Horobin RW, Borrell JI, et al. Porphycenes: facts and prospects in photodynamic therapy of cancer. Curr Med Chem 2007;14(9):997-1026.

[46] Bourre L, Rousset N, Thibaut S, Eleouet S, Lajat Y, Patrice T. PDT effects of m-THPC and ALA, phototoxicity and apoptosis. Apoptosis 2002 Jun;7(3):221-230.

[47] Thibaut S, Bourre L, Hernot D, Rousset N, Lajat Y, Patrice T. Effects of BAPTA-AM, Forskolin, DSF and Z.VAD.fmk on PDT-induced apoptosis and m-THPC phototoxicity on B16 cells. Apoptosis 2002 Apr;7(2):99-106.

[48] Szeimies RM, Karrer S, Radakovic-Fijan S, Tanew A, Calzavara-Pinton PG, Zane C, et al. Photodynamic therapy using topical methyl 5-aminolevulinate compared with cryotherapy for actinic keratosis: A prospective, randomized study. J Am Acad Dermatol 2002 Aug;47(2):258-262.

[49] Szeimies RM. Methyl aminolevulinate-photodynamic therapy for basal cell carcinoma. Dermatol Clin 2007 Jan;25(1):89-94.

[50] Szeimies RM, Morton CA, Sidoroff A, Braathen LR. Photodynamic therapy for non-melanoma skin cancer. Acta Derm Venereol 2005;85(6):483-490.

[51] Bolfarini GC, Siqueira-Moura MP, Demets GJ. In vitro evaluation of combined hyperthermia and photodynamic effects using magnetoliposomes loaded with cucurbituril zinc phthalocyanine complex on melanoma. 2012 Jun 5.

[52] Khurana M, Ulrich S, Kim A, Moriyama Y, Netchev G, Akens MK, et al. Biodistribution and Pharmacokinetic Studies of a Porphyrin Dimer Photosensitizer (Oxdime) by Fluorescence Imaging and Spectroscopy in Mice Bearing Xenograft Tumors. Photochem Photo 2012 Jun 23.

[53] Rapozzi V, Zorzet S, Zacchigna M, Drioli S, Xodo LE. The PDT activity of free and pegylated pheophorbide a against an amelanotic melanoma transplanted in C57/BL6 mice. Invest New Drugs 2012 Jun 12.

[54] Sharma KV, Davids LM. Depigmentation in melanomas increases the efficacy of hypericin-mediated photodynamic-induced cell death. Photodiagnosis Photodyn Ther 2012 Jun;9(2):156-163.

[55] Shrestha TB, Seo GM, Basel MT, Kalita M, Wang H, Villanueva D, et al. Stem cell-based photodynamic therapy. Photochem Photobiol Sci 2012 Jul;11(7):1251-1258.

[56] Conforti F, Menichini G, Zanfini L, Tundis R, Statti GA, Provenzano E, et al. Evaluation of phototoxic potential of aerial components of the fig tree against human melanoma. Cell Prolif 2012 Jun;45(3):279-285.

[57] Maduray K, Odhav B, Nyokong T. In vitro photodynamic effect of aluminum tetrasulfophthalocyanines on melanoma skin cancer and healthy normal skin cells. Photodiagnosis Photodyn Ther 2012 Mar;9(1):32-39.

[58] Slastnikova TA, Rosenkranz AA, Gulak PV, Schiffelers RM, Lupanova TN, Khramtsov YV, et al. Modular nanotransporters: a multipurpose in vivo working platform for targeted drug delivery. Int J Nanomedicine 2012;7:467-482.

[59] Wagner M, Suarez ER, Theodoro TR, Machado Filho CD, Gama MF, Tardivo JP, et al. Methylene blue photodynamic therapy in malignant melanoma decreases expression of proliferating cell nuclear antigen and heparanases. Clin Exp Dermatol 2012 Jul; 37(5):527-533.

[60] Dabrowski JM, Arnaut LG, Pereira MM, Urbanska K, Simoes S, Stochel G, et al. Combined effects of singlet oxygen and hydroxyl radical in photodynamic therapy with photostable bacteriochlorins: evidence from intracellular fluorescence and increased photodynamic efficacy in vitro. Free Radic Biol Med 2012 Apr 1;52(7):1188-1200.

[61] Yoshii H, Yoshii Y, Asai T, Furukawa T, Takaichi S, Fujibayashi Y. Photo-excitation of carotenoids causes cytotoxicity via singlet oxygen production. Biochem Biophys Res Commun 2012 Jan 6;417(1):640-645.

[62] Schmitt F, Barry NP, Juillerat-Jeanneret L, Therrien B. Efficient photodynamic therapy of cancer using chemotherapeutic porphyrin-ruthenium metalla-cubes. Bioorg Med Chem Lett 2012 Jan 1;22(1):178-180.

[63] Menichini G, Alfano C, Provenzano E, Marrelli M, Statti GA, Menichini F, et al. Cachrys pungens Jan inhibits human melanoma cell proliferation through photo-induced cytotoxic activity. Cell Prolif 2012 Feb;45(1):39-47.

[64] Radzi R, Osaki T, Tsuka T, Imagawa T, Minami S, Okamoto Y. Morphological study in B16F10 murine melanoma cells after photodynamic hyperthermal therapy with indocyanine green (ICG). J Vet Med Sci 2012 Apr;74(4):465-472.

[65] Rapozzi V, Umezawa K, Xodo LE. Role of NF-kappaB/Snail/RKIP loop in the response of tumor cells to photodynamic therapy. Lasers Surg Med 2011 Sep;43(7): 575-585.

[66] Dabrowski JM, Krzykawska M, Arnaut LG, Pereira MM, Monteiro CJ, Simoes S, et al. Tissue uptake study and photodynamic therapy of melanoma-bearing mice with a nontoxic, effective chlorin. ChemMedChem 2011 Sep 5;6(9):1715-1726.

[67] Kim MR, Morrison H, Mohammed SI. Effect of a photoactivated rhodium complex in melanoma. Anticancer Drugs 2011 Oct;22(9):896-904.

[68] You BJ, Wu YC, Wu CY, Bao BY, Chen MY, Chang YH, et al. Proteomics displays cytoskeletal proteins and chaperones involvement in Hedyotis corymbosa-induced photokilling in skin cancer cells. Exp Dermatol 2011 Aug;20(8):653-658.

[69] Sharma KV, Bowers N, Davids LM. Photodynamic therapy-induced killing is enhanced in depigmented metastatic melanoma cells. Cell Biol Int 2011 Sep;35(9): 939-944.

[70] Maduray K, Karsten A, Odhav B, Nyokong T. In vitro toxicity testing of zinc tetrasulfophthalocyanines in fibroblast and keratinocyte cells for the treatment of melanoma cancer by photodynamic therapy. J Photochem Photobiol B 2011 May 3;103(2):98-104.

[71] Grimm S, Mvondo D, Grune T, Breusing N. The outcome of 5-ALA-mediated photodynamic treatment in melanoma cells is influenced by vitamin C and heme oxygenase-1. Biofactors 2011 Jan;37(1):17-24.

[72] Tammela T, Saaristo A, Holopainen T, Yla-Herttuala S, Andersson LC, Virolainen S, et al. Photodynamic ablation of lymphatic vessels and intralymphatic cancer cells prevents metastasis. Sci Transl Med 2011 Feb 9;3(69):69ra11.

[73] Kastle M, Grimm S, Nagel R, Breusing N, Grune T. Combination of PDT and inhibitor treatment affects melanoma cells and spares keratinocytes. Free Radic Biol Med 2011 Jan 15;50(2):305-312.

[74] Robertson CA, Abrahamse H, Evans D. The in vitro PDT efficacy of a novel metallophthalocyanine (MPc) derivative and established 5-ALA photosensitizing dyes against human metastatic melanoma cells. Lasers Surg Med 2010 Dec;42(10):766-776.

[75] Moisenovich MM, Ol'shevskaya VA, Rokitskaya TI, Ramonova AA, Nikitina RG, Savchenko AN, et al. Novel photosensitizers trigger rapid death of malignant human cells and rodent tumor transplants via lipid photodamage and membrane permeabilization. PLoS One 2010 Sep 15;5(9):e12717.

[76] Otake E, Sakuma S, Torii K, Maeda A, Ohi H, Yano S, et al. Effect and mechanism of a new photodynamic therapy with glycoconjugated fullerene. Photochem Photobiol 2010 Nov-Dec;86(6):1356-1363.

[77] Dabrowski JM, Arnaut LG, Pereira MM, Monteiro CJ, Urbanska K, Simoes S, et al. New halogenated water-soluble chlorin and bacteriochlorin as photostable PDT sensitizers: synthesis, spectroscopy, photophysics, and in vitro photosensitizing efficacy. ChemMedChem 2010 Oct 4;5(10):1770-1780.

[78] Chen P, Jiang X, Wei DP, Li L. The effects of intense pulsed light and 5-aminolevulinic acid on the cultured B16 marine melanoma cells. Sichuan Da Xue Xue Bao Yi Xue Ban 2010 Mar;41(2):280-283.

[79] Mroz P, Huang YY, Szokalska A, Zhiyentayev T, Janjua S, Nifli AP, et al. Stable synthetic bacteriochlorins overcome the resistance of melanoma to photodynamic therapy. FASEB J 2010 Sep;24(9):3160-3170.

[80] Camerin M, Magaraggia M, Soncin M, Jori G, Moreno M, Chambrier I, et al. The in vivo efficacy of phthalocyanine-nanoparticle conjugates for the photodynamic therapy of amelanotic melanoma. Eur J Cancer 2010 Jul;46(10):1910-1918.

[81] Barbugli PA, Siqueira-Moura MP, Espreafico EM, Tedesco AC. In vitro phototoxicity of liposomes and nanocapsules containing chloroaluminum phthalocyanine on human melanoma cell line. J Nanosci Nanotechnol 2010 Jan;10(1):569-573.

[82] Serra A, Pineiro M, Santos CI, Gonsalves AM, Abrantes M, Laranjo M, et al. In vitro photodynamic activity of 5,15-bis(3-hydroxyphenyl)porphyrin and its halogenated derivatives against cancer cells. Photochem Photobiol 2010 Jan-Feb;86(1):206-212.

[83] Nikitina RG, Mardynskaja VP, Morozova TG, Drozhzhina VV. A method for improving the efficiency of therapy for melanoma. Bull Exp Biol Med 2009 Aug;148(2): 238-240.

[84] Ouedraogo M, De Maesschalck E, Soentjens-Werts V, Dubois J. In vitro cytotoxicity study of oxaziridines generated after chlordiazepoxide, demoxepam, and desmethylchlordiazepoxide UV irradiation. Drug Chem Toxicol 2009;32(4):417-423.

[85] Camerin M, Rello-Varona S, Villanueva A, Rodgers MA, Jori G. Metallo-naphthalocyanines as photothermal sensitisers for experimental tumours: in vitro and in vivo studies. Lasers Surg Med 2009 Nov;41(9):665-673.

[86] Krestyn E, Kolarova H, Bajgar R, Tomankova K. Photodynamic properties of ZnTPPS(4), ClAlPcS(2) and ALA in human melanoma G361 cells. Toxicol In Vitro 2009 Aug 29.

[87] Zhao B, Yin JJ, Bilski PJ, Chignell CF, Roberts JE, He YY. Enhanced photodynamic efficacy towards melanoma cells by encapsulation of Pc4 in silica nanoparticles. Toxicol Appl Pharmacol 2009 Dec 1;241(2):163-172.

[88] Mamoon AM, Gamal-Eldeen AM, Ruppel ME, Smith RJ, Tsang T, Miller LM. In vitro efficiency and mechanistic role of indocyanine green as photodynamic therapy agent for human melanoma. Photodiagnosis Photodyn Ther 2009 Jun;6(2):105-116.

[89] Davids LM, Kleemann B, Cooper S, Kidson SH. Melanomas display increased cytoprotection to hypericin-mediated cytotoxicity through the induction of autophagy. Cell Biol Int 2009 Oct;33(10):1065-1072.

[90] Kolarova H, Tomankova K, Bajgar R, Kolar P, Kubinek R. Photodynamic and sonodynamic treatment by phthalocyanine on cancer cell lines. Ultrasound Med Biol 2009 Aug;35(8):1397-1404.

[91] Tsai T, Ji HT, Chiang PC, Chou RH, Chang WS, Chen CT. ALA-PDT results in phenotypic changes and decreased cellular invasion in surviving cancer cells. Lasers Surg Med 2009 Apr;41(4):305-315.

[92] Chen Y, Zheng W, Li Y, Zhong J, Ji J, Shen P. Apoptosis induced by methylene-blue-mediated photodynamic therapy in melanomas and the involvement of mitochondrial dysfunction revealed by proteomics. Cancer Sci 2008 Oct;99(10):2019-2027.

[93] Hao E, Friso E, Miotto G, Jori G, Soncin M, Fabris C, et al. Synthesis and biological investigations of tetrakis(p-carboranylthio-tetrafluorophenyl)chlorin (TPFC). Org Biomol Chem 2008 Oct 21;6(20):3732-3740.

[94] Chang CJ, Yu JS, Wei FC. In vitro and in vivo photosensitizing applications of Photofrin in malignant melanoma cells. Chang Gung Med J 2008 May-Jun;31(3):260-267.

[95] Korbelik M, Cecic I. Complement activation cascade and its regulation: relevance for the response of solid tumors to photodynamic therapy. J Photochem Photobiol B 2008 Oct 16;93(1):53-59.

[96] Kolarova H, Nevrelova P, Tomankova K, Kolar P, Bajgar R, Mosinger J. Production of reactive oxygen species after photodynamic therapy by porphyrin sensitizers. Gen Physiol Biophys 2008 Jun;27(2):101-105.

[97] Skidan I, Dholakia P, Torchilin V. Photodynamic therapy of experimental B-16 melanoma in mice with tumor-targeted 5,10,15,20-tetraphenylporphin-loaded PEG-PE micelles. J Drug Target 2008 Jul;16(6):486-493.

[98] Davids LM, Kleemann B, Kacerovska D, Pizinger K, Kidson SH. Hypericin phototoxicity induces different modes of cell death in melanoma and human skin cells. J Photochem Photobiol B 2008 May 29;91(2-3):67-76.

[99] Schmitt F, Govindaswamy P, Suss-Fink G, Ang WH, Dyson PJ, Juillerat-Jeanneret L, et al. Ruthenium porphyrin compounds for photodynamic therapy of cancer. J Med Chem 2008 Mar 27;51(6):1811-1816.

[100] Ma LW, Nielsen KP, Iani V, Moan J. A new method for photodynamic therapy of melanotic melanoma -- effects of depigmentation with violet light photodynamic therapy. J Environ Pathol Toxicol Oncol 2007;26(3):165-172.

[101] Janczyk A, Wolnicka-Glubisz A, Urbanska K, Kisch H, Stochel G, Macyk W. Photodynamic activity of platinum(IV) chloride surface-modified TiO2 irradiated with visible light. Free Radic Biol Med 2008 Mar 15;44(6):1120-1130.

[102] Tomankova K, Kolarova H, Vujtek M, Bajgar R. Photodynamic effect on melanoma cells investigated by atomic force microscopy. Gen Physiol Biophys 2007 Sep;26(3): 200-206.

[103] Frank J, Lornejad-Schafer MR, Schoffl H, Flaccus A, Lambert C, Biesalski HK. Inhibition of heme oxygenase-1 increases responsiveness of melanoma cells to ALA-based photodynamic therapy. Int J Oncol 2007 Dec;31(6):1539-1545.

[104] Fabris C, Vicente MG, Hao E, Friso E, Borsetto L, Jori G, et al. Tumour-localizing and -photosensitising properties of meso-tetra(4-nido-carboranylphenyl)porphyrin (H2TCP). J Photochem Photobiol B 2007 Dec 14;89(2-3):131-138.

[105] Rijcken CJ, Hofman JW, van Zeeland F, Hennink WE, van Nostrum CF. Photosensitiser-loaded biodegradable polymeric micelles: preparation, characterisation and in vitro PDT efficacy. J Control Release 2007 Dec 20;124(3):144-153.

[106] Kolarova H, Nevrelova P, Bajgar R, Jirova D, Kejlova K, Strnad M. In vitro photodynamic therapy on melanoma cell lines with phthalocyanine. Toxicol In Vitro 2007 Mar;21(2):249-253.

[107] Dabrowski JM, Pereira MM, Arnaut LG, Monteiro CJ, Peixoto AF, Karocki A, et al. Synthesis, photophysical studies and anticancer activity of a new halogenated water-soluble porphyrin. Photochem Photobiol 2007 Jul-Aug;83(4):897-903.

[108] Ji HX, Zhang F, Gao LQ, Jia LY, Xiong Y, Liang C, et al. Photodynamic therapy of pigmented choroidal melanomas in rabbits using hematoporphyrin monomethyl ether. Zhonghua Yan Ke Za Zhi 2007 Mar;43(3):212-216.

[109] Kolarova H, Lenobel R, Kolar P, Strnad M. Sensitivity of different cell lines to phototoxic effect of disulfonated chloroaluminium phthalocyanine. Toxicol In Vitro 2007 Oct;21(7):1304-1306.

[110] Ferrario A, Rucker N, Wong S, Luna M, Gomer CJ. Survivin, a member of the inhibitor of apoptosis family, is induced by photodynamic therapy and is a target for improving treatment response. Cancer Res 2007 May 15;67(10):4989-4995.

[111] Korbelik M, Cooper PD. Potentiation of photodynamic therapy of cancer by complement: the effect of gamma-inulin. Br J Cancer 2007 Jan 15;96(1):67-72.

[112] Hiruma H, Katakura T, Takenami T, Igawa S, Kanoh M, Fujimura T, et al. Vesicle disruption, plasma membrane bleb formation, and acute cell death caused by illumination with blue light in acridine orange-loaded malignant melanoma cells. J Photochem Photobiol B 2007 Jan 3;86(1):1-8.

[113] Nowak-Sliwinska P, Karocki A, Elas M, Pawlak A, Stochel G, Urbanska K. Verteporfin, photofrin II, and merocyanine 540 as PDT photosensitizers against melanoma cells. Biochem Biophys Res Commun 2006 Oct 20;349(2):549-555.

[114] Schacht V, Szeimies RM, Abels C. Photodynamic therapy with 5-aminolevulinic acid induces distinct microcirculatory effects following systemic or topical application. Photochem Photobiol Sci 2006 May;5(5):452-458.

[115] Saji H, Song W, Furumoto K, Kato H, Engleman EG. Systemic antitumor effect of intratumoral injection of dendritic cells in combination with local photodynamic therapy. Clin Cancer Res 2006 Apr 15;12(8):2568-2574.

[116] Friso E, Roncucci G, Dei D, Soncin M, Fabris C, Chiti G, et al. A novel 10B-enriched carboranyl-containing phthalocyanine as a radio- and photo-sensitising agent for boron neutron capture therapy and photodynamic therapy of tumours: in vitro and in vivo studies. Photochem Photobiol Sci 2006 Jan;5(1):39-50.

[117] Saczko J, Kulbacka J, Chwilkowska A, Drag-Zalesiniska M, Wysocka T, Lugowski M, et al. The influence of photodynamic therapy on apoptosis in human melanoma cell line. Folia Histochem Cytobiol 2005;43(3):129-132.

[118] Kolarova H, Macecek J, Nevrelova P, Huf M, Tomecka M, Bajgar R, et al. Photodynamic therapy with zinc-tetra(p-sulfophenyl)porphyrin bound to cyclodextrin induces single strand breaks of cellular DNA in G361 melanoma cells. Toxicol In Vitro 2005 Oct;19(7):971-974.

[119] Camerin M, Rello S, Villanueva A, Ping X, Kenney ME, Rodgers MA, et al. Photothermal sensitisation as a novel therapeutic approach for tumours: studies at the cellular and animal level. Eur J Cancer 2005 May;41(8):1203-1212.

[120] Macecek J, Kolarova H, Psotova J, Bajgar R, Huf M, Nevrelova P, et al. Assessment of cellular damage by comet assay after photodynamic therapy in vitro. Acta Medica (Hradec Kralove) 2004;47(4):327-329.

[121] Posen Y, Kalchenko V, Seger R, Brandis A, Scherz A, Salomon Y. Manipulation of redox signaling in mammalian cells enabled by controlled photogeneration of reactive oxygen species. J Cell Sci 2005 May 1;118(Pt 9):1957-1969.

[122] Schastak S, Jean B, Handzel R, Kostenich G, Hermann R, Sack U, et al. Improved pharmacokinetics, biodistribution and necrosis in vivo using a new near infra-red photosensitizer: tetrahydroporphyrin tetratosylat. J Photochem Photobiol B 2005 Mar 1;78(3):203-213.

[123] Mazor O, Brandis A, Plaks V, Neumark E, Rosenbach-Belkin V, Salomon Y, et al. WST11, a novel water-soluble bacteriochlorophyll derivative; cellular uptake, pharmacokinetics, biodistribution and vascular-targeted photodynamic activity using melanoma tumors as a model. Photochem Photobiol 2005 Mar-Apr;81(2):342-351.

[124] Vena FC, Turchiello RF, Laville I, Pigaglio S, Blais J, Tedesco AC. 5-aminolevulinic acid ester-induced protoporphyrin IX in a murine melanoma cell line. Lasers Med Sci 2004;19(2):119-126.

[125] Karmakova T, Feofanov A, Nazarova A, Grichine A, Yakubovskaya R, Luk'yanets E, et al. Distribution of metal-free sulfonated phthalocyanine in subcutaneously transplanted murine tumors. J Photochem Photobiol B 2004 Jul 19;75(1-2):81-87.

[126] Ropp S, Guy J, Berl V, Bischoff P, Lepoittevin JP. Synthesis and photocytotoxic activity of new alpha-methylene-gamma-butyrolactone-psoralen heterodimers. Bioorg Med Chem 2004 Jul 1;12(13):3619-3625.

[127] Ickowicz Schwartz D, Gozlan Y, Greenbaum L, Babushkina T, Katcoff DJ, Malik Z. Differentiation-dependent photodynamic therapy regulated by porphobilinogen deaminase in B16 melanoma. Br J Cancer 2004 May 4;90(9):1833-1841.

[128] Lim DS, Ko SH, Lee WY. Silkworm-pheophorbide alpha mediated photodynamic therapy against B16F10 pigmented melanoma. J Photochem Photobiol B 2004 Mar 19;74(1):1-6.

[129] Barge J, Decreau R, Julliard M, Hubaud JC, Sabatier AS, Grob JJ, et al. Killing efficacy of a new silicon phthalocyanine in human melanoma cells treated with photodynamic therapy by early activation of mitochondrion-mediated apoptosis. Exp Dermatol 2004 Jan;13(1):33-44.

[130] Szurko A, Kramer-Marek G, Widel M, Ratuszna A, Habdas J, Kus P. Photodynamic effects of two water soluble porphyrins evaluated on human malignant melanoma cells in vitro. Acta Biochim Pol 2003;50(4):1165-1174.

[131] Kolarova H, Mosinger J, Lenobel R, Kejlova K, Jirova D, Strnad M. In vitro toxicity testing of supramolecular sensitizers for photodynamic therapy. Toxicol In Vitro 2003 Oct-Dec;17(5-6):775-778.

[132] Nagata S, Obana A, Gohto Y, Nakajima S. Necrotic and apoptotic cell death of human malignant melanoma cells following photodynamic therapy using an amphiphilic photosensitizer, ATX-S10(Na). Lasers Surg Med 2003;33(1):64-70.

[133] Babilas P, Schacht V, Liebsch G, Wolfbeis OS, Landthaler M, Szeimies RM, et al. Effects of light fractionation and different fluence rates on photodynamic therapy with 5-aminolaevulinic acid in vivo. Br J Cancer 2003 May 6;88(9):1462-1469.

[134] Haddad R, Kaplan O, Greenberg R, Siegal A, Skornick Y, Kashtan H. Photodynamic therapy of murine colon cancer and melanoma using systemic aminolevulinic acid as a photosensitizer. Int J Surg Investig 2000;2(3):171-178.

[135] Jezek P, Nekvasil M, Skobisova E, Urbankova E, Jirsa M, Zadinova M, et al. Experimental photodynamic therapy with MESO-tetrakisphenylporphyrin (TPP) in liposomes leads to disintegration of human amelanotic melanoma implanted to nude mice. Int J Cancer 2003 Feb 20;103(5):693-702.

[136] Hu L, Wu X, Song Y, Young LH, Gragoudas ES. Photodynamic therapy of pigmented choroidal melanomas in rabbits. Zhonghua Yan Ke Za Zhi 2002 Aug;38(8):491-494.

[137] Urbanska K, Romanowska-Dixon B, Matuszak Z, Oszajca J, Nowak-Sliwinsk P, Stochel G. Indocyanine green as a prospective sensitizer for photodynamic therapy of melanomas. Acta Biochim Pol 2002;49(2):387-391.

[138] Bourre L, Rousset N, Thibaut S, Eleouet S, Lajat Y, Patrice T. PDT effects of m-THPC and ALA, phototoxicity and apoptosis. Apoptosis 2002 Jun;7(3):221-230.

[139] Lang K, Bolsen K, Stahl W, Ruzicka T, Sies H, Lehmann P, et al. The 5-aminolevulinic acid-induced porphyrin biosynthesis in benign and malignant cells of the skin. J Photochem Photobiol B 2001 Dec 1;65(1):29-34.

[140] Drzewiecka A, Urbanska K, Matuszak Z, Pineiro M, Arnaut LG, Habdas J, et al. Tritolylporphyrin dimer as a new potent hydrophobic sensitizer for photodynamic therapy of melanoma. Acta Biochim Pol 2001;48(1):277-282.

[141] Pahernik S, Langer S, Botzlar A, Dellian M, Goetz AE. Tissue distribution and penetration of 5-ALA induced fluorescence in an amelanotic melanoma after topical application. Anticancer Res 2001 Jan-Feb;21(1A):59-63.

[142] Zilberstein J, Schreiber S, Bloemers MC, Bendel P, Neeman M, Schechtman E, et al. Antivascular treatment of solid melanoma tumors with bacteriochlorophyll-serine-based photodynamic therapy. Photochem Photobiol 2001 Mar;73(3):257-266.

[143] Rice L, Wainwright M, Phoemix DA. Phenothiazine photosensitizers. III. Activity of methylene blue derivatives against pigmented melanoma cell lines. J Chemother 2000 Feb;12(1):94-104.

[144] Busetti A, Soncin M, Reddi E, Rodgers MA, Kenney ME, Jori G. Photothermal sensitization of amelanotic melanoma cells by Ni(II)-octabutoxy-naphthalocyanine. J Photochem Photobiol B 1999 Nov-Dec;53(1-3):103-109.

[145] Soncin M, Busetti A, Fusi F, Jori G, Rodgers MA. Irradiation of amelanotic melanoma cells with 532 nm high peak power pulsed laser radiation in the presence of the photothermal sensitizer Cu(II)-hematoporphyrin: a new approach to cell photoinactivation. Photochem Photobiol 1999 Jun;69(6):708-712.

[146] Langer S, Abels C, Botzlar A, Pahernik S, Rick K, Szeimies RM, et al. Active and higher intracellular uptake of 5-aminolevulinic acid in tumors may be inhibited by glycine. J Invest Dermatol 1999 May;112(5):723-728.

[147] Decreau R, Richard MJ, Verrando P, Chanon M, Julliard M. Photodynamic activities of silicon phthalocyanines against achromic M6 melanoma cells and healthy human melanocytes and keratinocytes. J Photochem Photobiol B 1999 Jan;48(1):48-56.

[148] Busetti A, Soncin M, Jori G, Rodgers MA. High efficiency of benzoporphyrin derivative in the photodynamic therapy of pigmented malignant melanoma. Br J Cancer 1999 Feb;79(5-6):821-824.

[149] Klotz LO, Fritsch C, Briviba K, Tsacmacidis N, Schliess F, Sies H. Activation of JNK and p38 but not ERK MAP kinases in human skin cells by 5-aminolevulinate-photodynamic therapy. Cancer Res 1998 Oct 1;58(19):4297-4300.

[150] Busetti A, Soncin M, Jori G, Kenney ME, Rodgers MA. Treatment of malignant melanoma by high-peak-power 1064 nm irradiation followed by photodynamic therapy. Photochem Photobiol 1998 Sep;68(3):377-381.

[151] Haddad R, Blumenfeld A, Siegal A, Kaplan O, Cohen M, Skornick Y, et al. In vitro and in vivo effects of photodynamic therapy on murine malignant melanoma. Ann Surg Oncol 1998 Apr-May;5(3):241-247.

[152] Woodburn KW, Fan Q, Kessel D, Luo Y, Young SW. Photodynamic therapy of B16F10 murine melanoma with lutetium texaphyrin. J Invest Dermatol 1998 May; 110(5):746-751.

[153] Abels C, Szeimies RM, Steinbach P, Richert C, Goetz AE. Targeting of the tumor microcirculation by photodynamic therapy with a synthetic porphycene. J Photochem Photobiol B 1997 Oct;40(3):305-312.

[154] Mantareva V, Shopova M, Spassova G, Wohrle D, Muller S, Jori G, et al. Si(IV)-methoxyethylene-glycol-naphthalocyanine: synthesis and pharmacokinetic and photosensitizing properties in different tumour models. J Photochem Photobiol B 1997 Oct; 40(3):258-262.

[155] Abels C, Fritsch C, Bolsen K, Szeimies RM, Ruzicka T, Goerz G, et al. Photodynamic therapy with 5-aminolaevulinic acid-induced porphyrins of an amelanotic melanoma in vivo. J Photochem Photobiol B 1997 Aug;40(1):76-83.

[156] Kim RY, Hu LK, Flotte TJ, Gragoudas ES, Young LH. Digital angiography of experimental choroidal melanomas using benzoporphyrin derivative. Am J Ophthalmol 1997 Jun;123(6):810-816.

[157] Zilberstein J, Bromberg A, Frantz A, Rosenbach-Belkin V, Kritzmann A, Pfefermann R, et al. Light-dependent oxygen consumption in bacteriochlorophyll-serine-treated melanoma tumors: on-line determination using a tissue-inserted oxygen microsensor. Photochem Photobiol 1997 Jun;65(6):1012-1019.

[158] Blom DJ, Schuitmaker HJ, de Waard-Siebinga I, Dubbelman TM, Jager MJ. Decreased expression of HLA class I on ocular melanoma cells following in vitro photodynamic therapy. Cancer Lett 1997 Jan 30;112(2):239-243.

[159] Fritsch C, Abels C, Goetz AE, Stahl W, Bolsen K, Ruzicka T, et al. Porphyrins preferentially accumulate in a melanoma following intravenous injection of 5-aminolevulinic acid. Biol Chem 1997 Jan;378(1):51-57.

[160] Michailov N, Peeva M, Angelov I, Wohrle D, Muller S, Jori G, et al. Fluence rate effects on photodynamic therapy of B16 pigmented melanoma. J Photochem Photobiol B 1997 Jan;37(1-2):154-157.

[161] Kim RY, Hu LK, Foster BS, Gragoudas ES, Young LH. Photodynamic therapy of pigmented choroidal melanomas of greater than 3-mm thickness. Ophthalmology 1996 Dec;103(12):2029-2036.

[162] Hadjur C, Richard MJ, Parat MO, Jardon P, Favier A. Photodynamic effects of hypericin on lipid peroxidation and antioxidant status in melanoma cells. Photochem Photobiol 1996 Aug;64(2):375-381.

[163] VanderWerf QM, Saxton RE, Chang A, Horton D, Paiva MB, Anderson J, et al. Hypericin: a new laser phototargeting agent for human cancer cells. Laryngoscope 1996 Apr;106(4):479-483.

[164] Donaldson MJ, Lim L, Harper CA, Mackenzie J, G Campbell W. Primary treatment of choroidal amelanotic melanoma with photodynamic therapy. Clin Experiment Ophthalmol 2005 Oct;33(5):548-549.

[165] Sheleg SV, Zhavrid EA, Khodina TV, Kochubeev GA, Istomin YP, Chalov VN, et al. Photodynamic therapy with chlorin e(6) for skin metastases of melanoma. Photodermatol Photoimmunol Photomed 2004 Feb;20(1):21-26.

[166] Baldea I, Filip AG. Photodynamic therapy in melanoma--an update. J Physiol Pharmacol 2012 Apr;63(2):109-118.

[167] Tuncer S, Kir N, Shields CL. Dramatic regression of amelanotic choroidal melanoma with PDT following poor response to brachytherapy. Ophthalmic Surg Lasers Imaging 2012 May 3;43(3):e38-40.

[168] Canal-Fontcuberta I, Salomao DR, Robertson D, Cantrill HL, Koozekanani D, Rath PP, et al. Clinical and histopathologic findings after photodynamic therapy of choroidal melanoma. Retina 2012 May;32(5):942-948.

[169] Campbell WG, Pejnovic TM. Treatment of amelanotic choroidal melanoma with photodynamic therapy. Retina 2012 Jul;32(7):1356-1362.

[170] Li X, Naylor MF, Le H, Nordquist RE, Teague TK, Howard CA, et al. Clinical effects of in situ photoimmunotherapy on late-stage melanoma patients: a preliminary study. Cancer Biol Ther 2010 Dec 1;10(11):1081-1087.

[171] Fasanella KE, McGrath K. Successful palliative treatment of duodenal metastatic melanoma with photodynamic therapy. Gastrointest Endosc 2009 Jan;69(1):182-184.

[172] Zilidis G, Aziz F, Telara S, Eljamel MS. Fluorescence image-guided surgery and repetitive Photodynamic Therapy in brain metastatic malignant melanoma. Photodiagnosis Photodyn Ther 2008 Dec;5(4):264-266.

[173] Chetty NC, Osborne V, Harland C. Amelanotic melanoma in situ: lack of sustained response to photodynamic therapy. Clin Exp Dermatol 2008 Mar;33(2):204-206.

[174] Soucek P, Cihelkova I. Primary treatment of choroidal amelanotic melanoma with photodynamic therapy--comment. Clin Experiment Ophthalmol 2006 Sep-Oct;34(7): 721; author reply 721-2.

[175] Naylor MF, Chen WR, Teague TK, Perry LA, Nordquist RE. In situ photoimmunotherapy: a tumour-directed treatment for melanoma. Br J Dermatol 2006 Dec;155(6): 1287-1292.

[176] Wachtlin J, Bechrakis NE, Foerster MH. Photodynamic therapy with verteporfin for uveal melanoma. Ophthalmologe 2005 Mar;102(3):241-246.

[177] Liggett PE, Lavaque AJ, Chaudhry NA, Jablon EP, Quiroz-Mercado H. Preliminary results of combined simultaneous transpupillary thermotherapy and ICG-based photodynamic therapy for choroidal melanoma. Ophthalmic Surg Lasers Imaging 2005 Nov-Dec;36(6):463-470.

[178] Kubicka-Trzaska A, Starzycka M, Romanowska-Dixon B, Morawski K. Use of indocyanine green for photodynamic therapy of choroidal melanoma--preliminary report. Klin Oczna 2003;105(3-4):132-135.

[179] Barbazetto IA, Lee TC, Rollins IS, Chang S, Abramson DH. Treatment of choroidal melanoma using photodynamic therapy. Am J Ophthalmol 2003 Jun;135(6):898-899.

[180] Schlotzer-Schrehardt U, Viestenz A, Naumann GO, Laqua H, Michels S, Schmidt-Erfurth U. Dose-related structural effects of photodynamic therapy on choroidal and retinal structures of human eyes. Graefes Arch Clin Exp Ophthalmol 2002 Sep;240(9): 748-757.

[181] Favilla I, Favilla ML, Gosbell AD, Barry WR, Ellims P, Hill JS, et al. Photodynamic therapy: a 5-year study of its effectiveness in the treatment of posterior uveal mela-

noma, and evaluation of haematoporphyrin uptake and photocytotoxicity of melanoma cells in tissue culture. Melanoma Res 1995 Oct;5(5):355-364.

[182] Chen B, Xu Y, Agostinis P, De Witte PA. Synergistic effect of photodynamic therapy with hypericin in combination with hyperthermia on loss of clonogenicity of RIF-1 cells. Int J Oncol 2001 Jun;18(6):1279-1285.

[183] Wiegell SR, Fabricius S, Stender IM, Berne B, Kroon S, Andersen BL, et al. A randomized, multicentre study of directed daylight exposure times of 1(1/2) vs. 2(1/2) h in daylight-mediated photodynamic therapy with methyl aminolaevulinate in patients with multiple thin actinic keratoses of the face and scalp. Br J Dermatol 2011 May; 164(5):1083-1090.

[184] Alecu M, Ursaciuc C, Halalau F, Coman G, Merlevede W, Waelkens E, et al. Photodynamic treatment of basal cell carcinoma and squamous cell carcinoma with hypericin. Anticancer Res 1998 Nov-Dec;18(6B):4651-4654.

[185] Bublik M, Head C, Benharash P, Paiva M, Eshraghi A, Kim T, et al. Hypericin and pulsed laser therapy of squamous cell cancer in vitro. Photomed Laser Surg 2006 Jun; 24(3):341-347.

[186] Chung PS, Rhee CK, Kim KH, Paek W, Chung J, Paiva MB, et al. Intratumoral hypericin and KTP laser therapy for transplanted squamous cell carcinoma. Laryngoscope 2000 Aug;110(8):1312-1316.

[187] Chung PS, Saxton RE, Paiva MB, Rhee CK, Soudant J, Mathey A, et al. Hypericin uptake in rabbits and nude mice transplanted with human squamous cell carcinomas: study of a new sensitizer for laser phototherapy. Laryngoscope 1994 Dec;104(12): 1471-1476.

[188] Liu CD, Kwan D, Saxton RE, McFadden DW. Hypericin and photodynamic therapy decreases human pancreatic cancer in vitro and in vivo. J Surg Res 2000 Sep;93(1): 137-143.

[189] D'Hallewin MA, Kamuhabwa AR, Roskams T, De Witte PA, Baert L. Hypericin-based fluorescence diagnosis of bladder carcinoma. BJU Int 2002 May;89(7):760-763.

[190] D'Hallewin MA, De Witte PA, Waelkens E, Merlevede W, Baert L. Fluorescence detection of flat bladder carcinoma in situ after intravesical instillation of hypericin. J Urol 2000 Aug;164(2):349-351.

[191] Kubin A, Loew HG, Burner U, Jessner G, Kolbabek H, Wierrani F. How to make hypericin water-soluble. Pharmazie 2008 Apr;63(4):263-269.

[192] Sim HG, Lau WK, Olivo M, Tan PH, Cheng CW. Is photodynamic diagnosis using hypericin better than white-light cystoscopy for detecting superficial bladder carcinoma? BJU Int 2005 Jun;95(9):1215-1218.

[193] Kubin A, Meissner P, Wierrani F, Burner U, Bodenteich A, Pytel A, et al. Fluorescence diagnosis of bladder cancer with new water soluble hypericin bound to polyvinylpyrrolidone: PVP-hypericin. Photochem Photobiol 2008 Nov-Dec;84(6):1560-1563.

[194] Bhuvaneswari R, Gan YY, Yee KK, Soo KC, Olivo M. Effect of hypericin-mediated photodynamic therapy on the expression of vascular endothelial growth factor in human nasopharyngeal carcinoma. Int J Mol Med 2007 Oct;20(4):421-428.

[195] Olivo M, Du HY, Bay BH. Hypericin lights up the way for the potential treatment of nasopharyngeal cancer by photodynamic therapy. Curr Clin Pharmacol 2006 Sep; 1(3):217-222.

[196] Kacerovska D, Pizinger K, Majer F, Smid F. Photodynamic therapy of nonmelanoma skin cancer with topical hypericum perforatum extract--a pilot study. Photochem Photobiol 2008 May-Jun;84(3):779-785.

[197] Davids LM, Kleemann B, Cooper S, Kidson SH. Melanomas display increased cytoprotection to hypericin-mediated cytotoxicity through the induction of autophagy. Cell Biol Int 2009 Oct;33(10):1065-1072.

[198] Mosmann T. Rapid colorimetric assay for cellular growth and survival: application to proliferation and cytotoxicity assays. J Immunol Methods 1983 Dec 16;65(1-2):55-63.

[199] Cory AH, Owen TC, Barltrop JA, Cory JG. Use of an aqueous soluble tetrazolium/formazan assay for cell growth assays in culture. Cancer Commun 1991 Jul;3(7): 207-212.

[200] Davids LM, Kleemann B. Combating melanoma: The use of photodynamic therapy as a novel, adjuvant therapeutic tool. Cancer Treat Rev 2010 Dec 16.

[201] Davids LM, du Toit E, Kidson SH, Todd G. A rare repigmentation pattern in a vitiligo patient: a clue to an epidermal stem-cell reservoir of melanocytes? Clin Exp Dermatol 2009 Mar;34(2):246-248.

[202] Kroemer G, El-Deiry WS, Golstein P, Peter ME, Vaux D, Vandenabeele P, et al. Classification of cell death: recommendations of the Nomenclature Committee on Cell Death. Cell Death Differ 2005 Nov;12 Suppl 2:1463-1467.

[203] Golstein P, Kroemer G. Cell death by necrosis: towards a molecular definition. Trends Biochem Sci 2007 Jan;32(1):37-43.

[204] Galluzzi L, Vitale I, Abrams JM, Alnemri ES, Baehrecke EH, Blagosklonny MV, et al. Molecular definitions of cell death subroutines: recommendations of the Nomenclature Committee on Cell Death 2012. Cell Death Differ 2012 Jan;19(1):107-120.

[205] Hanahan D, Weinberg RA. Hallmarks of cancer: the next generation. Cell 2011 Mar 4;144(5):646-674.

[206] Wellbrock C, Weisser C, Geissinger E, Troppmair J, Schartl M. Activation of p59(Fyn) leads to melanocyte dedifferentiation by influencing MKP-1-regulated mitogen-activated protein kinase signaling. J Biol Chem 2002 Feb 22;277(8):6443-6454.

[207] Cohen C, Zavala-Pompa A, Sequeira JH, Shoji M, Sexton DG, Cotsonis G, et al. Mitogen-actived protein kinase activation is an early event in melanoma progression. Clin Cancer Res 2002 Dec;8(12):3728-3733.

[208] Tsao H, Goel V, Wu H, Yang G, Haluska FG. Genetic interaction between NRAS and BRAF mutations and PTEN/MMAC1 inactivation in melanoma. J Invest Dermatol 2004 Feb;122(2):337-341.

[209] Davies H, Bignell GR, Cox C, Stephens P, Edkins S, Clegg S, et al. Mutations of the BRAF gene in human cancer. Nature 2002 Jun 27;417(6892):949-954.

[210] Gray-Schopfer VC, da Rocha Dias S, Marais R. The role of B-RAF in melanoma. Cancer Metastasis Rev 2005 Jan;24(1):165-183.

[211] Tong Z, Singh G, Rainbow AJ. Sustained activation of the extracellular signal-regulated kinase pathway protects cells from photofrin-mediated photodynamic therapy. Cancer Res 2002 Oct 1;62(19):5528-5535.

[212] Mercurio F, Manning AM. NF-kappaB as a primary regulator of the stress response. Oncogene 1999 Nov 1;18(45):6163-6171.

[213] Ryter SW, Gomer CJ. Nuclear factor kappa B binding activity in mouse L1210 cells following photofrin II-mediated photosensitization. Photochem Photobiol 1993 Nov; 58(5):753-756.

[214] Danial NN, Korsmeyer SJ. Cell death: critical control points. Cell 2004 Jan 23;116(2): 205-219.

[215] Oleinick NL, Morris RL, Belichenko I. The role of apoptosis in response to photodynamic therapy: what, where, why, and how. Photochem Photobiol Sci 2002 Jan;1(1): 1-21.

[216] Agostinis P, Buytaert E, Breyssens H, Hendrickx N. Regulatory pathways in photodynamic therapy induced apoptosis. Photochem Photobiol Sci 2004 Aug;3(8):721-729.

[217] Buytaert E, Callewaert G, Vandenheede JR, Agostinis P. Deficiency in apoptotic effectors Bax and Bak reveals an autophagic cell death pathway initiated by photodamage to the endoplasmic reticulum. Autophagy 2006 Jul-Sep;2(3):238-240.

[218] Fisher DE. Apoptosis in cancer therapy: crossing the threshold. Cell 1994 Aug 26;78(4):539-542.

[219] Micheau O, Solary E, Hammann A, Martin F, Dimanche-Boitrel MT. Sensitization of cancer cells treated with cytotoxic drugs to fas-mediated cytotoxicity. J Natl Cancer Inst 1997 Jun 4;89(11):783-789.

[220] Ali SM, Chee SK, Yuen GY, Olivo M. Hypericin induced death receptor-mediated apoptosis in photoactivated tumor cells. Int J Mol Med 2002 Jun;9(6):601-616.

[221] Reiners JJ,Jr, Agostinis P, Berg K, Oleinick NL, Kessel D. Assessing autophagy in the context of photodynamic therapy. Autophagy 2010 Jan;6(1):7-18.

[222] Dewaele M, Maes H, Agostinis P. ROS-mediated mechanisms of autophagy stimulation and their relevance in cancer therapy. Autophagy 2010 Oct 19;6(7).

[223] Garg AD, Krysko DV, Vandenabeele P, Agostinis P. DAMPs and PDT-mediated photo-oxidative stress: exploring the unknown. Photochem Photobiol Sci 2011 May;10(5): 670-680.

[224] Garg AD, Nowis D, Golab J, Vandenabeele P, Krysko DV, Agostinis P. Immunogenic cell death, DAMPs and anticancer therapeutics: an emerging amalgamation. Biochim Biophys Acta 2010 Jan;1805(1):53-71.

[225] Green DR, Ferguson T, Zitvogel L, Kroemer G. Immunogenic and tolerogenic cell death. Nat Rev Immunol 2009 May;9(5):353-363.

[226] Zitvogel L, Kepp O, Kroemer G. Decoding cell death signals in inflammation and immunity. Cell 2010 Mar 19;140(6):798-804.

[227] Zitvogel L, Kepp O, Senovilla L, Menger L, Chaput N, Kroemer G. Immunogenic tumor cell death for optimal anticancer therapy: the calreticulin exposure pathway. Clin Cancer Res 2010 Jun 15;16(12):3100-3104.

[228] Demaria S, Pikarsky E, Karin M, Coussens LM, Chen YC, El-Omar EM, et al. Cancer and inflammation: promise for biologic therapy. J Immunother 2010 May;33(4): 335-351.

[229] Garg AD, Nowis D, Golab J, Agostinis P. Photodynamic therapy: illuminating the road from cell death towards anti-tumour immunity. Apoptosis 2010 Mar 10.

[230] Buytaert E, Callewaert G, Hendrickx N, Scorrano L, Hartmann D, Missiaen L, et al. Role of endoplasmic reticulum depletion and multidomain proapoptotic BAX and BAK proteins in shaping cell death after hypericin-mediated photodynamic therapy. FASEB J 2006 Apr;20(6):756-758.

[231] Ritz R, Roser F, Radomski N, Strauss WS, Tatagiba M, Gharabaghi A. Subcellular colocalization of hypericin with respect to endoplasmic reticulum and Golgi apparatus in glioblastoma cells. Anticancer Res 2008 Jul-Aug;28(4B):2033-2038.

[232] Galanou MC, Theodossiou TA, Tsiourvas D, Sideratou Z, Paleos CM. Interactive transport, subcellular relocation and enhanced phototoxicity of hypericin encapsulated in guanidinylated liposomes via molecular recognition. Photochem Photobiol 2008 Sep-Oct;84(5):1073-1083.

[233] Ali SM, Olivo M. Bio-distribution and subcellular localization of Hypericin and its role in PDT induced apoptosis in cancer cells. Int J Oncol 2002 Sep;21(3):531-540.

[234] Ali SM, Chee SK, Yuen GY, Olivo M. Hypericin induced death receptor-mediated apoptosis in photoactivated tumor cells. Int J Mol Med 2002 Jun;9(6):601-616.

[235] English DS, Doyle RT, Petrich JW, Haydon PG. Subcellular distributions and excited-state processes of hypericin in neurons. Photochem Photobiol 1999 Mar;69(3):301-305.

[236] Crnolatac I, Huygens A, Agostinis P, Kamuhabwa AR, Maes J, van Aerschot A, et al. In vitro accumulation and permeation of hypericin and lipophilic analogues in 2-D and 3-D cellular systems. Int J Oncol 2007 Feb;30(2):319-324.

[237] Theodossiou TA, Hothersall JS, De Witte PA, Pantos A, Agostinis P. The Multifaceted Photocytotoxic Profile of Hypericin. Mol Pharm 2009 Sep 24.

[238] Ho YF, Wu MH, Cheng BH, Chen YW, Shih MC. Lipid-mediated preferential localization of hypericin in lipid membranes. Biochim Biophys Acta 2009 Jun;1788(6): 1287-1295.

[239] Mojzisova H, Bonneau S, Brault D. Structural and physico-chemical determinants of the interactions of macrocyclic photosensitizers with cells. Eur Biophys J 2007 Nov; 36(8):943-953.

[240] Buytaert E, Matroule JY, Durinck S, Close P, Kocanova S, Vandenheede JR, et al. Molecular effectors and modulators of hypericin-mediated cell death in bladder cancer cells. Oncogene 2008 Mar 20;27(13):1916-1929.

[241] Verfaillie T, Salazar M, Velasco G, Agostinis P. Linking ER Stress to Autophagy: Potential Implications for Cancer Therapy. Int J Cell Biol 2010;2010:930509.

[242] Thomas C, MacGill RS, Miller GC, Pardini RS. Photoactivation of hypericin generates singlet oxygen in mitochondria and inhibits succinoxidase. Photochem Photobiol 1992 Jan;55(1):47-53.

[243] Miccoli L, Beurdeley-Thomas A, De Pinieux G, Sureau F, Oudard S, Dutrillaux B, et al. Light-induced photoactivation of hypericin affects the energy metabolism of human glioma cells by inhibiting hexokinase bound to mitochondria. Cancer Res 1998 Dec 15;58(24):5777-5786.

[244] Theodossiou TA, Papakyriakou A, Hothersall JS. Molecular modeling and experimental evidence for hypericin as a substrate for mitochondrial complex III; mitochondrial photodamage as demonstrated using specific inhibitors. Free Radic Biol Med 2008 Dec 1;45(11):1581-1590.

[245] Utsumi T, Okuma M, Kanno T, Takehara Y, Yoshioka T, Fujita Y, et al. Effect of the antiretroviral agent hypericin on rat liver mitochondria. Biochem Pharmacol 1995 Aug 25;50(5):655-662.

[246] Buytaert E, Callewaert G, Vandenheede JR, Agostinis P. Deficiency in apoptotic effectors Bax and Bak reveals an autophagic cell death pathway initiated by photodamage to the endoplasmic reticulum. Autophagy 2006 Jul-Sep;2(3):238-240.

[247] Castano AP, Mroz P, Hamblin MR. Photodynamic therapy and anti-tumour immunity. Nat Rev Cancer 2006 Jul;6(7):535-545.

[248] Panaretakis T, Kepp O, Brockmeier U, Tesniere A, Bjorklund AC, Chapman DC, et al. Mechanisms of pre-apoptotic calreticulin exposure in immunogenic cell death. EMBO J 2009 Mar 4;28(5):578-590.

[249] Young AR, Narita M, Ferreira M, Kirschner K, Sadaie M, Darot JF, et al. Autophagy mediates the mitotic senescence transition. Genes Dev 2009 Apr 1;23(7):798-803.

[250] Lu Z, Luo RZ, Lu Y, Zhang X, Yu Q, Khare S, et al. The tumor suppressor gene ARHI regulates autophagy and tumor dormancy in human ovarian cancer cells. J Clin Invest 2008 Dec;118(12):3917-3929.

[251] Gewirtz DA. Autophagy, senescence and tumor dormancy in cancer therapy. Autophagy 2009 Nov;5(8):1232-1234.

[252] Nystrom T. Role of oxidative carbonylation in protein quality control and senescence. EMBO J 2005 Apr 6;24(7):1311-1317.

[253] Pattingre S, Tassa A, Qu X, Garuti R, Liang XH, Mizushima N, et al. Bcl-2 antiapoptotic proteins inhibit Beclin 1-dependent autophagy. Cell 2005 Sep 23;122(6):927-939.

[254] Coussens LM, Werb Z. Inflammation and cancer. Nature 2002 Dec 19-26;420(6917): 860-867.

[255] Szatrowski TP, Nathan CF. Production of large amounts of hydrogen peroxide by human tumor cells. Cancer Res 1991 Feb 1;51(3):794-798.

[256] Toyokuni S, Okamoto K, Yodoi J, Hiai H. Persistent oxidative stress in cancer. FEBS Lett 1995 Jan 16;358(1):1-3.

[257] Sander CS, Chang H, Hamm F, Elsner P, Thiele JJ. Role of oxidative stress and the antioxidant network in cutaneous carcinogenesis. Int J Dermatol 2004 May;43(5): 326-335.

[258] Lincoln DT, Ali Emadi EM, Tonissen KF, Clarke FM. The thioredoxin-thioredoxin reductase system: over-expression in human cancer. Anticancer Res 2003 May-Jun; 23(3B):2425-2433.

[259] Cen D, Gonzalez RI, Buckmeier JA, Kahlon RS, Tohidian NB, Meyskens FL,Jr. Disulfiram induces apoptosis in human melanoma cells: a redox-related process. Mol Cancer Ther 2002 Jan;1(3):197-204.

[260] Cen D, Brayton D, Shahandeh B, Meyskens FL,Jr, Farmer PJ. Disulfiram facilitates intracellular Cu uptake and induces apoptosis in human melanoma cells. J Med Chem 2004 Dec 30;47(27):6914-6920.

[261] Huang P, Feng L, Oldham EA, Keating MJ, Plunkett W. Superoxide dismutase as a target for the selective killing of cancer cells. Nature 2000 Sep 21;407(6802):390-395.

[262] Dobos J, Timar J, Bocsi J, Burian Z, Nagy K, Barna G, et al. In vitro and in vivo antitumor effect of 2-methoxyestradiol on human melanoma. Int J Cancer 2004 Dec 10;112(5):771-776.

[263] Russo GL. Ins and outs of dietary phytochemicals in cancer chemoprevention. Biochem Pharmacol 2007 Aug 15;74(4):533-544.

[264] Tyagi AK, Singh RP, Agarwal C, Chan DC, Agarwal R. Silibinin strongly synergizes human prostate carcinoma DU145 cells to doxorubicin-induced growth Inhibition, G2-M arrest, and apoptosis. Clin Cancer Res 2002 Nov;8(11):3512-3519.

[265] De Larco JE, Park CA, Dronava H, Furcht LT. Paradoxical roles for antioxidants in tumor prevention and eradication. Cancer Biol Ther 2010 Mar 8;9(5).

[266] Farmer PJ, Gidanian S, Shahandeh B, Di Bilio AJ, Tohidian N, Meyskens FL,Jr. Melanin as a target for melanoma chemotherapy: pro-oxidant effect of oxygen and metals on melanoma viability. Pigment Cell Res 2003 Jun;16(3):273-279.

[267] Chen KG, Valencia JC, Lai B, Zhang G, Paterson JK, Rouzaud F, et al. Melanosomal sequestration of cytotoxic drugs contributes to the intractability of malignant melanomas. Proc Natl Acad Sci U S A 2006 Jun 27;103(26):9903-9907.

[268] Chen KG, Leapman RD, Zhang G, Lai B, Valencia JC, Cardarelli CO, et al. Influence of melanosome dynamics on melanoma drug sensitivity. J Natl Cancer Inst 2009 Sep 16;101(18):1259-1271.

[269] Raposo G, Marks MS. The dark side of lysosome-related organelles: specialization of the endocytic pathway for melanosome biogenesis. Traffic 2002 Apr;3(4):237-248.

[270] Hearing VJ. Biogenesis of pigment granules: a sensitive way to regulate melanocyte function. J Dermatol Sci 2005 Jan;37(1):3-14.

[271] Baldea I. Melanocyte pigmentation – friend or foe on the route to melanoma. In: Tanaka Y, editor. Breakthroughs in Melanoma Research Rijeka, Croatia: InTech; 2011. p. 183-217.

[272] Solano F, Martinez-Esparza M, Jimenez-Cervantes C, Hill SP, Lozano JA, Garcia-Borron JC. New insights on the structure of the mouse silver locus and on the function of the silver protein. Pigment Cell Res 2000;13 Suppl 8:118-124.

[273] Kwon BS, Chintamaneni C, Kozak CA, Copeland NG, Gilbert DJ, Jenkins N, et al. A melanocyte-specific gene, Pmel 17, maps near the silver coat color locus on mouse chromosome 10 and is in a syntenic region on human chromosome 12. Proc Natl Acad Sci U S A 1991 Oct 15;88(20):9228-9232.

[274] Theos AC, Truschel ST, Raposo G, Marks MS. The Silver locus product Pmel17/gp100/Silv/ME20: controversial in name and in function. Pigment Cell Res 2005 Oct;18(5):322-336.

[275] Orlow SJ. Melanosomes are specialized members of the lysosomal lineage of organelles. J Invest Dermatol 1995 Jul;105(1):3-7.

[276] Raposo G, Tenza D, Murphy DM, Berson JF, Marks MS. Distinct protein sorting and localization to premelanosomes, melanosomes, and lysosomes in pigmented melanocytic cells. J Cell Biol 2001 Feb 19;152(4):809-824.

[277] Valencia JC, Hoashi T, Pawelek JM, Solano F, Hearing VJ. Pmel17: controversial indeed but critical to melanocyte function. Pigment Cell Res 2006 Jun;19(3):250-2; author reply 253-7.

[278] Nelson JS, McCullough JL, Berns MW. Photodynamic therapy of human malignant melanoma xenografts in athymic nude mice. J Natl Cancer Inst 1988 Mar 2;80(1): 56-60.

[279] Meyskens FL,Jr, Farmer P, Fruehauf JP. Redox regulation in human melanocytes and melanoma. Pigment Cell Res 2001 Jun;14(3):148-154.

[280] Shackleton M, Quintana E, Fearon ER, Morrison SJ. Heterogeneity in cancer: cancer stem cells versus clonal evolution. Cell 2009 Sep 4;138(5):822-829.

[281] Marotta LL, Polyak K. Cancer stem cells: a model in the making. Curr Opin Genet Dev 2009 Feb;19(1):44-50.

[282] Al-Hajj M, Wicha MS, Benito-Hernandez A, Morrison SJ, Clarke MF. Prospective identification of tumorigenic breast cancer cells. Proc Natl Acad Sci U S A 2003 Apr 1;100(7):3983-3988.

[283] Bonnet D, Dick JE. Human acute myeloid leukemia is organized as a hierarchy that originates from a primitive hematopoietic cell. Nat Med 1997 Jul;3(7):730-737.

[284] O'Brien CA, Pollett A, Gallinger S, Dick JE. A human colon cancer cell capable of initiating tumour growth in immunodeficient mice. Nature 2007 Jan 4;445(7123): 106-110.

[285] Singh SK, Hawkins C, Clarke ID, Squire JA, Bayani J, Hide T, et al. Identification of human brain tumour initiating cells. Nature 2004 Nov 18;432(7015):396-401.

[286] Abel EV, Aplin AE. Finding the root of the problem: the quest to identify melanoma stem cells. Front Biosci (Schol Ed) 2011 Jun 1;3:937-945.

[287] Jones PM, George AM. The ABC transporter structure and mechanism: perspectives on recent research. Cell Mol Life Sci 2004 Mar;61(6):682-699.

[288] Frank NY, Margaryan A, Huang Y, Schatton T, Waaga-Gasser AM, Gasser M, et al. ABCB5-mediated doxorubicin transport and chemoresistance in human malignant melanoma. Cancer Res 2005 May 15;65(10):4320-4333.

[289] Keshet GI, Goldstein I, Itzhaki O, Cesarkas K, Shenhav L, Yakirevitch A, et al. MDR1 expression identifies human melanoma stem cells. Biochem Biophys Res Commun 2008 Apr 18;368(4):930-936.

[290] Monzani E, Facchetti F, Galmozzi E, Corsini E, Benetti A, Cavazzin C, et al. Melanoma contains CD133 and ABCG2 positive cells with enhanced tumourigenic potential. Eur J Cancer 2007 Mar;43(5):935-946.

[291] Robey RW, Steadman K, Polgar O, Bates SE. ABCG2-mediated transport of photosensitizers: potential impact on photodynamic therapy. Cancer Biol Ther 2005 Feb; 4(2):187-194.

[292] Tamura A, An R, Hagiya Y, Hoshijima K, Yoshida T, Mikuriya K, et al. Drug-induced phototoxicity evoked by inhibition of human ABC transporter ABCG2: development of in vitro high-speed screening systems. Expert Opin Drug Metab Toxicol 2008 Mar; 4(3):255-272.

[293] Liu W, Baer MR, Bowman MJ, Pera P, Zheng X, Morgan J, et al. The tyrosine kinase inhibitor imatinib mesylate enhances the efficacy of photodynamic therapy by inhibiting ABCG2. Clin Cancer Res 2007 Apr 15;13(8):2463-2470.

Chapter 23

Study of the Anti-Photoaging Effect of Noni (*Morinda citrifolia*)

Hideaki Matsuda, Megumi Masuda, Kazuya Murata,
Yumi Abe and Akemi Uwaya

Additional information is available at the end of the chapter

http://dx.doi.org/10.5772/53621

1. Introduction

During the aging process, morphological changes in the human skin appear most noticeably in areas of frequent exposure to ultraviolet (UV) light from the sun, such as the face and hands. Chronic UV exposure induces photoaging, characterized by pigmented spots and wrinkles in the skin. Gradual destruction of the ozonosphere has raised photoaging risk. This has led to rapid growth of the anti-photoaging cosmetic market, especially among women with young and fair skin. Sunscreen agents are a first choice for protection against photoaging. However, a certain amount of UV irradiation penetrates skin dermis, and adverse effect may occur with use of these agents. Because of this, a current trend is the development of safer cosmetic ingredients that effectively inhibit the UV signaling pathways leading to photoaging [1].

Therefore, in this chapter we discuss searching for novel cosmetic ingredients from natural resources which prevent the generation of pigmented spots and wrinkles *via* antagonistic activities against UV signaling pathways. We focused this search on plants growing along the coasts of South Pacific islands, as they may have developed specific self-defense systems against harmful UV radiation. Following this strategy, we selected "noni" (*Morinda citrifolia* L., Rubiaceae).

2. Subtropical plant noni

Selected *M. citrifolia* as a subject is commonly called "noni", which is a subtropical plant distributed widely in the tropical/ subtropical zone, including Tahiti and Hawaii. The tree is a rapidly growing evergreen that is resistant to drought and poor soil conditions.

Noni has been utilized for various reasons in many areas. The root was used as dye in Japan, and the leaves and the seeds, as well as the fruit, were eaten frequently in Southeast Asia and the Pacific islands. Currently, the fruit juice and leaf tea are sold in the functional foods market. Noni is also used as an herbal medicine to promote health and beauty. The whole plant, from the root to fruit, has been used without waste for more than 2000 years as a panacea [2]. Therefore, noni was considered a "gift from God" by generations of Pacific Islanders.

In the last decade, many papers have reported the chemical constituents and biological activities of noni including hypotensive [3], hypoglycemic [4], and anticancer activities [5], which scientifically support traditional claims of noni. Noni has been used traditionally for the treatment of dermatoses such as ringworm, dry skin, acne, pustule, and other skin troubles. Moreover, ripe noni fruit juice has been drunk for cosmetic reasons. In some areas, the dried immature noni fruit, the leaves, or the seeds mixed with coconut oil have been used as an external treatment [6]. But studies reporting potential cosmetic uses of noni, such as inhibition of melanogenesis and reduction of wrinkles, have only recently been completed. Noni fruit contains a large number of seeds throughout its flesh. But during the production of noni fruit juice, the seeds are removed and discarded. Considering the potential utility of all parts of the plant, we investigated extracts from the fruit flesh, leaves, and seeds for active anti-photoaging agents.

3. Skin whitening effect of noni

3.1. Screening tests for melanogenesis inhibitory effect of noni

During photoaging, UV rays trigger melanogenesis and chromatosis. These processes generate pigmented spots by UV activation of melanocyte tyrosinase (a melanin synthesis enzyme) which then converts L-tyrosine to L-DOPA, followed by conversion to dopaquinone. Dopaquinone subsequently forms melanin through several steps, including auto-oxidation. As such, tyrosinase inhibitors may be useful for prevention of pigmented spots.

Initial evaluation of the anti-melanogenesis activity of noni was carried out using an *in vitro* tyrosinase inhibition assay with 50% ethanol extracts of fruit flesh (Fruit-ext), leaves (Leaf-ext), and seeds (Seed-ext). As oxidative reactions also contribute to melanogenesis [7], the 1-diphenyl-2-picrylhydrazyl (DPPH) assay was also performed to find whether noni has antioxidant activity.

3.1.1. Tyrosinase inhibitory activities

The results of the *in vitro* tyrosinase inhibition assay are shown in Table 1. At 20 to 500 μg/ml, Seed-ext inhibited tyrosinase activity, in a concentration-dependent manner. Fruit-ext exhibited weak activity only at 500 μg/ml, and Leaf-ext did not inhibit enzyme activity at any concentration [8].

3.1.2. DPPH radical scavenging activities

As oxidative reactions contribute to melanogenesis, the DPPH assay was performed to measure the antioxidant activity of noni. As shown in Table 2, Seed-ext exhibited potent DPPH radical scavenging activity, with an IC_{50} value of 12 μg/ml. Leaf-ext and Fruit-ext exhibited weaker antioxidant activities, with IC_{50} values of 113 and 240 μg/ml, respectively [8].

The results of the two assays reveal that Seed-ext has stronger tyrosinase inhibitory and antioxidant activity than Fruit-ext and Leaf-ext.

Samples	Concentration	OD (×1000) [a)] at 475 nm	Inhibition (%)
Control		472±4	
Fruit-ext	20 (μg/ml)	471±3	0
	100 (μg/ml)	451±2	5
	500 (μg/ml)	419±9[i]	11
Leaf-ext	20 (μg/ml)	471±2	0
	100 (μg/ml)	460±2	3
	500 (μg/ml)	442±1[i]	6
Seed-ext	20 (μg/ml)	449±5[i]	5
	100 (μg/ml)	394±4[i]	17
	500 (μg/ml)	365±4[i]	23
Kojic acid	10 (μM)	207±3[i]	56
	50 (μM)	77±3[i]	84

Table 1. Tyrosinase Inhibitory Activities of Fruit-ext, Leaf-ext, Seed-ext and Kojic Acid ([a)] OD: optical density. Each value represents the mean±S.E. of 3 experiments. Significantly different from control group, [i]: $p<0.01$.)

Samples	Concentration	OD (×1000) [a)] at 520 nm	Inhibition (%)	IC_{50} value [b)]
Control		974±21		
Fruit-ext	100 (μg/ml)	759±3[i]	22	240 (μg/ml)
	200 (μg/ml)	536±5[i]	45	
	400 (μg/ml)	188±3[i]	81	
Leaf-ext	50 (μg/ml)	765±4[i]	22	113 (μg/ml)
	100 (μg/ml)	570±3[i]	42	
	200 (μg/ml)	301±6[i]	69	
Seed-ext	5 (μg/ml)	771±2[i]	21	12 (μg/ml)
	10 (μg/ml)	537±7[i]	45	
	20 (μg/ml)	121±5[i]	88	
L-Ascorbic acid	20 (μM)	570±4[i]	41	23 (μM)
	50 (μM)	79±2[i]	92	

Table 2. DPPH Radical Scavenging Activities of Fruit-ext, Leaf-ext, Seed-ext and L-Ascorbic Acid ([a)] OD: optical density. Each value represents the mean±S.E. of 3 experiments. Significantly different from control group, [i]: $p<0.01$. [b)] IC_{50} value represents the concentration of sample required to scavenge 50% of DPPH free radical.)

3.2. Inhibitory effect of noni seeds on melanogenesis and its active compounds

According to the *in vitro* the screenings, Seed-ext may have melanogenesis inhibitory properties. Further examination of Seed-ext involved the use of B16 murine melanoma cells as an *in vitro* melanogenesis test model. In this assay, cells were stimulated by α-melanocyte stimulating hormone (α-MSH) and incubated for 72 hrs with the vehicle or test material [9]. As shown in Table 3, vehicle control treated cells, stimulated with α–MSH, significantly promoted melanogenesis compared to control that was not stimulated with α-MSH. At concentrations ranging from 12.5 to 200 μg/ml, Seed-ext inhibited α-MSH-stimulated melanogenesis in a concentration dependent manner without any significant effects on cell proliferation [10].

The tyrosinase inhibitory activity of Seed-ext was not as potent as that of other well known skin whitening agents. But in the B16 melanoma cells culture system, it inhibited melanin production. Thus, noni seed may be useful as an anti-photoaging cosmetic ingredient which prevents pigmented spots by interacting with a different active site than existing general skin whitening agents.

Samples	**Concentration**	**α-MSH (μM)**	**Melanin content (μg/well)**	**Cell proliferation (%)**
Control			1.6±0.4	61.9±1.2
Vehicle control		1	42.8±1.6[ii]	100.0±1.2[ii]
Seed-ext	12.5 (μg/ml)	1	29.0±0.6[i]	100.6±1.1
	50 (μg/ml)	1	21.1±0.6[i]	105.9±1.2
	200 (μg/ml)	1	11.9±0.6[i]	103.5±2.5
Kojic acid	100 (μM)	1	13.5±0.4[i]	107.4±1.9
	200 (μM)	1	6.9±0.4[i]	103.2±2.4

Table 3. Effects of Seed-ext and Kojic Acid on α-MSH-Stimulated Melanogenesis in B16 Melanoma Cells (Each value in melanin content represents the mean±S.E. of 3 experiments. Significantly different from the control group, [ii]: $p<0.01$. Significantly different from the vehicle control group, [i]: $p<0.01$. Each value in cell proliferation represents the mean ±S.E. of 3 experiments.)

As Seed-ext was confirmed to potently inhibit melanogenesis, activity guided isolation of the active compounds was carried out. Two lignans, 3,3'-bisdemethylpinoresinol (**1**) and americanin A (**2**), were isolated from noni seeds and found to be active constituents. As shown in Table 4, 10 and 20 μM of **1** displayed weak inhibition of cell proliferation. But 1.25 to 5 μM of **1** inhibited melanogenesis in a concentration dependent without any significant effects on cell proliferation. Also, 100 and 200 μM of **2** inhibited melanogenesis [10]. **1** (IC_{50} value: 0.3 mM) and **2** (IC_{50} value: 2.7 mM) exhibited tyrosinase inhibition, and **1** (IC_{50} value: 4 μM) and **2** (IC_{50} value: 11 μM) exhibited potent DPPH radical scavenging properties [8].

http://dx.doi.org/10.5772/53621

Samples	Concentration (μM)	α-MSH (μM)	Melanin content (μg/well)	Cell proliferation (%)
Run 1				
Control			4.5±0.8	55.2±1.3
Vehicle control		1	37.5±1.5[ii]	100.0±1.1[ii]
1	1.25	1	29.9±0.6[i]	97.8±0.4
	2.5	1	21.6±0.8[i]	101.0±1.7
	5	1	18.5±1.2[i]	99.1±0.7
	10	1	15.2±0.2[i]	88.8±1.2[i]
	20	1	13.2±0.8[i]	88.5±0.3[i]
Kojic acid	100	1	17.2±1.1[i]	97.1±1.3
	200	1	6.4±0.4[i]	98.2±1.4
Run 2				
Control			7.3±2.5	58.8±2.4
Vehicle control		1	39.0±0.9[ii]	100.0±5.1[ii]
2	12.5	1	39.3±0.7	101.6±1.0
	25	1	36.7±0.7	107.1±0.4
	50	1	33.9±0.8	103.3±0.9
	100	1	25.5±1.5[i]	99.4±4.5
	200	1	13.9±1.0[i]	102.8±1.4
Kojic acid	100	1	15.7±1.0[i]	101.9±3.8
	200	1	8.6±0.6[i]	98.4±2.7

Table 4. Effects of 3,3'-Bisdemethylpinoresinol (1), Americanin A (2) and Kojic Acid on α-MSH-Stimulated Melanogenesis in B16 Melanoma Cells (Each value in melanin content represents the mean±S.E. of 3 experiments. Significantly different from the control group, [ii]: $p<0.01$. Significantly different from the vehicle control group, [i]: $p<0.01$. Each value in cell proliferation represents the mean±S.E. of 3 experiments.)

Compared to kojic acid, which is a common skin whitening ingredient, **1** exhibited more potent inhibition of melanogenesis. This suggested that the anti-melanogenesis effect of **1** may be due to the suppression of tyrosinase protein expression in the cells, rather than inhibiting tyrosinase itself.

3.3. Effects of noni compounds; 3,3'-bisdemethylpinoresinol and americanin A on inhibitory melanogenesis activity

As the anti-melanogenesis of Seed-ext may be due to **1** and **2**, the inhibitory mechanism of these two lignans was studied with α-MSH stimulated B16 melanoma cells.

3.3.1. Effects of 3,3′-bisdemethylpinoresinol and americanin A on tyrosinase expression in B16 melanoma cells

First, the effect of **1** and **2** on tyrosinase expression in α-MSH stimulated B16 melanoma cells was investigated by using Western blot analysis. As shown in Fig. 1, the tyrosinase expression of the control at 72 hrs was enhanced remarkably. But after 72 hrs of treatment with **1** (5 μM) or **2** (200 μM), the enhancement of expression was notably suppressed without any significant effect on cell proliferation [10].

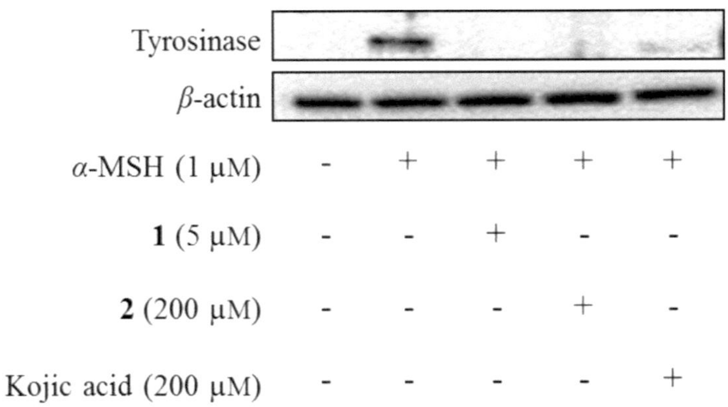

Figure 1. Effects of 3,3′-Bisdemethylpinoresinol (1), Americanin A (2) and Kojic Acid on Tyrosinase Expression in α-MSH-Stimulated B16 Melanoma Cells (The cells were treated with α-MSH (1 μM) in the presence of **1** (5 μM), **2** (200 μM) or kojic acid (200 μM) for 72 hrs. The level of tyrosinase expression was examined by Western blot analysis using specific antibody. Equal protein loading was confirmed by β-actin expression.)

3.3.2. Inhibition of tyrosinase in B16 melanoma cells by 3,3′-bisdemethyl-pinoresinol and americanin A

With suppressed expression of the enzyme, the activity of tyrosinase in the cell may decrease. Secondly, α-MSH stimulated B16 melanoma cells were cultivated during treatment with **1** or **2**. Next, the amount of melanin and tyrosinase activity in the cells were measured.

As shown in Fig. 2A, the intracellular melanin content of control group increased remarkably after cultivation for 24 to 72 hrs, whereas the content in cells treated with **1** (5 μM) or **2** (200 μM) decreased after 72 hrs. As shown in Fig. 2B, the tyrosinase activity in the α-MSH stimulated cells was also significantly inhibited by addition of **1** (5 μM) or **2** (200 μM) after 24 to 72 hrs incubation [10].

As just described, lignans **1** (5 μM) and **2** (200 μM) inhibited intracellular melanin contents induced by α-MSH. The results of Western blot analysis demonstrated that **1** and **2** remarkably inhibit tyrosinase stimulated by α-MSH. Moreover, as **1** and **2** reduced intracellular tyrosinase activity, it became clear that their melanogenesis inhibitory activity involved suppression of tyrosinase expression.

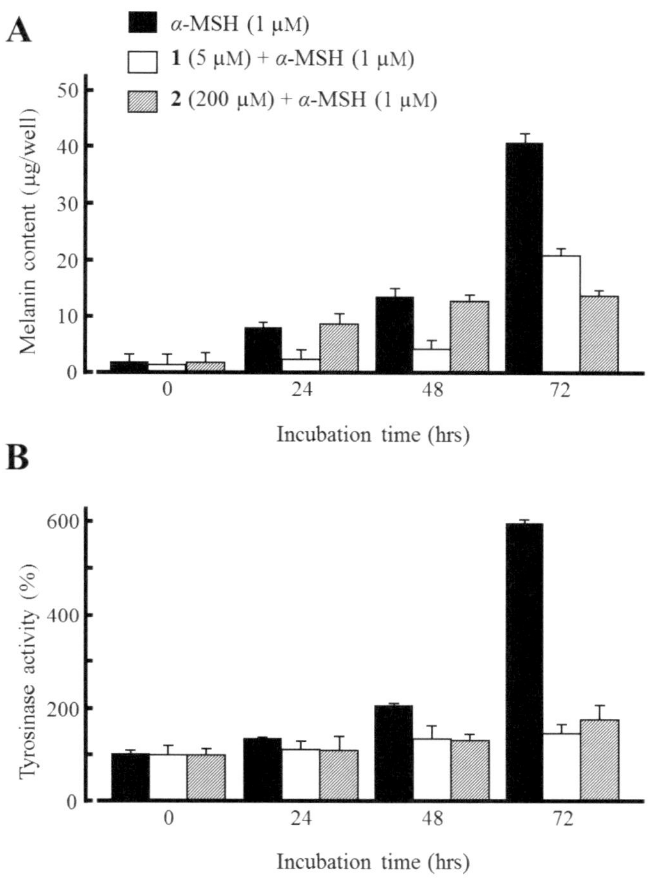

Figure 2. Effects of 3,3'-Bisdemethylpinoresinol (1) and Americanin A (2) on Melanogenesis and Tyrosinase Activity in α-MSH-Stimulated B16 Melanoma Cells (The cells were treated with α-MSH (1 μM, black column), **1** (5 μM, white column) and **2** (200 μM, slashed column) for the indicated times. (A) The melanin content was determined. (B) Tyrosinase activity was determined by measuring the formation of dopachrome. Data represent mean±S.E. of two different experiments each carried out in triplicate.)

3.3.3. *Effect of 3,3'-bisdemethylpinoresinol and americanin A on phosphorylation of p38 MAPK*

During melanogenesis in melanocytes, it is known that microphthalmia-associated transcription (MITF) is a transcription factor that regulates expression of the tyrosinase gene, and that melanins are produced by the activation of MITF [11]. Since mitogen-activated protein kinases (MAPKs) pathway is one of the intracellular signals that activates MITF, further research on this pathway was performed. It has been reported that phosphorylation of p38 MAPK activates MITF, whereas that of ERK1/2 and p70 S6K suppress MITF [12, 13]. The effects of **1** and **2** on the MAPK signaling activities of α-MSH-stimulated B16 melanoma cells were examined.

The levels of phosphorylation of p38 MAPK were compared, at 6 and 12 hrs after stimulation of B16 melanoma cells by α-MSH (1 μM). As shown in Fig. 3A, the analysis at 6 and 12 hrs reveals that the levels of phosphorylation of p38 MAPK in B16 cells were enhanced by α-MSH treatment in comparison to those without α-MSH. The treatment with lignan **1** (5 μM) or lignan **2** (200 μM) suppressed phosphorylation of p38 MAPK and enhanced that of ERK1/2 at 6 and 12 hrs after stimulated by α-MSH (Fig. 3B). However, both lignans had no effect on p70 S6K phosophorylation (Fig. 3B) [10].

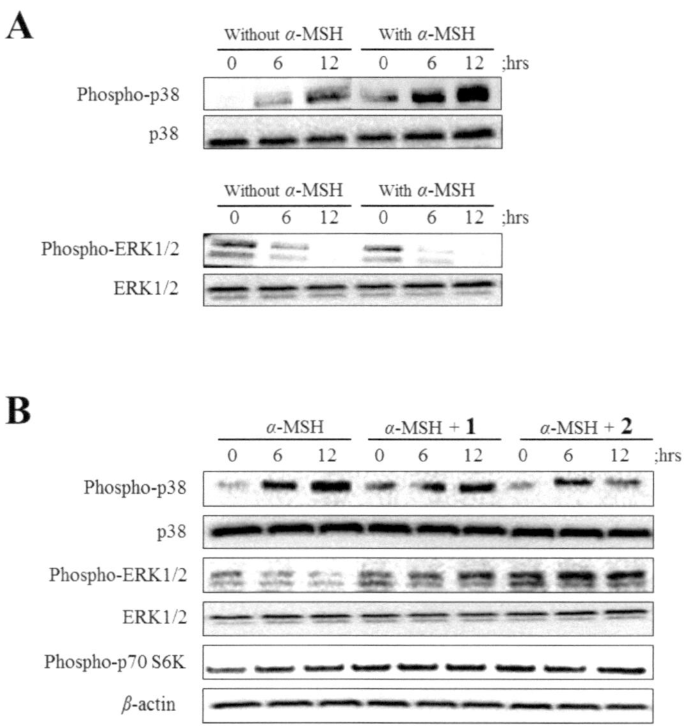

Figure 3. (A) Effect of α-MSH on Phosphorylation of p38 MAPK and ERK1/2 in B16 Melanoma Cells. (B) Effects of 3,3'-Bisdemethylpinoresinol (1) and Americanin A (2) on Phosphorylation of p38 MAPK, ERK1/2 and p70 S6K in α-MSH-Stimulated B16 Melanoma Cells ((A) The cells were treated with or without α-MSH (1 μM) for the indicated times. (B) The cells were treated with α-MSH (1 μM) in the presence of **1** (5 μM) or **2** (200 μM) for the indicated times. Phosphorylation of p38 MAPK, ERK1/2, and p70 S6K was assessed by Western blot analysis with using specific antibody for phosphorylated forms of p38 MAPK, ERK1/2, and p70 S6K. Equal protein loading was confirmed by β-actin expression.)

http://dx.doi.org/10.5772/53621

As the inhibitory mechanism of melanogenesis in α-MSH-stimulated B16 melanoma cells, These results strongly suggest that the lignans inhibit tyrosinase expression by suppressing p38 MAPK phosphorylation and enhancing ERK1/2, which then prevents activation of MITF.

4. Inhibitory effect of noni on wrinkle formation

It is thought that wrinkles form mainly by aging, but they are also caused by photoaging. The causes are degradation of moisture-retaining property of epidermis and transformation of dermal configuration due to altered elastic or collagen fibers in the cutis. Anti-wrinkle cosmetics are useful for comparatively slight wrinkles and fine lines. The main functions of anti-wrinkle cosmetics included normalization of moisture retention by the cornified layer, acceleration of keratinocyte turnover, and acceleration of collagen and elastin synthesis through proliferation and stimulation of fibroblasts. Recently, retinol and its analogs, so-called retinoids, have received increased attention and utilization as a cosmetic ingredient because they promote fibroblastic collagen production in the cutis and improve skin tension. Also, vitamin A reportedly accelerates turnover, which reduces hyperpigmented skin spots caused by melanin excreted by the epidermis, even though it has no inhibitory effects on activation of tyrosinase and melanogenesis. But retinoids irritate the skin and have adverse effects such as dermatitis. Therefore, safer reducing wrinkle ingredients are needed [1].

4.1. Wrinkle inhibition screening test of noni

One cause of photoaging wrinkle formation is the degradation of collagen, a main component of corium connective tissue [14]. The degradation of collagen is promoted by release of human leukocyte elastase (HLE) from infiltrated neutrophils into the skin by UV irradiation [15]. HLE cleaves the triple helix structure of type I collagen and degrades elastic fiber in human skin [16]. Thus, HLE inhibitors may be useful for the prevention of wrinkle formation.

4.1.1. Inhibitory effect of noni on HLE and its active compounds

The inhibitory effect of noni on wrinkle formation was investigated by measuring HLE inhibiting activity *in vitro*. As shown in Table 5, concentrations raging from 0.5 to 1.0 mg/ml of Seed-ext displayed HLE inhibitory activity in a concentration-dependent manner. Fruit-ext and Leaf-ext had no inhibitory activity at 1.0 mg/ml [8].

As Seed-ext exhibited potent HLE inhibitory activity compared with Fruit-ext and Leaf-ext, noni seeds appear to be the most source of cosmetic ingredients capable of preventing wrinkle formation during photoaging.

The active compounds in Seed-ext were isolated using the HLE inhibition bioassay as a fractionation guide. Ursolic acid (**3**) was isolated from Seed-ext and found to the active constituent. The IC_{50} value of **3** in the HLE inhibition assay was 0.07 mM. The IC_{50} value of phenylmethanesulfonyl fluoride (PMSF), the positive control, was 0.14 mM. Thus, **3** was more potent than the positive control (data not shown) [8].

Samples	Concentration	OD (×1000) [a] at 405 nm	Inhibition (%)	IC $_{50}$ value [b]
Control A [c]		946±23		
Fruit-ext	0.1 (mg/ml)	994±38 [i]	-8	
	0.5 (mg/ml)	1014±9 [i]	-10	
	1.0 (mg/ml)	1039±9 [i]	-12	
Leaf-ext	0.1 (mg/ml)	1014±16 [i]	-10	
	0.5 (mg/ml)	1023±18 [i]	-11	
	1.0 (mg/ml)	1042±36 [i]	-13	
Seed-ext	0.1 (mg/ml)	1052±20 [i]	-14	1.0 (mg/ml)
	0.5 (mg/ml)	722±21 [i]	22	
	1.0 (mg/ml)	467±30 [i]	50	
Control B [d]		925±9		
PMSF	0.08 (mM)	676±7 [ii]	29	0.14 (mM)
	0.15 (mM)	383±14 [ii]	60	
	0.50 (mM)	100±1 [ii]	90	

Table 5. HLE Inhibitory Activities of Fruit-ext, Leaf-ext, Seed-ext and PMSF ([a] OD: optical density. [b] IC_{50} value represents the concentration of sample required to inhibit 50% of HLE activity. [c] Control A is a control for extracts. [d] Control B is a control for PMSF. Each value represents the mean±S.E. of 3 experiments. Significantly different from control A group, [i]: $p<0.01$. Significantly different from control B group, [ii]: $p<0.01$.)

4.2. Inhibitory effect of noni seeds on matrix metalloproteinase-1 (MMP-1) secretion and its active compounds

Matrix metalloproteinases (MMPs) are matrix degrading enzymes associated with destructive processes including inflammation, tumor invasion and skin aging [1]. More than 20 subtypes of MMPs have been reported [17]. Among these, MMP-1, secreted from human skin fibroblasts, is mainly responsible for the degradation of dermal type I collagen in the photoaging process [18]. Also, HLE activates MMP-1 [19]. Thus, it is expected that MMP-1 and HLE inhibitors may be useful for the prevention of photoaging and subsequent wrinkle formation.

Since Seed-ext displayed strong HLE inhibitory activity, its ability to inhibit MMP-1 secretion was investigated in UV-irradiated normal human dermal fibroblasts (NHDFs). The amount of MMP-1 protein secreted from NHDFs into culture media was analyzed by Western blotting. UVA irradiation (5 J/cm^2) enhanced the secretion of MMP-1 from NHDFs in the vehicle control group at 9 to 48 hrs incubation, as compared to the control group without UVA-irradiation (Fig. 4). The group which was treated with Seed-ext (10 μg/ml) after UVA-irradiated NHDFs inhibited the secretion MMP-1 at 24 to 48 hrs, when compared to the vehicle control (Fig. 4) [20]. Seed-ext was not cytotoxic at 3 to 30 μg/ml.

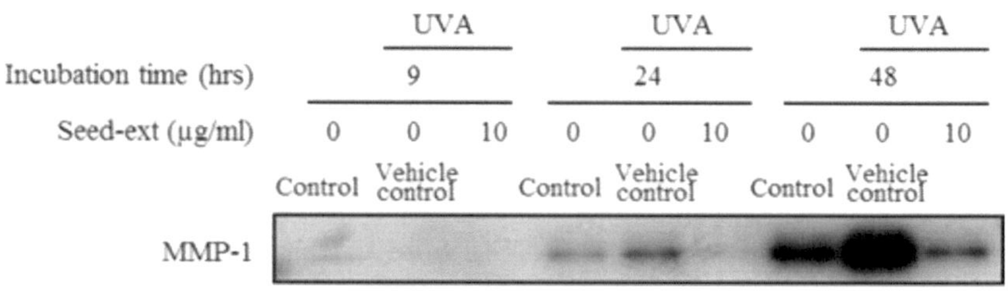

Figure 4. Effect of Seed-ext on MMP-1 Secretion from UVA-Irradiated NHDFs (Fibroblasts were exposed to UVA (5 J/cm^2) and then cultured in the serum free medium containing test samples for 9, 24, and 48 hrs. MMP-1 protein levels in the cultured medium at the indicated times were assessed by Western blot analysis using the antibody against human MMP-1. The blot is representative of three separate experiments and represents a single immunoblot.)

The active compounds responsible for the inhibitory effect of Seed-ext on MMP-1 secretion were searched for by following bioassay guided fractionation. As shown in Fig. 5A and 5B, 3,3'-bisdemethylpinoresinol (**1**), which is an active anti-melanogenesis compound, significantly inhibited the secretion MMP-1 at 3 μM. On the other hand, ursolic acid (**3**), which is an active anti-HLE compound, had no effect on MMP-1 secretion (data not shown). There was no cytotoxicity from **1** and **3** at 0.03, 0.1 and 0.3 μM [20].

It is clear that ursolic acid (**3**) inhibits HLE, whereas 3,3'-bisdemethylpinoresinol (**1**) inhibits MMP-1 secretion. Further, Seed-ext inhibits both MMP-1 secretion and HLE activity. There are very few plant extracts or compounds that have both inhibitory effects. Thus, noni seeds may be an ideal cosmetic ingredient to prevent wrinkle formation.

4.3. Inhibitory effect of 3,3′-bisdemethylpinoresinol on MMP-1 secretion

In UV irradiated skin, MMP-1 is a major collagenolytic enzyme responsible for collagen damage [21]. It has been reported that UV irradiation promotes expression of MMP-1 in NHDFs [22] and secretion into culture media [23]. It is also known that UV irradiation activates intracellular fibroblast signals, c-Jun-N-terminal kinase (JNK) and p38 mitogen-activated protein kinase (p38 MAPK) cascades, promotes phosphorylation of JNK and p38, enhances expression of c-Jun and c-Fos, followed by activation of activation protein-1 (AP-1), and, in the end, enhances expression of MMP-1 [14, 24]. In order to find the mechanism of inhibition of MMP-1, compound **1** was investigated for effects on intracellular MMP-1 expression and activation of MAPKs in UVA-irradiated NHDFs.

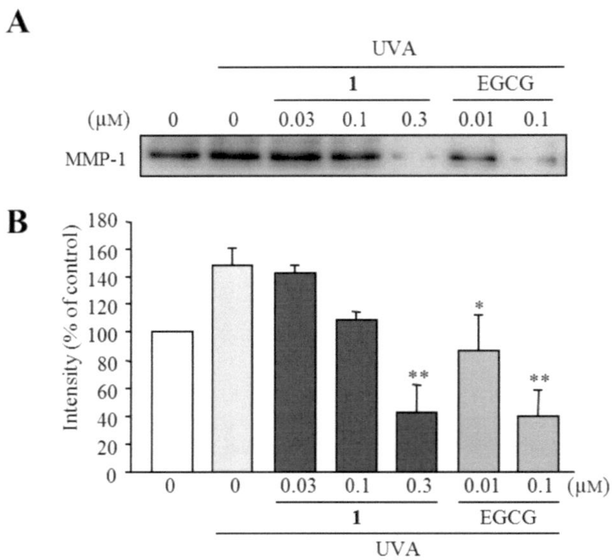

Figure 5. Effects of 3,3'-Bisdemethylpinoresinol (1) and and epigallocatechin-3-*O*-gallate (EGCG) on MMP-1 Secretion from UVA-Irradiated NHDFs (Fibroblasts were exposed to UVA (5 J/cm^2) and then cultured in the serum free medium containing test samples for 48 hrs. MMP-1 protein levels in the cultured medium were assessed by Western blot analysis using human MMP-1 specific antibody. (A) The blot is representative of three separate experiments and represents a single immunoblot. (B) All data is reported as mean±S.E. of three separate experiments. Significantly different from the vehicle control group, *: $p<0.05$, **: $p<0.01$.)

4.3.1. Effect of 3,3'-bisdemethylpinoresinol (1) on intracellular MMP-1 expression in UVA irradiation NHDFs

First, the effect of **1** on intracellular MMP-1 expression in UVA-irradiation was examined. In the vehicle control group, UVA irradiation enhanced the levels of intracellular MMP-1 expression at 24 and 48 hrs, with most of the MMP-1 expression being detected at 48 hrs (Fig. 6). But in the treatment group (addition of **1**, 0.3 μM), the expression was down-regulated at 48 hrs (Fig. 6A). The levels of MMP-1 secretion from UVA-irradiated NHDF into the culture medium increased at 48 hrs in the vehicle control group, whereas the treatment group (addition of **1**, 0.3 μM) obviously inhibited MMP-1 secretion (Fig. 6B) [20].

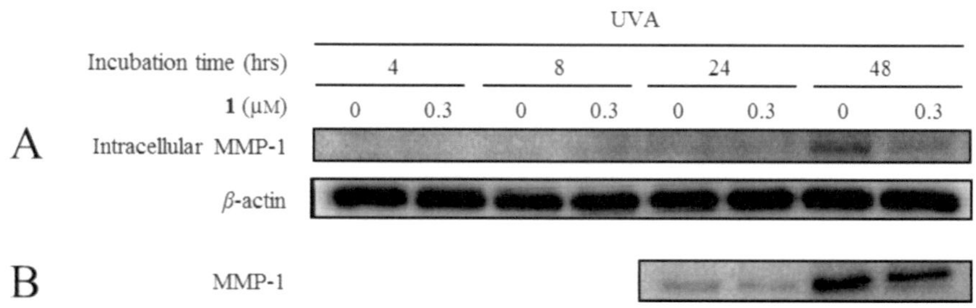

Figure 6. (A) Effect of 3,3'-Bisdemethylpinoresinol (1) on the Intracellular MMP-1 Expression in UVA-Irradiated NHDFs (B) Effect of 3,3'-Bisdemethylpinoresinol (1) on MMP-1 Secretion from UVA-Irradiated NHDFs ((A) Fibroblasts were exposed to UVA (5 J/cm^2) and then cultured in the serum free medium containing test samples for 4, 8, 24, and 48 hrs. Intracellular MMP-1 protein levels, at the indicated times, were assessed by Western blot analysis using human MMP-1 specific antibody. The blot is representative of two separate experiments and represents a single immunoblot. (B) Fibroblasts were exposed to UVA (5 J/cm^2) and then cultured in serum free medium containing test samples for 24 to 48 hrs. MMP-1 protein levels in cultured medium were assessed by Western blot analysis using human MMP-1 specific antibody. The blot is representative of two separate experiments and represents a single immunoblot.)

4.3.2. Effect of 3,3'-bisdemethylpinoresinol on MAPKs phosphorylation in UVA-irradiated NHDFs

The effect of **1** on activation of MAPKs was investigated by Western blot analysis. JNK and p38 MAPK phosophorylation in UVA irradiated NHDFs versus incubation time is shown in Fig. 7A. JNK phosophorylation was enhanced in a more rapid and transient manner at 0.5 to 1 hr after UVA irradiation, whereas that of p38 MAPK was enhanced at 0 to 1 hr. Therefore, the effect of **1** (0.1 and 0.3 μM) on JNK and p38 MAPK phosophorylation in UVA-irradiated NHDFs was examined at 0.5 hr after irradiation. As shown in Fig. 7B, **1** (0.1 μM) had no inhibitory effect of JNK and p38 MAPK, whereas **1** (0.3 μM) inhibited phosphorylation of both [20].

The results suggest that 1 inhibits MMP-1 secretion in UVA-irradiated NHDFs by decreasing JNK and p38 phosphorylation and suppressing c-Jun and c-Fos expression. This, subsequently, inhibits AP-1 and MMP-1 expression, resulting in a reduction in MMP- secretion.

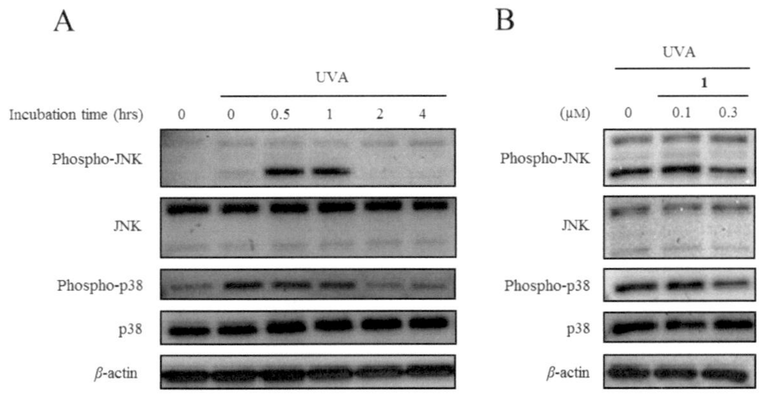

Figure 7. Time Course of MAPKs Phosphorylation in UVA-Irradiated NHDFs (B) Effect of 3,3'-Bisdemethylpinoresinol (1) on MAPKs Phosphorylation in UVA-Irradiated NHDFs ((A) Fibroblasts were exposed to UVA (5 J/cm^2) and then cultured in the serum free medium for the indicated time. Total cellular proteins were prepared for Western blot analysis of MAPKs and phospho-MAPKs proteins using the antibodies against phospho-form and total-form of JNK and p38. *β*-actin was used as an internal control. The blot is representative of three separate experiments and represents a single immunoblot. (B) Fibroblasts were exposed to UVA (5 J/cm^2) and then cultured in the serum free medium for 0.5 hr. Total cellular proteins were prepared for Western blot analysis of MAPKs and phospho-MAPKs proteins using the antibodies against phospho-form and total-form of JNK and p38. *β*-actin was used for internal control. The blot is representative of three separate experiments and represents a single immunoblot.)

5. Inhibitory effect of noni seeds on poor blood fluidity

In addition to melanogenesis and degradation of collagen by HLE and MMP-1, blood stagnation may also contribute to hyperpigmented spots on the skin. In oriental medicine, the clinical state of blood stasis in the venous system is called "Oketsu" in Japanese. Accumulation of wastes caused by blood stagnation in the skin leads to pigmentation. Degradation of blood flow, leading to dry skin and atrophy, also leads to wrinkle formation. Therefore, improved blood fluidity is likely to prevent formation of pigmented spots and wrinkles. As cosmetic ingredients that improve blood fluidity are desired for use in anti-photoaging products, the effect of noni seeds on poor blood fluidity was investigated.

5.1. Antithrombotic effect of noni seeds in a disseminated intravascular coagulation (DIC) rat model

The effect of noni seeds on excessive increased blood coagulation, accompanying poor blood fluidity, was examined by using a DIC rat model, induced by lipopolysaccharide (LPS) [25, 26].

Each Seed-ext (200 and 500 mg/kg) was administrated orally once a day to the rats for 7 successive days. LPS was injected on Day 7. Four hrs after injection, blood samples were collected from the abdominal great vein (vena cava). Whole blood passage time was measured by a micro channel array flow analyzer (MC-FAN). As shown in Table 6, the vehicle control group (LPS-induced) significantly prolonged blood passage time, in comparison with the control group. However, Seed-ext dose-dependently reduced passage time [27].

Platelet count, fibrinogen and fibrin degradation products (FDP) were also measured. Seed-ext had no effect on any of these hematological parameters (Table 6) [27].

Samples	Dose [a)]	Route [b)]	Blood passage time (s) [c)]	Platelets ($\times 10^4/\mu l$)	Fibrinogen (mg/dl)	FDP (μg/ml)
Control		*p.o.*	17±1	81.1±2.5	198.0±5.2	0.43±0.06
Vehicle control		*p.o.*	1813±34[ii]	18.4±1.1[ii]	96.6±3.9[ii]	2.06±0.17[ii]
Seed-ext	200 (mg/kg)	*p.o.*	1722±16[iii]	26.7±0.5[i]	96.7±2.9	1.86±0.11
	500 (mg/kg)	*p.o.*	1413±19[i]	22.5±0.8	105.2±2.7	1.75±0.07
Heparin	500 (U/kg)	i.v.	26±1[i]	46.1±2.8[i]	194.1±7.2[i]	0.52±0.15[iii]

Table 6. Effects of Seed-ext and Heparin on Blood Passage Time, Platelet Count, Fibrinogen, and FDP in Rats, after LPS Injection (Each value represents the mean±S.E. (*n*=7). Significantly different from the control group, [ii]: $p<0.01$. Significantly different from the vehicle control group, [iii]: $p<0.05$, [i]: $p<0.01$. [a)] For 7 successive days, 0.2% CMC-Na was administered orally to control and vehicle control groups. Each extract (200 and 500 mg/kg) was suspended with CMC-Na and administrated orally to each test group once daily for 7 successive days (Day 1-7). 1 hr after the final daily dose on Day 7, LPS (1 mg/kg, dissolved in saline, i.v.) was injected into the tail vein. Heparin (500 U/kg, dissolved in saline, i.v.) was administered intravenously to the rats 1 hr before LPS injection on Day 7 to the heparin group. [b)] *p.o.*: oral administration, i.v.: intravenous administration [c)] Blood passage time measured by MC-FAN as the time taken for the flow of 50 μl of sample mixture (1.8 ml of blood and 0.2 ml of 3.8% sodium citrate solution).

The results from the DIC rat model experiments suggest that Seed-ext improves poor blood fluidity. Therefore, noni seeds may help reduce pigmentation associated with blood stagnation.

5.2. Inhibitory effect of noni seeds, and active consituents, on platelet aggregation

Blood fluidity, as measured by using MC-FAN, is influenced by erythroid deformability, leukocytic adherence ability and thrombocytic agglutinability [28, 29]. Blood flow regulating factors in microcirculation have vascular systemic and blood component functions. Circulatory system function deteriorates with platelet aggregation induced coagulation, degradation of erythrocyte deformability, hemagglutination, elevation of plasma viscosity, and by degradation of fibrinolytic system activation [28, 29].

In order to examine the inhibitory effect of Seed-ext on blood coagulation, collagen-induced platelet aggregation [30] and polybrene-induced erythrocyte aggregation [31], *in vitro* tests were carried out. Seed-ext did not inhibit platelet aggregation (data not shown). But it did inhibit hemagglutination at concentrations ranging from 50 to 500 μg/ml (Table 7). As shown in Table 7, **3** inhibited platelet aggregation at 10 to 50 μM. Lingnans **1** and **2** had weak effects of platelet aggregation, when comparison to **3** [27].

The results suggest that one inhibitory mechanisms behind the effect of Seed-ext on poor blood fluidity in the DIC rat model may be anti-hemaggulatination by 1, 2, and 3.

Samples	**Concentration**	**Aggregation (%)**	**Inhibition (%)**
Control		45±1	
Seed-ext	50 (μg/ml)	27±1[i]	40
	200 (μg/ml)	8±1[i]	82
	500 (μg/ml)	9±1[i]	81
1	10 (μM)	42±1	7
	20 (μM)	39±1	13
	50 (μM)	34±1[i]	24
	100 (μM)	27±1[i]	41
2	10 (μM)	42±2	7
	20 (μM)	41±1	9
	50 (μM)	38±1	16
	100 (μM)	32±1[i]	29
3	5 (μM)	40±0	11
	10 (μM)	31±2[i]	31
	20 (μM)	10±5[i]	78
	50 (μM)	7±2[i]	84
Neuraminidase	7.8 (mU/ml)	36±2	19
	15.6 (mU/ml)	33±3[i]	27
	31.3 (mU/ml)	23±1[i]	48
	62.5 (mU/ml)	17±1[i]	63
	125 (mU/ml)	8±0[i]	82

Table 7. Effects of Seed-ext, **1**, **2**, **3** and Neuraminidase on Polybrene-Induced Erythrocyte Aggregation (Each value represents the mean±S.E. of 3 experiments. Significantly different from control group, [iii]: *p*<0.05, [i]: *p*<0.01.)

5.3. Fibrinolytic activity of noni seeds in rats

Activation of the fibrinolytic system improves blood flow by promoting the lysis of thrombi in blood vessel walls. To better understand the fibrinolytic potential of Seed-ext, as it relates to degradation of blood fluidity, the euglobulin lysis time (ELT) assay in normal rats was conducted. ELT is the time required for the disappearance of a fibrin clot produced by the addition of thrombin to the eugloblin fraction obtained from blood samples [32]. A reduction in ELT reveals activation of fibrinolysis activity, whereas an extension in ELT implies reduced activity [32].

Seed-ext was administrated orally, and 1 hr later, blood samples were collected. Then ELT was measured using eugloblin fractions from the sample. As shown in Table 8, Seed-ext significantly reduced ELT at dosages from 50 and 200 mg/kg in dose-dependent manner. This reveals that Seed-ext may have an enhancing effect on fibrinolysis activity [27].

Samples	Dose	Route	ELT (min)
Control A [a)]		*p.o.*	98±2
Seed-ext	50 (mg/kg)	*p.o.*	55±5[i]
	200 (mg/kg)	*p.o.*	42±7[i]
Control B [b)]		i.v.	97±2
Dextran sulphate sodium salt	5 (mg/kg)	i.v.	32±3[ii]

Table 8. Effects of Seed-ext and Dextran Sulphate Sodium Salt on ELT in Rats ([a)] Control A is a control for extracts. [b)] Control B is a control for dextran sulphate sodium salt. Each value represents the mean±S.E. of 7 rats. Significantly different from control A group, [i]: $p<0.01$. Significantly different from control B group, [ii]: $p<0.01$.)

Seed-ext has an inhibitory effect on hemagglutination. But it also activates fibrinolysis, suggesting that it may improve blood flow through anti-coagulation and fibrinolysis systems. As such, noni seeds may be a useful supplementary ingredient for the prevention of both pigmented spots and wrinkles caused by venous blood stagnation.

6. Conclusion

We are the first to investigate and find 4 inhibitory effects—namely tyrosinase, melanogenesis, HLE, and MMP-1—for noni seeds related to prevention of pigmented spots and wrinkles by photoaging. As a desirable anti-photoaging agent that is antagonistic to the UV signaling pathways of photoaging, Seed-ext may be a useful novel cosmetic ingredient for the prevention or treatment for pigmented spots and wrinkles. Since we found Seed-ext may improve blood fluidity, it may also be a useful supplemental ingredient aimed for beauty. However, further research, including clinical trials, is needed.

Noni fruit flesh and leaves have been used as functional foods, but the seeds have been discarded without utilization in most cases. Production of a cosmetic ingredient from noni seeds adds significant value to this largely unused natural resource.

Author details

Hideaki Matsuda[1], Megumi Masuda[1], Kazuya Murata[1], Yumi Abe[2] and Akemi Uwaya[2]

1 Faculty of Pharmacy, Kinki University, Japan

2 Research & Development, Morinda Worldwide, Inc., Japan

References

[1] Yaar M., Gilchrest B. A., Photoageing: mechanism, prevention and therapy., British Journal of Dermatology, 2007; 157, 874-887.

[2] Ross I. A., Medicinal Plants of the World Vol. II., Totowa: Humana press; 2001, p309-317.

[3] Youngken H. W., Jenkins H. J., Butler C. L., Studies on *Morinda citrifolia* L. II., Journal of the American Pharmaceutical Association, 1960; 49, 271-273.

[4] Kamiya K., Hamabe W., Harada S., Murakami R., Tokuyama S., Satake T., Chemical constituents of *Morinda citrifolia* roots exhibit hypoglycemic effects in streptozotocin-induced diabetic mice., Biological and Pharmaceutical Bulletin, 2008; 31(5), 935-938.

[5] Wang M. Y., Su C., Cancer preventive effect of *Morinda citrifolia* (Noni)., Annals of the New York Academy of Sciences, 2001; 952, 161-168.

[6] Pande M., Naiker M., Mills G., Singh N., Voro T., The Kura files: qualitative social survey., Pacific Health Dialog, 2005; 12(2), 85-93.

[7] Tobin D., Thody A. J., The superoxide anion may mediate short- but not long-term effects of ultraviolet radiation on melanogenesis., Experimental Dermatology, 1994; 3(3), 99-105.

[8] Masuda M., Murata K., Fukuhama A., Naruto S., Fujita T., Uwaya A., Isami F., Matsuda H., Inhibitory effects of constituents of *Morinda citrifolia* seeds on elastase and tyrosinase., Journal of Natural Medicines, 2009; 63(3), 267-273.

[9] Ohguchi K., Akao Y., Nozawa Y., Involvement of calpain in melanogenesis of mouse B16 melanoma cells., Molecular and Cellular Biochemistry, 2005; 275(1-2), 103-107.

[10] Masuda M., Itoh K., Murata K., Naruto S., Uwaya A., Isami F., Matsuda H., Inhibitory effects of *Morinda citrifolia* extract and its constituents on melanogenesis in murine B16 melanoma cells., Biological and Pharmaceutical Bulletin, 2012; 35(1), 78-83.

[11] Widlund H. R., Fisher D. E., Microphthalamia-associated transcription factor: a critical regulator of pigment cell development and survival., Oncogene, 2003; 22(20), 3035-3041.

[12] Kim D.-S., Hwang E.-S., Lee J.-E., Kim S.-Y., Kwon S.-B., Park K.-C., Sphingosine-1-phosphate decreases melanin synthesis via sustained ERK activation and subsequent MITF degradation., Journal of Cell Science, 2003; 116, 1699-1706.

[13] Smalley K., Eisen T., The involvement of p38 mitogen-activated protein kinase in the alpha-melanocyte stimulating hormone (alpha-MSH)-induced melanogenic and anti-proliferative effects in B16 murine melanoma cells., FEBS Letters, 2000; 476(3), 198-202.

[14] Rittié L., Fisher G. J., UV-light-induced signal cascades and skin aging., Ageing Research Reviews, 2002; 1(5), 705-720.

[15] Rijken F., Kiekens R. C. M., Bruijnzeel P. L. B., Skin-infiltrating neutrophils following exposure to solar-simulated radiation could play an important role in photoageing of human skin., British Journal of Dermatology, 2005; 152(2), 321-328.

[16] Kafienah W., Buttle D. J., Burnett D., Hollander A. P., Cleavage of native type I collagen by human neutrophil elastase., The Biochemical Journal, 1998; 330, 897-902.

[17] Grant G. M., Giambernardi T. A., Grant A. M., Klebe R. J., Overview of expression of matrix metalloproteinases (MMP-17, MMP-18, and MMP-20) in cultured human cells., Matrix Biology, 1999; 18(2), 145-148.

[18] Wang X.-Y., Bi Z.-G., UVB-irradiated human keratinocytes and interleukin-1alpha indirectly increase MAP kinase/AP-1 activation and MMP-1 production in UVA-irradiated dermal fibroblasts., Chinese Medical Journal, 2006; 119(10), 827-831.

[19] Takeuchi H., Gomi T., Shishido M., Watanabe H., Suenobu N., Neutrophil elastase contributes to extracellular matrix damage induced by chronic low-dose UV irradiation in a hairless mouse photoaging model., Journal of Dermatological Science, 2010; 60(3), 151-158.

[20] Masuda M., Murata K., Naruto S., Uwaya A., Isami F., Matsuda H., Matrix metalloproteinase-1 inhibitory activities of *Morinda citrifolia* seed extract and its constituents in UVA-irradiated human dermal fibroblasts., Biological and Pharmaceutical Bulletin, 2012; 35(2), 210-215.

[21] Brennan M., Bhatti H., Nerusu K. C., Bhagavathula N., Kang S., Fisher G. J., Varani J., Voorhees J. J., Matrix metalloproteinase-1 is the major collagenolytic enzyme responsible for collagen damage in UV-irradiated human skin., Photochemistry and Photobiology, 2003; 78(1), 43-48.

[22] Suganuma K., Nakajima H., Ohtsuki M., Imokawa G., Astaxanthin attenuates the UVA-induced up-regulation of matrix metalloproteinase-1 and skin fibroblast elastase in human dermal fibroblasts., Journal of Dermatological Science, 2010; 58(2), 136-142.

[23] Oh H.-I., Shim J.-S., Gwon S.-H., Kwon H.-J., Hwang J.-K., The effect of xanthorrhizol on the expression of matrix metalloproteinase-1 and type-I procollagen in ultraviolet-irradiated human skin fibroblasts., Phytotherapy Research, 2009; 23(9), 1299-1302.

[24] Fisher G. J., Talwar H. S., Lin J., Lin P., McPhillips F., Wang Z., Li X., Wan Y., Kang S., Voorhees J. J., Retinoic acid inhibits induction of c-Jun protein by ultraviolet radiation that occurs subsequent to activation of mitogen-activated protein kinase pathways in human skin *in vivo*., The Journal of Clinical Investigation, 1998; 101(6), 1432-1440.

[25] Schoendorf T. H., Rosenberg M., Beller F. K., Endotoxin-induced disseminated intravascular coagulation in nonpregnant rats. A new experimental model., The American Journal of Pathology, 1971; 65(1), 51-58.

[26] Chang G.-T., Min S.-Y., Kim J.-H., Kim S.-H., Kim J.-K., Kim C.-H., Anti-thrombic activity of Korean herbal medicine, Dae-Jo-Whan and its herbs., Vascular Pharmacology, 2005; 43(4), 283-288.

[27] Masuda M., Murata K., Itoh K., Naruto S., Uwaya A., Isami F., Matsuda H., Effects of *Morinda citrifolia* extract and its constituents on blood fluidity., Journal of Traditional Medicines, 2011, 28(2), 47-54.

[28] Seki K., Sumino H., Murakami M., Study on blood rheology measured by MC-FAN., Rinsho Byori, 2003; 51(8), 770-775.

[29] Itoh K., Masuda M., Naruto S., Murata K., Matsuda H., Effects of unripe *Citrus hassaku* fruits extract and its flavanone glycosides on blood fluidity., Biological and Pharmaceutical Bulletin, 2010; 33(4), 659-664.

[30] Born G. V. R., Cross M. J., The Aggregation of Blood Platelets., The Journal of Physiology, 1963; 168, 178-195.

[31] Sabio H., Levien M., Atkinson S., Continuous recording of red cell interactions., Thrombosis Research, 1983; 29(5), 537-540.

[32] Sakuragawa N., Euglobulin lysis time., Nihon Rinsho, 1997; 55, 139-144.

Chapter 24

Inhibiting S100B in Malignant Melanoma

Kira G. Hartman, Paul T. Wilder, Kristen Varney,
Alexander D. Jr. MacKerell, Andrew Coop,
Danna Zimmer, Rena Lapidus and David J. Weber

Additional information is available at the end of the chapter

http://dx.doi.org/10.5772/55176

1. Introduction

The development of new therapies for patients diagnosed with malignant melanoma is in high need. In this chapter, the design and testing of inhibitors are discussed for S100B, a calcium-binding protein that down-regulates the tumor suppressor p53. Because p53 is wild type in many malignant melanoma patients, the restoration of p53 with S100B inhibitors (SBiXs) represents a new and potentially effective strategy for sensitizing melanoma cells to p53-dependent apoptosis pathways and for targeting this deadly cancer. Such a strategy requires blocking of the S100B-p53 protein-protein interaction (PPI) and involves methods including computer aided drug design (CADD), screening technologies, nuclear magnetic resonance (NMR), X-ray crystallography, and medicinal chemistry approaches. The ultimate goal is to design a highly specific and potent inhibitor of S100B that has clinical value.

2. The S100 protein family

The S100 family of EF-hand calcium-binding proteins has more than 20 members, with the genes encoding these proteins present only in vertebrates [7]. S100 proteins (S100s) are expressed in both a cell type and tissue-specific manner to provide diverse functional roles including calcium homeostasis, cell-cell communication, cell proliferation, differentiation, cytoskeletal dynamics, and cell morphology [7-10]. On the other hand, dysregulation of S100 expression is observed in several types of cancers, including malignant melanoma [7-9]. They are also problematic when elevated in several cognitive disorders including those arising from traumatic brain injuries [12-16]. While S100 proteins themselves have no inherent enzymatic activity, they regulate important biological processes via specific Ca^{2+}-dependent protein-protein interactions [17,18].

The first members of the S100 family were discovered in 1965 in a subcellular fraction from bovine brain tissue and were named based on their solubility in 100% saturated ammonium sulfate. When this protein fraction was examined in detail, two similar, but distinct proteins were discovered and designated S100α and S100β that are now referred to as S100A1 and S100B, respectively [17,19]. As with S100A1 and S100B, other S100s have a similar molecular weight (9-12 kDa), have homologous amino acid sequences (>40%), and typically exist as symmetric homodimers, or as heterodimers, held together by noncovalent interactions as pairs of four-helix bundles [20,21]. Two EF-hand helix-loop-helix calcium-binding structural motifs, first defined using the "E" and "F" helices from the X-ray crystal structure of parvalbumin, are present in each S100 subunit [22]. The N-terminal "*S100*" or "*pseudo*" EF-hand (EF1) is comprised of 14 rather than the original 12 residues and this 14 amino acid sequence readily distinguishes S100s from other EF-hand calcium signaling proteins. The canonical EF-hand (EF2) is found at the C-terminus of each subunit and typically binds Ca^{2+} with a higher affinity than EF1. The two EF-hand domains are connected by a stretch of amino acid residues (<25 residues) termed the "hinge region". This "hinge" together with the C-terminal loop of the S100 protein contains the least amount of sequence homology and, therefore, represents the two regions that give each family member their individual target-binding specificity [7,8,23]. In addition to binding Ca^{2+}, several S100s bind Zn^{2+} at a separate site from the EF-hand calcium-binding domains. The Zn^{2+} site can also bind other metals (i.e. Mn^{2+}, Cu^{2+}, and others) and has two ligating residues contributed from each subunit at the dimer interface to provide tetrahedral coordination that is typical for Zn^{2+} [24]. However, for S100B, Zn^{2+}-binding is not sufficient to induce target binding on its own, but rather functions by increasing the affinity S100B has for Ca^{2+} and its target proteins [25,26].

Figure 1. Structures of apo- versus holo-S100B. Ribbon diagrams comparing the NMR solution structures of calcium-free (left) and calcium-bound S100B (right), illustrating the 90° reorientation of helices 3 and 3′ in each subunit of S100B. Shown in yellow on one subunit is the S100B target binding site that is exposed after the Ca^{2+}-dependent conformational change.

http://dx.doi.org/10.5772/55176

3. S100B structure & interactions with ions

As with most S100 proteins, each 91 amino acid subunit of S100B has four alpha helices arranged into two helix-loop-helix (HLH) calcium-binding motifs connected by the flexible "hinge" region. Helix 1 and 2 make up the S100 EF-hand, while helix 3 and 4 form the canonical EF-hand (Figure 1). Each S100B subunit, therefore, binds two molecules of calcium, though with significantly different affinities [27]. While the canonical EF-hand binds Ca^{2+} with moderate affinity (K_D = 20 – 50 μM), the weaker S100 EF-hand binds Ca^{2+} with a much lower affinity (K_D = 200 – 500 μM) [27-30]. Calcium binding induces a dramatic conformational change in S100B where helix 3 rotates by 90º to become perpendicular to helix 4 (Figure 1). This change in conformation exposes a unique binding pocket, which in turn, binds to targets specific for each S100 protein generating a biological response [23]. However, it is clear that the dissociation constants of calcium from most S100s *in vitro*, including S100B, are too weak to compete on their own for free Ca^{2+} typically present in the cytosol (100 to 500 nM). Interestingly, it is now understood that the affinity of S100s for Ca^{2+} is increased by as much as 300-fold when bound to biologically relevant target proteins (i.e. at 100 nM free Ca^{2+}) suggesting that S100s typically only sequester free Ca^{2+} when their biologically relevant targets are present at optimal levels within the cell [31-34]. While the mechanism for this allosteric tightening of Ca^{2+} is not completely understood, it is known that when a target peptide derived from CapZ (termed TRTK-12) is bound to S100B, a loss in μs-ms motions occurs throughout the protein including in the side chain of a Ca^{2+}-coordinating residues. These results were consistent with the hypotheses that stabilizing motions, particularly for Ca^{2+}-coordinating residue(s) in EF2, could be responsible for the significant increase in Ca^{2+}-ion binding affinity observed when a target is bound to Ca^{2+}-S100B [35]. Likewise, the binding of S100B to Zn^{2+} (K_D = 90 ± 20 nM) stabilizes residues in the C-terminus of the protein, resulting in an increase in both Ca^{2+}- and target-binding affinities [28,36].

Thus, as with many EF-hand proteins, S100 signaling proteins do not bind Ca^{2+} with high affinity unless they are bound to their biologically relevant protein target(s) [32-34,37,38]. In other words, in the absence of a bound target, the Ca^{2+}-binding affinity for most S100 proteins is relatively low (i.e. in the μM range [1,17,27,39], but when bound to peptides (i.e. TRTK-12) or full-length targets, the Ca^{2+}-binding affinity can be increased by 5- to 300-fold, respectively [32-34,37,38,40]. This property is physiologically necessary because while there are over 600 EF-hand Ca^{2+}-binding domains within any given cell, Ca^{2+} homeostasis must be maintained with sufficient free Ca^{2+} ion concentrations for proper signaling (i.e. 100 to 500 nM). Thus, as a physiological control mechanism, S100s and many other EF-hand proteins do not sequester significant amounts of free Ca^{2+} unless their functionally relevant molecular target is available [29,34,38]. It is especially important for drug design that we continue to investigate and understand this phenomenon at the molecular level because S100 inhibitor binding must mimic the EF-hand-target complex and allosterically tighten Ca^{2+} ion binding affinity upon complex formation to be effective inside the cell [35,37]. For S100B, this includes targets such as p53, hdm2, hdm4, Rsk1 and RAGE, among others, which subsequently contributes to a Ca^{2+}-mediated growth response in a cell-specific manner, including those in skin and brain (Table 1).

4. S100B pathology

The protein S100B is found in melanocytes, glial cells, chondrocytes, and adipocytes, exhibiting both intra- and extracellular functionality. The cellular responses elicited by S100B can vary depending on several factors, including concentration (nM or μM), cell type, and cellular location [8,9]. Of particular concern is the role of elevated S100B in melanoma (Figure 2), the most deadly of all skin cancers, notorious for its resistence to chemotherapy and radiation. Clinical studies have established S100B as an effective biomarker for melanoma; however, this is only the case when highly specific S100B antibodies are used [12]. For example, in one study, samples from 412 melanoma patients at varying stages were compared to those diagnosed with non-melanoma skin cancers and inflammatory cutaneous diseases. Using a cutoff value of 0.2 μg/l serum S100B, a positive correlation was observed for patients having S100B levels above the cutoff level and advancement of tumor stage, indicative of a contribution by S100B to micro- and/or macro-metastases [41-43]. Though elevated S100B cannot be used to identify tumor thickness or lympth node status, it is predictive of poor patient prognosis, increased tumor recurrence, and low overall survival [9,41-44]. Subsequent studies reinforce these findings and consistently show elevated levels of S100B to be a sensitive and specific marker of melanoma progression with the ability to detect metastases or relapse at much earlier timepoints. S100B levels can also be used to monitor treatment strategies for rapid identification of whether a particular therapy is promising or for deciding to take an alternative approach [9]. While S100B is a useful prognostic indicator for melanoma, its use as a biomarker for several other cancers with elevated S100B is still under investigation; including colorectal cancer [45-47], several gliomas [48,49], mengiomas [50], non-small cell lung cancer (NSCLC) [51], renal cell carcinoma (RCC) [52], and thyroid carcinoma [53]. In addition, these clinical observations underscore the need to fully understand the role of elevated S100B in cancer, which is ongoing [2-4,54].

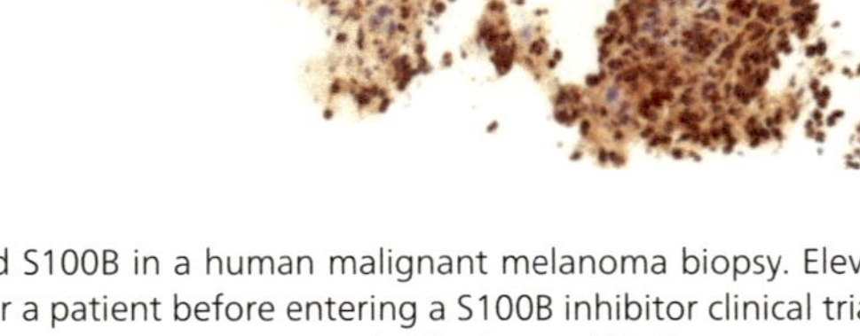

Figure 2. Staining for elevated S100B in a human malignant melanoma biopsy. Elevated S100B is stained brown in this human biopsy recorded for a patient before entering a S100B inhibitor clinical trial (SBi1). Patients are also tested for their p53 status and S100B:p53 ratio as recommended by Lin et al [2-4].

Although not considered in detail here, S100B also plays an important role in the brain, and as with cancer, several cognitive disorders show over-expression of S100B in brain tissue and are associated with pathological states including Alzheimer's disease (AD), Down's syndrome (DS), and schizophrenia [55-59]. One mechanism for this pathology is that elevated intracellular levels of S100B present in glial cells are excreted and regulate neighboring neuronal cell activity. At low levels, the presence of this extracellular S100B is sufficient to promote neurite extension and growth, while elevated S100B levels are toxic and lead to neuronal cell apoptosis [9,60]. As with skin cancer, the clinical utility of S100B as a marker to identify and characterize neurological diseases and traumas is complicated by overlapping expression of S100B and other S100s in several cell types, its multiple mechanisms of secretion, and its association with more than one neurodegenerative disorder [14]. However, as found for melanoma, lowering S100B levels upon drug delivery is one means used to evaluate drug efficacy for treating schizophrenia [16,61]. Furthermore, the development of S100B inhibitors themselves may be useful for the treatment of these neuropathies, making the identification of such compounds important for advancing efforts towards understanding and treating cancers and cognitive disorders in which S100B levels are at pathologically high levels [62].

Cellular Activity	Protein	References
Ca^{2+} Homeostasis	AHNAK*	[26]
Cell Cycle Regulation	Hdm2, Hdm4	[63]
	NDR	[64,65]
Cytoskeletal Regulation	Caldesmon*	[66]
	Calponin	[67]
	CapZα	[68]
	GFAP	[69]
	IQGAP1	[70]
	MARCKS*	[71]
	Src kinase	[26]
	τ-protein*	[72]
	Tubulin	[73]
Energy Metabolism	Fructose 1,6 bisphosphate aldolase	[74]
	Phosphoglucomutase	[75]
Growth & Survival	p53*	[1,28,76,77]

*PKC-mediated phosphorylation target proteins

Table 1. Targets of S100B

5. S100B targets

The ability of S100B to bind a diverse array of protein and enzyme targets is attributable to its broad consensus target-binding sequence [63]. S100B targets include proteins involved in calcium homeostasis, cell-cycle regulation, cytoskeletal regulation, energy metabolism, and growth/survival (Table 1). One common theme among several S100B-target interactions is that they regulate protein phosphorylation [78]. For example, S100B associates with nuclear Dbf2-related (NDR) protein by binding a region distinct from the active site and inducing a conformational change, which stimulates autophosphorylation, and ultimately activates the protein [64]. S100B also regulates phosphorylation by binding to kinase substrates such as those of protein kinase C (PKC) and sterically blocking phosphorylation [76,77,79] (Table 1). This includes the myristoylated alanine-rich C-kinase substrate (MARCKS), τ-protein, and caldesmon to name a few [66,80,81]. One noteable S100B target is the PKC substrate, p53, which is activated by phosphorylation in the C-terminal negative regulatory domain (NRD). In addition to blocking PKC-dependent phosphorylation, the S100B-p53 complex formation shifts the p53 tetramer to dimer to monomer equilibrium towards oligomer dissociation [76,78]. Thus, for p53, when S100B levels are too high, PKC-mediated activation of p53 is inhibited and p53 tetramers are dissociated. Consequently, p53 cannot bind DNA, which affects its transcriptional activity [2,28,76,77,82,83] and inhibits its ability to control cell cycle progression and apoptosis [2-4]. Other S100B targets include the E3 that designates p53 for ubiquitination, Hdm2, and the Hdm2 regulator, Hdm4 [63]. Thus, studies are underway to understand how S100B complexes involving Hdm2/Hdm4 contribute to lowering p53 levels in melanoma. Complicating this is the fact that both of these negative regulators of p53, Hdm2 and S100B, are themselves transcriptionally regulated by p53 [4,63]. This feedback regulatory mechanism results in time-dependent regulation of p53 that depends on having correct levels of all four proteins for proper regulation of cell cycle growth arrest and apoptosis [63]. Since elevated S100B disrupts the maintenance of p53 levels and promotes a cancerous phenotype, the development of small molecule inhibitors designed to target Ca^{2+}-bound S100B has become a high priority. Specifically, investigations are focused on the identification of compounds capable of blocking the Ca^{2+}-dependent S100B-p53 interaction in malignant melanoma (Figure 3). Ideally, administration of such compounds would reactivate p53 in malignant melanoma, as found for $siRNA^{S100B}$, to induce normal apoptosis pathways and reduce proliferation/survival of the cancer cells [2-4].

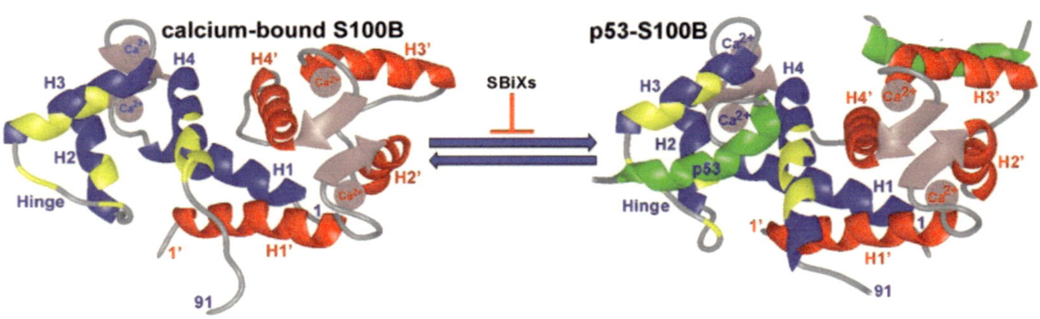

Figure 3. Illustration of the p53-binding site on S100B. Shown are ribbon diagrams Ca^{2+}-bound S100B (NMR), $p53^{367-388}$-bound Ca^{2+}-bound S100B (NMR, PDB entry 1DT7). The helices of S100B are colored in blue, while the $p53^{367-388}$ peptide is shown in red. Gray spheres represent the two calcium molecules per subunit. S100B inhibitors (SBiXs) are being developed to inhibit the Ca^{2+}-dependent formation of the S100B-p53 complex.

6. Targeting the S100B-p53 interaction

Binding of S100B to p53 blocks PKC-dependent phosphorylation, p53 tetramerization, and p53-dependent transcription activation [28,63,76,82,83]. Therefore, efforts to restore wild-type p53 activities in malignant melanoma are underway as part of a drug design strategy [28]. A combination of approaches is being used, including those involving target validation and screening, computer aided drug design, structural biology, medicinal chemistry, and *in vivo* biology and drug testing methods (Figure 4). In one case, a previously FDA approved drug was discovered to block the S100B-p53 interaction. The wealth of available data associated with this compound, including its use in animals and human clinical trials made repurposing it for use in malignant melanoma a fairly quick transition.

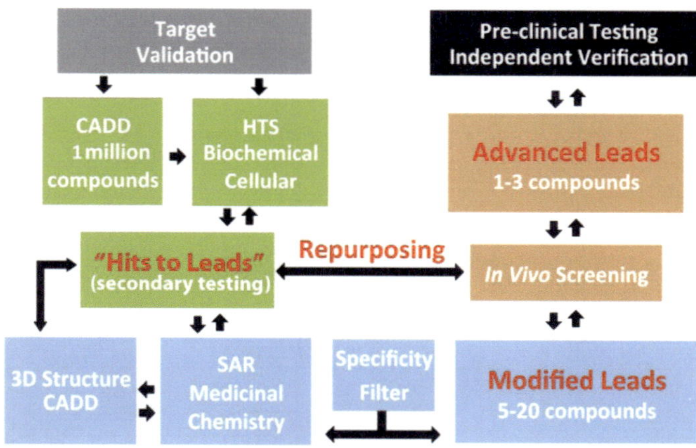

Figure 4. Summary of strategies for advancing hits from screening studies to leads, modified leads, and then advanced lead compounds. This schematic is a general guideline for the early stages of drug development. The data from these approaches is compiled and used to choose "candidate" compounds that are studied more extensively in humans for their toxicology and effectiveness in treating cancer. It is oftern advantageous to consider repurposing compounds that are already known to be safe in humans as a means to advance this process more quickly.

Screening for S100B inhibitors was initiated using computer-aided drug design methods (CADD) [28,84], and in all steps of identifying and prioritizing "hits" during these and other screens, the pharmacological activity of compounds was evaluated semi-quantitatively, providing an unbiased means of eliminating compounds that do not fulfill specific "drug-like" criteria [84,85]. Compounds identified in screens are also evaluated regarding their potential for absorption, distribution, and metabolism/excretion (ADME) properties [86]. Among many CADD approaches, a recent structure-based technique termed Site Identification by Ligand Competitive Saturation (SILCS) is now used extensively [87-89]. The simultaneous presence of benzene, propane and water in MD simulations of the target protein (ie. S100B) in this fragment-based computational approach identifies potential binding regions for aliphatic moieties, aromatic moieties and hydrogen bond donors and acceptors, while simultaneously allowing for increased flexibility and conformational changes to occur within the drug-binding site [87-89]. In addition, SILCS is very useful for strategically modifying "hits" or "lead compounds" to span a larger area of the protein surface [87,88]. CADD methods such as these are particularly important for blocking protein-protein interactions (PPIs) such as that for the S100B-p53 complex since at least three distinct target binding pockets have been identified on S100B (Figure 5) [27,29,30,37,63,68,90,91]. As a result, the drug pentamidine diisethionate (Pnt), which is referred to as SBi1 (designated SBiX, where 'X' is an arbitrary compound number), was identified at a very early stage of the screening process as an effective inhibitor of the S100B-p53 complex [84]. Pnt was approved by the FDA as an antimicrobial agent for the treatment of Pneumocystis carinii pneumonia (PCP), which allowed for repurposing of this drug for *in vivo* testing for efficacy in treating malignant melanoma (Figure 4). To this end, a clinical trial is ongoing at the University of Maryland Medical Center (UMMC) to determine the efficacy of Pnt in melanoma patients *(0794GCC: "Treatment of melanoma with wild-type p53 and detectable S100B using pentamidine (SBi1): a Phase II trial with correlative biomarker end-points";* CA135624; PI: Dr. Ed Sausville, M.D.; Co-PI: Dr. David J. Weber). Although, there are promising results for the use of Pnt for the treatment of malignant melanoma, efforts have continued with the goal of engineering a compound with higher efficacy and more specificity for targeting S100B (versus other S100 proteins).

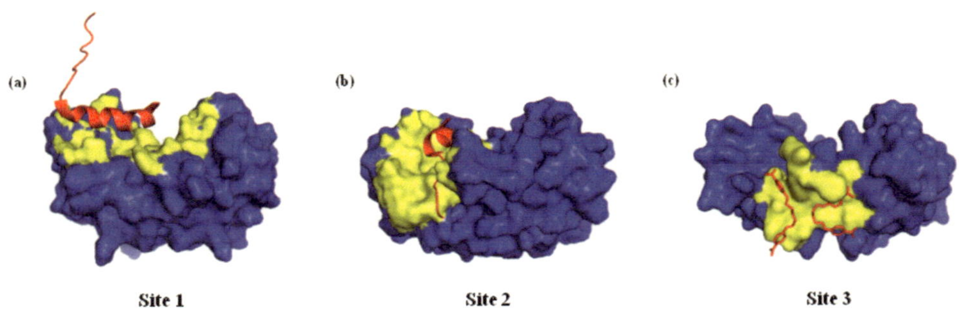

Figure 5. Three binding pockets are targeted on S100B. Surface representation of the structures of Ca^{2+}-S100B bound to (a) the C-terminal negative regulatory domain of p53 (PDB ID: 1DT7)(1), (b) TRTK-12 (PDB ID: 1MWN) [5], and (c) pentamidine, also referred to as SBi1 (PDB ID: 3CR4) [6]. Sites 1, 2, and 3 are labeled. The protein is depicted as a blue surface and the regions within 3 Å of the bound peptide or small molecule are colored yellow. TRTK-12, p53 peptide, and pentamidine are shown in red.

In addition to CADD, biochemical and cellular screening methods are continuously ongoing to identify "hits" that can be considered further as scaffolds for drug development (Figure 4). One sensitive method done *in vitro* is a fluorescence polarization competition assay (FPCA), which can identify PPI inhibitors in a high-throughput manner. This competition assay takes advantage of a small molecule inhibitor causing the dissociation of a small peptide-bound fluorophore from a larger protein-peptide complex. Specifically, SBiX inhibitors can readily be identified since the smaller, faster rotating free fluorophore-bound peptide will exhibit lower polarization when competed away by the SBiX and compared to the larger S100B-peptide complex. Importantly, the labeled-peptide must differ in molecular weight from the S100B-peptide complex to provide a reasonable dynamic range for the assay [92].

While it is important to show that an S100B-compound complex forms *in vitro*, it is also important to demonstrate that the SBiX has anti-cancer activity in cellular assays (i.e. growth inhibition, reduction in survival, increase apoptosis activity etc). In addition to showing compound efficacy in cells, these assays are important for providing information about other properties of the compound(s) including its membrane permeability and overall toxicity. One reliable method for identifying inhibitors of S100B-dependent pathways is via the creation of matched cell lines that only differ in S100B expression level. For example, MALME-3M melanoma cells were selected because they express elevated S100B protein levels and retain wild-type p53. Small interfering RNA (siRNA) was then stably transfected into the MALME-3M cells to give a scrambled siRNA control with high S100B levels and an isogenetically matched siRNA^{S100B} construct resulting in low S100B (unpublished data). These matched cell lines provided a means for a large-scale screen of compound libraries to identify SBiXs with potency and specificity towards pathways involving S100B. The "hits" in this cellular assay were then routinely tested for direct binding and secondary cellular assays were completed by comparing the effect of these hits on primary malignant melanoma cells side-by-side with normal melanocytes [84]. Compounds that result in indiscriminate cell death were considered toxic rather than from specific inhibition of S100B or an S100B-dependent pathway and highlighted the importance of including normal melanocytes in every screen. Preferential growth inhibition of melanoma with high S100B as compared to little or no effect on the melanocytes or cells containing siRNA^{S100B} was considered to be an early indication that the compound may have promising therapeutic value. This is exemplified with pentamidine, since treatment of C8146A primary melanoma cells resulted in significant cell growth inhibition, but little or no effect was noticed from this drug on normal melanocytes [84].

One of the most important requirements of any drug development program is to obtain physiological data at an early stage in the process to help determine whether a lead compound is effective and/or shows unanticipated toxicities *in vivo [93]*. This is particularly important for S100 inhibitors since there are over 20 structurally similar proteins in the S100 protein family, and they each regulate specific cellular pathway(s) [94,95]. To address these issues as quickly as possible, an *in vivo* screening assay was developed to test potential lead compounds for melanoma at an early stage in the drug development process. Once promising hits are designated as lead compounds via *in vitro* and cellular testing and secondary validation protocols, they need to be tested *in vivo*. Leads to be tested *in vivo* are chosen based on binding affinities (K_Ds) and/or specificity both in biochemical assays and in cellular assays. For the cellular assays, specificity and potential off-target effects are evaluated by comparing IC_{50} values of isogenic cell lines with or without S100B over-expression [96,97]. The vast majority of lead SBiXs are new chemical entities that require extensive optimization prior to entering *in vivo* testing, with the exception of those compounds that have been repurposed from other studies and trials. Animal models play a fundamental role in such *in vivo* testing. For example, a compound may need to be more lipophilic to pass through the cell membrane and reach its target or side groups may need to be added to allow for oral delivery or brain penetration. In the case of accessible tumors such as melanoma, drugs can be delivered directly to the tumor (intratumoral) without optimization for systemic delivery [93]. In addition, intratumoral delivery can achieve significantly higher drug concentrations at the site of action than can be obtained via systemic delivery. For this purpose a multi-allelic genetically engineered mouse model was chosen to test SBiX compounds since this model mimics spontaneous tumoriogenesis and heterogeneity as well as provide additional information necessary for additional target validation [98]. One such melanoma model is the RAS-induced INK4a/ARF$^{-/-}$ mouse [99], which was chosen for *in vivo* SBiX screening because it has: (i) an intact S100B-p53 signaling pathway (elevated S100B and wild type p53), (ii) an intact immune system, (iii) tumors which are amenable to intratumoral delivery, and (iv) a proven record in developing new melanoma therapies [99,100]. This screen utilizes 2-3 month old experimental Tyr::RAS^{G12V}/INK4a/ARF$^{-/-}$ male mice that develop spontaneous cutaneous melanomas in the pinna of the ears (30%), torso (23%), and tail (20%) without distant metastasis [99] and uses tumor proliferation rate as the primary outcome. Although the screen is not optimized for obtaining tolerability, PK or PD information, the gross/histological pathology, SBiX levels and p53 pathway reactivation in the tumors are monitored as is necessary to select more advanced leads that have potential for proceeding to pre-clinical testing (Table 2).

In the case of modified leads that have ADME properties favorable for systemic administration, concurrent tolerability (MTD) and pharmacokinetic (PK) assays are also conducted. MTD and PK trials are also performed to determine if a lead is suitable for pre-clinical testing or if it requires additional medicinal chemistry optimization and/or further evaluation prior to pre-clinical testing. If the compound is found to be toxic, then it is eliminated from further consideration. Should successful tumor shrinkage be observed in mice treated with the well-tolerated S100B inhibitors, an effort is then put in place to consider phase 1 or 2b human clinical trials.

Parameter	Leads	Modified Leads	Advanced Leads
K_D	<10 μM	<50 nM	<50 nM
IC_{50} in cells	<10 μM	<50 nM	<50 nM
Off target effects	$K_D \approx IC_{50}$	$K_D \approx IC_{50}$	$K_D \approx IC_{50}$
Activity in target (-/-) cells	<50%	<20%	<10%
CYP2D6 Metabolism	Not determined	No	No
P450 CYP induction	Not determined	<50% at 30 mM	<50% at 30 mM
Bioavailability	Not determined	Preferred oral	Preferred oral
Metabolic stability	Not determined	>80% after 1 hour	>80% after 1 hour
BSA Ligand K_D	Not determined	K_D> 10 mM	K_D> 10 mM
Specificity	>5:1	>50:1	>500:1

Table 2. Some criteria for leads, modified leads, and advanced leads

7. SBiX lead optimization

SBiX leads are typically optimized using structure-based drug design and by examining structure/activity relationships (SAR) using traditional medicinal chemistry approaches. Modified leads are also tested using cellular and *in vivo* assays described above to determine whether the modification improved efficacy, specificity, and other criteria listed in Table 2. Although several leads were identified for S100B and are undergoing optimization via a structure-based drug design approach, diverse scaffolds remain essential at this stage of development in case the existing lead compounds become intractable.

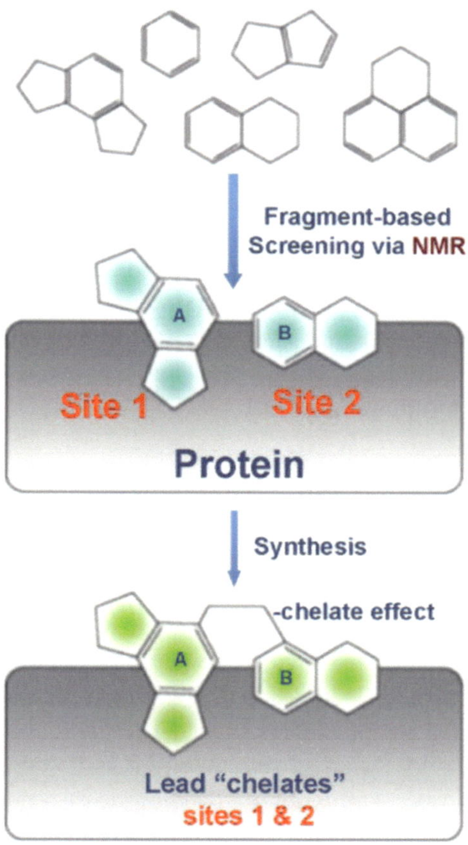

Figure 6. SAR by NMR [11]. NMR screens identify compounds that bind pockets "all over" the protein, which can be linked synthetically to obtain high affinity and specific SBiX inhibitors.

The availability of 3D structures of S100B-SBiX complexes allow for CADD to be used to select compounds from 3D chemical databases with an enhanced potential for binding to S100B [101-105] and/or to engineer compounds de novo via *in silico* methods [106,107]. In an iterative process, new S100B-drug complexes are solved, lead modifications to improve affinity predicted via CADD, predicted compounds synthesized and the resulting compounds experimentally evaluated. Work is also underway to develop novel inhibitors of S100B via a fragment-based approach that targets multiple binding sites on the protein identified by NMR, X-ray crystallography, and CADD techniques, including the new SILCS technique [87]. The SAR by NMR approach is now a standard method for quickly identifying ^{1}H-^{15}N and/or ^{1}H-^{13}C chemical shift perturbations in HSQC and/or TROSY spectra as a result of an S100B-small molecule interaction; this enables rapid, qualitative identification of binding site(s) on S100B for fragment-based design of new compounds that take advantage of the well-established "chelate effect" involved in linking fragments that bind neighboring sites [108,109] (Figure 6). For fast exchanging inhibitors, saturation transfer differences are collected to identify protons of the lead at the S100B-lead interface [84,110,111]. Thus, progress using a combination of functional-group optimization and the fragment-based approaches offers the potential for improvement in affinities/specificity, and for identifying novel leads. As new lead compounds are identified and structurally characterized (NMR, X-ray crystallography), SBiX affinity is considered as is scaffold diversity due to potential unforeseen problems with compounds that can occur during later-stage preclinical development (e.g. pharmacokinetic limitations, toxicity in humans). Therefore, as many as 3-6 chemical scaffolds are under consideration for development, and this number will be reduced as the project proceeds based on ADME properties, synthetic feasibility, and other pre-clinical/clinical information (Table 2). Such criteria include physiochemical properties related to bioavailability (molecular weight, clogP, TPSA, pKa, nitrogen atoms, carboxylates, H-bond donors, H-bond acceptors, rotatable bonds, H-bonds), and dose-limiting toxicities that may be predictive of the therapeutic index. Importantly, promising leads are routinely tested *in vivo* as early as possible to avoid wasted effort on toxic/ineffective compounds.

8. Summary

Ongoing collaborative efforts involving biology, structure determination, CADD and synthetic chemistry have lead to the development of a collection of inhibitors of S100B. These efforts include identification of the FDA approved compound pentamidine, which is currently being evaluated in human clinical trials. In addition, the work has identified several novel chemical scaffolds that are undergoing optimization and have laid the foundation for the application of fragment-based approaches to design additional novel scaffolds. Notably, while the goal of this research is to develop a potent inhibitor of S100B for the treatment of malignant melanoma, we anticipate that the knowledge gained to date will be of utility in designing specific inhibitors of other members of the S100 protein family for the treatment of a range of S100 associated disease states.

Acknowledgements

Support from the NIH (CA107331; to DJW), The Center for Biomolecular Therapeutics (CBT), and the University of Maryland Computer-Aided Drug Design Center is appreciated.

http://dx.doi.org/10.5772/55176

Author details

Kira G. Hartman[1], Paul T. Wilder[1,3,4], Kristen Varney[1,2,3], Alexander D. Jr. MacKerell[2,3,4], Andrew Coop[2,4], Danna Zimmer[1,3], Rena Lapidus[3,4] and David J. Weber[1,3,4*]

*Address all correspondence to: dweber@som.umaryland.edu

1 Department of Biochemistry and Molecular Biology, University of Maryland School of Medicine, Baltimore, MD, USA

2 Department of Pharmaceutical Sciences, University of Maryland School of Pharmacy, Baltimore, MD, USA

3 Center for Biomolecular Therapeutics, University of Maryland School of Medicine, Baltimore, MD, USA

4 University of Maryland Marlene and Stewart Greenebaum NCI Cancer Center, Baltimore, MD, USA

References

[1] Rustandi, R. R., Baldisseri, D. M., and Weber, D. J. (2000) *Nat Struct Biol* 7, 570-574

[2] Lin, J., Blake, M., Tang, C., Zimmer, D., Rustandi, R. R., Weber, D. J., and Carrier, F. (2001) *J Biol Chem* 276, 35037-35041

[3] Lin, J., Yang, Q., Wilder, P. T., Carrier, F., and Weber, D. J. (2010) *J Biol Chem* 285, 27487-27498

[4] Lin, J., Yang, Q., Yan, Z., Markowitz, J., Wilder, P. T., Carrier, F., and Weber, D. J. (2004) *J Biol Chem* 279, 34071-34077

[5] Rustandi, R. R., Baldisseri, D. M., Inman, K. G., Nizner, P., Hamilton, S. M., Landar, A., Zimmer, D. B., and Weber, D. J. (2002) *Biochemistry* 41, 788-796

[6] Charpentier, T. H., Wilder, P. T., Liriano, M. A., Varney, K. M., Pozharski, E., MacKerell, A. D., Jr., Coop, A., Toth, E. A., and Weber, D. J. (2008) *J Mol Biol* 382, 56-73

[7] Marenholz, I., Heizmann, C. W., and Fritz, G. (2004) *Biochem Biophys Res Commun* 322, 1111-1122

[8] Donato, R. (2001) *Int J Biochem Cell Biol* 33, 637-668

[9] Harpio, R., and Einarsson, R. (2004) *Clin Biochem* 37, 512-518

[10] Zimmer, D. B., Cornwall, E. H., Landar, A., and Song, W. (1995) *Brain Res Bull* 37, 417-429

[11] Fesik, S. W. (1993) *J Biomol NMR* 3, 261-269

[12] Gaynor, R., Herschman, H. R., Irie, R., Jones, P., Morton, D., and Cochran, A. (1981) *Lancet* 1, 869-871

[13] Van Eldik, L. J., and Griffen, W. S. T. (1994) *Biochimica et Biophysica Acta* 1223, 398-403

[14] Steiner, J., Bogerts, B., Schroeter, M. L., and Bernstein, H. G. (2011) *Clinical chemistry and laboratory medicine : CCLM / FESCC* 49, 409-424

[15] Steiner, J., Marquardt, N., Pauls, I., Schiltz, K., Rahmoune, H., Bahn, S., Bogerts, B., Schmidt, R. E., and Jacobs, R. (2011) *Brain Behav Immun* 25, 1233-1241

[16] Rothermundt, M., Ahn, J. N., and Jorgens, S. (2009) *Gen Physiol Biophys* 28 Spec No Focus, F76-81

[17] Kligman, D., and Hilt, D. C. (1988) *Trends in biochemical sciences* 13, 437-443

[18] Donato, R. (1991) *Cell Calcium* 12, 713-726

[19] Moore, B. W. (1965) *Biochemical and biophysical research communications* 19, 739-744

[20] Isobe, T., Ishioka, N., and Okuyama, T. (1981) *European Journal of Biochemistry* 115, 469-474

[21] Hunter, M. J., and Chazin, W. J. (1998) *J Biol Chem* 273, 12427-12435

[22] Kretsinger, R. H. (1979) *Adv Cyclic Nucleotide Res* 11, 1-26

[23] Drohat, A. C., Baldisseri, D. M., Rustandi, R. R., and Weber, D. J. (1998) *Biochemistry* 37, 2729-2740

[24] Baudier, J., Galsser, N., Haglid, K., and Gerard, D. (1984) *Biochimica et Biophysica Acta* 790, 164-173

[25] Barber, K. R., McClintock, K. A., Jamieson, G. A., Jr., Dimlich, R. V., and Shaw, G. S. (1999) *J Biol Chem* 274, 1502-1508

[26] Gentil, B. J., Delphin, C., Mbele, G. O., Deloulme, J. C., Ferro, M., Garin, J., and Baudier, J. (2001) *J Biol Chem* 276, 23253-23261

[27] Markowitz, J., Carrier, F., Varney, K. M., Mackerell, A. D., Jr., and Weber, D. J. (2005) *AACR Meeting Abstracts* 2005, 1140-a-

[28] Rustandi, R. R., Drohat, A. C., Baldisseri, D. M., Wilder, P. T., and Weber, D. J. (1998) *Biochemistry* 37, 1951-1960

[29] Markowitz, J., Rustandi, R. R., Varney, K. M., Wilder, P. T., Udan, R., Wu, S. L., Horrocks, W. D., and Weber, D. J. (2005) *Biochemistry* 44, 7305-7314

[30] Markowitz, J., Mackerell, A. D., Jr., Carrier, F., Charpentier, T. H., and Weber, D. J. (2005) *Curr Top Med Chem* 5, 1093-1108

[31] Ferreon, J. C., Lee, C. W., Arai, M., Martinez-Yamout, M. A., Dyson, H. J., and Wright, P. E. (2009) *Proc Natl Acad Sci U S A* 106, 6591-6596

[32] Wright, N. T., Cannon, B. R., Wilder, P. T., Morgan, M. T., Varney, K. M., Zimmer, D. B., and Weber, D. J. (2009) *Journal of molecular biology* 386, 1265-1277

[33] Wright, N. T., Inman, K. G., Levine, J. A., Cannon, B. R., Varney, K. M., and Weber, D. J. (2008) *J Biomol NMR* 42, 279-286

[34] Wright, N. T., Prosser, B. L., Varney, K. M., Zimmer, D. B., Schneider, M. F., and Weber, D. J. (2008) *J Biol Chem* 283, 26676-26683

[35] Liriano, M. A., Varney, K. M., Wright, N. T., Hoffman, C. L., Toth, E. A., Ishima, R., and Weber, D. J. (2012) *Journal of molecular biology*

[36] Wilder, P. T., Baldisseri, D. M., Udan, R., Vallely, K. M., and Weber, D. J. (2003) *Biochemistry* 42, 13410-13421

[37] Charpentier, T. H., Thompson, L. E., Liriano, M. A., Varney, K. M., Wilder, P. T., Pozharski, E., Toth, E. A., and Weber, D. J. (2010) *J Mol Biol* 396, 1227-1243

[38] Malashkevich, V. N., Varney, K. M., Garrett, S. C., Wilder, P. T., Knight, D., Charpentier, T. H., Ramagopal, U. A., Almo, S. C., Weber, D. J., and Bresnick, A. R. (2008) *Biochemistry* 47, 5111-5126

[39] Baudier, J., and Gerard, D. (1986) *J Biol Chem* 261, 8204-8212

[40] Wright, N. T., Cannon, B. R., Zimmer, D. B., and Weber, D. J. (2009) *Current chemical biology* 3, 138-145

[41] Hauschild, A., Engel, G., Brenner, W., Glaser, R., Monig, H., Henze, E., and Christophers, E. (1999) *The British journal of dermatology* 140, 1065-1071

[42] Hauschild, A., Engel, G., Brenner, W., Glaser, R., Monig, H., Henze, E., and Christophers, E. (1999) *Oncology* 56, 338-344

[43] Hauschild, A., Michaelsen, J., Brenner, W., Rudolph, P., Glaser, R., Henze, E., and Christophers, E. (1999) *Melanoma research* 9, 155-161

[44] Karnell, R., von Schoultz, E., Hansson, L. O., Nilsson, B., Arstrand, K., and Kagedal, B. (1997) *Melanoma Res* 7, 393-399

[45] Huang, M. Y., Wang, H. M., Chang, H. J., Hsiao, C. P., Wang, J. Y., and Lin, S. R. (2012) *DNA Cell Biol* 31, 43-49

[46] Huang, M. Y., Wang, H. M., Tok, T. S., Chang, H. J., Chang, M. S., Cheng, T. L., Wang, J. Y., and Lin, S. R. (2012) *DNA Cell Biol* 31, 625-635

[47] Hwang, C. C., Chai, H. T., Chen, H. W., Tsai, H. L., Lu, C. Y., Yu, F. J., Huang, M. Y., and Wang, J. Y. (2011) *Ann Surg Oncol* 18, 139-145

[48] Preusser, M., Hoischen, A., Novak, K., Czech, T., Prayer, D., Hainfellner, J. A., Baumgartner, C., Woermann, F. G., Tuxhorn, I. E., Pannek, H. W., Bergmann, M., Radl-

wimmer, B., Villagran, R., Weber, R. G., and Hans, V. H. (2007) *Am J Surg Pathol* 31, 1709-1718

[49] Gartner, W., Ilhan, A., Neziri, D., Base, W., Weissel, M., Wohrer, A., Heinzl, H., Waldhor, T., Wagner, L., and Preusser, M. (2010) *Neuro Oncol* 12, 1004-1008

[50] Hancq, S., Salmon, I., Brotchi, J., Gabius, H. J., Heizmann, C. W., Kiss, R., and Decaestecker, C. (2004) *Int J Oncol* 25, 1233-1240

[51] Pang, X., Min, J., Liu, L., Liu, Y., Ma, N., and Zhang, H. (2012) *Med Oncol*

[52] Yang, J. F., Zhang, X. Y., and Qi, F. (2004) *Zhong Nan Da Xue Xue Bao Yi Xue Ban* 29, 301-304

[53] Nagasaka, A., Umekawa, H., Hidaka, H., Iwase, K., Nakai, A., Ariyoshi, Y., Ohyama, T., Aono, T., Nakagawa, H., Ohtani, S., and et al. (1987) *Metabolism* 36, 388-391

[54] American Cancer Society. (2011)

[55] Van Eldik, L. J., and Wainwright, M. S. (2003) *Restor Neurol Neurosci* 21, 97-108

[56] Sorci, G., Bianchi, R., Riuzzi, F., Tubaro, C., Arcuri, C., Giambanco, I., and Donato, R. (2010) *Cardiovascular psychiatry and neurology* 2010

[57] Zimmer, D. B., Chaplin, J., Baldwin, A., and Rast, M. (2005) *Cell Mol Biol (Noisy-le-grand)* 51, 201-214

[58] Mori, T., Asano, T., and Town, T. (2010) *Cardiovascular psychiatry and neurology* 2010

[59] Mrak, R. E., and Griffin, W. S. (2004) *J Neuropathol Exp Neurol* 63, 679-685

[60] Castets, F., Griffin, W. S., Marks, A., and Van Eldik, L. J. (1997) *Brain Res Mol Brain Res* 46, 208-216

[61] Rothermundt, M., Ponath, G., and Arolt, V. (2004) *Int Rev Neurobiol* 59, 445-470

[62] Roltsch, E., Holcomb, L., Young, K. A., Marks, A., and Zimmer, D. B. (2010) *J Neuroinflammation* 7, 78

[63] Wilder, P. T., Lin, J., Bair, C. L., Charpentier, T. H., Yang, D., Liriano, M., Varney, K. M., Lee, A., Oppenheim, A. B., Adhya, S., Carrier, F., and Weber, D. J. (2006) *Biochim Biophys Acta* 1763, 1284-1297

[64] Millward, T. A., Heizmann, C. W., Schafer, B. W., and Hemmings, B. A. (1998) *Embo J* 17, 5913-5922

[65] Bhattacharya, S., Large, E., Heizmann, C. W., Hemmings, B., and Chazin, W. J. (2003) *Biochemistry* 42, 14416-14426

[66] Skripnikova, E. V., and Gusev, N. B. (1989) *FEBS Lett* 257, 380-382

[67] Wills, F. L., McCubbin, W. D., and Kay, C. M. (1993) *Biochemistry* 32, 2321-2328

[68] Inman, K. G., Yang, R., Rustandi, R. R., Miller, K. E., Baldisseri, D. M., and Weber, D. J. (2002) *J Mol Biol* 324, 1003-1014

[69] Bianchi, R., Garbuglia, M., Verzini, M., Giambanco, I., Ivanenkov, V. V., Dimlich, R. V., Jamieson, G. A., Jr., and Donato, R. (1996) *Biochimica et Biophysica Acta* 1313, 258-267

[70] Mbele, G. O., Deloulme, J. C., Gentil, B. J., Delphin, C., Ferro, M., Garin, J., Takahashi, M., and Baudier, J. (2002) *J Biol Chem* 277, 49998-50007

[71] Sheu, F. S., Huang, F. L., and Huang, K. P. (1995) *Arch Biochem Biophys* 316, 335-342

[72] Baudier, J., and Cole, R. D. (1988) *J. Biol. Chem.* 263, 5876-5883

[73] Donato, R. (1987) *Cell Calcium* 8, 283-297

[74] Zimmer, D. B., and Van Eldik, L. J. (1986) *J Biol Chem* 261, 11424-11428

[75] Landar, A., Caddell, G., Chessher, J., and Zimmer, D. B. (1996) *Cell Calcium* 20, 279-285

[76] Baudier, J., Delphin, C., Grunwald, D., Khochbin, S., and Lawrence, J. J. (1992) *Proc Natl Acad Sci U S A* 89, 11627-11631

[77] Wilder, P. T., Rustandi, R. R., Drohat, A. C., and Weber, D. J. (1998) *Protein Sci* 7, 794-798

[78] Donato, R., Cannon, B. R., Sorci, G., Riuzzi, F., Hsu, K., Weber, D. J., and Geczy, C. L. (2012) *Curr Mol Med*

[79] Brozzi, F., Arcuri, C., Giambanco, I., and Donato, R. (2009) *J Biol Chem* 284, 8797-8811

[80] Albert, K. A., Wu, W. C., Nairn, A. C., and Greengard, P. (1984) *Proc Natl Acad Sci U S A* 81, 3622-3625

[81] Baudier, J., Mochly-Rosen, D., Newton, A., Lee, S. H., Koshland, D. E., Jr., and Cole, R. D. (1987) *Biochemistry* 26, 2886-2893

[82] Sakaguchi, K., Sakamoto, H., Lewis, M. S., Anderson, C. W., Erickson, J. W., Appela, E., and Xie, D. (1997) *Biochemistry* 36, 10117-10124

[83] Sakaguchi, K., Sakamoto, H., Xie, D., Erickson, J. W., Lewis, M. S., Anderson, C. W., and Appella, E. (1997) *J Protein Chem* 16, 553-556

[84] Markowitz, J., Chen, I., Gitti, R., Baldisseri, D. M., Pan, Y., Udan, R., Carrier, F., MacKerell, A. D., Jr., and Weber, D. J. (2004) *J Med Chem* 47, 5085-5093

[85] Whitlow, J. L., Varughese, J. F., Zhou, Z., Bartolotti, L. J., and Li, Y. (2009) *Journal of molecular graphics & modelling* 27, 969-977

[86] Lipinski, C. A., Lombardo, F., Dominy, B. W., and Feeney, P. J. (2001) *Adv Drug Deliv Rev* 46, 3-26

[87] Guvench, O., and MacKerell Jr, A. D. (2009) *PLoS Comp. Biol.* 5, e1000435

[88] Raman, E. P., Yu, W., Guvench, O., and Mackerell, A. D. (2011) *J Chem Inf Model* 51, 877-896

[89] Foster, T. J., Mackerell, A. D., Jr., and Guvench, O. (2012) *J Comput Chem* 33, 1880-1891

[90] Charpentier, T. H., Wilder, P. T., Liriano, M. A., Varney, K. M., Zhong, S., Coop, A., Pozharski, E., MacKerell, A. D., Jr., Toth, E. A., and Weber, D. J. (2009) *Biochemistry* 48, 6202-6212

[91] Markowitz, J., MacKerell, A. D., Jr., and Weber, D. J. (2007) *Mini Rev Med Chem* 7, 609-616

[92] Wilder, P. T., Charpentier, T. H., Liriano, M. A., Gianni, K., Varney, K. M., Pozharski, E., Coop, A., Toth, E. A., Mackerell, A. D., and Weber, D. J. (2010) *International journal of high throughput screening* 2010, 109-126

[93] Zimmer, D. B., Lapidus, R.G., Weber, D.J. (2012) *Methods Mol Biol* in press

[94] Leclerc, E., and Heizmann, C. W. (2011) *Front Biosci (Schol Ed)* 3, 1232-1262

[95] Zimmer, D. B., and Weber, D. J. (2010) *Cardiovascular psychiatry and neurology* 2010

[96] Vitolo, M. I., Weiss, M. B., Szmacinski, M., Tahir, K., Waldman, T., Park, B. H., Martin, S. S., Weber, D. J., and Bachman, K. E. (2009) *Cancer Research* 69, 8275-8283

[97] Weiss, M. B., Vitolo, M. I., Mohseni, M., Rosen, D. M., Denmeade, S. R., Park, B. H., Weber, D. J., and Bachman, K. E. (2010) *Oncogene* 29, 4715-4724

[98] Singh, M., Lima, A., Molina, R., Hamilton, P., Clermont, A. C., Devasthali, V., Thompson, J. D., Cheng, J. H., Bou Reslan, H., Ho, C. C., Cao, T. C., Lee, C. V., Nannini, M. A., Fuh, G., Carano, R. A., Koeppen, H., Yu, R. X., Forrest, W. F., Plowman, G. D., and Johnson, L. (2010) *Nat Biotechnol* 28, 585-593

[99] Chin, L., Pomerantz, J., Polsky, D., Jacobson, M., Cohen, C., Cordon-Cardo, C., Horner, J. W., 2nd, and DePinho, R. A. (1997) *Genes & Development* 11, 2822-2834

[100] Larue, L., and Beermann, F. (2007) *Pigment Cell Res* 20, 485-497

[101] Lawrence, M. C., and Davis, P. C. (1992) *Proteins* 12, 31-41

[102] Martin, Y. C. (1992) *J Med Chem* 35, 2145-2154

[103] Ewing, T. J. A., and Kuntz, I. D. (1997) *J. Comput. Chem.* 18, 1175-1189

[104] Makino, S., and Kuntz, I. D. (1997) *J. Comp. Chem.* 18, 1812-1825

[105] Taylor, R. D., Jewsbury, P. J., and Essex, J. W. (2002) *J. Comp. Aided Mol. Des.* 16, 151-166

[106] Oprea, T. I., Ho, C. M. W., and Marshall, G. R. (1995) De Novo Design: Ligand construction and prediction of affinity, in computer-aided molecular design: Application

in agrochemicals, materials, and pharmaceuticals. (Reynolds, C. H., Holloway, M. K., and Cox, H. K. eds.), American Chem. Soc., Washington, D.C. pp 64-81

[107] Schneider, G., Lee, M. L., Stahl, M., and Schneider, P. (2000) *J Comput Aided Mol Des* 14, 487-494

[108] Hajduk, P. J., Dinges, J., Miknis, G. F., Merlock, M., Middleton, T., Kempf, D. J., Egan, D. A., Walter, K. A., Robins, T. S., Shuker, S. B., Holzman, T. F., and Fesik, S. W. (1997) *J Med Chem* 40, 3144-3150

[109] Hajduk, P. J., Meadows, R. P., and Fesik, S. W. (1997) *Science* 278, 497-499

[110] Mayer, M., and Meyer, B. (2001) *J Am Chem Soc* 123, 6108-6117

[111] Meinecke, R., and Meyer, B. (2001) *J Med Chem* 44, 3059-3065

Chapter 25

Immunomodulation

Konstantinos Arnaoutakis, Dorothy A. Graves,
Laura F. Hutchins and Thomas Kieber-Emmons

Additional information is available at the end of the chapter

http://dx.doi.org/10.5772/53667

1. Introduction

Immune treatment for melanoma has roots in clinical observations surrounding regression of normal nevi, the appearance of halo nevi, the correlation of vitiligo with outcome, the occurrence of spontaneous regression of primary melanomas, nodal metastases of unknown primary lesions and the occurrence of metastases many years after resection of a primary lesion. Coupling these observations with the observations on the power of the immune system to reject transplanted organs and control leukemia after allogeneic bone marrow transplant, the possibility of harnessing and directing this power has been a source of both excitement and disappointment.

In examining the natural history of normal nevi, it is noted that they undergo a life cycle in which growth occurs during childhood in the border of the epidermis and dermis (junctional nevi). With increasing age the melanocytes move deeper into the dermis. As adult life continues they regress in old age. It is not evident that this type of regression has an immune basis.

Another type of regression called halo nevi is more definitively tied to the immune system [1]. Akasu, et. al have described halo nevi regression in four stages characterized initially by pan-T lymphocytes in stage one and the addition of KP-1 positive cells as well as FX IIIa-positive cells in stage two. Stage three continues with increased numbers of FX IIIa-positive cells and the addition of Langerhans cells. Finally upon complete regression in stage four there is a moderate mononuclear infiltrate comprised predominantly of T cells [2]. The role of natural killer (NK) cells has been studied in normal and malignant melanocytic lesions. The highest concentration of NK cells was seen in regressing malignant lesions followed by regressing normal nevi [3]. This type of "spontaneous" regression is observed in other benign skin lesions such as keratoachanthomas, and the pathologic studies give insight into the possibility of stimulating similar immune action against malignancies [1, 2].

The autoimmune condition of vitiligo has been associated with regression of metastases as well as better outcomes associated with immunotherapy. Vitiligo is mediated through autoantibodies. Antibodies against tyrosinase have been observed in patients with melanoma as well as vitiligo not associated with melanoma. Other autoimmune effects are well documented with immunotherapeutic treatments, indicating the ability of the therapy to break tolerance to self-antigens [4-7].

Spontaneous regression is observed in primary melanoma [8, 9]. Statistics vary on the incidence but may be as high as 20%, especially if cases of unknown primary are included. When remnants of primary lesions are found, they frequently are partially regressed and show histologic evidence of infiltration by lymphocytes. Although some have observed a worse clinical outcome with partially regressed primary lesions, patients with nodal metastases and unknown primaries tend to have a better outcome. The latter observation is attributed to improved immune surveillance compared to patients with intact primaries [10-14]. Regression of metastases is less common and has anecdotally been tied to infections or surgeries. Regression of metastases seems to predict a better overall outcome [15, 16].

The issue of late metastases from primary melanoma is well documented but much harder to explain. Issues within the tumor microenvironment remain incompletely explored, but high on the list of explanations is the possibility that the immune system is able to control proliferation until some as yet undocumented effect allows escape [17, 18].

Early studies with nonspecific therapies described below produced enough positive results to keep interest in melanoma immunotherapy alive. However, progress in the clinic has been slow until very recently. Many issues have presented challenges to progress. Among them is an incomplete understanding of the normal immune system, including immune tolerance and the effects of the tumor microenvironment on the immune response. Drug development required technology to produce biologic agents, and that capability has only recently been perfected. Issues of study design also need to be kept in mind. Subject selection can be difficult since these studies require immune competence but disease advanced enough to answer the question in a reasonable time frame with a reasonable number of subjects.

2. Biomarkers and endpoints

Biomarkers and surrogate endpoints are tools to obtain information about disease status or response to interventions. The mainstay of efficacy determination in cancer therapeutic clinical trials has been the regression of known tumor masses listed as complete response (CR), partial response (PR), stable disease (SD) or progressive disease (PD) along with various survival endpoints: overall survival (OS), disease free survival (DFS) and progression free survival (PFS). Each of these endpoints is defined by the study. The response criteria have been standardized by various systems. The World Health Organization (WHO) developed the most commonly used system called response criteria for solid tumors (RECIST) [19]. Recent developments in assessing response during trials utilizing the drug, ipilimumab, have served to highlight differences in direct cytotoxic chemotherapy responses and those seen with immunotherapy. The responses in tumor measurement seen in the ipilimumab trials did not correspond to the survival endpoints. Subjects had prolonged survival with delayed or no tumor measurement changes. These observations have led to a new system for assessing immune based therapies called immune-related response criteria (irRC) [20].

Biomarkers can serve to assess efficacy, but it is difficult to find results that consistently correlate with clinical response. Some assays can serve as immunologic endpoints in addition to or instead of tumor regression, PFS and OS in clinical studies. The most frequent measurements include: antibody titers, delayed type hypersensitivity (DTH) skin tests, enzyme-linked immunosorbent assay (ELISA), enzyme-linked immunospot assay (ELISPOT), tetramer markers of antigen specific T cells and other assays indicating that the therapy induced a response toward its target [21-25].

All of these issues should be considered in assessing the past studies and in the planning of future studies. As we will discuss, progress has been made and enthusiasm is at an all-time high.

2.1. Patient selection

Predicting response to treatment is probably the best way to increase benefit from a variety of different immunotherapy agents that are currently approved or under investigation for the treatment of early stage (as adjuvant therapy) or advanced melanoma. Identifying patients that are likely to respond to these agents would spare patients unnecessary toxicities and encourage more research in the field.

Response to treatment may be determined by clinical characteristics or by the presence or level of biomarkers in the serum or tissue that predict a robust response to immunotherapy agents. Clinical characteristics such as ulcerated lesions appear to get more benefit from interferon (IFN) in the adjuvant setting [26]. In addition, Eastern Cooperative Oncology Group (ECOG) performance status, the number of involved organs and sites of metastases appear to be treatment factors predicting response to interleukin 2 (IL-2) in some studies [27].

The appearance of serum autoantibodies or clinical manifestations of autoimmunity during treatment with IFNα-2b was associated with improved outcomes in patients with melanoma [28]. In addition, multiplexed analysis of serum cytokines appeared to be potentially useful as a predictive marker of response to IFNα-2b in patients with high-risk operable melanoma [29]. A serum proteomic analysis has been found to possibly predict response to IL-2 treatment [30]. In this study, high pretreatment serum vascular endothelial growth factor (VEGF) and fibronectin levels were predictive of resistance to treatment. A marker of potential interest in ipilimumab therapy appears to be the absolute lymphocyte count [31]. Absolute lymphocyte counts that exceeded 1 x 10^9/L at the time of the third ipilimumab dose were associated with a survival benefit at one year. Immune responses to NY-ESO-1, a cancer-testis antigen, also appear to correlate with clinical benefit from ipilimumab [32].

Gene signatures within the tumor have also shown some correlation with clinical benefit both for IL-2 and vaccination [33, 34]. Little is known about some of the newer drugs such as the CTLA-4 antagonists (ipilimumab) or other checkpoint inhibitors. It has been suggested that the presence of PD-L1 expression detected by immunohistochemistry may predict response to PD-1 antibody therapy [35].

Undoubtedly, utilizing serum and tissue biomarkers for response to treatment is much more challenging for immunotherapy than in the field of molecular targeted therapies. For example V600E BRAF mutations predict treatment response in patients who receive vemurafenib, a BRAF inhibitor. In melanoma immunotherapy, however, no serum or tissue biomarkers have yet been prospectively studied in the context of a clinical trial.

3. Immunoregulatory barriers, immune tolerance and tumor microenvironment

The immune system is designed to protect our bodies from foreign agents. This protection is selective, such that host tissues are recognized as self and preserved (termed immunologic tolerance), while other agents are recognized as foreign and targeted for killing. Cancer cells, however, present the immune system with a unique challenge. While some, such as virally transformed cells, express foreign viral proteins on their surface, most tumors express normal proteins and carbohydrates. Efforts to understand how tumors survive immunosurveillance versus how and when they are targeted for killing have preoccupied scientists for well over half a century. This section explores what we currently know about the complex interplay between the immune system and cancer cells as it relates to immunotherapy.

We know now that tumor cells are immunogenic but efficacy is limited due to the lack of robustness of the response. There are two primary reasons for this: 1) due to the nature of the immunogens (self antigens) and 2) the active role-played by tumors to suppress the response. The mammalian anti-tumor response engages both the humoral and cell-mediated arms of the immune system through both specific (adaptive) and non-specific (innate) effectors. While cytotoxic T lymphocytes (CTLs), NK cells and T helper (TH) cells are viewed as the most significant players in the anti-tumor response, they are not alone [36]. Antigen presenting cells (APCs - macrophages and dendritic cells) are absolutely essential to stimulate a variety of anti-tumor responses across tumor types, and anti-tumor antibodies are often easily found in patients with melanoma and many other solid tumors, indicating a strong humoral response following stimulation by antigen specific TH cells [37]. There is accumulating evidence that the CD4+ T cell population is far more involved in the anti-tumor response than previously thought [38, 39]. When APCs present antigen to TH cells in the context of a major histocompatibility complex (MHC) molecule on their surface, TH cells become activated and can stimulate B cells to result in the proliferation of antibody-producing plasma cells and CTLs to result in direct killing of the tumor cells. NK cells and macrophages can also directly kill tumor cells alone or with the help of antibodies or complement.

3.1. Melanoma antigenicity

The goal of cancer immunotherapy is to provoke the immune system to generate a tumor cell rejection strength response and to prevent recurrence of cancer by establishing long-term effector cell memory. In order for the immune system to mount an attack against melanoma, it must first recognize the involved tumor cells as foreign or in need of clearing (a danger signal); it can then target them for killing. Tumor cells, like all cells, display a variety of proteins on their cell surface, and when antigen is presented in the context of MHC, the cell may be recognized by the T cell receptor (TCR) on an effector T lymphocyte. Tumor cells in general and melanoma tissues specifically, are antigenically diverse, and their ability to survive correlates with the ability of the tumor antigens to avoid detection by the immune system [40, 41]. Highly antigenic tumor cells are killed off rather quickly, due to the immune system's ability to recognize the tumor cells and mount an effective immune response, while poorly antigenic tumor cells thrive. Tumor specific transplantation antigens (TSTAs) generally convey strong immunogenicity. These are antigens expressed on the surface of tumor cells that are specific to that tumor or type of tumor. However, the majority of antigens associated with melanoma cells are tumor associated transplantation antigens, or TATAs. TATAs are antigens that are associated with tumor cells, but not unique to tumor cells. TATAs are far better at preserving a tumor cell under the radar of the immune system, because these antigens are not danger signals.

Within the tumor microenvironment, tolerance may be naturally overcome by antigen expression levels or the timing of antigen expression. Melanomas overexpress many antigens that are present in normal melanocytes but at lower levels, and expression of these antigens suggest a progression of differentiation from normal melanocytes to melanomas. For example, a melanoma expressing a mutant triosephosphate isomerase protein was discovered to bind MHC class II at five times greater affinity than the wild type oligopeptide, resulting in both a significant increase in surface expression and an increase in immunogenicity [42]. Some melanoma cells overexpress the transferrin receptor by a factor of 100 [43]. Some human melanomas overexpress the gangliosides relative to levels seen in normal melanocytes, illustrating that overexpression of carbohydrates can attract the attention of the immune system, similar to protein antigens [44].

Much of melanoma's antigenicity comes from the more than 100 identified melanoma TATAs. Melan-A/MART-1, gp100 and tyrosinase are well studied differentiation antigens expressed in both primary and metastatic melanoma [45-53].

Melanoma cells may also express oncofetal antigens which are normally displayed during embryogenesis but only expressed in select tissues, if at all, in adults. These include the cancer germ-line/cancer-testis (CT) antigens. MAGE-A family members and NY-ESO-1 are the most significant members of this group to date, and expression of MAGE-A1 and MAGE-A4 increases with tumor progression [47, 54, 55]. NY-ESO-1 is only expressed in adults in testis and placenta tissue, however, it is expressed in up to 40% of late stage melanomas and is highly immunogenic [56]. MAGE-6 is expressed in more than 70% of metastatic melanomas [57].

Identification of melanoma TATAs is crucial as a key strategy for immunotherapy. Administration of vaccines that deliver TATAs can push the immune system into overcoming tolerance. T cells specific for TATAs have been identified in melanoma patients, and spontaneously occurring circulating T cells reactive to Melan-A and NY-ESO-1 were recently found to be predictive of better survival [58]. A recent study reported an analysis of the human leukocyte antigen 1 (HLA-I) peptidomes from melanomas in four patients, and while finding that melanoma antigenicity was highly variable, the investigators also found that the peptidomes were highly immunogenic, identifying new potential peptides for melanoma vaccines [41].

3.2. Immunoevasion strategies

Tumor cells increase their odds of survival by lowering their immunological profiles. TH cells, CTLs and antibodies specific for TATAs are readily detectable in the blood, lymph nodes and tumors of cancer patients. Despite tolerance, the immune system can mount an immune response to these antigens, but tumors and/or tumor cells may persist, so all the efforts of the immune system are not enough to clear tumor cells. The immunoevasion strategies utilized by melanomas are impressive and generally include down-regulation of TATAs on the tumor cell surface, secretion of immunosuppressive cytokines that affect APCs and shedding of material that promotes the stimulation of the inhibitory regulatory T cells (Tregs). Together, these strategies create a toleragenic tumor microenvironment that is both adaptive to immune pressures and predictive of clinical outcomes.

Many tumor cells stop displaying TATAs or TSTAs on their surface to escape immune recognition [59]. Expression of MART-1, gp100 and tyrosinase generally decreases as melanoma progresses [60]. Following immunization with gp100 or MART-1 peptides, melanoma metastases lost expression of the corresponding TATA, suggesting that TATAs can be downregulated in direct response to a specific CTL anti-tumor response [45]. This strategy is specifically adaptive to removing known CTL targets from the tumor population and selects for proliferation of tumor cells that do not bear antigens yet targeted by the CTL response.

Tumor cells may additionally repress expression of MHC class I proteins by repressing MHC I gene expression or posttranslational modifications [59]. In fact, many human tumors demonstrate a decreased expression of MHC I, and the loss of MHC I expression is often associated with more invasive and metastatic tumors [61, 62]. In melanoma, MHC I expression correlates with disease progression, and the lack of HLA I expression and lack of response to T cell based immunotherapy may be linked to acquired β2-microglobulin gene defects [63-65]. C-myc oncogene overexpression in melanoma also correlates with HLA I downregulation [66]. The one caveat of this strategy, however, is that a total lack of MHC expression invites attack by NK cells [67]. To circumvent this, tumor cells often only lower MHC I expression, retaining some minimal expression to protect themselves while not alarming the immune system.

Tumors in general create microenvironments with depressed immune activity such that few functional cytotoxic cells are found near the developing tumor. One strategy for this involves the poorly understood regulation of lymphocyte types within the tumor microenvironment. Moderate to large numbers of tumor infiltrating lymphocytes (TILs) have been associated with improved survival in melanoma patients; however this has not been observed consistently [68, 69]. While most patients with melanoma have TILs, the mere presence of TILs is obviously not sufficient to mount an effective anti-tumor response [70]. Tumor cells are able to attract a particular type of T cell that is immunosuppressive. Tregs can directly inhibit and kill CTLs and TH cells, and they functionally drive the tumor's T helper Type 2 (Th-2) immune environment by producing the immunosuppressive cytokines IL-10 and tumor growth factor beta (TGF-β) while suppressing CTL production of immunostimulatory T helper Type 1 (Th-1) cytokines interferon gamma (IFN γ) and IL-2 [71]. Tregs also negatively regulate effector dendritic cells and NK cells. In melanoma, depletion of Tregs prior to infusion with activated T lymphocytes (adoptive cell therapy) measurably improves response rates [72].

Melanoma cells may also create an immunosuppressed microenvironment through galectin expression [73]. Deregulation of galectins is common in human tumors. Expression of galectin 3 correlates with melanoma metastasis and poorer disease outcomes, perhaps through induction of TIL apoptosis. Galectin 1 may also induce apoptosis of T cells and this may be an important mechanism of tumor evasion for melanoma. Additionally, galectins 1 and 3 convey resistance to apoptosis in tumor cells, though this is less studied in melanoma.

Immunosuppression similar to that found in the tumor microenvironment can also be found in the sentinel lymph node [71, 74]. Tregs are found in higher numbers in metastatic melanoma sentinel lymph nodes, and as in the tumor microenvironment, this appears to be mediated by Th-2 cytokines IL-6, IL-8, IL-10 and TGF-β, among others. This locoregional immunosupporession is thought to be necessary for metastasis and prepares the lymphatic environment for the arrival and survival of metastastic cells [75]. While dendritic cells are detectable in melanoma sentinel lymph nodes, they may be present in lower number and/or contain a higher percentage of immature dendritic cells that lack the costimulatory molecules necessary for effective T cell activation [74, 76].

IL-10 and TGF-β are immunosuppressive cytokines utilized by melanoma to create an immunosuppressive microenvironment and progress disease toward metastasis [77, 78]. Both cytokines can induce T cells to undergo apoptosis; TGF-β can additionally induce apoptosis in dendritic cells and macrophages. Normal melanocytes are subject to TGF-β anti-proliferative regulation, and loss of this phenotype is thought to be a crucial step toward melanoma development [77]. Neutrophils from patients with melanoma constitutively and spontaneously synthesize IL-10 through activation by serum amyloid A 1 (SAA-1) which is enriched in melanoma tissue [79].

There are a variety of other general tumor microenvironment conditions and immunoevasion strategies that melanomas employ to ensure their survival. Hypoxia occurs in solid tumor masses and is well known to create an immunosuppressive tumor microenvironment [80]. Tumor cells can also alter the expression of stress proteins that bind NK cells for targeted killing. Melanoma cells predominantly express the MICA and ULBP2 stress proteins, and a correlation has been found between poor prognosis and expression of soluble ULBP2 that is competitive for NK cell binding [81, 82]. Heat shock proteins are well known to promote tumor growth, invasion and metastasis through a variety of mechanisms [83]. Expression of heat shock proteins 90 and 40 (hsp90 and hsp40) in melanoma tissue correlates with advanced disease and patient survival, in the case of hsp40 [84].

It is important to remember that while immune evasion and creation of an immunsuppressive tumor microenvironment is highly variable among melanomas, the ability of the tumor to effectively create a strong toleragenic microenvironment correlates with clinical outcome. Toleragenic tumor microenvironments are associated with sentinel lymph node involvement and more advanced disease [74]. Efforts to overcome this tolerance and re-capitulate the balance of immune system regulators to a state of anti-tumor effectiveness comprise the field of immunotherapy, and success in this therapeutic approach holds tremendous promise for not only halting tumor progression but for turning back the clock to ultimately result in tumor clearance.

3.3. Immunotherapy strategies

Most immunotherapy efforts strive to activate T cells and specifically CTLs. Therapeutic melanoma vaccines may enhance antigen presentation directly through peptides or DNA. A synthetic peptide vaccine targeted to the melanoma gp100 TATA, for example, has resulted in good objective clinical responses [85]. Vaccines may also rely on the assistance of dendritic cells, a key stimulator of immune cells [86-88]. The goal is to utilize TSTA or TATA antigens to provoke the development and proliferation of cytotoxic cells directed against tumor cells, thereby overcoming tolerance.

Adoptive cell transfer or therapy (ACT) is a passive immunotherapeutic approach in which a patient's antigen-specific cells are expanded and activated *ex vivo* and then reintroduced following radiation or chemotherapy [89]. TILs, autologous T cell clones, donor anti-tumor lymphocytes and genetically engineered lymphocytes have all been used in this strategy. Some encouraging results have been seen in melanoma patients with advanced disease [90]. In three separate trials, autologous TILs provided through ACT and administered with IL-2 to metastatic melanoma patients resulted in up to a 72% objective response rate, and 22% of the 93 subjects had complete tumor regression [91]. ACT employing autologous T cells targeting NY-ESO-1 resulted in objective responses in five of 11 metastatic melanoma patients and two complete regressions at one-year post-procedure [92]. While it is argued that ACT is more effective in metastatic melanoma than ipilimumab (see below), it is practically more complex to administer and less accessible for a majority of patients [90].

Cytokines have shown efficacy in high risk local and metastatic melanoma patients as well. IL-2 and IFNα-2b have been investigated the most. IL-2 alone produces a durable remission in some patients, though it is often associated with significant side effects, and better outcomes may be obtained by combining it with other therapeutic approaches [93]. A pooled analysis of nearly 2,000 stage IIB and III melanoma patients indicated that adjuvant high dose IFNα-2b prolongs relapse free survival in patients [94].

At present, the greatest promise for metastatic melanoma patients lies in immunomodulatory antibody therapy against immunological checkpoints. Immunotherapies that employ this targeting strategy are recent and have yielded some of the most promising clinical responses in decades. Immunological checkpoints are negative regulators of the immune system. Cytotoxic T lymphocyte antigen 4 (CTLA4) is found on naïve T cells and Tregs; upon activation it turns off TCR signaling and serves to stop activation of targeted T cells. Antibodies to CTLA4 prevent this from happening and prolong and intensify T cell activation [36]. Ipilimumab was approved by the U.S. Food and Drug Administration (FDA) in 2012 for the treatment of metastatic melanoma owing to the overall survival benefit observed in a phase III study that has now resulted in durable responses lasting 8 years and beyond [95]. Although ipilimumab is the only FDA-approved checkpoint inhibitor indicated for treatment of melanoma, there are others in the pipeline [96]. Tremelimumab is another CTLA4 antibody, and there are several programmed death ligand 1 (PD-1) antibodies undergoing clinical development as well [97, 98]. Though both CTLA4 and PD-1 antibodies have demonstrated significant improvement in clinical outcome for metastatic melanoma patients, they are not effective in all patients and cause a new and unique spectrum of side effects termed "immune-related adverse events."

4. Nonspecific immune therapy and adjuvants

The success of anti-tumor and antiviral vaccines often requires the use of an adjuvant, a substance that significantly enhances the immune response to a coadministered antigen. Only a handful of adjuvants have both sufficient potency and acceptable toxicity for clinical investigation. The critical roles of vaccine adjuvants lie in their ability to: (1) enable the use of otherwise impotent antigens; (2) extend the benefits of vaccination to poor responders (e.g., older or immune-compromised patients); and (3) effect dose-sparing of rare and expensive antigens in short supply (e.g., during an epidemic) [99]. Vaccine adjuvants for the most part can be evaluated as such only when they are associated with a vaccine. Early therapies were nonspecific and were thought to produce a general immune response. Many current vaccine trials utilize nonspecific immune stimulants as adjuncts.

4.1. BCG

Adjuvant therapy of melanoma assumes that treatment will be more effective when the tumor burden is small. Mycobacterium bovis bacillus Calmette-Guérin (BCG) is an old vaccine/adjuvant used in countries where tuberculosis is widespread. First used in humans in 1921, BCG is made from a strain of weakened bovine tuberculosis bacterium. The local and systemic effect of BCG has been known for decades and is an immunomodulating agent for melanoma. BCG therapy induces a massive local immune response characterized by the expression of multiple cytokines. A significant correlation between a reduced risk of melanoma and BCG and vaccinia vaccination in early childhood or infectious diseases later in life has already been reported from the FEBrile Infections and Melanoma (FEBIM) multicenter case-control study [100]. Such observations suggest that BCG can augment immune responses and be used in adjuvant therapy strategies.

Phase II trials indicate that active specific immunotherapy can alter the natural course of American Joint Committee on Cancer [AJCC] Stage III and IV melanoma following surgical resection of nodal or distant metastases. Initial adjuvant immunotherapy trials demonstrated a greater disease-free interval in patients treated with BCG compared with historical controls [101]. In one study 149 patients at high risk of recurrence after surgical treatment of local or regional malignant melanoma were given BCG for 2 years and were followed up for a median of 28 months from the start of immunotherapy [101]. Studies such as these suggest that improved survival rates following recurrence might be explained by the pattern of recurrence; suggesting local or regional sites might be more responsive to treatment. Mechanistic studies suggest that tumor necrosis factor (TNF)-related apoptosis-inducing ligand (TRAIL) is induced by BCG treatment. Subsequently, BCG and components of the mycobacterial cell wall can directly stimulate the release of soluble TRAIL through toll-like receptor-2 (TLR2) recognition that is augmented by IFN. Based on the need for a Th-1 cytokine response to BCG therapy for therapeutic results, it might be proposed that cells migrating in response to BCG treatment release TRAIL. In addition, IFN acts to augment and prolong the amount of TRAIL released by effector cells, resulting in an effective therapeutic outcome.

Early trials of BCG-based immunotherapy for melanoma consistently showed a trend toward improved clinical outcomes in patients treated with BCG compared with observation alone (reviewed by [102]). However, mature results of a phase III randomized trial of BCG versus observation and BCG plus dacarbazine versus BCG in the adjuvant therapy of AJCC stage I-III melanoma (E1673: an ECOG trial) ascribes no benefit for BCG for this patient population [103]. As early as 1976 BCG was tested as an immunotherapy systemic adjunct to surgery in malignant melanoma [104]. In 1984 a polyvalent BCG formulation along with Canvaxin began testing in phase II trials as postsurgical adjuvant therapy for stage III melanoma [105], with results from such trials summarized as no apparent benefit from vaccination [106, 107].

Although experiments with animals have demonstrated that BCG mediates anti-tumor activity, most randomized adjuvant clinical trials have failed to show significant benefit to patients with malignant melanoma. This may be because there is no accepted clinical technique for monitoring *in vivo* BCG activity. As a result the optimal route of administration and dose of BCG have not been truly determined as well as the optimal BCG strain. Attempts to improve the efficacy of BCG therapy have been made. One approach introduced the gene encoding the 65 kDa hsp of Mycobacterium tuberculosis into a mouse malignant melanoma cell line (B16) as proof of principle [108].The 65 kDa hsp was expressed after gene transduction and significantly enhanced the anti-tumor effect of BCG immunotherapy, further indicating that CD4+ T cells play an important role in this anti-tumor effect.

4.2. DETOX

Many adjuvants currently under evaluation for use in cancer vaccines activate relevant APCs, such as dendritic cells and macrophages, via TLRs and promote effective uptake,

http://dx.doi.org/10.5772/53667

processing and presentation of antigen to T-cells in draining lymph nodes. The Gram-negative bacterial cell constituent lipopolysaccharide (LPS) is known to possess strong immunostimulatory properties and has been evaluated as an adjuvant for promoting immune responses to minimally immunogenic antigens, including TATAs. The relatively recent discovery of TLRs and the identification of TLR4, in particular, as the signaling receptor for lipid A have allowed for a better understanding of how this immunostimulant functions with regard to induction of innate and adaptive immune responses. Local TLR stimulation is an attractive approach to induce anti-tumor immunity. Tumor cells respond to TLR ligands with an increase in MHC class I expression and induce IL-6 secretion *in vitro*. Melanoma cells are typically characterized as having low expression of MHC I. Consequently TLR ligands interacting with melanoma cells might enhance MHC class I expression, along with their targeting by melanoma specific CTLs. Although several lipid A species, including LPS and synthetic analogs, have been developed and tested as monotherapeutics for the treatment of cancer, monophosphoryl lipid A (MPL), a ligand for TLR4 has been evaluated as a cancer vaccine adjuvant in published human clinical trials. MPL comprises the lipid A portion of Salmonella minnesota LPS [109]. LPS and MPL induce similar cytokine profiles, but MPL is at least 100-fold less toxic.

DETOX, an adjuvant consisting of MPL and purified mycobacterial cell-wall skeleton (CWS) is another vaccine potentiating agent. MPL (Corixa Corp., Seattle, Washington, USA) adjuvant is a chemically modified LPS derivative that displays greatly reduced toxicity while maintaining most of the immunostimulatory activity of LPS [110] signaling through TLR4 to stimulate the innate immune system. MPL adjuvant has been used extensively in clinical trials as a component in prophylactic and therapeutic vaccines targeting infectious disease, cancer and allergies. MPL has been administered to more than 300,000 human subjects in studies of next-generation vaccines, emerging as a safe and effective vaccine adjuvant. In one study DETOX markedly potentiated antibody but had little effect on DTH responses to melanoma vaccine immunization. It did not appear to improve DFS in comparison to alum in this non-randomized study [111]. DETOX has been formulated into Melacine (Corixa Corp.), a vaccine prepared from the lysate of two melanoma cell lines adjuvanted with DETOX. In clinical trials with Melacine, tumor progression is delayed in the vaccine-treated patients, although this was only observed in patients with certain HLA phenotypes.

The potency of local TLR treatment in therapy demonstrates that local treatment with TLR adjuvants like MPL might effectively restore anti-tumor immunity. Melacine is available for sale in Canada.

4.3. QS-21

Saponins are natural glycosides of steroid or triterpene which exhibit many different biological and pharmacological activities [112]. Notably, saponins can activate the mammalian immune system, and this has led to significant interest in their potential as vaccine adjuvants. The most widely used saponin-based adjuvants are Quil A and its derivative QS-21, isolated from the bark of the Quillaja saponaria Molina (Chilean soap bark tree); these have been evaluated in numerous clinical trials [113]. Their unique capacity to stimulate both the Th-1 immune response and the production of CTLs against exogenous antigens makes them ideal for use in subunit vaccines and vaccines directed against intracellular pathogens as well as cancer.

QS-21 possesses an ability to clinically augment significant antibody and T cell responses to vaccine antigens against a variety of infectious diseases, degenerative disorders and cancers. Currently, there exists no rapid *in vitro* biological screen for assessing the potential efficacy of saponin vaccine adjuvants, given that the mechanism by which saponins augment the immune response is unknown. As a result, evaluation of novel saponins as immunostimulants typically proceed directly to preclinical studies involving mouse vaccination with antigens [99, 112-114].

QS-21 appears to augment both Th-1 and Th-2 type responses and to favor the *in vivo* priming of antigen-specific CD8+ cytotoxic cells. QS-21 has been used in a variety of melanoma targeting vaccines [115]. QS-21 has been shown to be superior to some vaccine formulations such as GM2-KLH plus QS-21 vaccine compared to GM2/BCG vaccine [115]. Efforts to further advance QS-21 in the clinic, as well as to illuminate its unknown mechanism of action, require access to adjuvant-active samples of known composition [114]. The recent synthesis of active molecules of QS-21 has provided a robust method to produce this leading vaccine adjuvant in high purity as well as to produce novel synthetic QS-21 congeners designed to induce increased immune responsiveness and decreased toxicity [99, 112-114].

4.4. Montanide

Mineral oils are known to be very efficient adjuvants but can sometimes induce local reactions with reactive antigens. In contrast, non-mineral oils are well tolerated but less effective with poor immunogens. Mineral oils stay at the injection site and are progressively eliminated by competent cells like the macrophages. They can also be partially metabolized into fatty acids, triglycerides, phospholipids or sterols. Water in oil emulsions represent one of the new promising generations of adjuvants for immunotherapy [116-118]. In this class both Montanide ISA 51 and 720 have been tested in animals and thousands of individuals and found to be safe. Nevertheless, the proper antigen concentration has yet to be established [116-118]. Adverse effects usually depend on the concentration and nature of the antigen.

The mechanistic premise of emulsions is the "depot" effect, in which the adjuvant protects the antigen from both dilution and rapid degradation and elimination by the host. By localizing and slowly releasing intact antigen, the adjuvant permits a slow, prolonged exposure of the immune system cells to a low level of antigen. This prolonged exposure results in continued stimulation of antibody producing cells, resulting in the production of high levels of antibody by the host.

MONTANIDE™ ISA 51 VG has been used in Phase I and II clinical trials for vaccines against malaria, HIV, and various cancers. MONTANIDE™ ISA 51 VG, has been tested in AIDS and cancer vaccine trials which together represent more than 10,000 patients and around 100,000 injections. A survey of ongoing clinical trials listed in ClinicalTrials.gov revealed 36 trials currently accruing patients that are using the olive-derived Montanide ISA

51 IFA. The formulation is generally well-tolerated and induces transient local reactions. Some transient general reactions such as flu-like symptoms are also observed. The results suggest that numerous repeated vaccine doses can be safely administered. Immunization with tumor associated antigen peptides in combination with montanide expands tumor antigen-specific CD8+ T cells in melanoma patients [119-122].

4.5. Cyclophosphamide

High-dose cyclophosphamide (CY) has long been used as an anti-cancer agent, a conditioning regimen for hematopoietic stem cell transplantation and a potent immunosuppressive agent in autoimmune diseases including aplastic anemia. High-dose CY is highly toxic to lymphocytes but spares hematopoietic stem cells because of their abundant levels of aldehyde dehydrogenase, the major mechanism of CY inactivation. CY has emerged as a clinically feasible agent that can suppress Tregs and allow more effective induction of anti-tumor immune responses [123]. Tregs have become an important player in regulating anti-cancer immune responses, with poor prognoses often ascribed to their action [124].

Studies using low dose CY in combination with vaccine components and IL-12 continue to suggest that CY is a viable addition to affect immune responses [125]. Low-dose CY is found to selectively deplete CD4+CD25+ T cells (Tregs) and impede tolerance allowing for a more active immune response. CY preconditioning can enhance the CD8+ T cell response to peptide vaccination, thus leading to enhanced anti-tumor effects against pre-existing tumors [126]. CY markedly enhanced the magnitude of secondary but not primary CTL response induced by vaccines and synergized with vaccine in therapy but not in prophylaxis tumor models [127].

4.6. Conclusions

The major issues that need to be addressed are designing more effective melanoma vaccines with a mix of melanoma-associated antigens that can stimulate clinically beneficial anti-tumor immune responses and finding an adjuvant that can safely, easily and powerfully boost the frequency and magnitude of these responses.

5. Cytokine therapy

Cytokine therapy has had an important position in the treatment of melanoma in the adjuvant and metastatic settings. Various cytokines have been studied with variable success. The most important cytokines in melanoma treatment thus far have been IFN, IL-2, IL-21 and GM-CSF.

5.1. IFN

Interferon IFN is a pleotropic cytokine that exerts anti-tumor activity through numerous mechanisms. High-dose IFNα-2b was approved by the FDA in 1995 for adjuvant therapy of resected stage IIB and III melanoma based on the results of ECOG E1684 [128]. This was a randomized controlled study of IFNα-2b administered at doses of 20 megaunits/m^2/d intravenously (IV) 5 days per week for 1 month and 10 megaunits/m^2 3 times per week subcutaneously (s.c.) for 48 weeks versus observation in 287 patients. Through this study IFNα-2b was the first agent to show a significant benefit in relapse-free survival (RFS) and OS of high-risk melanoma patients in a randomized controlled trial. A subsequent study [129] (E1690) with a total of 642 patients evaluated the efficacy of high-dose IFNα-2b for 1 year (20 megaunits/m^2/d IV 5 days/week for 4 weeks; 10 megaunits/m^2 s.c. TIW for 48 weeks) and low-dose IFNα-2b (3 megaunits/d TIW) for 2 years versus observation in high-risk (stage IIB and III) melanoma with RFS and OS as end points. The results of the intergroup E1690 trial demonstrated a RFS benefit of IFNα-2b that was dose-dependent and significant for the high-dose INFα-2b. Neither high-dose nor low dose IFNα-2b demonstrated an OS benefit compared with observation at the time.

Pooled data from E1684 and E1690 showed that RFS, but not OS, was significantly prolonged for patients treated with high dose IFN versus observation [94]. Long term OS data from E1684 also shows a diminishing level of statistical significance (P=.02 at 7 years, but P=.09 at 12.6 years' median follow-up) [94]. Additional studies by the Eastern Organisation for Research and Treatment of Cancer (EORTC) [130] with adjuvant pegylated IFNα-2b (6 μg/kg per week for 8 weeks followed by 3 μg/kg per week for an intended duration of 5 years) showed a similarly significant and sustained effect on RFS.

The effect of IFNα on OS has been criticized strongly since only two studies (E1684 and E1694) have shown a survival benefit. In contrast, several other studies mentioned above have shown RFS as the only benefit. A recent meta-analysis [131] showed statistically significant improvement in both RFS and OS. The meta-analysis included 14 randomized controlled trials published between 1990 and 2008 and involved 8,122 patients, of which 4,362 were allocated to the IFNα arm. Subgroup analysis and meta-regression did not identify an optimal IFNα dose, the optimal treatment duration or a subset of patients more responsive than others to the adjuvant therapy. Therefore, the role of IFN in the adjuvant setting remains controversial by many. The National Comprehensive Cancer Network (NCCN) has a 2B recommendation for the use of IFN as an adjuvant treatment, and enrollment in clinical trials is encouraged.

Single-agent IFN has demonstrated modest activity in patients with metastatic malignant melanoma with response rates between 10%-20% [132]. Most of the responses were transient and usually restricted to cutaneous metastases [133]. Therefore, its use in the metastatic setting has been employed more frequently in combination with chemotherapy (biochemotherapy) with improved response rates but without a well documented survival benefit [134]. Other cytokines have been subsequently evaluated, and the interest in IFN has been shifted to the adjuvant setting as mentioned above.

5.2. IL-2

One of the most promising immune stimulating cytokines has been interleukin 2 (IL-2). High dose IL-2 produces not only PRs but also CRs. Overall objective response rates (ORR) are approximately 16% with IL-2 with a 6% CR rate [93]. Importantly, some patients achieved durable CRs which led to the approval of high-dose IL-2 for patients with metastatic melanoma. Responses occurred with all sites of disease and in patients with large tumor burdens (unlike previously with IFN). Disease progression was not observed in any patient responding for longer than 30 months, and in some cases where disease progression was observed, durable disease free status was achieved with metastasectomy.

The use of high-dose IL-2, however, is limited by its severe toxicity; 2.2% of the patients in the National Cancer Institute (NCI) trial series died from treatment-related toxicities with bacterial sepsis being the predominant cause of death. No deaths were observed in the NCI series when antibiotic prophylaxis was implemented. However, the incidence of grade 3-4 toxicities remains high, ranging between 1-64%. Alternate regimens have been employed including low dose IL-2 alone or in combination with IFN-α or chemotherapy. However, there is evidence that suggests that high dose IL-2 is a more efficacious regimen. A phase II study showed durable CRs with high-dose bolus IL-2 in patients with metastatic melanoma who have experienced progression after biochemotherapy [135]. In addition, IL-2 based biochemotherapy regimens have not shown significantly better results than chemotherapy alone, presumptively due to the fact that high dose IL-2 is not utilized [136].

5.3. IL-21

The role of other cytokines has also been explored. IL-21 has recently emerged as a promising cytokine [137]. In an open-label, multicenter phase II study, IL-21 was given as a bolus injection on days 1 through 5 on alternate weeks using three different dosing regimens in 40 patients with malignant melanoma. Cohort 1 received 50 μg/kg per day by outpatient IV bolus injection for 5 days of each week during weeks 1, 3, and 5 of an 8-week cycle. Cohort 2 received 30 μg/kg per day on the same schedule, and cohort 3 received 50 μg/kg per day for 5 days of each week during weeks 1 and 3 of a 6-week cycle. The primary objective of the study was to assess efficacy (ORR and PFS) of IL-21 in this population. The ORR to IL-21 was 22.5%. The median PFS was 4.3 months and the median OS was 12.4 months, suggesting that this is an active agent that warrants further investigation. The 30 μg/kg per day dose and schedule was generally well tolerated as an outpatient regimen, with the most common adverse events being flu-like symptoms and rash, most of which were grade 1 or 2.

5.4. GM-CSF

Granulocyte macrophage-colony stimulating factor (GM-CSF) has also been studied mostly in the adjuvant setting. Forty-eight patients with stage III or IV melanoma were treated in a phase II trial with long-term, chronic, intermittent GM-CSF after complete surgical resection of disease [138]. The median survival duration was 37.5 months in the study patients versus 12.2 months in the matched controls. OS and DFS were significantly prolonged in patients who received GM-CSF compared with matched historical controls, and treatment was well tolerated with acceptable toxicity. A phase III prospective, randomized, placebo-controlled study (E4697) failed to show an OS benefit but improved DFS in patients with completely resected high-risk melanoma with minimal toxicity [139].

5.5. Conclusions

Immune stimulating cytokines have historically been an important part of the therapeutic armamentarium for early stage and metastatic melanoma due to the importance of the immune system in this disease. The currently approved IFN and IL-2 treatments in the adjuvant and metastatic settings, respectively, provide modest but reproducible clinical benefits. Their use is limited by toxicity and the lack of clearly defined predictive-to-treatment tools. In the near future, the development of novel molecular and immune treatments might limit their role. However, the durable responses that we see in some patients should not be ignored, and the search for predictive biomarkers should continue.

6. Vaccine therapy

The purpose of cancer vaccines is to evoke an immune response against malignant cells. One of the earliest approaches was taken more than 100 years ago when Dr. William Coley treated patients with Coley's Toxin derived from bacteria [22]. Although clinical success in individual trials has been uncommon, a meta-analysis of 56 clinical trials showed that evidence of an immune response predicted a better outcome [140]. Vaccines are of various types, each with advantages and disadvantages. The following discussion will be divided by the vaccine type, and when available, clinical data in advanced and adjuvant settings.

6.1. Autologous whole cell vaccines

Vaccines derived from the patient's own cancer should have the advantage of presenting the complete array of tumor antigens, both internal and external. There should be less chance of the remaining tumor mutating sufficiently to avoid detection. These vaccines should be able to produce both humoral and cellular immunity [141]. Autologous vaccines are produced by irradiating resected tumors or by establishing cell lines from resected specimens [22]. This approach is difficult from a technical and regulatory standpoint. It is further hampered by limiting eligible patients to those with accessible cancer and those who can wait for the vaccine development [141]. These vaccines have used the cells themselves with adjuvants or cells modified to produce cytokines.

An autologous whole cell vaccine is exemplified in work done by Berd, et. al. Early reports demonstrated clinical response to an irradiated autologous tumor cell vaccine given with BCG as an adjuvant. Subsequently, low dose CY preceded vaccination. In that study there were 5 responses in the 40 subjects assessable for response. The responses were associated with DTH responses [142]. In the next series of studies the vaccine was modified by the hapten, dinitrophenyl (DNP), and BCG and CY were maintained. Sixty two subjects with resected nodal metastases were vaccinated and compared to historical controls. There was a perceived benefit in disease progression and survival, especially in subjects over the age of

50 years [143]. In an expansion of this initial trial to 214 subjects, there was an improvement in OS in patients who developed a positive DTH response (59.3% vs 29.3%; $p < 0.001$). Forty-seven percent of subjects had a DTH response [144].

Work done by the National Biotherapy Study Group utilizing patient specific autologous tumor cell lines in patients with melanoma has been summarized [145]. This series of studies utilized different adjuvants including BCG, IFNγ and GM-CSF. Once again, benefit was seen in groups developing a positive DTH response [145-147]. Additional non-randomized studies show positive outcomes as well, but without randomization, the results are difficult to weigh [148-151]. Some studies have genetically modified the tumor cells to secret cytokines. These trials have also been non-randomized but have shown positive results [152, 153]. A randomized trial using an autologous tumor vaccine processed to extract hsps compared to physician's choice was conducted in 322 patients with metastatic disease. There was no difference between the two groups overall, but subjects with M1a disease had longer survival when treated with vaccine [154].

6.2. Allogeneic whole cell vaccines

Allogeneic whole cell vaccines are produced by a cell line or cell lines. Other features are similar to the autologous cell vaccines. The advantage of this approach is that it is more readily available and would prevent delays in treatment that are necessitated by the autologous vaccines. However the antigens may not match those of the patient's melanoma [141].

A vaccine developed by Dr. Donald Morton beginning in 1984 from three irradiated melanoma cell lines has been studied the most extensively. It is named Canvaxin (CancerVax Corp., Carlsbad, California, USA). There were extensive phase II trials done in patients with stage IV disease demonstrating response to therapy. However, when tested in randomized multicenter trials in resected stage III and IV melanoma patients, there was no benefit noted. However, the trials were stopped prior to their planned accrual by the data safety monitoring board for futility [141, 155-157]. Other allogeneic vaccines including VACCIMEL (produced from three melanoma cell lines) have had less mature study and similar biomarker results [158].

6.3. Tumor lysate vaccines

Tumor lysate vaccines have similar advantages and disadvantages of allogeneic vaccines. The vaccinia melanoma oncolysate (VMO) vaccine is prepared from four allogeneic cell lines infected with the vaccinia virus to increase immunogenicity. The cells are then lysed by sonication prior to administration. VMO yielded encouraging phase II results, however, there was no statistically significant increase in DFS when studied in an adjuvant setting [157, 159].

A second tumor lysate vaccine, called Melacine (Corixa Corp., Seattle Washington, USA) is also a cell lysate vaccine which has been tested in two large randomized trials. One adjuvant trial conducted by the Southwest Oncology Group (SWOG) studied 600 eligible patients treated with Melacine along with the adjuvant DETOX versus observation. To be eligible the subjects had to have intermediate thickness lesions and negative nodes; however, sentinel lymph node biopsy was not required, and therefore, the staging in this trial would be considered inadequate by today's standards. Survival in the overall analysis showed no difference between treatment and observation, however, a subgroup of patients expressing certain MHC classes showed a five-year survival rate of 83% compared to 59% in the observation group. This subset analysis was statistically significant [160-163]. An Ad Hoc Melanoma Working Group reported a separate study in stage III resected patients comparing high dose IFN for one year versus low lose IFN plus Melacine with DETOX for 2 years. Six hundred subjects were registered. There was no difference in outcome [164]. As described above, high dose IFN had been shown previously to be superior to observation.

6.4. Protein vaccines

Protein vaccines using purified proteins have the potential for a broader spectrum of antigens, but they can be more complex to manufacture and monitor for response [157]. The use of hsps, which have a normal function in chaperoning proteins as they are processed into peptides, has also been explored with peptide vaccines [154] and may have a role in identifying new antigenic targets [165]. A trial using NY-ESO was found to produce a strong immunologic response after vaccination. There were better clinical outcomes compared to placebo in those given the protein vaccine compared to placebo. The adjuvant used in the trial was ISCOMATRIX [166].

6.5. Ganglioside antigen vaccines

Gangliosides are non-protein antigens (glycosphingolipids containing sialic acids) that have been shown to elicit antibodies. They are present on melanoma cells (GM2, GD2, GD3) [157, 167]. The GM2 antigen plus BCG versus BCG alone was studied in stage III resected patients. There was no difference in DFS, but subjects with IgM antibodies against the antigen had better outcome [167]. GM2 conjugated to a keyhole limpet hemocyanin (KLH) and administered with the adjuvant QS-21 had better immunogenicity [168]. This same vaccine was compared to high dose IFN in an Intergroup adjuvant trial in patients with resected stage IIB or III melanoma. The trial ended when an interim analysis showed therapeutic inferiority in the vaccine arm [169].

6.6. Peptide vaccines

Peptide vaccines have the advantage of being easy to manufacture and have an excellent safety record. However, there are challenges that impact their effectiveness. These include the identification of epitopes that stimulate a T cell response, selecting an appropriate adjuvant, breaking tolerance without causing limiting autoimmunity, handling MHC restriction and assessing the need for multi-epitope vaccines [170]. Peptide vaccines have been reported to increase survival following resection of metastatic lesions [171] and have been shown to have increased immune efficacy with various adjuvants [172, 173]. Use of multiple peptides has been another strategy [121, 174, 175]. An ECOG study testing a multi-epitope vaccine with GM-CSF and/or IFNα-2b showed that an immune response to the vaccine correlated with outcome but that the cytokines did not affect outcome [176].

One of the most studied peptide vaccines is a modified gp100 peptide antigen. This vaccine has been studied in locally advanced stage III or stage IV patients comparing IL-2 to IL-2 plus vaccine. The results showed a statistically significant improvement in response rate and PFS in the vaccine arm [177]. This is in contrast to a report from the Cytokine Working Group analysis of three phase II trials looking at a similar vaccine with IL-2 showing no benefit to the addition of the vaccine [178]. Another phase III study comparing ipilimumab plus gp100 vaccine versus gp100 plus placebo versus ipilimumab plus placebo failed to show a benefit to the addition of the vaccine, and the vaccine alone was inferior [95].

6.7. Monoclonal antibodies

Anti-idiotype vaccines consist of monoclonal antibodies that mimic an antigen. The theoretical hypothesis is sound [179-181], but trials have been limited [182-184]. These vaccines have not been tested prospectively.

6.8. Viral vaccines

Viral vectors can boost the immunogenicity of the vaccines they carry [141, 185]. However the presence of neutralizing antibodies in the host could play a role [186]. Novel methods of utilizing this mode of immune stimulation are still being explored [187, 188]. A randomized trial in stage III resected patients utilizing a vaccinia viral lysate vaccine failed to show benefit [189]. Transduction of cell lines to produce expression of B7-1and IL-2 have been accomplished and show promising immunostimulatory effects [190, 191]. These techniques are difficult to pursue from a technical and regulatory standpoint. Recombinant viral vaccines have also been used to prime dendritic cells [192].

6.9. DNA vaccines

DNA vaccines have the advantage of specificity for the target for which they encode, which can simplify monitoring, but in general they have not done well in breaking tolerance [141, 193-195]. Two groups have reported on vaccines that rely on production of GM-CSF. Dranoff has reported on a vaccine utilizing melanoma cell lines engineered to produce GM-CSF and has noted improved anti-tumor effects [196]. A different approach using an intralesional vaccination with an oncolytic herpesvirus encoding GM-CSF has been developed and has had initial positive results [197, 198]. Another agent called Allovectin-7 consists of a plasmid containing DNA encoding for the MHC class I gene, HLA-B7. It was administered by intralesional injection. Early studies showed evidence of biologic activity [199]. Subsequent phase II studies showed efficacy locally as well as systemically [200-203]. A phase III study has not yet been reported.

7. Cellular therapy

The transfer of immunologically competent white blood cells or their precursors into the host (cellular adoptive immunotherapy, adoptive cell treatment, adoptive cell therapy [ACT]) has been studied extensively in patients with melanoma over the last 30 years. Since it was thought that the effect of IL-2 is potentiated by this form of therapy, various studies examined the role of combination regimens with lymphokine-activated killer cells (LAK cells) or TILs with or without lymphodepletion with mixed results.

7.1. TILs

Earlier studies with LAK cells [204] showed promise, improving the responses with IL-2. A randomized study [205] with IL-2 and LAK cells compared to IL-2 alone failed to show significant improvement in survival which tempered the initial enthusiasm. Subsequent studies with Tumor Infiltrating Lymphocytes (TILs) [206] showed some response to treatment (overall ORR in these patients was 34%) when combined with IL-2. Interestingly, there was no significant difference in the ORR in patients whose therapy with high-dose IL-2 had failed (32%) compared with patients not previously treated with IL-2 (34%). However, the responses appeared to be short-lived, probably due to the transient persistence of the transferred TILs [207].

The addition of lymphodepletion has been thought to promote the persistence of the transferred TILs by eliminating the regulatory cells. Pooled data from three clinical trials employing three different lymphodepleting regimens [91] showed high responses between 49-72%. Ninety-five percent of these patients had progressive disease following a prior systemic treatment. Twenty of the 93 patients (22%) achieved complete tumor regression, and 19 have ongoing complete regressions beyond 3 years. The actuarial 3- and 5-year survival rates for the entire group were 36% and 29%, respectively, but for the 20 complete responders were 100% and 93%. Factors associated with objective response included longer telomeres of the infused cells, the number of CD8+ CD27+ cells infused and the persistence of the infused cells in the circulation at one month. This treatment appears to also be helpful in the treatment of intracranial disease [208].

At this point, there is reserved enthusiasm about the role of TILs with lymphodepletion regimens. There are several programs within the United States [209] outside of the NCI, where this work was pioneered, and internationally more groups are starting to employ similar strategies.

7.2. Dendritic cells

Another form of ACT is the infusion of dendritic cells. There is a lot of interest in developing dendritic cell based immunotherapy strategies since the approval of sipuleucel-T, an autologous dendritic cell based immunotherapy in hormone refractory prostate cancer. Dendritic cells are believed to induce a Th-1 response which activates CTLs through processing and presenting of peptides derived from the tumor protein antigens. In a study that evaluated the role of dendritic cells pulsed with Mage-3A1 tumor peptide and a recall antigen, tetanus toxoid or tuberculin, 6 of 11 patients with advanced stage IV melanoma experienced significant regression of their metastases [210]. Resolution of skin metastases in two of the patients was accompanied by $CD8^+$ T cell infiltration, whereas nonregressing lesions lacked $CD8^+$ T cells.

In another trial [211] 16 patients with metastatic stage IV melanoma were treated with dendritic cells derived from incubation of peripheral blood mononuclear cells with IL-4 and GM-CSF and overnight pulsing with several peptides (tyrosinase, gp100 and MART-1). One patient had a complete remission of lung and pleural disease after two cycles of therapy. Two additional patients had SD, and two patients had mixed responses. In general, reviewing over 30 studies that employed dendritic cell-based treatments [212], it appears that clinical response (defined as CR, PR or SD) was significantly correlated with the use of peptide antigens, use of helper antigen or adjuvant and induction of tumor antigen specific T cells.

Although there appears to be a real effect of these treatments on tumor response in a subset of the treated patients, undoubtedly the success has not been universal and convincing [213]. This could be due to Tregs that counteract the effect of dendritic cells. In addition, melanoma can also mediate dendritic cell suppression possibly through the activation of the MEK1/2-p44/42 axis [214]. Finally, little is known about optimal dendritic cell generation, administration and immune monitoring which could hamper progress in this field.

8. Enhancement of cellular immunity

8.1. Checkpoint inhibitors

Monoclonal antibodies targeted against a number of regulatory immune system checkpoints are being evaluated in patients with advanced melanoma. The recently approved ipilimumab remains the prototype, but others are currently being evaluated in several trials.

8.2. Ipilimumab

Ipilimumab is a monoclonal antibody against cytotoxic T-lymphocyte antigen 4 (CTLA-4). In two phase III trials ipilimumab showed improved OS in patients with advanced melanoma. In the first one [95], 676 HLA-A*0201–positive patients with unresectable stage III or IV melanoma, whose disease had progressed while they were receiving therapy for metastatic disease were studied. More than 70% of the patients had M1c disease (presence of visceral metastases), and more than 36% had elevated lactate dehydrogenase levels. The patients were randomly assigned, in a 3:1:1 ratio, to receive ipilimumab plus gp100, ipilimumab alone or gp100 alone. Ipilimumab, at a dose of 3 mg/kg of body weight, was administered with or without gp100 every three weeks for up to four treatments. HLA-A*0201–positivity was required because of the use of the gp100 vaccine. Certain patients were allowed to have another course of treatment upon progression. The primary end point was OS.

The median OS was 10.0 months among patients receiving ipilimumab plus gp100, as compared with 6.4 months among patients receiving gp100 alone (hazard ratio for death, 0.68; P<0.001). The median OS with ipilimumab alone was 10.1 months (hazard ratio for death in comparison with gp100 alone, 0.66; P=0.003). No difference in OS was detected between the ipilimumab groups (hazard ratio with ipilimumab plus gp100, 1.04; P=0.76). The best OR or SD was seen in the ipilimumab-alone group (10.9%) and a disease control rate (the proportion of patients with a PR, CR or SD) of 28.5%. In the ipilimumab-alone group, 60.0% maintained an OR for at least two years. Responses to ipilimumab continued to improve beyond week 24: in the ipilimumab-alone group, two patients with SD improved to a PR, and three with a PR improved to a CR. Interestingly, among 31 patients given reinduction therapy with ipilimumab, a PR, CR or SD was achieved by 21 weeks. Grade 3 or 4 immune-related adverse events occurred in 10 to 15% of patients treated with ipilimumab and in 3% treated with gp100 alone. There were 14 deaths related to the study drugs (2.1%), and seven were associated with immune-related adverse events.

In the second phase III study [215], 502 patients with previously untreated metastatic melanoma were assigned in a 1:1 ratio to receive 10 mg/kg ipilimumab plus 850 mg/m^2 dacarbazine or 850 mg/m^2 dacarbazine plus placebo, given at weeks 1, 4, 7 and 10, followed by 850 mg/m^2 dacarbazine alone every three weeks through week 22. Patients with SD or an OR and no dose-limiting toxic effects received ipilimumab or placebo every 12 weeks thereafter as maintenance therapy. Similarly with the previous study a significant number of patients had poor prognosis based on the presence of visceral metastases and increased lactate dehydrogenase. The primary end point was OS.

OS was significantly longer in the group receiving ipilimumab plus dacarbazine than in the group receiving dacarbazine plus placebo (11.2 months vs. 9.1 months), with higher survival rates in the ipilimumab–dacarbazine group at one year (47.3% vs. 36.3%), two years (28.5% vs. 17.9%), and three years (20.8% vs. 12.2%) (hazard ratio for death, 0.72; P<0.001). The rate of disease control (PR, CR or SD) did not differ significantly between the two groups: 33.2% in the ipilimumab–dacarbazine group and 30.2% in the dacarbazine group (P=0.41). The rate of best OR (PR or CR) was 15.2% in the ipilimumab–dacarbazine group and 10.3% in the dacarbazine group (P=0.09). However, the median duration of response among all patients with a PR or CR was 19.3 months (95% CI, 12.1 to 26.1) in the ipilimumab–dacarbazine group and 8.1 months (95% CI, 5.19 to 19.8) in the dacarbazine group (P=0.03). In addition, some patients in the study who were receiving ipilimumab had an improvement from PR to CR after six months. Grade 3 or 4 adverse events occurred in 56.3% of patients treated with ipilimumab plus dacarbazine, as compared with 27.5% treated with dacarbazine and placebo (P<0.001). No drug-related deaths or gastrointestinal perforations occurred in the ipilimumab–dacarbazine group.

Patients with untreated brain metastases were excluded from both phase III studies. However, phase II data indicate that ipilimumab has activity in patients with brain metastases [216]. The currently approved dose is 3 mg/kg based on the registration trial [95], however other doses and schedules [217] have been used that do not appear to produce significantly different results but appear to increase toxicity.

The experience with ipilimumab has shown that a subgroup of patients may experience a late response and more interestingly, some patients exhibit apparent disease progression after 12 weeks of ipilimumab followed by subsequent disease regression [218]. Therefore, traditional criteria (e.g. RECIST) may not apply in the evaluation of patients who receive ipilimumab or similar treatments, and different criteria may need to be established in the interpretation of efficacy data in clinical trials [20].

Based on the favorable results from the ipilimumab studies, other anti-CTLA4 antibodies are currently being evaluated such as tremelimumab. Tremelimumab has a longer half-life than ipilimumab and is dosed less frequently. Phase II data showed results similar to ipilimumab with durable responses suggesting a potential role for tremelimumab in melanoma [219]. However, a phase III trial comparing tremelimumab and chemotherapy failed to demonstrate an improvement in OS [220].

8.3. Toxicity with ipilimumab

The toxicity of ipilimumab appears to be related to the increased activation of the immune system. A variety of immune mediated adverse events have been observed. Some of them are life-threatening and the most common are enterocolitis, hepatitis, dermatitis and endocrinopathies, but others such as neurologic complications, ocular symptoms, hematologic manifestations, vasculitis, et al are also observed.The prompt administration of corticosteroids is paramount when these are observed, and in some cases treatment interruption or permanent discontinuation is required. A relationship between the development of side effects and anti-tumor activity has been proposed by several investigators [218].

8.4. PD-1

Another regulatory checkpoint is Programmed Death-1 receptor (PD-1). Its inhibition is currently being evaluated in clinical trials. The PD-1 and PD ligand-1 (PD-L1) interaction is believed to affect T cell anti-tumor immunity. Many tumors express high levels of PD-L1. When PD-L1 interacts with the PD-1 receptor on T cells, T cell function is impaired through a variety of mechanisms including induction of apoptosis, suppression of proliferation and inhibition of T cell cytokine production [96]. There are several ways to target PD-1; one way is targeting the PD-1 receptor and another is targeting the PD-1 ligand. There are several molecules currently under investigation that target the PD-1 receptor directly (BMS-936558, CT-011, MK-3475). In a recent study [98], BMS-936558 showed significant anti-tumor activity in a variety of solid tumors. In melanoma patients response rates were 28% and appeared to be durable. Interestingly, of 17 patients with PD-L1–negative tumors, none had an OR while 9 of 25 patients (36%) with PD-L1–positive tumors had an OR (P=0.006). CT-011 has demonstrated favorable results in hematologic malignancies but has not been well studied in melanoma patients yet [221], although there is an ongoing phase I study being conducted at present. The role of MK-3475 in melanoma is also currently being evaluated in a phase I trial. Another molecule which is not probably directly targeting the PD-1 is AMP-224; it is a fusion protein of B7-DC and an antibody Fc portion. It is not a monoclonal antibody like the three checkpoint agents mentioned previously, and no data has been reported yet regarding its efficacy in human trials. PD-L1 monoclonal antibodies have emerged as another strategy to affect the PD-1/PD L-1 pathway. A multi-center phase I study evaluating the role of BMS-936559 in patients with advanced cancers including melanoma showed a 17% response rate in melanoma patients with some of those being durable responses [97].

8.5. Co-stimulatory agonists

4-1BB or CD137 is a member of the TNF receptor (TNFR) family and provides a costimulatory signal important to the effective generation of many types of T cell responses. A completed phase I study in melanoma with BMS-663513, a fully human anti-CD137 agonist monoclonal antibody, showed that this agent was well tolerated and three PRs were seen [222].

OX-40 is another member of the TNFR family. An agonist molecule is also under investigation, but mature data are not yet available [223].

8.6. Conclusions

Checkpoint inhibitors and co-stimulatory agonists are improving anti-tumor cellular immunity. In a similar way to the more non-specific activation through cytokines, responses are durable but are not seen in all patients. This brings up issues such as appropriate patient selection, biomarker development and optimization of the dose, frequency and administration in order to optimize efficacy.

9. Combination approaches

Combination approaches have been traditionally used in the treatment of melanoma (for example different cytokines together or cytokines with chemotherapy). It is quite interesting that the results of this strategy have not been yet as successful as expected. While new agents are developed and we understand more about their function, these strategies may become more successful. At this point there is a lot of interest combining checkpoint inhibitors with other checkpoint blocking agents, co-stimulatory agonists, chemotherapy, targeted agents (such as B-type Raf kinas [BRAF] inhibitors) and radiotherapy. Interestingly, the BRAF inhibitors appear to improve T cell recognition of melanoma [224] which reinforces a rational combination of targeted therapy and immunotherapy. The results are not yet mature and studies are ongoing, but there is preclinical and retrospective data that support this model of treatment [224-227]. The following combination strategies have shown some recent benefit and promise.

9.1. Anti-CTLA4 and IFNa

A phase II study [227] combining tremelimumab and high dose IFN in patients with advanced melanoma showed an ORR of 24% with 4 patients obtaining a CR. Toxicity was acceptable and the median OS was 21 months. The University of Pittsburgh group is now contemplating a neoadjuvant and adjuvant therapy that employs an anti-CTLA4 and IFN-α combination strategy.

9.2. Anti-CTLA4 and GM-CSF

A phase II study through ECOG combining ipilimumab and GM-CSF is currently ongoing. Previous studies [228] with periodic infusions of anti-CTLA-4 antibodies after vaccination with irradiated, autologous tumor cells engineered to secrete GM-CSF have yielded favorable results with acceptable toxicity.

9.3. IL-2 and gp-100

A phase III trial evaluated the combination of IL-2 and the gp100 peptide vaccine in advanced melanoma. This combination therapy increased the response rate (16% vs. 6%) with more CRs in the combination arm and a trend toward increased OS [177]. Interestingly, the single arm responses were lower than expected. A similarly designed study employing ipilimumab did not show significant benefit in the combination arm [95].

10. Conclusion

Immunotherapy holds the promise of "the cure" for cancer. Glimpses of this outcome have been seen throughout the past century but may be best exemplified in melanoma therapy. Although attempts in the past have not had satisfactory results, the knowledge gained along with the ability to develop biologically active drugs is bearing fruit in the current generation of clinical trials. The few positive results have kept the interest for cancer immunotherapy alive which has also helped us to achieve a better understanding of the immune system in relationship to cancer treatment. The improvement in outcome seen with gp100 plus IL-2 is impressive, and the power of the anti-cancer and autoimmune toxicities seen with ipilimumab is dramatic. The excitement stems not only from the clinical results that were obtained but also by our ability to successfully manipulate the complex immune system in a different way than before. Undoubtedly, there are a lot of unanswered questions including why are there still a large number of patients who do not achieve responses with immunotherapy and eventually die from advanced disease? However, unlike immunotherapy applied to other advanced setting solid tumors, immunotherapy in advanced melanoma has resulted in some durable responses and possibly cures.

The future of immunotherapy in melanoma and other tumor types would ideally involve research in a broad range of directions. An optimization of the IL-2 based treatments is needed to improve the number of durable responses. Results from the current work at NCI augmenting IL-2 treatment with lymphodepletion are quite encouraging. Identification of serum or tissue biomarkers is also urgently needed. Biomarker research is often complex, but this work should reveal a better understanding of the tumor itself as well as the host. The checkpoint inhibitors such as ipilimumab and tremelimumab have opened the door for research into other immunologic checkpoints such as PD-1 and co-stimulatory signals. The need for a reliable melanoma biomarker is again paramount, and the significance of PD-L1 expression that is currently under investigation is anticipated with interest. Studying mechanisms of resistance in all cancer immunotherapeutics is equally important.

The combination of different immunotherapeutics with each other, with molecularly targeted agents or with conventional treatments such as chemotherapy or radiation therapy, may not be the simple process that combination strategies with vaccines were in the past, but this approach is quite attractive and rational and will help us further understand the role of the immune system in this disease. In a similar fashion, sequential therapy, using different agents at different times might improve clinical response and survival. Appropriate first line selection is also quite challenging since there are currently three approved agents in BRAF V600E mutated patients (high does IL-2, ipilimumab and vemurafenib) and two for BRAF wild type patients (high dose IL-2 and ipilimumab). A randomized clinical trial of ipilimumab followed by vemurafenib versus vemurafenib followed by ipilimumab is planned through the NCI Cooperative Group mechanisms [218]. Future clinical trials will hopefully provide some answers to these questions. In the design of clinical trials, the importance of refining the RECIST criteria for immunotherapy agents cannot be overemphasized. Overall, this is an exciting time for cancer immunologists and clinicians who treat patients with melanoma. The future for innovative trials of new agents and combinations is brighter than ever before.

Acknowledgements

The authors would like to thank Linda Ray for her invaluable administrative support.

Author details

Konstantinos Arnaoutakis, Dorothy A. Graves, Laura F. Hutchins and
Thomas Kieber-Emmons

Division of Hematology/Oncology and Department of Pathology University of Arkansas for Medical Sciences, Little Rock, AR, Winthrop P. Rockefeller Cancer Institute, USA

References

[1] I. B. Bayer-Garner, D. Ivan, M. R. Schwartz and J. A. Tschen, "The immunopathology of regression in benign lichenoid keratosis, keratoacanthoma and halo nevus," *Clin. Med. Res.*, vol. 2, pp. 89-97, May, 2004.

[2] R. Akasu, L. From and H. J. Kahn, "Characterization of the mononuclear infiltrate involved in regression of halo nevi," *J. Cutan. Pathol., vol. 21, pp. 302-311, Aug, 1994.*

[3] K. McKay, P. C. Moore, B. R. Smoller and K. M. Hiatt. Association between natural killer cells and regression in melanocytic lesions. Hum. *Pathol. [All @ UAMS; LRVA (latest 10 years)].* 42(12), pp. 1960-1964. 2011. Available: http://ovidsp.ovid.com/ovidweb.cgi?T=JS&CSC=Y&NEWS=N&PAGE=fulltext&D=medl&AN=21676435.

[4] N. Arpaia, N. Cassano and G. A. Vena. Regressing cutaneous malignant melanoma and vitiligo-like depigmentation. Int. J. Dermatol. [Part @ UAMS (Click Library Holdings)]. 45(8), pp. 952-956. 2006. Available: http://ovidsp.ovid.com/ovidweb.cgi?T=JS&CSC=Y&NEWS=N&PAGE=fulltext&D=med4&AN=16911383.

[5] M. G. Bouwhuis, A. Gast, A. Figl, A. M. Eggermont, K. Hemminki, D. Schadendorf and R. Kumar. Polymorphisms in the CD28/CTLA4/ICOS genes: Role in malignant melanoma susceptibility and prognosis?. Cancer Immunology, Immunotherapy [Not locally available; ask about Interlibrary Loan]. *59(2),* pp. 303-312. 2010. Available: http://ovidsp.ovid.com/ovidweb.cgi?T=JS&CSC=Y&NEWS=N&PAGE=fulltext&D=medl&AN=19672595.

[6] P. Fishman, O. Merimski, E. Baharav and Y. Shoenfeld. Autoantibodies to tyrosinase: The bridge between melanoma and vitiligo. *Cancer* [All @ UAMS; LRVA (latest 10 years)]. 79(8), pp. 1461-1464. 1997. Available: http://ovidsp.ovid.com/ovidweb.cgi?T=JS&CSC=Y&NEWS=N&PAGE=fulltext&D=med4&AN=9118024.

[7] K. A. Chianese-Bullock, E. M. Woodson, H. Tao, S. A. Boerner, M. Smolkin, W. W. Grosh, P. Y. Neese, P. Merrill, G. R. Petroni and C. L. Slingluff Jr. Autoimmune toxicities associated with the administration of antitumor vaccines and low-dose interleukin-2. *Journal of Immunotherapy* [All @ UAMS]. 28(4), pp. 412-419. 2005. Available: http://ovidsp.ovid.com/ovidweb.cgi?T=JS&CSC=Y&NEWS=N&PAGE=fulltext&D=medc&AN=16000961.

[8] C. Printz, "Spontaneous regression of melanoma may offer insight into cancer immunology," *J. Natl. Cancer Inst.,* vol. 93, pp. 1047-1048, Jul 18, 2001.

[9] W. A. High, D. Stewart, C. R. Wilbers, C. J. Cockerell, M. P. Hoang and J. E. Fitzpatrick, "Completely regressed primary cutaneous malignant melanoma with nodal and/or visceral metastases: a report of 5 cases and assessment of the literature and diagnostic criteria," *J. Am. Acad. Dermatol.,* vol. 53, pp. 89-100, Jul, 2005.

[10] K. K. Anbari, L. M. Schuchter, L. P. Bucky, R. Mick, M. Synnestvedt, D. Guerry 4th, R. Hamilton and A. C. Halpern, "Melanoma of unknown primary site: presentation, treatment, and prognosis--a single institution study. University of Pennsylvania Pigmented Lesion Study Group," *Cancer,* vol. 79, pp. 1816-1821, May 1, 1997.

[11] B. Schlagenhauff, W. Stroebel, U. Ellwanger, F. Meier, C. Zimmermann, H. Breuninger, G. Rassner and C. Garbe, "Metastatic melanoma of unknown primary origin shows prognostic similarities to regional metastatic melanoma: recommendations for initial staging examinations," *Cancer,* vol. 80, pp. 60-65, Jul 1, 1997.

[12] G. H. Baab and C. M. McBride. Malignant melanoma: The patient with an unknown site of primary origin. *Archives of Surgery* [All @ UAMS; LRVA (latest 10 years)].

110(8), pp. 896-900. 1975. Available: http://ovidsp.ovid.com/ovidweb.cgi?T=JS&CSC=Y&NEWS=N&PAGE=fulltext&D=med1&AN=1156155.

[13] M. F. Demierre. Thin melanomas and regression, thick melanomas and older men: Prognostic implications and perspectives on secondary prevention. *Arch. Dermatol.* [All @ UAMS; Part @ ACH(Click Lib.Holdings) & LRVA(10 yrs)]. *138(5),* pp. 678-682. 2002. Available: http://ovidsp.ovid.com/ovidweb.cgi?T=JS&CSC=Y&NEWS=N&PAGE=fulltext&D=med4&AN=12020232.

[14] J. K. O'Neill, R. Khundar, L. Knowles, N. Scott-Young and A. Orlando. Melanoma with an unknown primary--a case series. Journal of Plastic, Reconstructive & Aesthetic Surgery: JPRAS [Online Access Only (Click E Journal Holdings for Information)]. *63(12),* pp. 2071-2080. 2010. Available: http://ovidsp.ovid.com/ovidweb.cgi?T=JS&CSC=Y&NEWS=N&PAGE=fulltext&D=medl&AN=20335085.

[15] M. King, D. Spooner and D. C. Rowlands. Spontaneous regression of metastatic malignant melanoma of the parotid gland and neck lymph nodes: A case report and a review of the literature. *Clinical Oncology (Royal College of Radiologists)* [Online Access Only (Click E Journal Holdings for Information)]. 13(6), pp. 466-469. 2001. Available: http://ovidsp.ovid.com/ovidweb.cgi?T=JS&CSC=Y&NEWS=N&PAGE=fulltext&D=med4&AN=11824888.

[16] L. V. Kalialis, K. T. Drzewiecki and H. Klyver. Spontaneous regression of metastases from melanoma: Review of the literature. *Melanoma Res.* [Online Access Only (Click E Journal Holdings for Information)]. 19(5), pp. 275-282. 2009. Available: http://ovidsp.ovid.com/ovidweb.cgi?T=JS&CSC=Y&NEWS=N&PAGE=fulltext&D=medl&AN=19633580.

[17] N. J. Crowley and H. F. Seigler, "Late recurrence of malignant melanoma. Analysis of 168 patients," *Ann. Surg.,* vol. 212, pp. 173-177, Aug, 1990.

[18] M. H. Schmid-Wendtner, J. Baumert, M. Schmidt, B. Konz, D. Holzel, G. Plewig and M. Volkenandt, "Late metastases of cutaneous melanoma: an analysis of 31 patients," *J. Am. Acad. Dermatol.,* vol. 43, pp. 605-609, Oct, 2000.

[19] E. A. Eisenhauer, P. Therasse, J. Bogaerts, L. H. Schwartz, D. Sargent, R. Ford, J. Dancey, S. Arbuck, S. Gwyther, M. Mooney, L. Rubinstein, L. Shankar, L. Dodd, R. Kaplan, D. Lacombe and J. Verweij, "New response evaluation criteria in solid tumours: revised RECIST guideline (version 1.1)," *Eur. J. Cancer,* vol. 45, pp. 228-247, Jan, 2009.

[20] J. D. Wolchok, A. Hoos, S. O'Day, J. S. Weber, O. Hamid, C. Lebbe, M. Maio, M. Binder, O. Bohnsack, G. Nichol, R. Humphrey and F. S. Hodi, "Guidelines for the evaluation of immune therapy activity in solid tumors: immune-related response criteria," *Clin. Cancer Res.,* vol. 15, pp. 7412-7420, Dec 1, 2009.

[21] J. Weber and A. Aparicio. Novel immunologic approaches to the management of malignant melanoma. Curr. *Opin. Oncol. 13(2),* pp. 124-128. 2001.

[22] Faries and D. L. Morton. Therapeutic vaccines for melanoma - current status. Biodrugs [Not locally available; ask about Interlibrary Loan]. *19(4),* pp. 247-260. 2005. Available: http://ovidsp.ovid.com/ovidweb.cgi?T=JS&CSC=Y&NEWS=N&PAGE=fulltext&D=ipab&AN=42-19506.

[23] L. A. DiFronzo, R. K. Gupta, R. Essner, L. J. Foshag and D. L. Morton. Enhanced humoral immune response correlates with improved disease-free and overall survival in american joint committee on cancer stage II melanoma patients receiving adjuvant polyvalent vaccine. *Journal of Clinical Oncology* [All @ UAMS; LRVA (latest 10 years)]. *20(15),* pp. 3242-3248. 2002. Available: http://ovidsp.ovid.com/ovidweb.cgi?T=JS&CSC=Y&NEWS=N&PAGE=fulltext&D=ipab&AN=39-16839.

[24] E. Hsueh, R. Gupta, K. Qi and D. Morton. Correlation of specific immune responses with survival in melanoma patients with distant metastases receiving polyvalent melanoma cell vaccine. Journal of Clinical Oncology 16(9), pp. 2913-2920. 1998.

[25] K. Shafer-Weaver, S. Rosenberg, S. Strobl, W. Gregory Alvord, M. Baseler and A. Malyguine. Application of the granzyme B ELISPOT assay for monitoring cancer vaccine trials. Journal of Immunotherapy [All @ UAMS]. 29(3), pp. 328-335. 2006. Available: http://ovidsp.ovid.com/ovidweb.cgi?T=JS&CSC=Y&NEWS=N&PAGE=fulltext&D=medc&AN=16699376.

[26] A. Eggermont, S. Suciu, A. Testori, P. Patel and A. Spatz, "Ulceration of primary melanoma and responsiveness to adjuvant interferon therapy: analysis of the adjuvant trials EORTC 18952 and EORTC 18991 in 2,644 patients," *J. Clin. Oncol., vol. 27, pp. 9007, 2009.*

[27] D. Schadendorf, S. M. Algarra, L. Bastholt, G. Cinat, B. Dreno, A. M. Eggermont, E. Espinosa, J. Guo, A. Hauschild, T. Petrella, J. Schachter and P. Hersey. Immunotherapy of distant metastatic disease. Annals of Oncology [Online Access Only (Click E Journal Holdings for Information)]. 20(Suppl 6), pp. 41-50. 2009. Available: http://ovidsp.ovid.com/ovidweb.cgi?T=JS&CSC=Y&NEWS=N&PAGE=fulltext&D=medl&AN=19617297.

[28] H. Gogas, J. Ioannovich, U. Dafni, C. Stavropoulou-Giokas, K. Frangia, D. Tsoutsos, P. Panagiotou, A. Polyzos, O. Papadopoulos, A. Stratigos, C. Markopoulos, D. Bafaloukos, D. Pectasides, G. Fountzilas and J. M. Kirkwood, "Prognostic significance of autoimmunity during treatment of melanoma with interferon," *N. Engl. J. Med.,* vol. 354, pp. 709-718, Feb 16, 2006.

[29] Z. R. Yurkovetsky, J. M. Kirkwood, H. D. Edington, A. M. Marrangoni, L. Velikokhatnaya, M. T. Winans, E. Gorelik and A. E. Lokshin, "Multiplex analysis of serum cytokines in melanoma patients treated with interferon-alpha2b," *Clin. Cancer Res.,* vol. 13, pp. 2422-2428, Apr 15, 2007.

[30] M. Sabatino, S. Kim-Schulze, M. C. Panelli, D. Stroncek, E. Wang, B. Taback, D. W. Kim, G. Deraffele, Z. Pos, F. M. Marincola and H. L. Kaufman, "Serum vascular en-

dothelial growth factor and fibronectin predict clinical response to high-dose interleukin-2 therapy," *J. Clin. Oncol., vol. 27, pp. 2645-2652, Jun 1, 2009.*

[31] G. Y. Ku, J. Yuan, D. B. Page, S. E. Schroeder, K. S. Panageas, R. D. Carvajal, P. B. Chapman, G. K. Schwartz, J. P. Allison and J. D. Wolchok, "Single-institution experience with ipilimumab in advanced melanoma patients in the compassionate use setting: lymphocyte count after 2 doses correlates with survival," *Cancer,* vol. 116, pp. 1767-1775, Apr 1, 2010.

[32] J. Yuan, M. Adamow, B. A. Ginsberg, T. S. Rasalan, E. Ritter, H. F. Gallardo, Y. Xu, E. Pogoriler, S. L. Terzulli, D. Kuk, K. S. Panageas, G. Ritter, M. Sznol, R. Halaban, A. A. Jungbluth, J. P. Allison, L. J. Old, J. D. Wolchok and S. Gnjatic. Integrated NY-ESO-1 antibody and CD8+ T-cell responses correlate with clinical benefit in advanced melanoma patients treated with ipilimumab. *Proc. Natl. Acad. Sci. U. S. A.* [All @ UAMS; LRVA (latest 10 years)]. *108(40),* pp. 16723-16728. 2011. Available: http://ovidsp.ovid.com/ovidweb.cgi?T=JS&CSC=Y&NEWS=N&PAGE=fulltext&D=medl&AN=21933959.

[33] T. F. Gajewski, J. Louahed and V. G. Brichard. Gene signature in melanoma associated with clinical activity: A potential clue to unlock cancer immunotherapy. *Cancer Journal* [Online Access Only (Click E Journal Holdings for Information)]. 16(4), pp. 399-403. 2010. Available: http://ovidsp.ovid.com/ovidweb.cgi?T=JS&CSC=Y&NEWS=N&PAGE=fulltext&D=medl&AN=20693853.

[34] R. J. Sullivan, Y. Hoshida, J. Brunet, S. Tahan, J. Aldridge, C. Kwabi, E. Gardiner, D. McDermott, T. Golub and M. B. Atkins, "A single center experience with high-dose (HD) IL-2 treatment for patients with advanced melanoma and pilot investigation of a novel gene expression signature as a predictor of response," *J. Clin. Oncol., vol. 27, pp. 9003, 2009.*

[35] J. R. Brahmer, C. G. Drake, I. Wollner, J. D. Powderly, J. Picus, W. H. Sharfman, E. Stankevich, A. Pons, T. M. Salay, T. L. McMiller, M. M. Gilson, C. Wang, M. Selby, J. M. Taube, R. Anders, L. Chen, A. J. Korman, D. M. Pardoll, I. Lowy and S. L. Topalian. Phase I study of single-agent anti-programmed death-1 (MDX-1106) in refractory solid tumors: Safety, clinical activity, pharmacodynamics, and immunologic correlates. *Journal of Clinical Oncology* [All @ UAMS; LRVA (latest 10 years)]. *28(19),* pp. 3167-3175. 2010. Available: http://ovidsp.ovid.com/ovidweb.cgi?T=JS&CSC=Y&NEWS=N&PAGE=fulltext&D=medl&AN=20516446.

[36] I. Mellman, G. Coukos and G. Dranoff, "Cancer immunotherapy comes of age," *Nature,* vol. 480, pp. 480-489, Dec 21, 2011.

[37] M. G. Lewis, R. L. Ikonopisov, R. C. Nairn, T. M. Phillips, G. H. Fairley, D. C. Bodenham and P. Alexander, "Tumour-specific antibodies in human malignant melanoma and their relationship to the extent of the disease," *Br. Med. J.,* vol. 3, pp. 547-552, Sep 6, 1969.

[38] F. Avogadri and J. D. Wolchok, "Selecting antigens for cancer vaccines," *Nat. Biotechnol.,* vol. 30, pp. 328-329, Apr 10, 2012.

[39] P. Muranski, A. Boni, P. A. Antony, L. Cassard, K. R. Irvine, A. Kaiser, C. M. Paulos, D. C. Palmer, C. E. Touloukian, K. Ptak, L. Gattinoni, C. Wrzesinski, C. S. Hinrichs, K. W. Kerstann, L. Feigenbaum, C. C. Chan and N. P. Restifo, "Tumor-specific Th17-polarized cells eradicate large established melanoma," *Blood,* vol. 112, pp. 362-373, Jul 15, 2008.

[40] F. S. Hodi, "Well-defined melanoma antigens as progression markers for melanoma: insights into differential expression and host response based on stage," *Clin. Cancer Res.,* vol. 12, pp. 673-678, Feb 1, 2006.

[41] S. Jarmalavicius, Y. Welte and P. Walden, "High immunogenicity of the HLA peptidomes of melanoma tumor cells," *J. Biol. Chem.,* Aug 6, 2012.

[42] R. Pieper, R. E. Christian, M. I. Gonzales, M. I. Nishimura, G. Gupta, R. E. Settlage, J. Shabanowitz, S. A. Rosenberg, D. F. Hunt and S. L. Topalian, "Biochemical identification of a mutated human melanoma antigen recognized by CD4(+) T cells," *J. Exp. Med.,* vol. 189, pp. 757-766, Mar 1, 1999.

[43] J. P. Brown, R. G. Woodbury, C. E. Hart, I. Hellstrom and K. E. Hellstrom, "Quantitative analysis of melanoma-associated antigen p97 in normal and neoplastic tissues," *Proc. Natl. Acad. Sci. U. S. A.,* vol. 78, pp. 539-543, Jan, 1981.

[44] P. Fredman, K. Hedberg and T. Brezicka, "Gangliosides as therapeutic targets for cancer," *BioDrugs,* vol. 17, pp. 155-167, 2003.

[45] E. Jager, M. Ringhoffer, J. Karbach, M. Arand, F. Oesch and A. Knuth, "Inverse relationship of melanocyte differentiation antigen expression in melanoma tissues and CD8+ cytotoxic-T-cell responses: evidence for immunoselection of antigen-loss variants in vivo," *Int. J. Cancer,* vol. 66, pp. 470-476, May 16, 1996.

[46] E. Jager, M. Ringhoffer, H. P. Dienes, M. Arand, J. Karbach, D. Jager, C. Ilsemann, M. Hagedorn, F. Oesch and A. Knuth. Granulocyte-macrophage-colony-stimulating factor enhances immune responses to melanoma-associated peptides in vivo. *International Journal of Cancer* [All @ UAMS]. 67(1), pp. 54-62. 1996. Available: http://ovidsp.ovid.com/ovidweb.cgi?T=JS&CSC=Y&NEWS=N&PAGE=fulltext&D=med4&AN=8690525.

[47] C. Barrow, J. Browning, D. MacGregor, I. D. Davis, S. Sturrock, A. A. Jungbluth and J. Cebon, "Tumor antigen expression in melanoma varies according to antigen and stage," *Clin. Cancer Res.,* vol. 12, pp. 764-771, Feb 1, 2006.

[48] Y. Kawakami, S. Eliyahu, C. Jennings, K. Sakaguchi, X. Kang, S. Southwood, P. F. Robbins, A. Sette, E. Appella and S. A. Rosenberg, "Recognition of multiple epitopes in the human melanoma antigen gp100 by tumor-infiltrating T lymphocytes associated with in vivo tumor regression," *J. Immunol.,* vol. 154, pp. 3961-3968, Apr 15, 1995.

[49] T. Boon, P. G. Coulie, B. J. Van den Eynde and P. van der Bruggen, "Human T cell responses against melanoma," *Annu. Rev. Immunol.*, vol. 24, pp. 175-208, 2006.

[50] R. F. Wang and S. A. Rosenberg, "Human tumor antigens for cancer vaccine development," *Immunol. Rev.*, vol. 170, pp. 85-100, Aug, 1999.

[51] D. Valmori, M. J. Pittet, C. Vonarbourg, D. Rimoldi, D. Lienard, D. Speiser, R. Dunbar, V. Cerundolo, J. C. Cerottini and P. Romero, "Analysis of the cytolytic T lymphocyte response of melanoma patients to the naturally HLA-A*0201-associated tyrosinase peptide 368-376," *Cancer Res.*, vol. 59, pp. 4050-4055, Aug 15, 1999.

[52] K. S. Lang, C. C. Caroli, A. Muhm, D. Wernet, A. Moris, B. Schittek, E. Knauss-Scherwitz, S. Stevanovic, H. G. Rammensee and C. Garbe, "HLA-A2 restricted, melanocyte-specific CD8(+) T lymphocytes detected in vitiligo patients are related to disease activity and are predominantly directed against MelanA/MART1," *J. Invest. Dermatol., vol. 116, pp. 891-897, Jun, 2001.*

[53] P. P. Lee, C. Yee, P. A. Savage, L. Fong, D. Brockstedt, J. S. Weber, D. Johnson, S. Swetter, J. Thompson, P. D. Greenberg, M. Roederer and M. M. Davis, "Characterization of circulating T cells specific for tumor-associated antigens in melanoma patients," *Nat. Med.*, vol. 5, pp. 677-685, Jun, 1999.

[54] E. Zorn and T. Hercend, "A MAGE-6-encoded peptide is recognized by expanded lymphocytes infiltrating a spontaneously regressing human primary melanoma lesion," *Eur. J. Immunol.*, vol. 29, pp. 602-607, Feb, 1999.

[55] M. Monte, M. Simonatto, L. Y. Peche, D. R. Bublik, S. Gobessi, M. A. Pierotti, M. Rodolfo and C. Schneider, "MAGE-A tumor antigens target p53 transactivation function through histone deacetylase recruitment and confer resistance to chemotherapeutic agents," *Proc. Natl. Acad. Sci. U. S. A.*, vol. 103, pp. 11160-11165, Jul 25, 2006.

[56] S. Gnjatic, H. Nishikawa, A. A. Jungbluth, A. O. Gure, G. Ritter, E. Jager, A. Knuth, Y. T. Chen and L. J. Old, "NY-ESO-1: review of an immunogenic tumor antigen," *Adv. Cancer Res.*, vol. 95, pp. 1-30, 2006.

[57] V. Vantomme, P. Boel, E. De Plaen, T. Boon and P. van der Bruggen, "A new tumor-specific antigenic peptide encoded by MAGE-6 is presented to cytolytic T lymphocytes by HLA-Cw16," *Cancer. Immun.*, vol. 3, pp. 17, Dec 10, 2003.

[58] B. Weide, H. Zelba, E. Derhovanessian, A. Pflugfelder, T. K. Eigentler, A. M. Di Giacomo, M. Maio, E. H. Aarntzen, I. J. de Vries, A. Sucker, D. Schadendorf, P. Buttner, C. Garbe and G. Pawelec, "Functional T cells targeting NY-ESO-1 or Melan-A are predictive for survival of patients with distant melanoma metastasis," *J. Clin. Oncol., vol. 30, pp. 1835-1841, May 20, 2012.*

[59] H. T. Khong and N. P. Restifo, "Natural selection of tumor variants in the generation of "tumor escape" phenotypes," *Nat. Immunol.*, vol. 3, pp. 999-1005, Nov, 2002.

[60] T. J. de Vries, A. Fourkour, T. Wobbes, G. Verkroost, D. J. Ruiter and G. N. van Muijen, "Heterogeneous expression of immunotherapy candidate proteins gp100,

MART-1, and tyrosinase in human melanoma cell lines and in human melanocytic lesions," *Cancer Res.*, vol. 57, pp. 3223-3229, Aug 1, 1997.

[61] F. Garrido, F. Ruiz-Cabello, T. Cabrera, J. J. Perez-Villar, M. Lopez-Botet, M. Duggan-Keen and P. L. Stern, "Implications for immunosurveillance of altered HLA class I phenotypes in human tumours," *Immunol. Today,* vol. 18, pp. 89-95, Feb, 1997.

[62] I. Algarra, A. Collado and F. Garrido, "Altered MHC class I antigens in tumors," *Int. J. Clin. Lab. Res.*, vol. 27, pp. 95-102, 1997.

[63] M. Bernal, F. Ruiz-Cabello, A. Concha, A. Paschen and F. Garrido, "Implication of the beta2-microglobulin gene in the generation of tumor escape phenotypes," *Cancer Immunol. Immunother., vol. 61, pp. 1359-1371, Sep, 2012.*

[64] N. P. Restifo, F. M. Marincola, Y. Kawakami, J. Taubenberger, J. R. Yannelli and S. A. Rosenberg, "Loss of functional beta 2-microglobulin in metastatic melanomas from five patients receiving immunotherapy," *J. Natl. Cancer Inst.*, vol. 88, pp. 100-108, Jan 17, 1996.

[65] K. Taniguchi, M. Petersson, P. Hoglund, R. Kiessling, G. Klein and K. Karre, "Interferon gamma induces lung colonization by intravenously inoculated B16 melanoma cells in parallel with enhanced expression of class I major histocompatibility complex antigens," *Proc. Natl. Acad. Sci. U. S. A.*, vol. 84, pp. 3405-3409, May, 1987.

[66] R. Versteeg, K. M. Kruse-Wolters, A. C. Plomp, A. van Leeuwen, N. J. Stam, H. L. Ploegh, D. J. Ruiter and P. I. Schrier, "Suppression of class I human histocompatibility leukocyte antigen by c-myc is locus specific," *J. Exp. Med.*, vol. 170, pp. 621-635, Sep 1, 1989.

[67] K. Karre, "NK cells, MHC class I molecules and the missing self," *Scand. J. Immunol.*, vol. 55, pp. 221-228, Mar, 2002.

[68] R. J. Tuthill, J. M. Unger, P. Y. Liu, L. E. Flaherty, V. K. Sondak and Southwest Oncology Group, "Risk assessment in localized primary cutaneous melanoma: a Southwest Oncology Group study evaluating nine factors and a test of the Clark logistic regression prediction model," *Am. J. Clin. Pathol., vol. 118, pp. 504-511, Oct, 2002.*

[69] D. A. Oble, R. Loewe, P. Yu and M. C. Mihm Jr, "Focus on TILs: prognostic significance of tumor infiltrating lymphocytes in human melanoma," *Cancer. Immun.*, vol. 9, pp. 3, Apr 2, 2009.

[70] C. M. Balch, S. J. Soong, J. E. Gershenwald, J. F. Thompson, D. S. Reintgen, N. Cascinelli, M. Urist, K. M. McMasters, M. I. Ross, J. M. Kirkwood, M. B. Atkins, J. A. Thompson, D. G. Coit, D. Byrd, R. Desmond, Y. Zhang, P. Y. Liu, G. H. Lyman and A. Morabito, "Prognostic factors analysis of 17,600 melanoma patients: validation of the American Joint Committee on Cancer melanoma staging system," *J. Clin. Oncol., vol. 19, pp. 3622-3634, Aug 15, 2001.*

[71] T. E. Grotz, A. S. Mansfield, J. W. Jakub and S. N. Markovic, "Regional lymphatic immunity in melanoma," *Melanoma Res.*, vol. 22, pp. 9-18, Feb, 2012.

[72] M. E. Dudley, J. C. Yang, R. Sherry, M. S. Hughes, R. Royal, U. Kammula, P. F. Robbins, J. Huang, D. E. Citrin, S. F. Leitman, J. Wunderlich, N. P. Restifo, A. Thomasian, S. G. Downey, F. O. Smith, J. Klapper, K. Morton, C. Laurencot, D. E. White and S. A. Rosenberg, "Adoptive cell therapy for patients with metastatic melanoma: evaluation of intensive myeloablative chemoradiation preparative regimens," *J. Clin. Oncol., vol. 26, pp. 5233-5239, Nov 10, 2008.*

[73] R. R. Braeuer, E. Shoshan, T. Kamiya and M. Bar-Eli, "The sweet and bitter sides of galectins in melanoma progression," *Pigment Cell. Melanoma Res.*, vol. 25, pp. 592-601, Sep, 2012.

[74] M. W. Ma, R. C. Medicherla, M. Qian, E. Vega-Saenz de Miera, E. B. Friedman, R. S. Berman, R. L. Shapiro, A. C. Pavlick, P. A. Ott, N. Bhardwaj, Y. Shao, I. Osman and F. Darvishian, "Immune response in melanoma: an in-depth analysis of the primary tumor and corresponding sentinel lymph node," *Mod. Pathol., vol. 25, pp. 1000-1010, Jul, 2012.*

[75] A. S. Mansfield, S. G. Holtan, T. E. Grotz, J. B. Allred, J. W. Jakub, L. A. Erickson and S. N. Markovic, "Regional immunity in melanoma: immunosuppressive changes precede nodal metastasis," *Mod. Pathol., vol. 24, pp. 487-494, Apr, 2011.*

[76] M. E. Polak, P. Johnson, S. Di Palma, B. Higgins, J. Hurren, N. J. Borthwick, M. J. Jager, D. Mccormick and I. A. Cree, "Presence and maturity of dendritic cells in melanoma lymph node metastases," *J. Pathol.*, vol. 207, pp. 83-90, Sep, 2005.

[77] A. Busse and U. Keilholz, "Role of TGF-beta in melanoma," *Curr. Pharm. Biotechnol.*, vol. 12, pp. 2165-2175, Dec, 2011.

[78] K. Asadullah, W. Sterry and H. D. Volk, "Interleukin-10 therapy--review of a new approach," *Pharmacol. Rev.*, vol. 55, pp. 241-269, Jun, 2003.

[79] C. De Santo, R. Arscott, S. Booth, I. Karydis, M. Jones, R. Asher, M. Salio, M. Middleton and V. Cerundolo, "Invariant NKT cells modulate the suppressive activity of IL-10-secreting neutrophils differentiated with serum amyloid A," *Nat. Immunol.*, vol. 11, pp. 1039-1046, Nov, 2010.

[80] A. Facciabene, X. Peng, I. S. Hagemann, K. Balint, A. Barchetti, L. P. Wang, P. A. Gimotty, C. B. Gilks, P. Lal, L. Zhang and G. Coukos, "Tumour hypoxia promotes tolerance and angiogenesis via CCL28 and T(reg) cells," *Nature*, vol. 475, pp. 226-230, Jul 13, 2011.

[81] N. Schwinn, D. Vokhminova, A. Sucker, S. Textor, S. Striegel, I. Moll, N. Nausch, J. Tuettenberg, A. Steinle, A. Cerwenka, D. Schadendorf and A. Paschen, "Interferon-gamma down-regulates NKG2D ligand expression and impairs the NKG2D-mediated cytolysis of MHC class I-deficient melanoma by natural killer cells," *Int. J. Cancer*, vol. 124, pp. 1594-1604, Apr 1, 2009.

[82] A. Paschen, A. Sucker, B. Hill, I. Moll, M. Zapatka, X. D. Nguyen, G. C. Sim, I. Gutmann, J. Hassel, J. C. Becker, A. Steinle, D. Schadendorf and S. Ugurel, "Differential

clinical significance of individual NKG2D ligands in melanoma: soluble ULBP2 as an indicator of poor prognosis superior to S100B," *Clin. Cancer Res.,* vol. 15, pp. 5208-5215, Aug 15, 2009.

[83] S. K. Calderwood, M. A. Khaleque, D. B. Sawyer and D. R. Ciocca, "Heat shock proteins in cancer: chaperones of tumorigenesis," *Trends Biochem. Sci.,* vol. 31, pp. 164-172, Mar, 2006.

[84] C. Shipp, B. Weide, E. Derhovanessian and G. Pawelec, "Hsps are up-regulated in melanoma tissue and correlate with patient clinical parameters," *Cell Stress Chaperones,* Aug 8, 2012.

[85] S. A. Rosenberg, J. C. Yang, D. J. Schwartzentruber, P. Hwu, F. M. Marincola, S. L. Topalian, N. P. Restifo, M. E. Dudley, S. L. Schwarz, P. J. Spiess, J. R. Wunderlich, M. R. Parkhurst, Y. Kawakami, C. A. Seipp, J. H. Einhorn and D. E. White, "Immunologic and therapeutic evaluation of a synthetic peptide vaccine for the treatment of patients with metastatic melanoma," *Nat. Med.,* vol. 4, pp. 321-327, Mar, 1998.

[86] J. C. Yang, "Melanoma vaccines," *Cancer J.,* vol. 17, pp. 277-282, Sep-Oct, 2011.

[87] W. J. Lesterhuis, E. H. Aarntzen, I. J. De Vries, D. H. Schuurhuis, C. G. Figdor, G. J. Adema and C. J. Punt, "Dendritic cell vaccines in melanoma: from promise to proof?" *Crit. Rev. Oncol. Hematol., vol. 66, pp. 118-134, May, 2008.*

[88] J. Banchereau and R. M. Steinman, "Dendritic cells and the control of immunity," *Nature,* vol. 392, pp. 245-252, Mar 19, 1998.

[89] M. E. Dudley and S. A. Rosenberg, "Adoptive-cell-transfer therapy for the treatment of patients with cancer," *Nat. Rev. Cancer.,* vol. 3, pp. 666-675, Sep, 2003.

[90] S. Lee and K. Margolin, "Tumor-Infiltrating Lymphocytes in Melanoma," *Curr. Oncol. Rep.,* Aug 10, 2012.

[91] S. A. Rosenberg, J. C. Yang, R. M. Sherry, U. S. Kammula, M. S. Hughes, G. Q. Phan, D. E. Citrin, N. P. Restifo, P. F. Robbins, J. R. Wunderlich, K. E. Morton, C. M. Laurencot, S. M. Steinberg, D. E. White and M. E. Dudley, "Durable complete responses in heavily pretreated patients with metastatic melanoma using T-cell transfer immunotherapy," *Clin. Cancer Res.,* vol. 17, pp. 4550-4557, Jul 1, 2011.

[92] P. F. Robbins, R. A. Morgan, S. A. Feldman, J. C. Yang, R. M. Sherry, M. E. Dudley, J. R. Wunderlich, A. V. Nahvi, L. J. Helman, C. L. Mackall, U. S. Kammula, M. S. Hughes, N. P. Restifo, M. Raffeld, C. C. Lee, C. L. Levy, Y. F. Li, M. El-Gamil, S. L. Schwarz, C. Laurencot and S. A. Rosenberg, "Tumor regression in patients with metastatic synovial cell sarcoma and melanoma using genetically engineered lymphocytes reactive with NY-ESO-1," *J. Clin. Oncol., vol. 29, pp. 917-924, Mar 1, 2011.*

[93] M. B. Atkins, M. T. Lotze, J. P. Dutcher, R. I. Fisher, G. Weiss, K. Margolin, J. Abrams, M. Sznol, D. Parkinson, M. Hawkins, C. Paradise, L. Kunkel and S. A. Rosenberg, "High-dose recombinant interleukin 2 therapy for patients with metastatic melano-

ma: analysis of 270 patients treated between 1985 and 1993," *J. Clin. Oncol., vol. 17, pp. 2105-2116, Jul, 1999.*

[94] J. M. Kirkwood, J. Manola, J. Ibrahim, V. Sondak, M. S. Ernstoff, U. Rao and Eastern Cooperative Oncology Group, "A pooled analysis of eastern cooperative oncology group and intergroup trials of adjuvant high-dose interferon for melanoma," *Clin. Cancer Res.,* vol. 10, pp. 1670-1677, Mar 1, 2004.

[95] F. S. Hodi, S. J. O'Day, D. F. McDermott, R. W. Weber, J. A. Sosman, J. B. Haanen, R. Gonzalez, C. Robert, D. Schadendorf, J. C. Hassel, W. Akerley, A. J. van den Eertwegh, J. Lutzky, P. Lorigan, J. M. Vaubel, G. P. Linette, D. Hogg, C. H. Ottensmeier, C. Lebbe, C. Peschel, I. Quirt, J. I. Clark, J. D. Wolchok, J. S. Weber, J. Tian, M. J. Yellin, G. M. Nichol, A. Hoos and W. J. Urba, "Improved survival with ipilimumab in patients with metastatic melanoma," *N. Engl. J. Med.,* vol. 363, pp. 711-723, Aug 19, 2010.

[96] M. A. Postow, J. Harding and J. D. Wolchok, "Targeting immune checkpoints: releasing the restraints on anti-tumor immunity for patients with melanoma," *Cancer J.,* vol. 18, pp. 153-159, Mar-Apr, 2012.

[97] J. R. Brahmer, S. S. Tykodi, L. Q. Chow, W. J. Hwu, S. L. Topalian, P. Hwu, C. G. Drake, L. H. Camacho, J. Kauh, K. Odunsi, H. C. Pitot, O. Hamid, S. Bhatia, R. Martins, K. Eaton, S. Chen, T. M. Salay, S. Alaparthy, J. F. Grosso, A. J. Korman, S. M. Parker, S. Agrawal, S. M. Goldberg, D. M. Pardoll, A. Gupta and J. M. Wigginton, "Safety and activity of anti-PD-L1 antibody in patients with advanced cancer," *N. Engl. J. Med.,* vol. 366, pp. 2455-2465, Jun 28, 2012.

[98] S. L. Topalian, F. S. Hodi, J. R. Brahmer, S. N. Gettinger, D. C. Smith, D. F. McDermott, J. D. Powderly, R. D. Carvajal, J. A. Sosman, M. B. Atkins, P. D. Leming, D. R. Spigel, S. J. Antonia, L. Horn, C. G. Drake, D. M. Pardoll, L. Chen, W. H. Sharfman, R. A. Anders, J. M. Taube, T. L. McMiller, H. Xu, A. J. Korman, M. Jure-Kunkel, S. Agrawal, D. McDonald, G. D. Kollia, A. Gupta, J. M. Wigginton and M. Sznol, "Safety, activity, and immune correlates of anti-PD-1 antibody in cancer," *N. Engl. J. Med.,* vol. 366, pp. 2443-2454, Jun 28, 2012.

[99] M. M. Adams, P. Damani, N. R. Perl, A. Won, F. Hong, P. O. Livingston, G. Ragupathi and D. Y. Gin, "Design and synthesis of potent Quillaja saponin vaccine adjuvants," *J Am Chem Soc,* vol. 132, pp. 1939-45, Feb 17, 2010.

[100] B. Krone, K. F. Kolmel, J. M. Grange, G. Mastrangelo, B. M. Henz, I. N. Botev, M. Niin, C. Seebacher, D. Lambert, R. Shafir, E. M. Kokoschka, U. R. Kleeberg, O. Gefeller and A. Pfahlberg, "Impact of vaccinations and infectious diseases on the risk of melanoma--evaluation of an EORTC case-control study," *Eur J Cancer,* vol. 39, pp. 2372-8, Nov, 2003.

[101] H. K. Silver, E. M. Ibrahim, J. A. Evers, J. W. Thomas, R. N. Murray and J. J. Spinelli, "Adjuvant BCG immunotherapy for stage I and II malignant melanoma," *Can Med Assoc J,* vol. 128, pp. 1291-5, Jun 1, 1983.

[102] J. H. Stewart 4th and E. A. Levine. Role of bacillus calmette-guerin in the treatment of advanced melanoma. Expert Review of Anticancer Therapy [Not locally available; ask about Interlibrary Loan]. *11(11),* pp. 1671-1676. 2011. Available: http://ovidsp.ovid.com/ovidweb.cgi?T=JS&CSC=Y&NEWS=N&PAGE=fulltext&D=medl&AN=22050015.

[103] S. S. Agarwala, D. Neuberg, Y. Park and J. M. Kirkwood, "Mature results of a phase III randomized trial of bacillus Calmette-Guerin (BCG) versus observation and BCG plus dacarbazine versus BCG in the adjuvant therapy of American Joint Committee on Cancer Stage I-III melanoma (E1673): a trial of the Eastern Oncology Group," *Cancer,* vol. 100, pp. 1692-8, Apr 15, 2004.

[104] D. L. Morton, F. R. Eilber, E. C. Holmes, F. C. Sparks and K. Ramming, "BCG immunotherapy as a systemic adjunct to surgery in malignant melanoma," *Med Clin North Am,* vol. 60, pp. 431-9, May, 1976.

[105] D. L. Morton, L. J. Foshag, D. S. Hoon, J. A. Nizze, E. Famatiga, L. A. Wanek, C. Chang, D. G. Davtyan, R. K. Gupta and R. Elashoff, "Prolongation of survival in metastatic melanoma after active specific immunotherapy with a new polyvalent melanoma vaccine," *Ann Surg,* vol. 216, pp. 463-82, Oct, 1992.

[106] D. L. Morton, E. C. Hsueh, R. Essner, L. J. Foshag, S. J. O'Day, A. Bilchik, R. K. Gupta, D. S. Hoon, M. Ravindranath, J. A. Nizze, G. Gammon, L. A. Wanek, H. J. Wang and R. M. Elashoff, "Prolonged survival of patients receiving active immunotherapy with Canvaxin therapeutic polyvalent vaccine after complete resection of melanoma metastatic to regional lymph nodes," *Ann Surg,* vol. 236, pp. 438-48; discussion 448-9, Oct, 2002.

[107] S. Hoshimoto, M. B. Faries, D. L. Morton, T. Shingai, C. Kuo, H. J. Wang, R. Elashoff, N. Mozzillo, M. C. Kelley, J. F. Thompson, J. E. Lee and D. S. Hoon, "Assessment of prognostic circulating tumor cells in a phase III trial of adjuvant immunotherapy after complete resection of stage IV melanoma," *Ann Surg,* vol. 255, pp. 357-62, Feb, 2012.

[108] I. Hara, N. Sato, H. Miyake, M. Muramaki, S. Hikosaka and S. Kamidono, "Introduction of 65 kDa antigen of Mycobacterium tuberculosis to cancer cells enhances antitumor effect of BCG therapy," *Microbiol Immunol,* vol. 48, pp. 289-95, 2004.

[109] C. W. Cluff, "Monophosphoryl lipid A (MPL) as an adjuvant for anti-cancer vaccines: clinical results," *Adv Exp Med Biol,* vol. 667, pp. 111-23, 2010.

[110] J. T. Evans, C. W. Cluff, D. A. Johnson, M. J. Lacy, D. H. Persing and J. R. Baldridge, "Enhancement of antigen-specific immunity via the TLR4 ligands MPL adjuvant and Ribi.529," *Expert Rev Vaccines,* vol. 2, pp. 219-29, Apr, 2003.

[111] N. Schultz, R. Oratz, D. Chen, A. Zeleniuch-Jacquotte, G. Abeles and J. C. Bystryn, "Effect of DETOX as an adjuvant for melanoma vaccine," *Vaccine,* vol. 13, pp. 503-8, Apr, 1995.

[112] H. X. Sun, Y. Xie and Y. P. Ye, "Advances in saponin-based adjuvants," *Vaccine,* vol. 27, pp. 1787-96, Mar 13, 2009.

[113] G. Ragupathi, J. R. Gardner, P. O. Livingston and D. Y. Gin, "Natural and synthetic saponin adjuvant QS-21 for vaccines against cancer," *Expert Rev Vaccines,* vol. 10, pp. 463-70, Apr, 2011.

[114] K. Deng, M. M. Adams, P. Damani, P. O. Livingston, G. Ragupathi and D. Y. Gin, "Synthesis of QS-21-xylose: establishment of the immunopotentiating activity of synthetic QS-21 adjuvant with a melanoma vaccine," *Angew Chem Int Ed Engl,* vol. 47, pp. 6395-8, 2008.

[115] P. O. Livingston, "Approaches to augmenting the immunogenicity of melanoma gangliosides: from whole melanoma cells to ganglioside-KLH conjugate vaccines," *Immunol Rev,* vol. 145, pp. 147-66, Jun, 1995.

[116] J. Aucouturier, L. Dupuis, S. Deville, S. Ascarateil and V. Ganne, "Montanide ISA 720 and 51: a new generation of water in oil emulsions as adjuvants for human vaccines," *Expert Rev Vaccines,* vol. 1, pp. 111-8, Jun, 2002.

[117] J. Aucouturier, S. Ascarateil and L. Dupuis, "The use of oil adjuvants in therapeutic vaccines," *Vaccine,* vol. 24 Suppl 2, pp. S2-44-5, Apr 12, 2006.

[118] E. J. Huijbers, J. Femel, K. Andersson, H. Bjorkelund, L. Hellman and A. K. Olsson, "The non-toxic and biodegradable adjuvant Montanide ISA 720/CpG can replace Freund's in a cancer vaccine targeting ED-B--a prerequisite for clinical development," *Vaccine,* vol. 30, pp. 225-30, Jan 5, 2012.

[119] J. Fourcade, P. Kudela, P. A. Andrade Filho, B. Janjic, S. R. Land, C. Sander, A. Krieg, A. Donnenberg, H. Shen, J. M. Kirkwood and H. M. Zarour, "Immunization with analog peptide in combination with CpG and montanide expands tumor antigen-specific CD8+ T cells in melanoma patients," *J Immunother,* vol. 31, pp. 781-91, Oct, 2008.

[120] J. Karbach, S. Gnjatic, A. Bender, A. Neumann, E. Weidmann, J. Yuan, C. A. Ferrara, E. Hoffmann, L. J. Old, N. K. Altorki and E. Jager, "Tumor-reactive CD8+ T-cell responses after vaccination with NY-ESO-1 peptide, CpG 7909 and Montanide ISA-51: association with survival," *Int J Cancer,* vol. 126, pp. 909-18, Feb 15, 2010.

[121] K. A. Chianese-Bullock, J. Pressley, C. Garbee, S. Hibbitts, C. Murphy, G. Yamshchikov, G. R. Petroni, E. A. Bissonette, P. Y. Neese, W. W. Grosh, P. Merrill, R. Fink, E. M. Woodson, C. J. Wiernasz, J. W. Patterson and S. C. L. Jr, "MAGE-A1-, MAGE-A10-, and gp100-derived peptides are immunogenic when combined with granulocyte-macrophage colony-stimulating factor and montanide ISA-51 adjuvant and administered as part of a multipeptide vaccine for melanoma," *J Immunol,* vol. 174, pp. 3080-6, Mar 1, 2005.

[122] S. N. Markovic, V. J. Suman, J. N. Ingle, J. S. Kaur, H. C. Pitot, C. L. Loprinzi, R. D. Rao, E. T. Creagan, M. R. Pittelkow, J. B. Allred, W. K. Nevala and E. Celis, "Peptide vaccination of patients with metastatic melanoma: improved clinical outcome in pa-

tients demonstrating effective immunization," *Am J Clin Oncol,* vol. 29, pp. 352-60, Aug, 2006.

[123] D. T. Le and E. M. Jaffee, "Regulatory T-cell modulation using cyclophosphamide in vaccine approaches: a current perspective," *Cancer Res,* vol. 72, pp. 3439-44, Jul 15, 2012.

[124] E. Elkord, E. M. Alcantar-Orozco, S. J. Dovedi, D. Q. Tran, R. E. Hawkins and D. E. Gilham, "T regulatory cells in cancer: recent advances and therapeutic potential," *Expert Opin Biol Ther,* vol. 10, pp. 1573-86, Nov, 2010.

[125] Q. Y. Guo, M. Yuan, J. Peng, X. M. Cui, G. Song, X. Sui and S. B. Lu, "Antitumor activity of mixed heat shock protein/peptide vaccine and cyclophosphamide plus interleukin-12 in mice sarcoma," *J Exp Clin Cancer Res,* vol. 30, pp. 24, 2011.

[126] F. Ghiringhelli, N. Larmonier, E. Schmitt, A. Parcellier, D. Cathelin, C. Garrido, B. Chauffert, E. Solary, B. Bonnotte and F. Martin, "CD4+CD25+ regulatory T cells suppress tumor immunity but are sensitive to cyclophosphamide which allows immunotherapy of established tumors to be curative," *Eur J Immunol,* vol. 34, pp. 336-44, Feb, 2004.

[127] M. L. Salem, A. N. Kadima, S. A. El-Naggar, M. P. Rubinstein, Y. Chen, W. E. Gillanders and D. J. Cole, "Defining the ability of cyclophosphamide preconditioning to enhance the antigen-specific CD8+ T-cell response to peptide vaccination: creation of a beneficial host microenvironment involving type I IFNs and myeloid cells," *J Immunother,* vol. 30, pp. 40-53, Jan, 2007.

[128] J. M. Kirkwood, M. H. Strawderman, M. S. Ernstoff, T. J. Smith, E. C. Borden and R. H. Blum, "Interferon alfa-2b adjuvant therapy of high-risk resected cutaneous melanoma: the Eastern Cooperative Oncology Group Trial EST 1684," *J. Clin. Oncol., vol. 14, pp. 7-17, Jan, 1996.*

[129] J. M. Kirkwood, J. G. Ibrahim, V. K. Sondak, J. Richards, L. E. Flaherty, M. S. Ernstoff, T. J. Smith, U. Rao, M. Steele and R. H. Blum, "High- and low-dose interferon alfa-2b in high-risk melanoma: first analysis of intergroup trial E1690/S9111/C9190," *J. Clin. Oncol., vol. 18, pp. 2444-2458, Jun, 2000.*

[130] A. M. Eggermont, S. Suciu, M. Santinami, A. Testori, W. H. Kruit, J. Marsden, C. J. Punt, F. Sales, M. Gore, R. Mackie, Z. Kusic, R. Dummer, A. Hauschild, E. Musat, A. Spatz, U. Keilholz and EORTC Melanoma Group, "Adjuvant therapy with pegylated interferon alfa-2b versus observation alone in resected stage III melanoma: final results of EORTC 18991, a randomised phase III trial," *Lancet,* vol. 372, pp. 117-126, Jul 12, 2008.

[131] S. Mocellin, S. Pasquali, C. R. Rossi and D. Nitti, "Interferon alpha adjuvant therapy in patients with high-risk melanoma: a systematic review and meta-analysis," *J. Natl. Cancer Inst.,* vol. 102, pp. 493-501, Apr 7, 2010.

[132] C. I. Falkson, G. Falkson and H. C. Falkson, "Improved results with the addition of interferon alfa-2b to dacarbazine in the treatment of patients with metastatic malignant melanoma," *J. Clin. Oncol., vol. 9, pp. 1403-1408, Aug, 1991.*

[133] E. T. Creagan, D. L. Ahmann, S. J. Green, H. J. Long, S. Frytak, J. R. O'Fallon and L. M. Itri, "Phase II study of low-dose recombinant leukocyte A interferon in disseminated malignant melanoma," *J. Clin. Oncol., vol. 2, pp. 1002-1005, Sep, 1984.*

[134] N. J. Ives, R. L. Stowe, P. Lorigan and K. Wheatley, "Chemotherapy compared with biochemotherapy for the treatment of metastatic melanoma: a meta-analysis of 18 trials involving 2,621 patients," *J. Clin. Oncol., vol. 25, pp. 5426-5434, Dec 1, 2007.*

[135] A. A. Tarhini, J. M. Kirkwood, W. E. Gooding, C. Cai and S. S. Agarwala, "Durable complete responses with high-dose bolus interleukin-2 in patients with metastatic melanoma who have experienced progression after biochemotherapy," *J. Clin. Oncol., vol. 25, pp. 3802-3807, Sep 1, 2007.*

[136] D. F. McDermott and M. B. Atkins, "More support for the judicious use of high-dose interleukin-2 in patients with advanced melanoma," *J. Clin. Oncol., vol. 25, pp. 3791-3793, Sep 1, 2007.*

[137] T. M. Petrella, R. Tozer, K. Belanger, K. J. Savage, R. Wong, M. Smylie, S. Kamel-Reid, V. Tron, B. E. Chen, N. N. Hunder, L. Hagerman, W. Walsh and E. A. Eisenhauer, "Interleukin-21 Has Activity in Patients With Metastatic Melanoma: A Phase II Study," *J. Clin. Oncol., Aug 20, 2012.*

[138] L. E. Spitler, M. L. Grossbard, M. S. Ernstoff, G. Silver, M. Jacobs, F. A. Hayes and S. J. Soong, "Adjuvant therapy of stage III and IV malignant melanoma using granulocyte-macrophage colony-stimulating factor," *J. Clin. Oncol., vol. 18, pp. 1614-1621, Apr, 2000.*

[139] D. H. Lawson, S. J. Lee, A. A. Tarhini, K. A. Margolin, M. S. Ernstoff and J. M. Kirkwood, "Phase III cooperative group study of yeast-derived granulocyte macrophage colony-stimulating factor (GM-CSF) versus placebo as adjuvant treatment of patients with completely resected stage III-IV melanoma," *J Clin Oncol,* vol. 28, pp. 8504, 2010.

[140] M. Chi and A. Z. Dudek. Vaccine therapy for metastatic melanoma: Systematic review and meta-analysis of clinical trials. *Melanoma Res. 21(3),* pp. 165-174. 2011.

[141] A. M. Terando, M. B. Faries and D. L. Morton. Vaccine therapy for melanoma: Current status and future directions. *Vaccine 25*pp. B4-B16. 2007.

[142] D. BERD, H. MAGUIRE, P. MCCUE and M. MASTRANGELO. Treatment of metastatic melanoma with an autologous tumor-cell vaccine - clinical and immunological results in 64 patients. *Journal of Clinical Oncology 8(11),* pp. 1858-1867. 1990.

[143] D. Berd, H. Maguire, L. Schuchter, R. Hamilton, W. Hauck, T. Sato and M. Mastrangelo. Autologous hapten-modified melanoma vaccine as postsurgical adjuvant treatment after resection of nodal metastases. Journal of Clinical Oncology 15(6), pp. 2359-2370. 1997.

[144] D. Berd, T. Sato, H. C. Maguire, J. Kairys and M. J. Mastrangelo. Immunopharmacologic analysis of an autologous, hapten-modified human melanoma vaccine. Journal of Clinical Oncology [All @ UAMS; LRVA (latest 10 years)]. *22(3),* pp. 403-415. 2004. Available: http://ovidsp.ovid.com/ovidweb.cgi?T=JS&CSC=Y&NEWS=N&PAGE=fulltext&D=ipab&AN=41-07931.

[145] R. O. Dillman, C. DePriest, C. DeLeon, N. M. Barth, L. S. Schwartzberg, L. D. Beutel, P. M. Schiltz and S. K. Nayak. Patient-specific vaccines derived from autologous tumor cell lines as active specific immunotherapy: Results of exploratory phase I/II trials in patients with metastatic melanoma. *Cancer Biotherapy and Radiopharmaceuticals 22(3),* pp. 309-321. 2007.

[146] R. Dillman, S. Selvan, P. Schiltz, C. Peterson, K. Allen, C. DePriest, E. McClay, N. Barth, P. Sheehy, C. de Leon and L. Beutel. Phase I/II trial of melanoma patient-speciric vaccine of proliferating autologous tumor cells, dendritic cells, and GM-CSF: Planned interim analysis. *Cancer Biotherapy and Radiopharmaceuticals 19(5),* pp. 658-665. 2004.

[147] R. O. Dillman, L. D. Beutel, N. M. Barth, C. de Leon, A. A. O'Connor, C. DePriest and S. K. Nayak. Irradiated cells from autologous tumor cell lines as patient-specific vaccine therapy in 125 patients with metastatic cancer: Induction of delayed-type hypersensitivity to autologous tumor is associated with improved survival. *Cancer Biother. Radiopharm. [Not locally available; ask about Interlibrary Loan]. 17(1),* pp. 51-66. 2002. Available: http://ovidsp.ovid.com/ovidweb.cgi?T=JS&CSC=Y&NEWS=N&PAGE=fulltext&D=med4&AN=11915174.

[148] A. Anichini, C. Vegetti and R. Mortarini. The paradox of T-cell-mediated antitumor immunity in spite of poor clinical outcome in human melanoma. Cancer Immunology, Immunotherapy [Not locally available; ask about Interlibrary Loan]. *53(10),* pp. 855-864. 2004. Available: http://ovidsp.ovid.com/ovidweb.cgi?T=JS&CSC=Y&NEWS=N&PAGE=fulltext&D=med4&AN=15175905.

[149] E. G. Elias, C. M. Suter and D. S. Fabian. Adjuvant immunotherapy in melanoma with irradiated autologous tumor cells and low dose cyclophosphamide. J. Surg. Oncol. [Part @ UAMS (Click Library Holdings)]. 64(1), pp. 17-22. 1997. Available: http://ovidsp.ovid.com/ovidweb.cgi?T=JS&CSC=Y&NEWS=N&PAGE=fulltext&D=med4&AN=9040795.

[150] E. G. Elias, J. L. Zapas, E. C. McCarron, S. L. Beam, J. H. Hasskamp and W. J. Culpepper. Sequential administration of GM-CSF (sargramostim (R)) and IL-2 +/- autologous vaccine as adjuvant therapy in cutaneous melanoma: An interim report of a phase II clinical trial. *Cancer Biotherapy and Radiopharmaceuticals 23(3),* pp. 285-291. 2008.

[151] O. Eton, D. Kharkevitch, M. Gianan, M. Ross, K. Itoh, M. Pride, C. Donawho, A. Buzaid, P. Mansfield, J. Lee, S. Legha, C. Plager, N. Papadopoulos, A. Bedikian, R. Benjamin and C. Balch. Active immunotherapy with ultraviolet B-irradiated autologous

whole melanoma cells plus DETOX in patients with metastatic melanoma. *Clinical Cancer Research 4(3),* pp. 619-627. 1998.

[152] R. Soiffer, T. Lynch, M. Mihm, K. Jung, C. Rhuda, J. C. Schmollinger, F. S. Hodi, L. Liebster, P. Lam, S. Mentzer, S. Singer, K. K. Tanabe, A. B. Cosimi, R. Duda, A. Sober, A. Bhan, J. Daley, D. Neuberg, G. Parry, J. Rokovich, L. Richards, J. Drayer, A. Berns, S. Clift, L. K. Cohen, R. C. Mulligan and G. Dranoff, "Vaccination with irradiated autologous melanoma cells engineered to secrete human granulocyte-macrophage colony-stimulating factor generates potent antitumor immunity in patients with metastatic melanoma," *Proc. Natl. Acad. Sci. U. S. A.,* vol. 95, pp. 13141-13146, Oct 27, 1998.

[153] S. Nawrocki, P. Murawa, J. Malicki, M. Kapcinska, K. Gryska, D. Izycki, A. Kaczmarek, M. Laciak, A. Czapczyk, A. Karczewska, S. Rose-John and A. Mackiewicz, "Genetically modified tumour vaccines (GMTV) in melanoma clinical trials," *Immunol. Lett., vol. 74, pp. 81-86, Sep 15, 2000.*

[154] A. Testori, J. Richards, E. Whitman, G. B. Mann, J. Lutzky, L. Camacho, G. Parmiani, G. Tosti, J. M. Kirkwood, A. Hoos, L. Yuh, R. Gupta and P. K. Srivastava. Phase III comparison of vitespen, an autologous tumor-derived heat shock protein gp96 peptide complex vaccine, with physician's choice of treatment for stage IV melanoma: The C-100-21 study group. *Journal of Clinical Oncology 26(6),* pp. 955-962. 2008.

[155] V. Sondak, M. Sabel and J. Mule. Allogeneic and autologous melanoma vaccines: Where have we been and where are we going? *Clinical Cancer Research 12(7),* pp. 2337S-2341S. 2006.

[156] E. Hsueh and D. Morton. Antigen-based immunotherapy of melanoma: Canvaxin therapeutic polyvalent cancer vaccine. *Semin. Cancer Biol. 13(6),* pp. 401-407. 2003.

[157] D. Berd and G. Parmiani. Human tumor vaccines go molecular. summary of american association for cancer research symposium, march 20,1995. *Cancer Immunology, Immunotherapy* [Not locally available; ask about Interlibrary Loan]. *41(3),* pp. 199-200. 1995. Available: http://ovidsp.ovid.com/ovidweb.cgi?T=JS&CSC=Y&NEWS=N&PAGE=fulltext&D=med3&AN=7553690.

[158] M. M. Barrio, P. T. de Motta, J. Kaplan, E. M. von Euw, A. I. Bravo, R. D. Chacon and J. Mordoh, "A phase I study of an allogeneic cell vaccine (VACCIMEL) with GM-CSF in melanoma patients," *J. Immunother.,* vol. 29, pp. 444-454, Jul-Aug, 2006.

[159] M. K. Wallack, S. D. Scoggin and M. Sivanandham, "Active specific immunotherapy with vaccinia melanoma oncolysate," *Mt. Sinai J. Med.,* vol. 59, pp. 227-233, May, 1992.

[160] M. S. Mitchell, W. Harel, J. Kan-Mitchell, L. G. LeMay, P. Goedegebuure, X. Q. Huang, F. Hofman and S. Groshen. Active specific immunotherapy of melanoma with allogeneic cell lysates. rationale, results, and possible mechanisms of action. *Ann. N. Y. Acad. Sci.* [Part @ UAMS (Click Library Holdings)]. *690*pp. 153-166. 1993.

Available: http://ovidsp.ovid.com/ovidweb.cgi?T=JS&CSC=Y&NEWS=N&PAGE=fulltext&D=med3&AN=8368734.

[161] V. K. Sondak, P. Y. Liu, R. J. Tuthill, R. A. Kempf and L. E. Flaherty. Adjuvant immunotherapy of resected, intermediate-thickness, node-negative melanoma with an allogeneic tumor vaccine: Overall results of a randomized trial of the southwest oncology group. *Journal of Clinical Oncology* [All @ UAMS; LRVA (latest 10 years)]. *20(8),* pp. 2058-2066. 2002. Available: http://ovidsp.ovid.com/ovidweb.cgi?T=JS&CSC=Y&NEWS=N&PAGE=fulltext&D=ipab&AN=39-11023.

[162] V. K. Sondak, J. Sosman, J. M. Unger, P. Y. Liu, J. Thompson, R. Tuthill, R. Kempf and L. Flaherty. Significant impact of HLA class I allele expression on outcome in melanoma patients treated with an allogeneic melanoma cell lysate vaccine. final analysis of SWOG-9035 [abstract]. *Annual Meeting Proceedings of the American Society of Clinical Oncology 707p*2004. Available: http://ovidsp.ovid.com/ovidweb.cgi?T=JS&CSC=Y&NEWS=N&PAGE=fulltext&D=cctr&AN=CN-00544014.

[163] J. A. Sosman, J. M. Unger, P. Y. Liu, L. E. Flaherty and SW Oncology Grp. Adjuvant immunotherapy of resected, intermediate-thickness, node-negative melanoma with an allogeneic tumor vaccine: Impact of HLA class I antigen expression on outcome. *Journal of Clinical Oncology* [All @ UAMS; LRVA (latest 10 years)]. *20(8),* pp. 2067-2075. 2002. Available: http://ovidsp.ovid.com/ovidweb.cgi?T=JS&CSC=Y&NEWS=N&PAGE=fulltext&D=ipab&AN=39-10980.

[164] M. S. Mitchell, J. Abrams, J. A. Thompson, M. Kashani-Sabet, R. C. DeConti, W. Hwu, M. B. Atkins, E. Whitman, M. S. Ernstoff, F. G. Haluska, J. G. Jakowatz, T. K. Das Gupta, J. M. Richards, W. E. Samlowski, J. J. Costanzi, F. R. Aronson, A. B. Deisseroth, A. Z. Dudek and V. E. Jones. Randomized trial of an allogeneic melanoma lysate vaccine with low-dose interferon alfa-2b compared with high-dose interferon alfa-2b for resected stage III cutaneous melanoma. *Journal of Clinical Oncology 25(15),* pp. 2078-2085. 2007.

[165] J. D. Wolchok and P. O. Livingston. Vaccines for melanoma: Translating basic immunology into new therapies. *Lancet Oncology* [Part @ UAMS (Click Library Holdings)]. 2(4), pp. 205-211. 2001. Available: http://ovidsp.ovid.com/ovidweb.cgi?T=JS&CSC=Y&NEWS=N&PAGE=fulltext&D=med4&AN=11905765.

[166] I. D. Davis, W. Chen, H. Jackson, P. Parente, M. Shackleton, W. Hopkins, Q. Chen, N. Dimopoulos, T. Luke, R. Murphy, A. M. Scott, E. Maraskovsky, G. McArthur, D. MacGregor, S. Sturrock, T. Y. Tai, S. Green, A. Cuthbertson, D. Maher, L. Miloradovic, S. V. Mitchell, G. Ritter, A. A. Jungbluth, Y. T. Chen, S. Gnjatic, E. W. Hoffman, L. J. Old and J. S. Cebon, "Recombinant NY-ESO-1 protein with ISCOMATRIX adjuvant induces broad integrated antibody and CD4(+) and CD8(+) T cell responses in humans," *Proc. Natl. Acad. Sci. U. S. A.,* vol. 101, pp. 10697-10702, Jul 20, 2004.

[167] P. O. Livingston, G. Y. Wong, S. Adluri, Y. Tao, M. Padavan, R. Parente, C. Hanlon, M. J. Calves, F. Helling and G. Ritter. Improved survival in stage III melanoma pa-

tients with GM2 antibodies: A randomized trial of adjuvant vaccination with GM2 ganglioside. *Journal of Clinical Oncology : Official Journal of the American Society of Clinical Oncology* [All @ UAMS; LRVA (latest 10 years)]. *12(5),* pp. 1036-1044. 1994. Available: http://ovidsp.ovid.com/ovidweb.cgi?T=JS&CSC=Y&NEWS=N&PAGE=fulltext&D=cctr&AN=CN-00100781.

[168] F. Helling, S. Zhang, A. Shang, S. Adluri and M. Calves. GM2-KLH conjugate vaccine: Increased immunogenicity in melanoma patients after administration with immunological adjuvant QS-21. *Cancer Res.* [All @ UAMS; LRVA (latest 10 years)]. *55(Jul 1),* pp. 2783-2788. 1995. Available: http://ovidsp.ovid.com/ovidweb.cgi?T=JS&CSC=Y&NEWS=N&PAGE=fulltext&D=ipab&AN=33-06593.

[169] J. M. Kirkwood, J. G. Ibrahim, J. A. Sosman, V. K. Sondak, S. S. Agarwala, M. S. Ernstoff and U. Rao. High-dose interferon alfa-2b significantly prolongs relapse-free and overall survival compared with the GM2-KLH/QS-21 vaccine in patients with resected stage IIB-III melanoma: Results of intergroup trial E1694/S9512/C509801. *Journal of Clinical Oncology* [All @ UAMS; LRVA (latest 10 years)]. *19(9),* pp. 2370-2380. 2001. Available: http://ovidsp.ovid.com/ovidweb.cgi?T=JS&CSC=Y&NEWS=N&PAGE=fulltext&D=med4&AN=11331315.

[170] C. Buteau, S. Markovic and E. Celis. Challenges in the development of effective peptide vaccines for cancer. Mayo Clin. *Proc. 77(4),* pp. 339-349. 2002.

[171] S. Tagawa, E. Cheung, W. Banta, C. Gee and J. Weber. Survival analysis after resection of metastatic disease followed by peptide vaccines in patients with stage IV melanoma. *Cancer 106(6),* pp. 1353-1357. 2006.

[172] P. Lee, F. Wang, J. Kuniyoshi, V. Rubio, T. Stuges, S. Groshen, C. Gee, R. Lau, G. Jeffery, K. Margolin, V. Marty and J. Weber. Effects of interleukin-12 on the immune response to a multipeptide vaccine for resected metastatic melanoma. *Journal of Clinical Oncology 19(18),* pp. 3836-3847. 2001.

[173] F. O. Smith, S. G. Downey, J. A. Klapper, J. C. Yang, R. M. Sherry, R. E. Royal, U. S. Kammula, M. S. Hughes, N. P. Restifo, C. L. Levy, D. E. White, S. M. Steinberg and S. A. Rosenberg. Treatment of metastatic melanoma using interleukin-2 alone or in conjunction with vaccines. Clinical Cancer Research 14(17), pp. 5610-5618. 2008.

[174] C. L. Slingluff, G. R. Petroni, K. A. ChianeseBullock, M. E. Smolkin, S. Hibbitts, C. Murphy, N. Johansen, W. W. Grosh, G. V. Yamshchikov, P. Y. Neese, J. W. Patterson, R. Fink and P. K. Rehm. Immunologic and clinical outcomes of a randomized phase II trial of two multipeptide vaccines for melanoma in the adjuvant setting. Clinical Cancer *Research : An Official Journal of the American Association for Cancer Research* [All @ UAMS]. *13(21),* pp. 6386-6395. 2007. Available: http://ovidsp.ovid.com/ovidweb.cgi?T=JS&CSC=Y&NEWS=N&PAGE=fulltext&D=cctr&AN=CN-00620609.

[175] V. Corbiere, J. Chapiro, V. Stroobant, W. Ma, C. Lurquin, B. Lethe, N. van Baren, B. J. Van den Eynde, T. Boon and P. G. Coulie. Antigen spreading contributes to MAGE

vaccination-induced regression of melanoma metastases. *Cancer Res. 71(4),* pp. 1253-1262. 2011.

[176] J. M. Kirkwood, S. Lee, S. J. Moschos, M. R. Albertini, J. C. Michalak, C. Sander, T. Whiteside, L. H. Butterfield and L. Weiner. Immunogenicity and antitumor effects of vaccination with peptide vaccine+/-granulocyte-monocyte colony-stimulating factor and/or IFN-alpha2b in advanced metastatic melanoma: Eastern cooperative oncology group phase II trial E1696. *Clinical Cancer Research : An Official Journal of the American Association for Cancer Research* [All @ UAMS]. *15(4),* pp. 1443-1451. 2009. Available: http://ovidsp.ovid.com/ovidweb.cgi?T=JS&CSC=Y&NEWS=N&PAGE=fulltext&D=cctr&AN=CN-00688685.

[177] D. J. Schwartzentruber, D. H. Lawson, J. M. Richards, R. M. Conry, D. M. Miller, J. Treisman, F. Gailani, L. Riley, K. Conlon, B. Pockaj, K. L. Kendra, R. L. White, R. Gonzalez, T. M. Kuzel, B. Curti, P. D. Leming, E. D. Whitman, J. Balkissoon, D. S. Reintgen, H. Kaufman, F. M. Marincola, M. J. Merino, S. A. Rosenberg, P. Choyke, D. Vena and P. Hwu, "Gp100 Peptide Vaccine and Interleukin-2 in Patients with Advanced Melanoma," *N. Engl. J. Med.,* vol. 364, pp. 2119-2127, Jun 2, 2011.

[178] J. A. Sosman, C. Carrillo, W. J. Urba, L. Flaherty and Ernstoff. Three phase II cytokine working group trials of gp100 (210M) peptide plus high-dose interleukin-2 in patients with HLA-A2-positive advanced melanoma. *Journal of Clinical Oncology* [All @ UAMS; LRVA (latest 10 years)]. *26(14),* pp. 2292-2298. 2008. Available: http://ovidsp.ovid.com/ovidweb.cgi?T=JS&CSC=Y&NEWS=N&PAGE=fulltext&D=ipab&AN=45-13437.

[179] M. Bhattacharya-Chatterjee, S. K. Chatterjee and K. A. Foon. Anti-idiotype vaccine against cancer. Immunol. *Lett. [Part @ UAMS (Click Library Holdings)].* 74(1), pp. 51-58. 2000. Available: http://ovidsp.ovid.com/ovidweb.cgi?T=JS&CSC=Y&NEWS=N&PAGE=fulltext&D=med4&AN=10996628.

[180] S. Ferrone. Anti-idiotypes in melanoma. Hybridoma [Online Access Only (Click E Journal Holdings for Information)]. 12(5), pp. 509-514. 1993. Available: http://ovidsp.ovid.com/ovidweb.cgi?T=JS&CSC=Y&NEWS=N&PAGE=fulltext&D=med3&AN=8300123.

[181] R. L. Metheringham, V. A. Pudney, B. Gunn, M. Towey, I. Spendlove and L. G. Durrant. Antibodies designed as effective cancer vaccines. *MAbs 1(1),* pp. 71-85. 2009. Available: http://ovidsp.ovid.com/ovidweb.cgi?T=JS&CSC=Y&NEWS=N&PAGE=fulltext&D=medl&AN=20046577.

[182] K. A. Foon, G. Sen, L. Hutchins, O. L. Kashala, R. Baral, M. Banerjee, M. Chakraborty, J. Garrison, R. A. Reisfeld and M. Bhattacharya-Chatterjee. Antibody responses in melanoma patients immunized with an anti-idiotype antibody mimicking disialoganglioside GD2. *Clinical Cancer Research* [All @ UAMS]. *4(5),* pp. 1117-1124. 1998. Available: http://ovidsp.ovid.com/ovidweb.cgi?T=JS&CSC=Y&NEWS=N&PAGE=fulltext&D=med4&AN=9607568.

[183] K. A. Foon, J. Lutzky, R. N. Baral, J. R. Yannelli, L. Hutchins, A. Teitelbaum, O. L. Kashala, R. Das, J. Garrison, R. A. Reisfeld and M. Bhattacharya-Chatterjee. Clinical and immune responses in advanced melanoma patients immunized with an anti-idiotype antibody mimicking disialoganglioside GD2. *Journal of Clinical Oncology* [All @ UAMS; LRVA (latest 10 years)]. *18(2),* pp. 376-384. 2000. Available: http://ovidsp.ovid.com/ovidweb.cgi?T=JS&CSC=Y&NEWS=N&PAGE=fulltext&D=med4&AN=10637253.

[184] P. B. Chapman, D. Wu, G. Ragupathi, S. Lu, L. Williams, W. J. Hwu, D. Johnson and P. O. Livingston. Sequential immunization of melanoma patients with GD3 ganglioside vaccine and anti-idiotypic monoclonal antibody that mimics GD3 ganglioside. Clinical Cancer *Research : An Official Journal of the American Association for Cancer Research* [All @ UAMS]. *10(14),* pp. 4717-4723. 2004. Available: http://ovidsp.ovid.com/ovidweb.cgi?T=JS&CSC=Y&NEWS=N&PAGE=fulltext&D=cctr&AN=CN-00502094.

[185] S. A. Rosenberg, J. C. Yang, D. J. Schwartzentruber, P. Hwu, S. L. Topalian, R. M. Sherry, N. P. Restifo, J. R. Wunderlich, C. A. Seipp, L. Rogers-Freezer, K. E. Morton, S. A. Mavroukakis, L. Gritz, D. L. Panicali and D. E. White. Recombinant fowlpox viruses encoding the anchor-modified gp100 melanoma antigen can generate antitumor immune responses in patients with metastatic melanoma. *Clinical Cancer Research* [All @ UAMS]. *9(8),* pp. 2973-2980. 2003. Available: http://ovidsp.ovid.com/ovidweb.cgi?T=JS&CSC=Y&NEWS=N&PAGE=fulltext&D=medc&AN=12912944.

[186] S. A. Rosenberg, Y. Zhai, J. C. Yang, D. J. Schwartzentruber and D. E. White. Immunizing patients with metastatic melanoma using recombinant adenoviruses encoding MART-1 or gp100 melanoma antigens. J. Natl. Cancer Inst. [All @ UAMS; LRVA (latest 10 years)]. *90(Dec 16),* pp. 1894-1900. 1998. Available: http://ovidsp.ovid.com/ovidweb.cgi?T=JS&CSC=Y&NEWS=N&PAGE=fulltext&D=ipab&AN=37-00699.

[187] M. Adamina, R. Rosenthal, W. P. Weber, D. M. Frey, C. T. Viehl, M. Bolli, R. W. Huegli, A. L. Jacob, M. Heberer, D. Oertli, W. Marti, G. C. Spagnoli and P. Zajac. Intranodal immunization with a vaccinia virus encoding multiple antigenic epitopes and costimulatory molecules in metastatic melanoma. Molecular Therapy 18(3), pp. 651-659. 2010.

[188] B. W. Bridle, J. E. Boudreau, B. D. Lichty, J. Brunelliere, K. Stephenson, S. Koshy, J. L. Bramson and Y. Wan. Vesicular stomatitis virus as a novel cancer vaccine vector to prime antitumor immunity amenable to rapid boosting with adenovirus. Molecular Therapy: The Journal of the American Society of Gene Therapy [Online Access Only (Click E Journal Holdings for Information)]. *17(10),* pp. 1814-1821. 2009. Available: http://ovidsp.ovid.com/ovidweb.cgi?T=JS&CSC=Y&NEWS=N&PAGE=fulltext&D=medl&AN=19603003.

[189] P. Hersey, A. S. Coates, W. H. McCarthy, J. F. Thompson and R. J. Simes. Adjuvant immunotherapy of patients with high-risk melanoma using vaccinia viral lysates of melanoma: Results of a randomized trial. *Journal of Clinical Oncology* [All @ UAMS; LRVA (latest 10 years)]. *20(20),* pp. 4181-4190. 2002. Available: http://

ovidsp.ovid.com/ovidweb.cgi?T=JS&CSC=Y&NEWS=N&PAGE=fulltext&D=ipab&AN=40-02647.

[190] A. Mazzocchi, C. Melani, L. Rivoltini, C. Castelli, M. Del Vecchio, C. Lombardo, M. Colombo and G. Parmiani. Simultaneous transduction of B7-1 and IL-2 genes into human melanoma cells to be used as vaccine: Enhancement of stimulatory activity for autologous and allogeneic lymphocytes. *Cancer Immunology Immunotherapy 50(4),* pp. 199-211. 2001.

[191] H. Kaufman, G. DeRaffele, J. Mitcham, D. Moroziewicz, S. Cohen, K. Hurst-Wicker, K. Cheung, D. Lee, J. Divito, M. Voulo, J. Donovan, K. Dolan, K. Manson, D. Panicali, E. Wang, H. Horig and F. Marincola. Targeting the local tumor microenvironment with vaccinia virus expressing B7.1 for the treatment of melanoma. J. Clin. Invest. 115(7), pp. 1903-1912. 2005.

[192] C. J. Kim, J. Cormier, M. Roden, L. Gritz, G. P. Mazzara, P. Fetsch, Y. Hijazi, K. H. Lee, S. A. Rosenberg and F. M. Marincola. Use of recombinant poxviruses to stimulate anti-melanoma T cell reactivity. Annals of Surgical Oncology [Part @ UAMS (Click Library Holdings)]. *5(1),* pp. 64-76. 1998. Available: http://ovidsp.ovid.com/ovidweb.cgi?T=JS&CSC=Y&NEWS=N&PAGE=fulltext&D=med4&AN=9524710.

[193] Sabel and V. K. Sondak. Tumor vaccines - A role in preventing recurrence in melanoma? American Journal of Clinical Dermatology [Not locally available; ask about Interlibrary Loan]. *3(9),* pp. 609-616. 2002. Available: http://ovidsp.ovid.com/ovidweb.cgi?T=JS&CSC=Y&NEWS=N&PAGE=fulltext&D=ipab&AN=40-06431.

[194] G. J. Prud'homme. DNA vaccination against tumors. J. Gene Med. [Not locally available; ask about Interlibrary Loan]. *7(1),* pp. 3-17. 2005. Available: http://ovidsp.ovid.com/ovidweb.cgi?T=JS&CSC=Y&NEWS=N&PAGE=fulltext&D=med4&AN=15538731.

[195] D. B. Lowe, M. H. Shearer, C. A. Jumper and R. C. Kennedy. Towards progress on DNA vaccines for cancer. Cellular and Molecular Life Sciences 64(18), pp. 2391-2403. 2007.

[196] G. Dranoff. GM-CSF-secreting melanoma vaccines. Oncogene [Part @ UAMS (Click Library Holdings)]. 22(20), pp. 3188-3192. 2003. Available: http://ovidsp.ovid.com/ovidweb.cgi?T=JS&CSC=Y&NEWS=N&PAGE=fulltext&D=med4&AN=12789295.

[197] H. L. Kaufman, D. W. Kim, G. DeRaffele, J. Mitcham, R. S. Coffin and S. Kim-Schulze. Local and distant immunity induced by intralesional vaccination with an oncolytic herpes virus encoding GM-CSF in patients with stage IIIc and IV melanoma. *Annals of Surgical Oncology 17(3),* pp. 718-730. 2010.

[198] H. L. Kaufman and S. D. Bines, "OPTIM trial: a Phase III trial of an oncolytic herpes virus encoding GM-CSF for unresectable stage III or IV melanoma," *Future Oncol.,* vol. 6, pp. 941-949, Jun, 2010.

[199] A. T. Stopeck, E. M. Hersh, E. T. Akporiaye, D. T. Harris, T. Grogan, E. Unger, J. Warneke, S. F. Schluter and S. Stahl, "Phase I study of direct gene transfer of an allogeneic histocompatibility antigen, HLA-B7, in patients with metastatic melanoma," *J. Clin. Oncol., vol. 15, pp. 341-349, Jan, 1997.*

[200] A. T. Stopeck, A. Jones, E. M. Hersh, J. A. Thompson, D. M. Finucane, J. C. Gutheil and R. Gonzalez. Phase II study of direct intralesional gene transfer of allovectin-7, an HLA-B7/beta2-microglobulin DNA-liposome complex, in patients with metastatic melanoma. *Clinical Cancer Research* [All @ UAMS]. *7(8),* pp. 2285-2291. 2001. Available: http://ovidsp.ovid.com/ovidweb.cgi?T=JS&CSC=Y&NEWS=N&PAGE=fulltext&D=med4&AN=11489803.

[201] R. Gonzalez, L. Hutchins, J. Nemunaitis, M. Atkins and P. O. Schwarzenberger, "Phase 2 trial of Allovectin-7 in advanced metastatic melanoma," *Melanoma Res.,* vol. 16, pp. 521-526, Dec, 2006.

[202] A. Y. Bedikian, J. Richards, D. Kharkevitch, M. B. Atkins, E. Whitman and R. Gonzalez, "A phase 2 study of high-dose Allovectin-7 in patients with advanced metastatic melanoma," *Melanoma Res.,* vol. 20, pp. 218-226, Jun, 2010.

[203] R. Chowdhery and R. Gonzalez, "Immunologic therapy targeting metastatic melanoma: allovectin-7," *Immunotherapy,* vol. 3, pp. 17-21, Jan, 2011.

[204] S. A. Rosenberg, M. T. Lotze, L. M. Muul, A. E. Chang, F. P. Avis, S. Leitman, W. M. Linehan, C. N. Robertson, R. E. Lee and J. T. Rubin, "A progress report on the treatment of 157 patients with advanced cancer using lymphokine-activated killer cells and interleukin-2 or high-dose interleukin-2 alone," *N. Engl. J. Med.,* vol. 316, pp. 889-897, Apr 9, 1987.

[205] S. A. Rosenberg, M. T. Lotze, J. C. Yang, S. L. Topalian, A. E. Chang, D. J. Schwartzentruber, P. Aebersold, S. Leitman, W. M. Linehan and C. A. Seipp, "Prospective randomized trial of high-dose interleukin-2 alone or in conjunction with lymphokine-activated killer cells for the treatment of patients with advanced cancer," *J. Natl. Cancer Inst.,* vol. 85, pp. 622-632, Apr 21, 1993.

[206] S. A. Rosenberg, J. R. Yannelli, J. C. Yang, S. L. Topalian, D. J. Schwartzentruber, J. S. Weber, D. R. Parkinson, C. A. Seipp, J. H. Einhorn and D. E. White, "Treatment of patients with metastatic melanoma with autologous tumor-infiltrating lymphocytes and interleukin 2," *J. Natl. Cancer Inst.,* vol. 86, pp. 1159-1166, Aug 3, 1994.

[207] A. I. Riker, S. Radfar, S. Liu, Y. Wang and H. T. Khong, "Immunotherapy of melanoma: a critical review of current concepts and future strategies," *Expert Opin. Biol. Ther.,* vol. 7, pp. 345-358, Mar, 2007.

[208] J. J. Hong, S. A. Rosenberg, M. E. Dudley, J. C. Yang, D. E. White, J. A. Butman and R. M. Sherry, "Successful treatment of melanoma brain metastases with adoptive cell therapy," *Clin. Cancer Res.,* vol. 16, pp. 4892-4898, Oct 1, 2010.

[209] Anonymous NCI. Available: http://www.cancer.gov/ncicancerbulletin/050112/page4.

[210] B. Thurner, I. Haendle, C. Roder, D. Dieckmann, P. Keikavoussi, H. Jonuleit, A. Bender, C. Maczek, D. Schreiner, P. von den Driesch, E. B. Brocker, R. M. Steinman, A. Enk, E. Kampgen and G. Schuler, "Vaccination with mage-3A1 peptide-pulsed mature, monocyte-derived dendritic cells expands specific cytotoxic T cells and induces regression of some metastases in advanced stage IV melanoma," *J. Exp. Med.*, vol. 190, pp. 1669-1678, Dec 6, 1999.

[211] R. Lau, F. Wang, G. Jeffery, V. Marty, J. Kuniyoshi, E. Bade, M. E. Ryback and J. Weber, "Phase I trial of intravenous peptide-pulsed dendritic cells in patients with metastatic melanoma," *J. Immunother.*, vol. 24, pp. 66-78, Jan-Feb, 2001.

[212] L. Engell-Noerregaard, T. H. Hansen, M. H. Andersen, P. Thor Straten and I. M. Svane, "Review of clinical studies on dendritic cell-based vaccination of patients with malignant melanoma: assessment of correlation between clinical response and vaccine parameters," *Cancer Immunol. Immunother., vol. 58, pp. 1-14, Jan, 2009.*

[213] D. Schadendorf, S. Ugurel, B. Schuler-Thurner, F. O. Nestle, A. Enk, E. B. Brocker, S. Grabbe, W. Rittgen, L. Edler, A. Sucker, C. Zimpfer-Rechner, T. Berger, J. Kamarashev, G. Burg, H. Jonuleit, A. Tuttenberg, J. C. Becker, P. Keikavoussi, E. Kampgen, G. Schuler and DC study group of the DeCOG, "Dacarbazine (DTIC) versus vaccination with autologous peptide-pulsed dendritic cells (DC) in first-line treatment of patients with metastatic melanoma: a randomized phase III trial of the DC study group of the DeCOG," *Ann. Oncol.*, vol. 17, pp. 563-570, Apr, 2006.

[214] D. T. Alexandrescu, T. E. Ichim, N. H. Riordan, F. M. Marincola, A. Di Nardo, F. D. Kabigting and C. A. Dasanu, "Immunotherapy for melanoma: current status and perspectives," *J. Immunother.*, vol. 33, pp. 570-590, Jul-Aug, 2010.

[215] R. Thomas, J. Padmanabha, M. Chambers, S. McFadyen, E. Walpole, G. Nielssen and M. Smithers. Metastatic lesions in the joint associated with acute inflammatory arthritis after dendritic cell immunotherapy for metastatic melanoma. *Melanoma Res.* [Online Access Only (Click E Journal Holdings for Information)]. 11(2), pp. 167-173. 2001. Available: http://ovidsp.ovid.com/ovidweb.cgi?T=JS&CSC=Y&NEWS=N&PAGE=fulltext&D=med4&AN=11333127.

[216] D. P. Lawrence, O. Hamid, D. F. McDermott, I. Puzanov, M. Sznol, J. Clark, T. Logan, F. S. Hodi, K. N. Heller and K. A. Margolin, "Phase II trial of ipilimubab monotherapy in melanoma patients with brain metastasis," *J. Clin. Oncol., vol. 28, pp. 8523, 2010.*

[217] J. D. Wolchok, B. Neyns, G. Linette, S. Negrier, J. Lutzky, L. Thomas, W. Waterfield, D. Schadendorf, M. Smylie, T. Guthrie Jr, J. J. Grob, J. Chesney, K. Chin, K. Chen, A. Hoos, S. J. O'Day and C. Lebbe, "Ipilimumab monotherapy in patients with pretreated advanced melanoma: a randomised, double-blind, multicentre, phase 2, dose-ranging study," *Lancet Oncol.*, vol. 11, pp. 155-164, Feb, 2010.

[218] K. T. Flaherty, J. A. Sosman and M. B. Atkins, "New options and new questions: How to select sequence therapies for patients with metastatic melanoma," *ASCO Educational Book*, pp. 524-530, 2012.

[219] J. M. Kirkwood, P. Lorigan, P. Hersey, A. Hauschild, C. Robert, D. McDermott, M. A. Marshall, J. Gomez-Navarro, J. Q. Liang and C. A. Bulanhagui, "Phase II trial of tremelimumab (CP-675,206) in patients with advanced refractory or relapsed melanoma," *Clin. Cancer Res.,* vol. 16, pp. 1042-1048, Feb 1, 2010.

[220] A. Ribas, A. Hauschild, R. Kefford, C. J. Punt, J. B. Haanen, M. Marmol, C. Garbe, J. Gomez-Navarro, D. Pavlov and M. Marshall, "Phase III, open-label, randomized, comparative study of tremelimumab (CP-675,206) and chemotherpay (temozolomide or dacarbazine) in patiens with advanced melanoma," *J. Clin. Oncol., vol. 26, pp. LBA9011, 2008.*

[221] D. M. Benson Jr, C. E. Bakan, A. Mishra, C. C. Hofmeister, Y. Efebera, B. Becknell, R. A. Baiocchi, J. Zhang, J. Yu, M. K. Smith, C. N. Greenfield, P. Porcu, S. M. Devine, R. Rotem-Yehudar, G. Lozanski, J. C. Byrd and M. A. Caligiuri, "The PD-1/PD-L1 axis modulates the natural killer cell versus multiple myeloma effect: a therapeutic target for CT-011, a novel monoclonal anti-PD-1 antibody," *Blood,* vol. 116, pp. 2286-2294, Sep 30, 2010.

[222] M. Sznol, F. S. Hodi, K. Margolin, D. F. McDermott, M. S. Ernstoff, J. M. Kirkwood, C. Wojtaszek, D. Feltquate and T. Logan, "Phase I study of BMS-663513, a fully human anti-CD137 agonist monoclonal antibody in patients with advanced cancer," *J. Clin. Oncol., vol. 26, pp. 3007, 2008.*

[223] B. Curti, A. Weinberg and N. Morris, "A phase I trial of monoclonal antibody to OX40 in patients with advanced cancer," *International Society for Biological Therapy of Cancer Annual Meeting,* 2007.

[224] A. Boni, A. P. Cogdill, P. Dang, D. Udayakumar, C. N. Njauw, C. M. Sloss, C. R. Ferrone, K. T. Flaherty, D. P. Lawrence, D. E. Fisher, H. Tsao and J. A. Wargo, "Selective BRAFV600E inhibition enhances T-cell recognition of melanoma without affecting lymphocyte function," *Cancer Res.,* vol. 70, pp. 5213-5219, Jul 1, 2010.

[225] M. A. Curran, W. Montalvo, H. Yagita and J. P. Allison, "PD-1 and CTLA-4 combination blockade expands infiltrating T cells and reduces regulatory T and myeloid cells within B16 melanoma tumors," *Proc. Natl. Acad. Sci. U. S. A.,* vol. 107, pp. 4275-4280, Mar 2, 2010.

[226] M. A. Curran, M. Kim, W. Montalvo, A. Al-Shamkhani and J. P. Allison, "Combination CTLA-4 blockade and 4-1BB activation enhances tumor rejection by increasing T-cell infiltration, proliferation, and cytokine production," *PLoS One,* vol. 6, pp. e19499, Apr 29, 2011.

[227] A. A. Tarhini, J. Cherian, S. J. Moschos, H. A. Tawbi, Y. Shuai, W. E. Gooding, C. Sander and J. M. Kirkwood, "Safety and efficacy of combination immunotherapy with interferon alfa-2b and tremelimumab in patients with stage IV melanoma," *J. Clin. Oncol., vol. 30, pp. 322-328, Jan 20, 2012.*

[228] F. S. Hodi, M. Butler, D. A. Oble, M. V. Seiden, F. G. Haluska, A. Kruse, S. Macrae, M. Nelson, C. Canning, I. Lowy, A. Korman, D. Lautz, S. Russell, M. T. Jaklitsch, N.

Ramaiya, T. C. Chen, D. Neuberg, J. P. Allison, M. C. Mihm and G. Dranoff, "Immunologic and clinical effects of antibody blockade of cytotoxic T lymphocyte-associated antigen 4 in previously vaccinated cancer patients," *Proc. Natl. Acad. Sci. U. S. A.*, vol. 105, pp. 3005-3010, Feb 26, 2008.